NUTRITIONAL QUALITY
INDEX OF FOODS

CHEDDAR CHEESE, BREAD, SALAD`

Nutrient	Amount	INQ	% STD	0% 50% 100%
ENERGY	303.13 kcal	1.00	15	BBBCCS
VITAMIN A	3203.60 IU	5.28	80	CCCCS * SSSSSSSSSSSSSSSSSSSSSSSSSSS
VITAMIN C	27.94 mg	3.07	47	SSSSS * SSSSSSSSSSSSS
THIAMIN	0.22 mg	1.42	22	BBBBB * SS
CALCIUM	295.79 mg	2.17	33	BBCCC * CCCCOSS
IRON	2.81 mg	1.16	18	BBBCS * S
POTASSIUM	439.06 mg	0.58	9	BSSS *
SODIUM	479.17 mg	1.05	16	BBBCC *
CHOLESTEROL	29.22 mg	0.55	8	CCC *
FAT-TOTAL	15.29 g	1.29	20	BCCCC * SS
SATURATED FATTY ACIDS	5.99 g	1.39	21	BCCCC * CCS
UNSATURATED FATTY ACIDS	2.64 g	0.88	13	CSSSS *

NUTRITIONAL QUALITY INDEX OF FOODS

R. Gaurth Hansen, Ph.D.
Professor of Nutrition and Biochemistry

Bonita W. Wyse, Ph.D., R.D.
Associate Professor of Nutrition
Utah State University
Logan, Utah

Ann W. Sorenson, Ph.D.
Adjunct Professor of Nutrition
Utah State University
Logan, Utah
and
Assistant Professor of Family
and Community Medicine
University of Utah
Salt Lake City, Utah

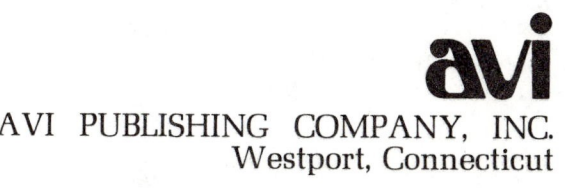

AVI PUBLISHING COMPANY, INC.
Westport, Connecticut

Library of Congress Cataloging in Publication Data

Hansen, Roger Gaurth, 1920–
    Nutritional quality index of foods.

    Includes indexes.
    1. Food.   2. Nutrition.   3. Food—Composition
—Tables.   I.   Wyse, Bonita W., joint author.
II.   Sorenson, Ann W., joint author.   III.   Title.
TX353.H174   641.1   79–17505
ISBN 0–87055–320–8

Printed in the United States of America by Eastern Graphics, Inc.

Preface

Since the turn of the century, important changes have taken place in the types and amounts of food consumed by individuals in the United States. In particular, the increased consumption of refined sugar and fat in various segments of the population has raised important questions regarding the nutritional adequacy of the average diet. Such questions are pertinent because there has been a concomitant decrease in consumption of cereals, especially whole grain cereals and potatoes. The equally well documented decrease in per capita consumption of milk and eggs and, during the last decade or two, of fruits is less important from a calorie standpoint, but certainly significant from a nutritional point of view.

Fat now typically supplies 40 to 45 percent of a person's total calories. This represents about a 15 percent increase in the fat-contributed proportion of calories since 1900, and is primarily from vegetable oils. Sugar intake, while holding relatively constant in recent years, went up substantially between 1900 and 1925. Fat and sugar nutrient sources may be described as "calorie dense."

Along with the changes in diet composition, we have seen calorie needs dramatically reduced as the prevailing life style involved less and less physical activity. At the turn of the century, a 3,000 calorie diet would probably have been adequate for anyone engaged in the then typically substantial physical activity. Today a 2,000 calorie diet may exceed the needs of the characteristically sedentary U.S. adult. The combination of our tending to meet our energy needs with calorie-dense foods and our declining physical activity has made it critical that we choose appropriate foods, with appropriateness being evaluated in terms of adequate intakes of all the essential nutrients. Obviously, those with minimal calorie needs must use the most care in selecting among their available food options.

The need for sound consumer judgments in making food choices has led us to consider how best to describe the nutritional values of foods in terms that could be understood by consumers, industry, and government alike. The purpose of this book is to describe a means of evaluating the nutritional qualities of all foods and food combinations in an uncomplicated and useful way.

The descriptive terms, "calorie dense" and "nutrient dense," have virtually opposite meanings. Foods rich in refined sugar and fat exemplify the calorie-dense designation and often are poor in other nutrients. Antithetically, a food that contains substantial quantities of various nutrients compared to its calorie content is nutrient dense.

Nutrient density (expressed as a ratio) can be used to describe nutritional quality. The numerator is the nutrient composition of the food supply or the diet, or the meal, or even the individual food. The denominator, the other parameter in the ratio, is human needs or allowances for individual nutrients. Both parameters are expressed on a common kilocalorie basis. Our knowledge of these parameters is growing, but the research base is incomplete.

The U.S. Department of Agriculture is attempting to assemble all available data on the nutrient composition of foods. The procedure is to computerize such information and make it accessible to everyone. The other factor, the nutrient allowances of humans, has been developed largely by the Food and Nutrition Board of the National Academy of Sciences and is presented periodically in its documents describing Recommended Dietary Allowances. The RDAs have become a standard of reference throughout the world. Information in the RDA Handbook is routinely used to define (and redefine) allowances for nutrients as research data expands. The 9th edition of this invaluable reference work is being prepared and is expected to recommend intakes for nutrients heretofore not considered. Eventually, dietary allowances for all nutrients essential to a totally adequate diet will probably be defined.

Comparisons of the nutrient composition of foods and the recommended dietary allowances of nutrients are meaningful only if made on a standard calorie basis (usually 100 or 1,000 calories). With computer technology, such comparisons are easily accomplished and can be responsive to new data as it emerges. With our system, the capacity of a food supply or a diet to meet human nutritional needs can be readily evaluated. For example, the "nutrient profile" in the figure of three specific food items—cheddar cheese, bread made from a mixture of whole wheat and enriched flour, and a salad has been adapted from a graphical computerized printout based on the above parameters.

When examined for representative or "leader nutrients," the nutrient profile shown in the figure reflects a highly nutritious combination of foods. We ignored protein as a "leader nutrient" because most people in the U.S. consume adequate quantities of high quality protein. Since amounts of the calcium and riboflavin in dairy products tend to be correlated, calcium was specified since there is thought to be more of a problem with a nutritional deficit of calcium, especially in the young, and also in some females. Vitamins A and C and thiamin were chosen because these three may be in short supply for some individuals. Potassium is considered primarily based upon availability of data on food composition. As more is learned about magnesium and zinc distribution in foods, one of them may be a more appropriate representative mineral element. Iron is notorious as the nutrient most difficult to obtain from the usual U.S. food supply, especially for those whose needs are greatest—the developing child and the premenopausal woman.

The sodium, cholesterol, and fatty acid contents of a diet are important to many. They are included in our analysis (based on unavoidably arbitrary standards) to illustrate the usefulness of the nutrient density system. To apply the system, two things must be known: 1) the composition of the foods consumed, and 2) the standards accepted as recommended allowances. As these two components become known in more detail, the definition of nutritional quality of our foods will improve.

CHEDDAR CHEESE, BREAD, SALAD*

Nutrient	Amount	INQ	% STD	0% 50% 100%
ENERGY	303.13 kcal	1.00	15	BBBCCS
VITAMIN A	3203.60 IU	5.28	80	CCCCS * SSSSSSSSSSSSSSSSSSSSSSSSSS
VITAMIN C	27.94 mg	3.07	47	SSSSS * SSSSSSSSSSSSS
THIAMIN	0.22 mg	1.42	22	BBBBB*SS
CALCIUM	295.79 mg	2.17	33	BBCCC * CCCCCSS
IRON	2.81 mg	1.16	18	BBBCS *S
POTASSIUM	439.06 mg	0.58	9	BSSS *
SODIUM	479.17 mg	1.05	16	BBBCC *
CHOLESTEROL	29.22 mg	0.55	8	CCC *
FAT-TOTAL	15.29 g	1.29	20	BCCCC*SS
SATURATED FATTY ACIDS	5.99 g	1.39	21	BCCCC * CCS
UNSATURATED FATTY ACIDS	2.64 g	0.88	13	CSSSS *

*Composite profile for 28g of CHEDDAR CHEESE (C), 25g each of whole wheat and enriched white flour BREAD (B) and a SALAD (S) composed of ½ c each iceberg lettuce and spinach, 1 tomato wedge, 1 tsp. of corn oil and 1 tsp. of vinegar.

The composite analysis is based upon the following daily intake values:
Energy 2000 kcal, Vitamin A 4000 IU, Vitamin C 60 mg, Thiamin 1 mg, Calcium 900 mg, Iron 16 mg, Sodium 3000 mg, Potassium 5000 mg, Cholesterol 350 mg, Fat-Total 78 g, Saturated Fatty Acids 28.5 g, Unsaturated Fatty Acids 20 g.

The three foods in the above figure in the proportions shown contribute about 300 calories of energy, or 15 percent of a 2,000 daily calorie need. A nutrient line on the graph that reaches or exceeds the length of the energy line represents a nutrient in an adequate balance to calorie content. In the illustration, "B" denotes the contribution of the bread,

"C" the contribution of the cheddar cheese, and "S" the salad. Obviously all three contribute to the energy supply. The vitamin A is derived largely from the salad, but some comes from the cheese. In total, 80 percent of the average daily need for vitamin A is supplied from these two foods. Practically all of the vitamin C is contributed by the salad, and the thiamin is largely derived from the bread and the salad. Whereas calcium comes from all three foods, cheese is an especially good source. Even though the standard for iron is high, i.e., 16 mg/2000 calories, this food combination provides iron in proportion to the calories supplied, largely because of the whole wheat and iron-enriched flour used to make the bread. For vitamin A, vitamin C, thiamin, calcium, and iron, it is important that, over a day, or, at least, in a week's time, the nutrient proportions balance the energy intake, as they do in this combination of foods.

While it is important to obtain an adequate amount of the above nutrients in relation to calories, some individuals may wish to limit the intake of other nutrients. This would be the situation for anyone wanting to reduce salt (sodium) intake. Since there is no RDA for sodium, the arbitrary standard chosen by the authors is 3 g of sodium, or about 7.5 g of salt. This is less than the average amount of salt consumed in the U.S., and probably a useful goal for many. For the foods in the above figure, the salt value is less than the energy content when measured against the 7.5 g daily standard. Although there has been no standard set for potassium, some feel that, on a molecular basis, potassium should about balance sodium, as it does in this diet.

The amount of cholesterol used as a standard for a 2,000 calorie intake is 350 mg, which was the upper limit recommended by the U.S. Dietary Goals. Thus for those concerned with cholesterol intake, this snack is well within the cholesterol standard. The amount of energy to be derived from fat according to the standard is 35 percent of calories. This is a reasonable guide, since diets planned within this standard using food readily available from the supermarkets are palatable. In our three foods, the fat is slightly in excess compared to the energy content and the source is the cheese and the salad dressing. As an average, in the United States, the proportion of polyunsaturated (P) to saturated (S) fatty acids is currently about 0.25, which many regard as appropriate. For purposes of our calculations, the P/S ratio of 0.70 has been chosen. Since there is no RDA for polyunsaturated fatty acids, the lower limit suggested in the U.S. Dietary Goals was selected. For those who wish to increase the ratio of polyunsaturated to saturated fatty acids, this system of food analysis can readily give direction. From the figure it is obvious that the unsaturated fatty acids intake (and consequently the P/S ratio) can be increased by adding more oil to the salad dressing. Of course, this would also increase the total fat in the diet and its calorie density. Oils provide largely calories with few other nutrients, although they do often contain appreciable quantities of vitamin E and sometimes vitamin A.

The combination illustrated and analyzed may be regarded as a prototype for use of the appendix of the book. There the individual nutrient profiles are displayed for foods for which data is available, and are derived from USDA Handbook 72. Starting with those foods that form an interesting or attractive part of the meal, it is possible, by using the erasable plastic ruler, to examine the balance of nutrients in any combination of foods or in any diet. School children grade K through 6, and also numerous adult groups, have been shown to readily understand and use the system. All have found it possible, even with a minimum amount of reading skills, to examine the balance of nutrients in food choices which are made. This suggests to us that, while the primary target for the book is the nutrition professional, it should have some interest to all consumers who are conscious of the nutritional quality of food.

The authors are grateful to Arthur Wittwer, Guen Brown and the other students who have through discussion contributed to the nutrient density concept. The computer analyses were performed by Mary Farley. The editorial assistance of Lois Cox and the secretarial skills of Kathy Daugherty, Alice Nelson and Carole Pattee were most appreciated.

Many of the chapters in this book have appeared in somewhat modified versions as articles in professional journals. The authors acknowledge the assistance and support of Mark Hegsted, *Nutrition Reviews*, Helen Ullrich, *Journal Nutrition Education,* Dorothea Turner, *Journal American Dietetic Association,* John Klis, *Food Technology*, and Adina Reinhardt and Mildred Quinn, *Family and Community Health.*

The authors also wish to express their appreciation to Dr. Norman W. Desrosier and the AVI Publishing Company for encouragement and assistance in bringing this book into being.

R. Gaurth Hansen
Bonita W. Wyse
Ann Sorenson
Logan, Utah

April 15, 1979

Contents

PART I
INDEX OF FOOD QUALITY

Need for An Index
of Nutritional Quality

What people eat and why depends upon such individual variables as income and "learned" preferences, as well as awareness of and access to information about nutritional values.

The individual variables that affect food choices are largely beyond influence by the scientific community, but they are important enough to warrant brief citation.

INCOME

The average American family is currently estimated to spend only about 16 percent of its income for food, as compared with 25 to 40 percent in Western Europe and 75 to 90 percent in many underdeveloped countries. By coupling reasonable food costs with an increase in real income, many (but not all) families in the United States have realized nutritional benefits. Families in middle to high income brackets consume more meat, poultry, fish, milk and milk products, fruits, and vegetables than do lower-income families. Poor people eat more breads and cereals. A recent national survey revealed that up to 15 percent of the population sampled consumed inadequate quantities of one or more of the nutrients measured.

Some of the deficiencies could be due to habits and personal preferences rather than economic constraints. In addition, any 24-hour history of food consumed may tend to exaggerate the estimates of overall dietary inadequacies. Regardless of the lack of precision of the estimates of deficiencies derived from dietary recall, however, the general conclusion is substantiated by biochemical analysis.

NEW PRODUCTS

Even the specialist has trouble assessing how today's continual changes in food production and processing affect the availability and quantities of individual nutrients consumed. Yet the choices the consumer makes inevitably parallel the availability of new products on the market, and these choices seem to be favoring what may be categorized as snack or convenience foods. As a proportion of calories consumed, snack or convenience foods will probably become increasingly prominent. Appropriate raw materials, whether isolated from plants or chemically prepared, coupled with advancing technology, will undoubtedly continue to change the character of the food supply. Food product analogs thus will be joining the ranks of convenience and substituted foods. What traditional foods these analogs displace in the consumers' market baskets could vitally affect their nutrition status.

FAMILY STRUCTURE

Even if the proper selection is made at the grocery store, individuals within each household will vary greatly in the amounts of specific foods they consume. Breakfast and lunch are vanishing as a family experience, leaving only the evening meal with social significance for the family. Many people prefer not to eat breakfast, while others take very limited quantities of food for breakfast. Lunches are frequently eaten away from the home by all members of the family. As a result, every member must know and practice the basic principles of good nutrition.

TOWARD A PRACTICABLE INDEX

Consumers, food processors, regulatory agencies, and nutritional scie i tists would all benefit from a properly defined index of food quality. The nutritional quality of any food is obviously a function of its chemical composition as related to the specific nutrient needs of the human. Unfortunately, human needs for nutrients and the composition of foods are (at best) incompletely known.

The basic need of any individual, however, is for energy. The National Research Council Food and Nutrition Board states: "Calorie allowances are established with the objective of providing energy in amounts sufficient to maintain body weight at a rate of growth at levels most conducive to well-being and health." For energy, it is obviously important to just meet the needs of the individual. For the other nutrients, however, the Board and others concerned with the adequacy of the diet have allowed for biological variability and increased needs during common stresses, while trying to permit full realization of growth and productive potentials. Admittedly, the requirement for nutrients cannot be strictly related to calorie needs in all cases because: "The margin above normal physiological requirement varies for each nutrient because of the differences in body storage capacity and individual requirements and the precision of assessing requirements and the hazard of excessive intake of certain nutrients." Nevertheless, individual nutrient and calorie needs can be related to the capacity of a food to satisfy them, and for many useful applications additional precision is not essential.

TABLE 1.1.

Standard recommended daily allowances (RDA) for nutrition labeling

Energy	(2800)*	1,000 kcal
Protein	65 g	23 g
Vitamin A	5,000 i.u.	1,780 i.u.
Vitamin B₁	1.5 mg	0.53 mg
Vitamin B₂	1.7 mg	0.61 mg
Vitamin C	60 mg	21.4 mg
Calcium	1,000 mg	357 mg
Iron	18 mg	6.4 mg

*The allowances for the individual nutrients used in Table 1 were derived from the published food labeling recommendations of the FDA, Federal Register, Volume 37, page 6497 A, March, 1972. While the calorie proportion is not specifically considered in the Federal Register, a personal communication with the FDA indicated 2800 kcal as an appropriate base for comparison of calories to other nutrients. Hence, Figures 2 through 7 were calculated using 2800 kcal as the common base. A food enrichment subcommittee of the Food and Nutrition Board has a study underway from which a standarized RDA may emerge. Further analysis may indicate that a lesser amount such as 2300 kcal is more appropriate. If so, the nutrient density comparisons presented here would have to be adjusted accordingly.

A standardized, recommended dietary allowance (RDA) is essential to the expression of food quality. For labeling purposes the Food and Drug Administration (FDA) has circulated a standardized RDA that indicates the recommended nutrient levels per 2,800 calories (Table 1.1). The derivation of the standardized RDA is obviously somewhat arbitrary, but it attempts to represent published allowances as modified for age and sex. For present purposes and for graphical presentations in this chapter, the FDA standardized RDA has been used without further attempts to justify each value.

Current handbooks on food composition are limited in content to a few of the essential nutrients for humans. In many cases, relevant data are still in private files or, at best, in widely scattered publications. Then, too, the nutrient content of any food is dependent on such factors as plant variety, time of harvest, and conditions of processing or storage prior to consumption. Further, such factors as availability of the nutrient in the food and the synergistic effect of various food combinations limit the precision of data on individual foods. The following discussion utilizes, for the most part, nutrient content information from C.F. Bowes and H.N. Church, and data derived from the USDA, and is related to human requirements for nutrients based on the FDA's standardized RDA for nutrients.

NUTRIENT DENSITY

For present purposes nutrient density of a food is defined as the ratio of the nutrient composition of food to nutrient requirements of the human. To compare the two parameters, calories have been used as the common denominator. Ratios of "1" would indicate that when calorie needs are met, those for individual nutrients are also satisfied. A food with a substantial number of the important nutrients in excess of calories is obviously of good quality, and its nutrient density (also nutrient: calorie ratio) will be greater than "1" in proportion to the supply of excess nutrients. Food containing calories in excess of nutrients will have nutrient densities less than "1," and a person would have to consume excessive calories from these foods to obtain the recommended quantities of nutrients. Existing information about the composition of foods and human nutrient needs permits evaluation in terms of nutrient density for only some of the key nutrients. But the nutrient density system of defining food quality reveals how incomplete our understanding of human requirements for the individual nutrients is, and further emphasizes our need for more detailed knowledge of food composition. What emerges is a qualitative (and somewhat quantitative) evaluation of a food in terms of human needs for nutrients.

TABLE 1.2.

Composition of milk in relation to nutrient needs of the infant

		A Composition of Milk*	B RDA/ 1,000 kcal**	Ratio A/B
Energy	kcal	1,000	1,000	1.0
Protein	g	54	18	3.0
Vitamin A	i.u.	2,100	1,700	1 2
Vitamin D	i.u.	630	450	1.4
Vitamin E	i.u.	1.4	10	0.1
Ascorbic Acid	mg	15.4	40	0.4
Folacin	mg	3.4	0.1	34
Niacin Eq.	mg	14	9.0	1.6
Vitamin B₁	mg	0.46	0.5	0.9
Vitamin B₂	mg	2.6	0.7	3.7
Vitamin B₆	mg	0.73	0.4	1 8
Vitamin B₁₂	ug	8 3	2.0	4.1
Calcium	g	1.8	0.7	2 6
Phosphorus	g	1.4	0.6	2 3
Iron	mg	1.4	17	0.1

*Cow's milk fortified with vitamin D
**Six to 12 months (Recommended Dietary Allowances
Seventh Revised Edition, 1968)

For purposes of illustrating the nutrient density concept, whole cows' milk as an infant food has been chosen for several reasons: (1) the chemical composition is known in adequate detail to illustrate the point, (2) the recommended dietary allowances have stated the requirements for infants, age six months to one year, more completely than for other age groups, and (3) the principal source of calories for children from six months to a year has been repeatedly shown to be milk. The data are first placed in tabular form to illustrate their derivation (Table 1.2). For most ordinary purposes, however, graphical presentations are more meaningful (Figure 1.1). In Table 1.2 and Figure 1.1 (which is derived from Table 1.2), the RDA information is taken directly from the recommendations of the Food and Nutrition Board for a child from six to 12 months. This permits correlation with the extensive analysis for the composition of milk. For the general discussion and purposes of this chapter, however, the FDA standardized RDA is more meaningful and is used in subsequent graphical presentations. The table and chart indicate that, for the child of between six months and one year, milk is a good, but not a complete, food. With respect to protein, vitamin A, riboflavin, thiamin, and calcium, when calorie needs are met, the intake of these nutrients is adequate or more than adequate. For vitamin C and iron, supplemental sources need to be sought to compensate for the deficit in

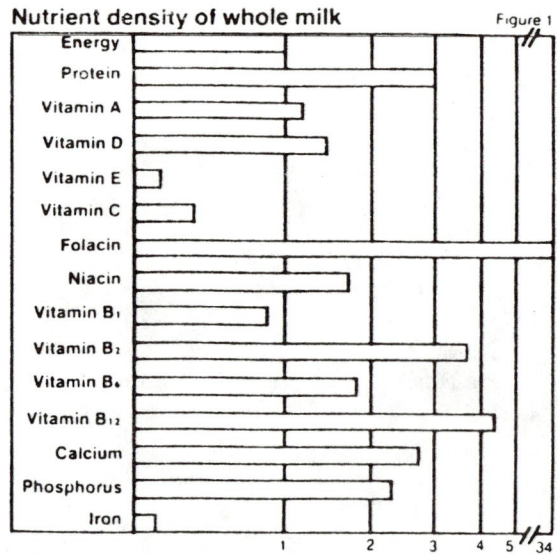

FIGURE 1.1. NUTRIENT DENSITY OF WHOLE MILK

deficit in milk. Quantitative needs of humans for vitamin E are less certain, but cows' milk appears to contain smaller quantities of this vitamin than does human milk.

Since foods differ widely in their chemical composition, and thus vary greatly from one another in their ability to supply essential nutrients to the individual, a balanced diet requires proper choice. Each particular food generally should not be expected to contain all of the nutrients required by man. Describing a food on the basis of its ratio of nutrient density illustrates this principle vividly and should encourage the practice of selecting a variety of foods to balance the diet.

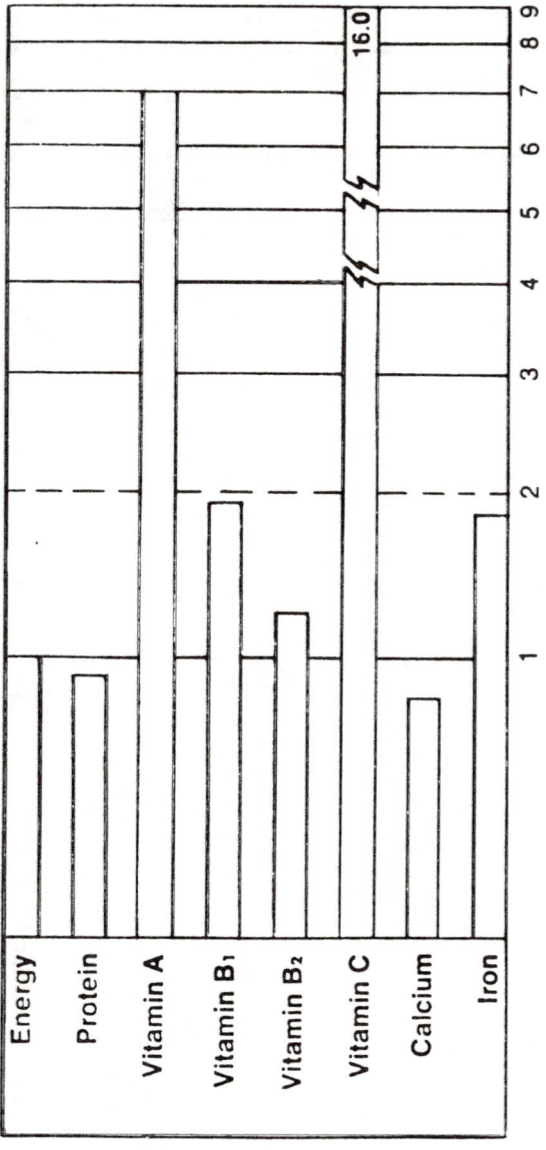

FIGURE 1.2. NUTRIENT DENSITY OF FRUIT AND VEGETABLES

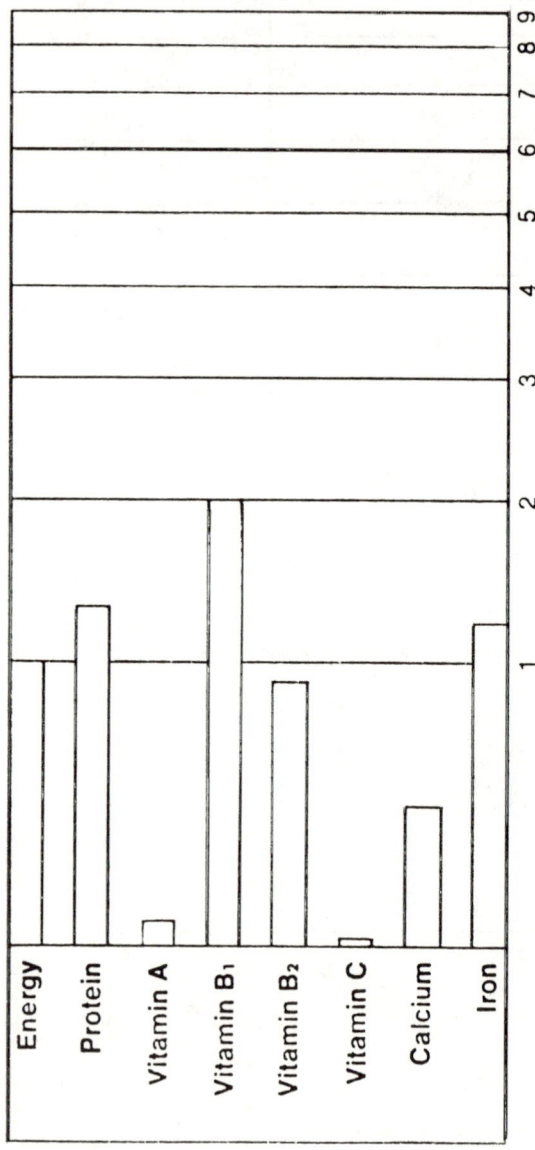

FIGURE 1.3.   NUTRIENT DENSITY OF BREAD AND CEREALS

SOME SPECIFIC RATIOS

Figure 1.2 (and all subsequent figures) utilizes the FDA's standardized RDA (Table 1.1). Fruits and vegetables as consumed in aggregate in the United States are obviously important supplementary sources of vitamin A, thiamin (B^1), and vitamin C, with nutrient densities of 7.0, 2.0, and 16.0, respectively. Fruits and vegetables are also important sources of protein, riboflavin, and iron. The nutritional quality of proteins of plant origin is improved when supplemented with foods of animal origin; nevertheless, fruits and vegetables can contribute valuable quantities of protein. In general, fruits and vegetables have high nutrient-calorie ratios but low caloric contents; hence, their potential contribution to a balanced diet may be overstated by this system.

With the exception of thiamin, the nutrients provided by the breads and cereals (Figure 1.3) on the basis of the ratio of nutrients to calories are not particularly notable. Foods in this group are almost devoid of vitamins A and C, but they do constitute low-cost sources of calories, protein, thiamin, calcium, and iron, and therefore are important to the diet.

Foods in the meat group (Figure 1.4) provide an abundance of protein, thiamin, riboflavin, and iron. The protein is of excellent quality with the ratio of protein to calories about 3 to 1. Thiamin, riboflavin, and iron are obtained from foods in the meat group in an excess of calories in a ratio of 1.5 or more. Foods in the milk group (Figure 1.5) contribute nutrients in excess of calories for the following items: proteins in a ratio of 2.2, riboflavin and calcium in a ratio of 3.5. Foods in this group have limited quantities of vitamin C and iron.

Since the FDA has abandoned the use of the expression "minimum daily requirement," the nutrient density system should reinforce the RDA as a guideline to good food choices. Perhaps the limit to which we can go with most consumers is to give them some qualitative idea of why a balanced diet is important. The USDA Basic Four classification system, which is the basis for the preceding charts, should be useful to consumers interested in achieving good nutrition through a varied diet. They can assure themselves of an adequate diet by selecting, daily, four or more servings of bread and cereals, which include some whole grain, enriched, or restored flour; four or more servings from the vegetable and fruit group, which includes a dark green or deep yellow vegetable, a citrus, or other fruit; two or more servings from the meat group, which includes beef, veal, pork, lamb, poultry, fish and eggs, with dry beans, peas and nuts as alternatives; and three or more servings from the milk group, which includes milk, cheese, ice cream, and foods derived principally from milk.

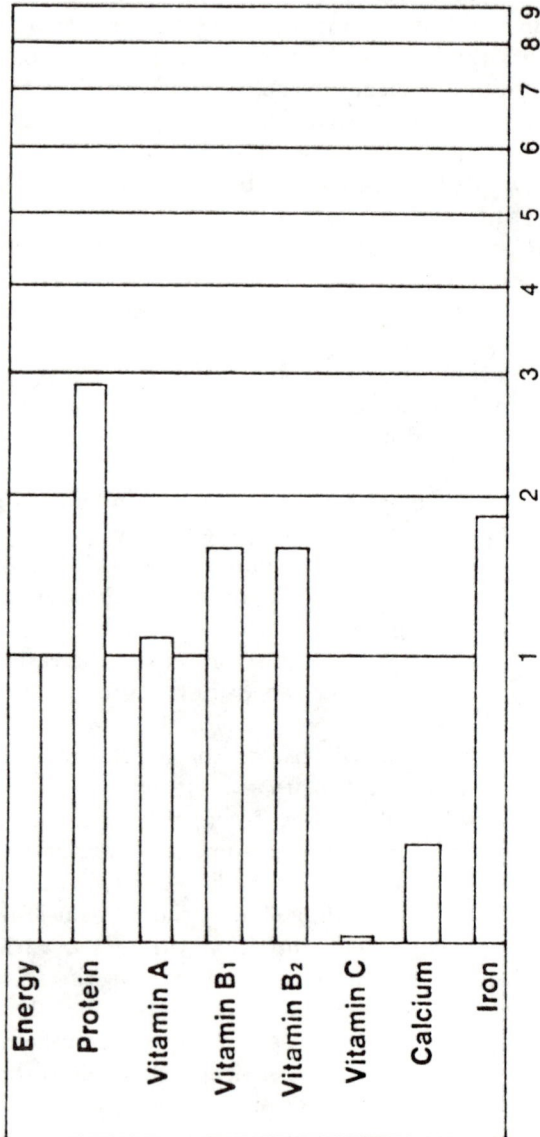

FIGURE 1.4. NUTRIENT DENSITY OF MEAT GROUP

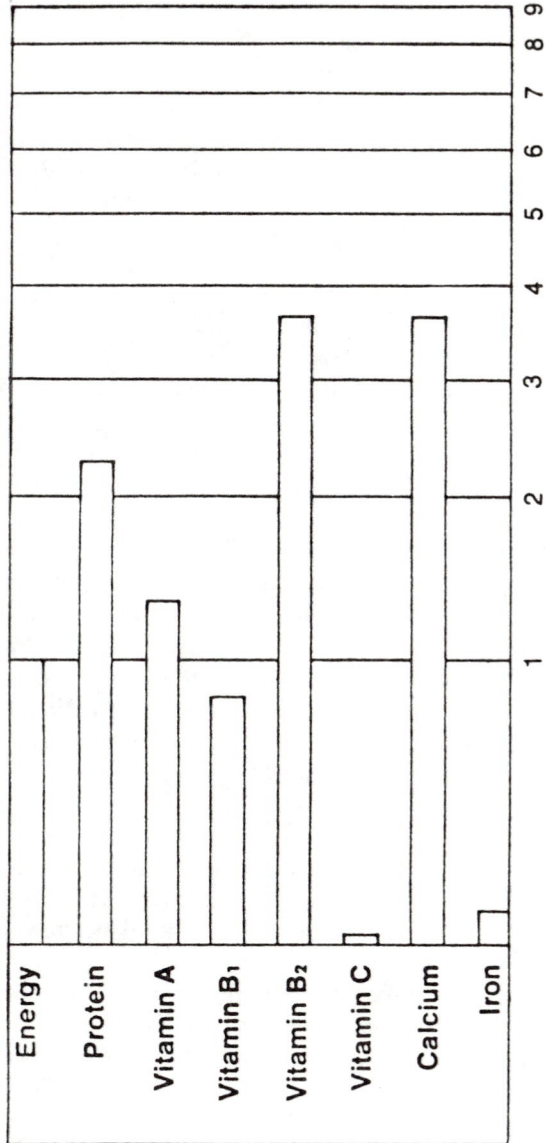

FIGURE 1.5. NUTRIENT DENSITY OF MILK AND MILK PRODUCTS

NUTRITIONAL DEFICITS

Based upon chemical composition data for the total food supply (Figure 1.6), as reported in the 1965-66 Household Food Consumption Survey (USDA, 1972), the most difficult requirement to meet is that for iron. The total U.S. food supply has enough iron to balance out the calories, placing a heavy emphasis on the proper selection of foods, especially for those whose needs for iron are greatest. The national nutrition survey, however, discovered widespread iron-deficiency anemia, especially in infants, young children, and women, and the American Medical Association Council on Foods and Nutrition and the National Research Council -Food and Nutrition Board are in favor of increasing iron supplementation of foods.

Findings from the U.S. ten-state survey suggest significant nutrient deficits that limit physical stature, particularly among the lower-income groups. While frank deficiency symptoms were rarely encountered in the survey in severe form, biochemical tests revealed less than desirable levels of several nutrients. In addition to a protein-calorie inadequacy, blood tests revealed low intakes of vitamin A and vitamin C, folic acid, and iodine. The excretion of thiamin and riboflavin indicated less than adequate intakes of these vitamins.

The recent nationwide survey, coupled with the survey of households by the United States Department of Agriculture, indicates that many people are consuming food that furnishes less than the recommended dietary allowances for one or more basic nutrients. Only about half of the American households had food supplies that were described as good by the USDA. Awareness of and access to nutrient-calorie ratio information among those who administer school lunch programs or are concerned with total national planning could do much to insure an adequate diet for the malnourished segment of the American public.

Currently, about 30 percent of the food each of us consumes provides calories almost devoid of other nutrient value. If the rest of the food we eat had greater than the ideal nutrient density of 1, which is rarely the case, that 30 percent deficit of some of the individual nutrients would be partially offset.

Educational advertising campaigns and adequate labeling are essential if consumers are to understand whether a diet is balanced in both caloric and nutrient content. Most consumers could be expected to welcome an index of food quality defined in relation to human needs for nutrients, making their quest for good nutrition easier.

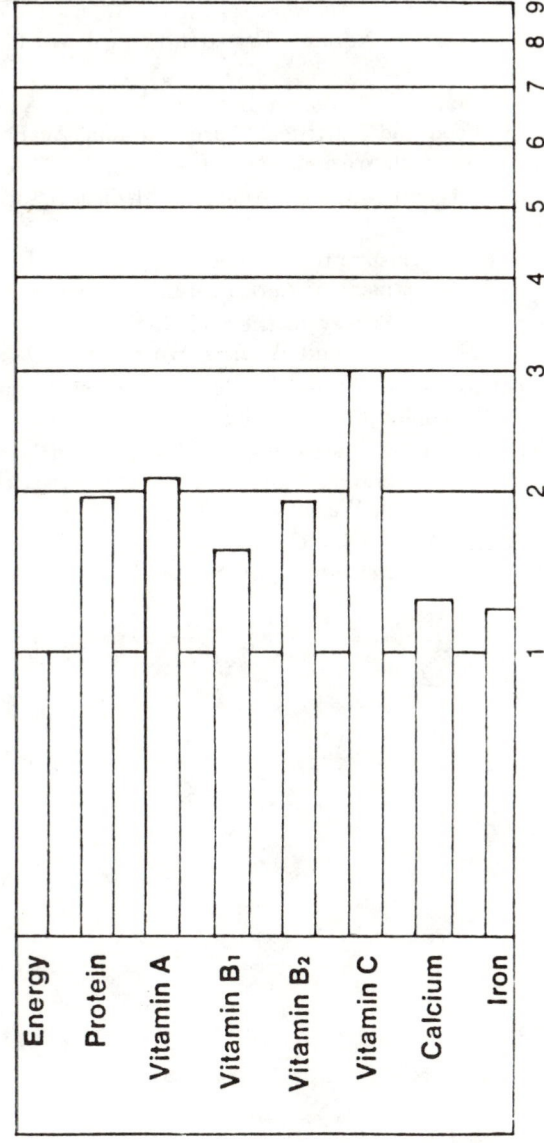

FIGURE 1.6. NUTRIENT DENSITY OF AGGREGATE FOOD AVAILABLE

*Based on data from the 1965-66 Household Food Consumption Survey (USDA, 1972). All data bars adjusted to an energy value of 1.0.

REFERENCES

ANON. 1974. Recommended Dietary Allowances, Eighth Revised Edition, p. 8   National Academy of Sciences-National Research Council, Washington, D.C.

ANON. 1969. Recommendations for Increased Iron Levels in the American Diet: A Statement of the Food and Nutrition Board. National Academy of Sciences-National Research Council, Washington, D.C.

ANON. 1972. Council on Foods and Nutrition, American Medical Association, *J. Am. Med. Assn.* 220:855.

ANON. 1972. Household Food Consumption Survey, Agricultural Research Service Report No. 11, U.S. Department of Agriculture, Washington, D.C.

ANON. 1972. Ten-State Nutrition Survey in the United States, 1968-1970, U.S. Department of Health, Education, and Welfare, Washington, D.C.

BOWES, C.F. and CHURCH, H.N. 1970. Food Values of Portions Commonly Used, Eleventh Edition. J.P. Lippincott, Philadelphia.

PAGE, L. and PHIPARD, E.F. 1957. Essentials of Adequate Diet-Facts for Nutrition Programs, Home Economics Report No. 3, Agricultural Research Service, U.S. Department of Agriculture, Washington, D.C.

WATT, B.K. and MERRILL, A.L. 1963. Composition of Foods: raw, processed, prepared. Agricultural Research Service, U.S. Department of Agriculture, Washington, D.C.

2

Standards for Evaluating Food Quality

The Food and Nutrition Board of the National Academy of Sciences-National Research Council, (NAS/NRC) is currently in the process of revising its Recommended Daily Dietary Allowances (RDAs). In the 8th edition NAS/NRC the RDAs are expressed in terms of total amounts of nutrients that children and adults in various sex and age groups should consume daily (Table 2.1). This format is most appropriate for use by nutrition professionals, but for many uses, such as planning food supplies for the general population, formulating new products, interpreting nutrition labeling, evaluating food consumption patterns of groups composed of children and adults, and educating the consumer, a way of stating the nutrient allowances in a simpler manner is needed.

NUTRIENT DENSITY APPROACH

Food is eaten largely to satisfy energy requirements. In order to achieve and maintain proper weight for age, the amount of food consumed over a period of time must reflect energy needs fairly precisely. Obviously, for all age groups, when energy requirements are met the foods must include the allowances for all other nutrients. Admittedly, requirements, and therefore allowances, for the various nutrients are not strictly related to energy in some cases; however, expressing dietary allowances in terms of energy permits a number of useful considerations.

Expressing dietary allowances and nutrient content of food on the same basis, i.e., nutrients per 1,000 kcal, makes possible a direct comparison between the two parameters from which quality judgments may be derived. For example, 1,000 kcal of fluid whole milk contains 54 g of protein, while 25 g is the suggested allowance for protein per 1,000 kcal. The resultant nutrient density ratio, or "Index of Nutritional Quality" (INQ), for milk protein, i.e., 2.2 (54/25), is independent of serving size.

TABLE 2.1. RECOMMENDED DAILY DIETARY ALLOWANCES OF THE FOOD AND NUTRITION BOARDS, NATIONAL ACADEMY OF SCIENCES—NATIONAL

	Age (years)	Weight (lb)	Height (in)	Energy (kcal)	Protein (g)	Fat-soluble vitamins			Water-soluble vitamins						
						Vita-min A Activity (IU)	Vita-min D (IU)	Vita-min E Activity (IU)	Ascor-bic Acid (mg)	Fola-cin (µg)	Nia-cin[b] (mg)	Ribo-flavin (mg)	Thia-min (mg)	Vita-min B₆ (mg)	Vita-min B₁₂ (µg)
Infants	0.0-0.5	14	24	kg × 117	kg × 2.2	1,400	400	4	35	50	5	0.4	0.3	0.3	0.3
	0.5-1.0	20	28	kg × 108	kg × 2.0	2,000	400	5	35	50	8	0.6	0.5	0.4	0.3
Children	1-3	28	34	1,300	23	2,000	400	7	40	100	9	0.8	0.7	0.6	1.0
	4-6	44	44	1,800	30	2,500	400	9	40	200	12	1.1	0.9	0.9	1.5
	7-10	66	54	2,400	36	3,300	400	10	40	300	16	1.2	1.2	1.2	2.0
Males	11-14	97	63	2,800	44	5,000	400	12	45	400	18	1.5	1.4	1.6	3.0
	15-18	134	69	3,000	54	5,000	400	15	45	400	20	1.8	1.5	2.0	3.0
	19-22	147	69	3,000	54	5,000	400	15	45	400	20	1.8	1.5	2.0	3.0
	23-50	154	69	2,700	56	5,000		15	45	400	18	1.6	1.4	2.0	3.0
	51+	154	69	2,400	56	5,000		15	45	400	16	1.5	1.2	2.0	3.0
Females	11-14	97	62	2,400	44	4,000	400	12	45	400	16	1.3	1.2	1.6	3.0
	15-18	119	65	2,100	48	4,000	400	12	45	400	14	1.4	1.1	2.0	3.0
	19-22	128	65	2,100	46	4,000	400	12	45	400	14	1.4	1.1	2.0	3.0
	23-50	128	65	2,000	46	4,000		12	45	400	13	1.2	1.0	2.0	3.0
	51+	128	65	1,800	46	4,000		12	45	400	12	1.1	1.0	2.0	3.0
	Pregnant			+300	+30	5,000	400	15	60	800	+2	+0.3	+0.3	2.5	4.0
	Lactating			+500	+20	6,000	400	15	80	600	+4	+0.5	+0.3	2.5	4.0

[a]The allowances are intended to provide for individual variations among most normal persons as they live in the United States under usual environmental stresses. Diets should be based on a variety of common foods in order to provide other nutrients for which human requirements have been less well defined.

[b]Although allowances are expressed as niacin, it is recognized that on the average 1 mg of niacin is derived from each 60 mg of dietary tryptophan.

[c]This increased requirement cannot be met by ordinary diets; therefore, the use of supplemental iron is recommended.

TABLE 2.2. NUTRIENT ALLOWANCES PER 1,000 KCAL DERIVED FROM RECOMMENDED DAILY DIETARY ALLOWANCES (NAS/NRC, 1974)

	Age (years)	Energy (kcal)	Protein (g)	Fat-soluble vitamins			Ascorbic Acid (mg)	Folacin (μg)	Niacin (mg)	Water-soluble vitamins			
				Vitamin A Activity (RE)	Vitamin D (IU)	Vitamin E Activity (IU)				Riboflavin (mg)	Thiamin (mg)	Vitamin B_6 (mg)	Vitamin B_{12} (μg)
Children	1-3	1,300	17.7	308	308	5.4	30.8	76.9	6.9	0.62	0.54	0.46	0.80
	4-6	1,800	16.7	278	220	5.0	22.0	111	6.7	0.61	0.50	0.50	0.83
	7-10	2,400	15.0	292	167	4.2	16.7	125	6.7	0.50	0.50	0.50	0.83
Males	11-14	2,800	15.7	357	143	4.3	16.1	143	6.4	0.54	0.50	0.57	1.1
	15-18	3,000	18.0	333	133	5.0	15.0	133	6.7	0.60	0.50	0.67	1.0
	19-22	3,000	18.0	333	133	5.0	15.0	133	6.7	0.60	0.50	0.67	1.0
	23-50	2,700	20.7	370		5.6	16.8	148	6.7	0.59	0.52	0.74	1.1
	51+	2,400	23.3	417		6.3	18.8	167	6.7	0.63	0.50	0.83	1.3
Females	11-14	2,400	18.3	333	167	5.0	18.8	167	6.7	0.54	0.50	0.67	1.3
	15-18	2,100	22.9	381	191	5.7	21.4	191	6.7	0.67	0.52	0.95	1.4
	19-22	2,100	21.9	381	191	5.7	21.4	191	6.7	0.67	0.52	0.95	1.4
	23-50	2,000	23.0	400		6.0	22.5	200	6.5	0.60	0.50	1.0	1.5
	51+	1,800	25.6	444		6.7	25.0	222	6.7	0.61	0.56	1.11	1.7

By exploiting the resulting ratio, an assessment of a food supply's ability to meet dietary allowances becomes possible, and food manufacturers, government agencies, and consumers have an easy means of understanding the nutritional contributions of a food to a balanced diet. Hence, food may be examined with respect to its ability to meet dietary allowances relative to the calories provided.

The distinctions among the dietary allowances for males, females, different age groups, and pregnancy and lactation, as shown in Table 2.1, are all vital and should be maintained for nutrition professionals such as the dietitian and clinician. However, expressing the allowances per 1,000 kcal in terms of a single value for each nutrient rather than different values for each sex and age group is a simplification for alternate uses; it should not be confused with or substituted for those traditional and important uses of the RDAs.

The utility of expressing nutrient allowances per 1,000 kcal was also an important consideration at a recent European conference (Wretlind 1977).

In order to obtain a single-value allowance for each nutrient, it is first necessary to convert the RDAs shown in Table 2.1 into allowances per 1,000 kcal by dividing each RDA by the calorie allowance and multiplying by 1,000; the results are shown in Table 2.2.

This table shows that for some nutrients, the allowances per 1,000 kcal are approximately constant, thus simplifying the choice of the single value for each of these nutrients. For those nutrients whose values are not constant, the single-value allowances should be largely based on the allowances for those persons whose nutrient-to-calorie needs are greatest, e.g., those with the lowest calorie needs, since they find it most difficult to meet other dietary allowances. A review of Table 2.2 shows the following: thiamin, riboflavin, niacin, and probably protein and iodine allowances per 1,000 kcal are constant, within error of calculation. Allowances for these nutrients per 1,000 kcal change somewhat with age and sex, but for practical considerations are a constant (see also Hegsted 1975). For example, the protein allowance per 1,000 kcal for children 1-3 years of age is 17.7 g, but varies from 15 to 25.6 g for the other age and sex categories.

The vitamin A allowance per 1,000 kcal ranges from 292 retinol equivalents (RE) for the 7-to 10-year-old child to 444 RE for the aged female. The rationale for this variation may not be completely defensible. An allowance of 400 RE per 1,000 kcal is probably justified.

The vitamin E allowance per 1,000 kcal varies from 4.2 to 6.7 international units (IU). An allowance of 5 mg per 1,000 kcal is therefore suggested.

The vitamin C allowance per 1,000 kcal could be stated as 30 mg. The recommended allowance for vitamin C has tended to decrease with recent editions of the RDAs. Both Canada and England recommend less than 20 mg per 1,000 kcal. Some recent reports suggest that vitamin C may enhance iron absorption and that a slightly higher allowance might be warranted. The present allowance is practically a constant per 1,000 kcal, and any change could be rationalized on a kilocalorie basis.

Vitamin B_{12} and folacin allowances are very nearly constants per 1,000 kcal. Under certain definable circumstances, folic acid supplementation should be prescribed by a physician. For example, the symptoms of pernicious anemia may be masked if too much folacin is consumed.

Magnesium and zinc allowances are also probably constant per 1,000 kcal within determinable limits.

The remainder of the nutrients need special consideration:

Vitamin D. The RDA for vitamin D, where listed, is 400 IU for each category of age and sex; this amount is used to fortify 1 qt. of milk. Interestingly the assumption has been made that the 23- to 50-year-old female does not require supplementary vitamin D (Anon. 1974). The literature concerning osteoporosis in women suggests that this recommendation needs reexamination. In any event, new methodological approaches for more precisely determining the vitamin D requirement for all age groups will undoubtedly emerge from recent discoveries (DeLuca 1976). At this point, nothing would be lost by stating the allowance per 1,000 kcal.

Calcium and Phosphorus. The allowances for calcium and phosphorus are similarly given in increments of 400 mg, implying enough uncertainty about the requirement for each that stating an allowance per 1,000 kcal is reasonable. Recent data indicate that the Ca/P ratio in the American diet is lower than the ideal ratio of 1.0. Phosphate consumption may be greater than is nutritionally desirable, so perhaps upper limits of intake should be defined as well. The uncertainties are sufficient, however, to suggest that it may be appropriate for many purposes to state calcium and phosphorus allowances per 1,000 kcal of food.

Vitamin B_6. Understandably, the requirement for vitamin B_6 is most directly related to protein intake. This is becoming increasingly more evident, and careful thought needs to be given in the food selection process to insure an adequate intake of Vitamin B_6. Practically, an allowance of vitamin B_6 per 1,000 kcal should be easier for the consumer to implement than one related directly to protein intake.

Iron. The difficulties of establishing an iron allowance have been discussed by Munro (1977). An intake as high as 9 mg per 1,000 kcal may be justified, with the lowest calorie intake per unit of body weight being that for women, who also have the greatest need for dietary iron. People eat foods, not just nutrients, and women in the household generally eat the same foods as the men and children. It is difficult to derive a selection of foods that would meet an allowance of 6 mg per 1,000 kcal and almost impossible to meet an allowance of 9 mg per 1,000 kcal. Regardless of the iron intake at which the allowance per 1,000 kcal is set, it will be difficult to satisfy it from the food supply.

Table 2.3 summarizes these recommended single-value allowances per 1,000 kcal. These allowances become broad guidelines to describe the nutritional quality of food and permit the comparison between calorie

TABLE 2.3. SINGLE-VALUE nutrient allowances per 1,000 kcal

Protein	25 g
Vitamin A	400 RE
Vitamin D	5 μg
Vitamin E	5 mg
Vitamin C	30 mg
Folacin	200 μg
Niacin	7 mg
Riboflavin	0.6 mg
Thiamin	0.5 mg
Vitamin B_6	1.0 mg
Vitamin B_{12}	1.5 μg
Calcium	500 mg
Phosphorus	500 mg
Iodine	75 μg
Iron	6–8 mg
Magnesium	150 mg
Zinc	7 mg

allowance and that for other nutrients. For those whose energy needs are least, it is obviously more critical for food to be selected to include a balanced supply of all the nutrients. The variety of food available and, therefore, the choices consumers must make probably will not be reduced. However, for many the total consumption should be reduced, making it imperative that all nutrient allowances should be included with as few calories as practical.

"PROVISIONAL" RDAs

To further assist consumers and professional nutritionists, provisional recommended dietary allowances to supplement the RDAs should also be considered by the Subcommittee on Dietary Allowances of the Food and Nutrition Board for inclusion in the next edition. There is an underlying assumption, with the use of the RDAs, that food selection will be made from a wide-enough variety of choices to ensure that nutrients which are known to be required by human beings, but for which no allowance has been established, will be consumed in adequate quantities.

Limitation of information regarding nutrient content of many foods and an inadequate knowledge of requirements for those nutrients prevents their being listed in the general summary table (Table 2.1). A need is emerging for establishing allowances for some nutrients not listed in the summary table; therefore, the Food and Nutrition Board should consider available evidence and, where it is insufficient to warrant establishing an allowance in the traditional sense, use such terminology as "provisional recommended dietary allowance." Such allowances obviously will be less well documented by research and observation and may be regarded as somewhat tentative and evolutionary in nature. As more research information becomes available, provisional allowances may expect to assume the status of those listed in the summary table. Table 2.4 is a suggested list of provisional RDAs, given, for the reasons discussed earlier in this article, in terms of nutrients per 1,000 kcal.

TABLE 2.4. PROVISIONAL
Recommended Dietary Allowances per
1,000 kcal

Pantothenic acid	3.0 mg
Biotin	0.05 mg
Vitamin K	15 μg
Potassium	0.50–3.0 g
Sodium	0.25–1.6 g
Copper	1.0 mg
Manganese	1.0
Chromium	0.025 mg
Selenium	0.025 mg
Molybdenum	0.07 mg
Fluoride	(1 mg /l of water)

There is reason to suggest that a provisional allowance should be established for pantothenic acid and biotin. Requirements for pantothenic acid and biotin, as well as their occurrence in foods, are known with less certainty than for other vitamins; hence, it is appropriate that an allowance for them imply more of a "provisional" status.

The function of vitamin K in human metabolism has been well established; however, a dietary need has not been well defined except in newborn infants prior to establishment of intestinal flora. However, provisional allowance for vitamin K probably can be made.

Many nutritionists feel that our consumption of sodium is too high;

therefore, a provisional RDA for sodium is suggested to help in controlling the amount consumed. Since sodium and potassium are important in maintaining proper electrolyte balance, a provisional RDA for potassium is also suggested.

Perhaps the most cogent argument for provisional RDA can be developed relative to requirements for trace elements which are not listed in the general table; namely, copper, manganese, chromium, selenium, and molybdenum. Suggested values for these trace elements are included in Table 2.4 (Mertz 1977).

Fluoride is clearly recognized as needed to promote growth of experimental animals being fed purified diets. It is becoming increasingly evident that the function of fluoride in bone and teeth development in human beings is positive and fundamental. To reduce the incidence of dental caries, it has become customary to add fluoride to the water supply. Therefore, it is appropriate to state the "allowance" for fluoride as parts per million or milligrams per liter of water.

Requirements of humans for sulfur and cobalt are met with sulfur-containing amino acids and vitamin B_{12} respectively. There is sometimes an exogenous need for choline and inositol for animals and microorganisms; there is not evidence, however, of special needs in humans beyond their biosynthetic capacity. Claims of unusual nutritional benefits for inositol and choline consumption are unfounded, and a provisional allowance for either compound is unwarranted.

Finally, elements such as tin, vanadium, silicon, and arsenic are probably nutritionally important for some species, but data for human need are not available.

REFERENCES

DeLUCA, H.F. 1976. Metabolism of vitamin D; current status   Am. J. Clin. Nutr. 29:1258.

EEGERDINGK, W. 1977. Personal Communication, The Albert Heijn Supermart, B.V., Zaandam, The Netherlands.

HANSEN, R.G. 1970. Malnutrition and the affluent society. Utah Science, 31:67.

HANSEN, R.G. 1971. Caloric requirements in relation to micronutrient intake. In AMA symp on Vitamins and Minerals in Processed Foods, New Orleans, La., March, . 180. Am. Med. Assn., Chicago, Ill.

HANSEN, D.M. 1975. Dietary standards. J. Am. Dietet, Assn. 66:13.

MERTZ, W. 1977. Personal communication. Beltsville Agricultural Research Center, Beltsville, Md.

MUNRO, H.N. 1977. How well recommended are the RDAs? J. Am. Dietet. Assn. 71:490.

NAS/NRC. 1974. "Recommended Dietary Allowances." 8th ed. Natl. Acad. of Sciences—Natl. Res. Council, Washington, D.C.

USDA. 1972. Food and nutrient intake of individuals in the United States, Spring 1965. Household Food Consumption Survey 1965-66, Report No. 11, U.S. Dept. of Agriculture—Agric. Res. Service, Washington, D.C.

WATT, B.K. and MERRILL, A.L. 1972. "Composition of Foods—Raw, Processed, Prepared." Agriculture Handbook No. 8., computer tapes. U. S. Dept. of Agriculture, Washington, D.C.

WRETLIND, A. 1977. Introduction—general aspects of recommended dietary allowances. Nutr. Metab. 21:210.

WYSE, B.W., SORENSON, A.W., WITTWER, A.J., and HANSEN, R.G. 1976. Nutritional quality index identifies consumer nutrient needs. Food Technol. 30(1):22.

3

Nutritional Attributes of Foods and Food Combinations

QUANTITY AND QUALITY

In the United States, because of the abundant supply of good food, the dietary choices available to consumers may surpass their average discriminatory capability. It is therefore not surprising that inappropriate or inadequate food selections are made. The Ten-State Nutrition Survey identified certain nutrient deficits and indicated that the diet of many of those surveyed needed to be improved (Anon. 1972). This conclusion was supported by dietary and biochemical assessments. In our opinion, some of the desired improvement can be achieved by providing better nutrition education to producers, processors, distributors and consumers of food.

THE USE OF INQs

INQs were calculated for all foods in Handbook No. 8:
- meat, poultry, fish, and eggs
- grains and grain products
- nuts, soybeans, and miscellaneous seeds
- fruits
- vegetables
- milk and milk products
- fats and oils
- sugars and sweets

Each food category was examined with reference to the distribution of the nutrients for which data are available. The U.S. RDAs were used as the standard for nutrient consumption throughout, with an arbitrary 2300 kcal energy base.

Table 3.1 can be examined from the point of view of either food

TABLE 3.1. PERCENTAGE OF FOODS FROM HANDBOOK NO. 8 WITH INDEX OF NUTRITIONAL QUALITY OF 1.0 OR HIGHER

Food Classification	Number of Foods	Protein[1]	Calcium	Phosphorus	Iron	Vitamin A	Thiamin	Riboflavin	Niacin[2]	Vitamin C
Fruits	307	3.0	14.2	11.9	41.7	44.7	38.0	20.9	22.6	79.5
Vegetables	414	81.3	60.3	92.2	86.3	63.9	82.8	73.7	79.0	93.0
Grains and grain products[3]	547	36.3	10.3	47.1	28.6	2.8	40.7	12.2	26.7	2.7
Nuts, soybeans and seeds	65	73.9	32.2	86.2	56.9	6.2	58.6	32.3	33.7	9.1
Meat, fish and egg products	921	91.7	8.2	87.1	57.2	13.8	36.5	58.0	82.4	6.3
Milk products	57	84.2	85.8	85.8	0.0	61.4	20.9	84.1	0.0	5.3
Sweets and sugars	80	12.5	18.6	30.8	21.1	0.0	2.6	15.0	11.3	1.3
Fats and oils	35	9.1	11.3	11.2	2.7	22.8	0.0	8.6	0.0	8.7

[1]Protein calculated on a standard of 45 g for milk, meat, fish and egg products, 65 g otherwise.
[2]Preformed niacin
[3]Includes pies, cakes and cookies.

classification and the nutrient strengths of each, or of a specific nutrient and the important food sources of that nutrient. Each approach has some value. The table shows the percentage of food items within each food classification in Handbook No. 8 that have INQs of 1.0 or greater for each of the nutrients examined. For example, 74% of foods in the nuts, soybeans, and miscellaneous seed group have INQs of 1.0 or greater for protein (based on a U.S. RDA of 65 g for this group of foods). This supports the idea that, on the average, this food group is a desirable source of protein. It can also be noted that most foods in this category provide substantial amounts of several nutrients except vitamins A and C.

The foods in the vegetable category provide in general more nutrients per calorie than do those in any other group. The vegetables are exceptionally good sources of vitamin C, with only 7% of the items with a lower proportion of the vitamin than of energy, in relation to human need. Since protein ratings are based on nitrogen determinations in food, the nutritional value of the protein in vegetables tends to be overstated and for that matter, the potential nutrient contribution of vegetables to the average diet may tend to be overstated because normally the percent of the total energy requirement derived from vegetables is not high. It is also clear from Table 3.1 that most other food categories have certain deficits.

A comparison of the iron and calcium contributions of the various food categories in Table 3.1 raises some interesting questions. Iron normally has been considered the nutrient most likely to be lacking in the U.S. diet for some segments of the population. Examination of the food categories, however, suggests that except for the milk products classification, iron allowances may be better met than calcium. (Iron INQs are calculated using the 18 mg U.S. RDA). Perhaps the calcium allowances are overstated, and/or undefined calcium deficiencies may be more common than previously thought. The latter possibility seems to be supported by the apparent increasing incidence of geriatric osteoporosis (Lutwak 1974).

Cereals contain many nutrients in significant amounts, but in proportion to the calories frequently below an INQ of 1.0. To illustrate, the bread and cereal category is normally thought to contribute substantial amounts of iron, thiamin, riboflavin, and niacin to the diet. Table 3.1 illustrates that only 29, 41, 12 and 27% of the foods in that category are adequate sources (INQs of 1.0) of iron, thiamin, riboflavin and niacin, respectively. The INQs for these nutrients for white enriched flour are iron = 1.0, thiamin = 1.9, riboflavin = 1.0 and niacin = 1.1, reflecting that white enriched flour "carries its own" for those B vitamins and iron.

The INQ concept as applied to food may be better communicated in graphic form. In Figure 3.1 the INQ, increasing from left to right, is

GRAINS AND GRAIN PRODUCTS

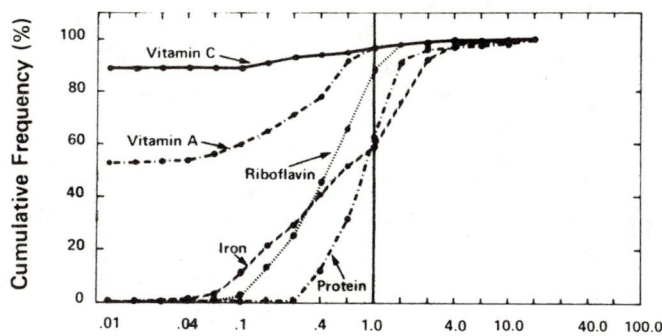

FIG. 3.1. INDEX OF NUTRITIONAL QUALITY

On the abscissa the Index of Nutritional Quality is recorded on a log scale. On the ordinate the frequency is a cumulative distribution in INQ values with 1 as a reference point. Each point on the curves includes the percentage of foods in the category with a given INQ plus those with less than that INQ. Thus they are cumulative moving from left to right on the chart, or with increasing INQ. INQ calculated from U.S. RDA values and an arbitrary 2300 kcal standard.

recorded on a log scale on the abscissa. On the ordinate, the percentage of foods at any point, 1.0 for example, includes all foods of INQ value between 0 and 1.0 for a particular food group. Thus the reference values on the ordinate are cumulative with increasing INQ values on the abscissa. Plotted at the left end of the scale is the percentage of grains and grain products that have an INQ of 0.01 or less for each of the listed nutrients. About 90% of them have little or no vitamin C, and nearly half have small amounts of vitamin A, yielding an INQ of 0.01. For the other three nutrients the mininum INQ is 0.04 or above, with most grain products falling in the region of 0.1 to 2.5. By this criterion, the grain products are not "outstanding" sources of any nutrients. Grain products are "fair" or "good" sources of protein, none of them having an INQ of less than 0.25, about 60% having an INQ between 0.25 and 1.0, with the remaining 40% having an INQ between 1.0 and 2.5. At the extreme right all lines approach 100% and include all foods in the category.

All products made from either whole wheat or enriched wheat flour, including quick breads, pastries, pies, cakes and cookies, are included in the grain products group. Unless the other ingredients in flour products are good sources of these vitamins and iron, nutrient "dilution" occurs, meaning that excess calories would have to be consumed to obtain adequate quantities of some of the nutrients. Most cereal-grain products in the U.S. are made with shortening and sugar, which contain virtually none of the B vitamins and iron.

Grain and grain products are important carriers of many of the nutrients for which knowledge of human requirements and food consumption data are incomplete. These nutrients are partially lost in the milling process and are not adequately restored. As often consumed, the cereal products do not contain large quantities of any particular nutrient when combined in many popular baked goods. Probably this should emphasize the importance of either revisions of the milling program or more realistic restoration of many of the nutritional elements lost, for example, zinc, manganese, copper, pyridoxine, pantothenic acid, etc. (Anon. 1974). Such a restoration program is probably economically feasible in the United States.

FIBER

The use of INQs as a way to explain the potential of various foods to contribute to a diet can be further illustrated with fiber. The current nutritional or medical claims for fiber eventually may or may not prove valid. But certainly the INQ approach clarifies the distribution of fiber in the diet and, for those who may be interested, how to select foods of high fiber content. The composition of food was constructed from our computer file of Handbook No. 8 data for crude fiber. It should be noted that fiber is not easily defined chemically, nor are analytical methods for fiber adequate (Trowell 1976, Hellendoorn et al. 1975). Furthermore, the "allowance" is an arbitrarily defined standard of 7 g, which corresponds to a suggested intake of 100 mg fiber per kg of body weight for a 70 kg individual (Cowgill and Anderson 1932). Thus a portion of a food that provides 2300 kcal and contains 7 g of fiber will have an INQ for fiber of 1.0.

Very few vegetables have an INQ of less than 1.0 (see Figure 3.2). In fact, about 45% of the vegetables have 70 g or more of fiber per 2300 kcal, i.e., INQ = 10.0. This means that 230-kcal portions of any of these vegetables would provide the 7 g of fiber. Some fruits and vegetables have INQs of 20.0 (140 g of fiber per 2300 kcal); a 115 kcal portion of any of these would supply 7 g of fiber, the assumed daily fiber "allowance" (Cowgill and Anderson 1932).

According to INQ analyses, grains and grain products have a trimodal distribution in fiber content (see Figure 3.3). The first modality (0.04-0.1) encompasses sweet bakery products. The refined cereals are in the middle (0.1-0.6). The unrefined cereals (0.6-4.0), however, can provide fiber in proportion to their energy contribution, based on the arbitrary 7 g daily allowance.

FIBER

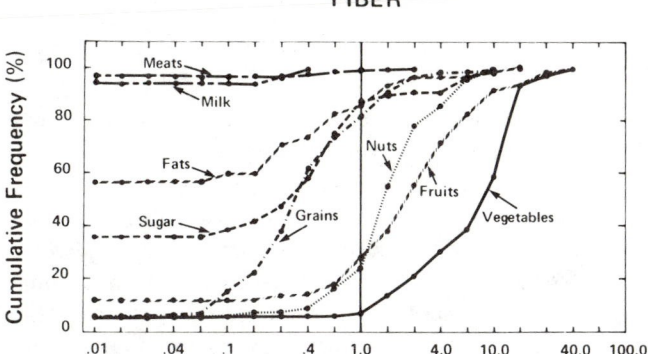

FIG. 3.2. INDEX OF NUTRITIONAL QUALITY

Fiber distribution in foods is in relation to energy content. An intake of 7 g for a 70 kilogram man has been assumed to be the standard.

FIBER

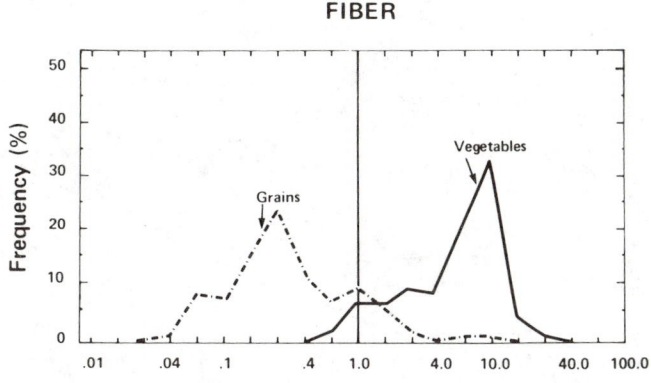

FIG. 3.3. INDEX OF NUTRITIONAL QUALITY

Distribution of fiber in foods with respect to energy content within two different food groups: grains and grain products, and vegetables. The trimodal distribution of the grain products results from categorical differences in fiber content between the unrefined cereals (INQ about 0.25), and the sweetened bakery products (INQ about 0.06).

As expected, almost 100% of the milk and meat products have fiber INQs of .01 or less, showing they contain virtually no fiber (Figure 3.2). In contrast, the unrefined cereals, with their INQs of 1.0 or slightly greater, require little or no supplementation relative to fiber to meet the assumed "allowance." When supplementary fiber is desired, vegetables, fruits, and nuts are obviously the prime food sources.

NUTRITION TERMINOLOGY

Textbooks of nutrition for use by professional educators, more popular articles aimed at the consumer, and certainly advertisements designed to sell food, all use such qualitative terms as "poor," "fair," "adequate," "good," "excellent," to describe nutritive potency of foods. A survey of popular nutrition texts using nutrient density criteria showed that these subjective modifiers are not used consistently either among textbook writers or within a textbook when referring to different nutrients (Anon 1976). There is an obvious need for adjectives that can have quantitative or semiquantitative meaning (Howard 1972). In practice, for educational and promotional purposes, statements are made and ideas are conveyed using words and phrases which attempt to imply quantitative significance, but at best they are only weakly qualitative and somewhat confusing.

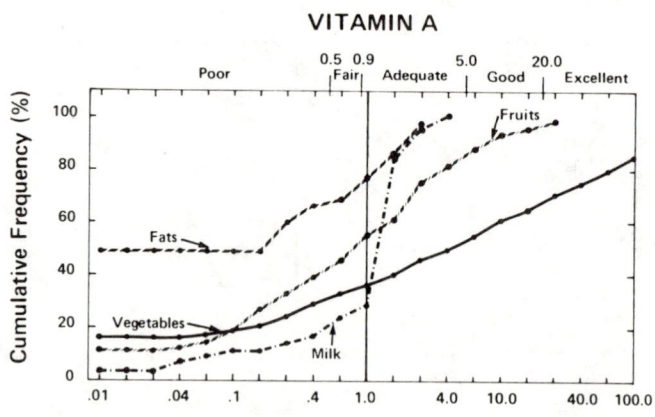

FIG. 3.4. INDEX OF NUTRITIONAL QUALITY

Vitamin A distribution in foods is in relation to energy content. The U.S. RDA for vitamin A (5,000 IU) per 2300 kcal is the standard.

If agreement could be reached on educationally desirable terms and suggested limits for their implication and use, a basis and point of reference could be the INQ as illustrated by the vitamin A example in Figure 3.4. The limits are readily definable. Of course, this assumes that the nutrient composition of foods and the allowances for nutrients are adequately known. Obviously there is a need for more information in both of these categories. A range of INQ values is suggested in Table 3.2 as a possible guideline to circumscribe these commonly used nutritional

TABLE 3.2. SUGGESTED QUANTITATIVE BASIS FOR NUTRITIONALLY DESCRIPTIVE ADJECTIVES

	Poor	Fair	Adequate	Good	Excellent
INQ for vitamins A & C	<0.5	0.5–0.89	0.9–4.9	5.0 –19.9	>20
INQ for other nutrients	<0.5	0.5–0.89	0.9–1.5	1.51– 4.9	>5

adjectives. Since the U.S. RDAs used in calculating INQs are derived from the Food and Nutrition Board's RDAs and the RDAs have a margin of safety, suggested guidelines follow. A food having an INQ of less than 0.5 for any nutrient should be considered a "poor" source for that nutrient, while an INQ between 0.5-0.9 should be considered as a "fair" nutrient source. INQs between 0.9-4.9 for vitamins A and C and between 0.9-1.5 for all other nutrients could be considered to be "adequate" sources since a similar proportion of nutrient and energy requirements is provided.

It may be questioned if the same nutrient density number can serve as the descriptive limits for the term "good" or "excellent" source of vitamin A or vitamin C on one hand, and protein on the other. For instance, there is some protein in most foods, while a more limited number of foods is relied upon to supply vitamin A and vitamin C in the diet. Figure 3.4 shows graphically the disparity of vitamin A distribution, with vegetables and some fruits being the major food sources with supplementary amounts of this nutrient. It might, therefore, be appropriate to expect a higher INQ for vitamin C and vitamin A in order for food to be termed an "excellent" source of that nutrient.

The single-value allowances per 1,000 kcal as discussed in Chapter 2 can provide a basis for evaluating the potential of foods to meet nutritional allowances. Figure 3.5 was constructed from a computer file of data from Agricultural Handbook No. 8 (Watt and Merrill 1973) for calcium using a standard of 450 mg per 1,000 kcal. Each food in Handbook No. 8 is assigned to a food category, i.e., milk and milk products meat, poultry, fish and eggs; grains and grain products; nuts, soybeans, and miscellaneous seeds; fruits; vegetables; fats and oils; and sugar and sweets. The abscissa of Figure 3.5 represents nutrient density ratios, plotted on a logarithmic scale. The ordinate represents the cumulative percentage of foods in a particular category that has a given nutrient density ratio plus those that have a lower ratio.

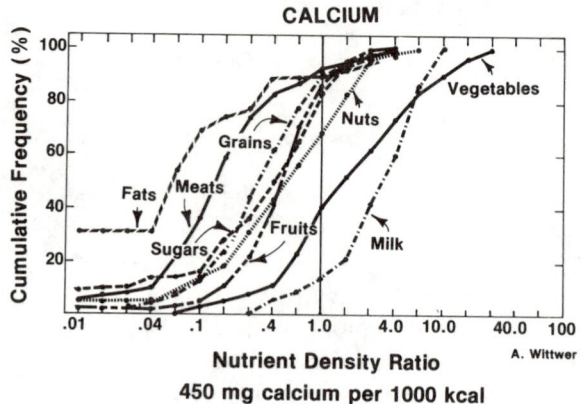

Fig. 3.5. NUTRIENT DENSITY ANALYSIS OF CALCIUM
DISTRIBUTION IN FOODS IN AGRICULTURE HANDBOOK NO.
8, BASED ON 450 MG OF CALCIUM PER 1,000 KCAL

For example, reading the milk curve at the point at which it crosses the vertical line representing a nutrient density ratio of 1.0 shows that 14% of the foods in the milk and milk products category have nutrient density ratios of 1.0 or less. Put antithetically, 86% of the foods in this group have calcium nutrient density ratios of 1.0 or higher, and 40% have calcium ratios of 4.0 or greater. Assuming a 2,000 kcal diet, a 500 kcal serving of food with a nutrient density ratio of 4.0 would provide 900 mg of calcium, which is the total allowance. A 500 kcal serving of food with a nutrient density ratio of 1.0 would provide 225 mg of calcium, one-fourth of the allowance. Using any food composition table and the simplified RDA values, the nutrient density ratio for any food or nutrient can be calculated. (Hansen 1973, Wyse *et al.* 1976).

The difficulty of meeting the iron allowance from foods is shown in Figure 3.6. The solid vertical line in the center of the graph represents a nutrient density ratio of 1.0 when 6 mg of iron per 1,000 kcal is the standard, while the dashed vertical line to the right of center represents the same ratio when 9 mg of iron per 1,000 kcal serves as the standard. When 6 mg per 1,000 kcal serves as the standard, 72% of the foods in the meat group have nutrient density ratios of 1.0 or greater; however, when the standard is adjusted to 9 mg per 1,000 kcal, only 44% of the foods comply.

Nutrient allowances per 1,000 kcal have been used in Figure 3.7 to evaluate the adequacy of a 1,000 kcal portion of a composite diet based on data from the 1965-66 Household Food Consumption Survey (Anon. 1972). The graph represents data from 9,935 males and females 18-55 years of age, who consumed on the average 2,157 kcal. The data indicate that in 1965, 1,000 kcal of consumed diet met and exceeded the allowance per 1,000 kcal for protein, vitamins A and C, thiamin and riboflavin but provided, only 70% and 80% of the calcium and iron allowances, respectively (using 8 mg per 1,000 kcal as the standard for iron). Professionals interested in developing nutrition education programs to correct these problem areas would do well to consult Figures 3.5 and 3.6 for appropriate food choices for increasing dietary calcium and iron.

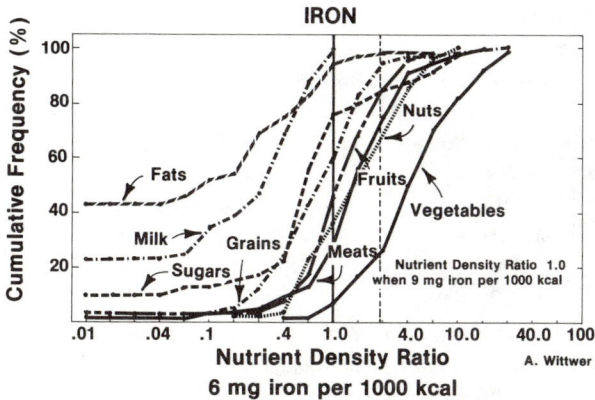

FIG. 3.6. NUTRIENT DENSITY ANALYSIS OF IRON DIS-TRIBUTION in foods in Agriculture Handbook No. 8, based on 6 mg (solid vertical line) and 9 mg (dashed vertical line) of iron per 1,000 kcal. On the abscissa the nutrient density is recorded on a log scale. On the ordinate the frequency is a cumulative distribution of nutrient density values with 1 as a reference point. Each point on the curves includes the percentage of foods in the category with a given nutrient density plus those with less than that nutrient density. Thus they are cumulative moving from left to right on the chart, or with increasing nutrient density.

NUTRIENT DENSITY ANALYSIS OF 1000-KCAL COMPOSITE
1965-66 HOUSEHOLD FOOD CONSUMPTION SURVEY DATA

Nutrient	INQ	Amount	% Standard	0	10	20	30	40	50	60	70	80	90	100
Energy	1.0	1000 kcal	100											
Protein	1.6	40 gm	163											
Vitamin A	1.4	564 R.E.	141											
Vitamin C	1.2	30 mg	120											
Thiamin	1.1	0.56 mg	111											
Riboflavin	1.3	0.80 mg	133											
Calcium	0.7	313 mg	70											
Iron	0.8	6.4 mg	80											

Standards per 1000-kcal: Protein - 25 gm; Vitamin A - 400 retinal equivalents; Vitamin C - 25 mg; Thiamin - 0.5 mg; Riboflavin - 0.6 mg; Calcium - 450 mg; Iron - 8 mg.

FIG. 3.7. NUTRIENT DENSITY ANALYSIS OF 1000–KCAL COMPOSITE 1965–66 HOUSEHOLD FOOD CONSUMPTION SURVEY DATA

REFERENCES

ANON. 1971. USDA Agricultural Research Service, Progress Report of the Consumer and Food Economics Division, Marketing and Nutrition Research, July 1, 1971, Agricultural Research Service, Washington, D.C.

ANON. 1972. Ten-State Nutrition Survey, 1968-1970. Highlights. U.S. Department of Health, Education and Welfare. Health Services and Mental Health Administration. Center for Disease Control. DHEW Publication No. (HSN) 72-8134, Atlanta, Georgia.

ANON. 1973. Federal Register. 38 (No.49):6960. March 14.

ANON. 1974A. Food and Nutrition Board, National Research Council. Proposed Fortification Policy for Cereal-Grain Products. National Academy of Sciences, Washington, D.C.

ANON. 1974B. Food and Nutrition Board, Recommended Dietary Allowances. 8th ed., National Academy of Sciences, Washington, D.C.

ANON. 1976. Society for Nutrition Education, Nutritional Claims for Food, Berkeley Calif. p. 22.

COWGILL, G.R., and Anderson, W.E. 1932. Laxative effects of wheat bran and "washed bran" in healthy men. J. Am. Med. Assn., 98:1866.

EMERSON, D.N. 1970. Potassium therapy and gastrointestinal lesions. Missouri Med., 67:310.

HANSEN, R.G. 1971. Caloric Requirements in Relation to Micronutrient Intake. Symposium on Vitamins and Minerals in Processed Foods. American Medical Assn., New Orleans, La., March 1971. p. 180.

HANSEN, R.G. 1973. An Index of Food Quality. Nutr. Rev. 31:1.

HELLENDOORN, E.W., NOORDHOFF, M.G. and J. SLAGMAN. 1975. Enzymatic determination of the indigestible residue (dietary fibre) content of human food. J. Sci. Fd. Agri., 26:1461.

HOWARD, H.W. 1972. Some Technical and Nutritional Aspects of Fabricated Foods. Unpublished paper presented before the Industry and Business Section. American Dairy Science Assn., 67th Annual Meeting. Blacksburg, Va., July, 1972.

LEVERTON, R.M. 1974. Fats in Food and Diet. USDA Agriculture Information Bulletin No. 361.

LUTWAK, L. 1974. Continuing need for calcium throughout life. Geriatrics. 29:171.

MENEELY, G.R. and BATTARBEE, H.D. 1976. Sodium and potassium. Nutr. Rev., 34:225.

SORENSON, A.W. and HANSEN, R.G. 1975. An Index of Food Quality. J. Nutr. Ed., 7:53.

SORENSON, A.W., WYSE, B.W., WITTWER, A.J. and HANSEN, R.G. 1976. An Index of Nutritional Quality for a balanced diet. J. Amer. Dietet. Assn., 68:236.

TROWELL, H. 1976. Definition of dietary fiber and hypotheses that it is a protective factor in certain diseases. Am. J. Clin. Nutr., 29:417.

WATT, B.K. and MERRILL, A.C. 1963. Compositions of Foods—Raw, Processed, Prepared. Agriculture Handbook No. 8 Rev. ed., USDA. Washington, D.C.

WRETLIND, A. 1974. World Sugar Production and Usage in Europe. Sugars in Nutrition. Ed., H.L. Sipple and K.W. McNutt. Academic Press, New York. pp. 88-90.

WYSE, B.W., SORENSON, A.W., WITTWER, A.J. and HANSEN, R.G. 1976. Nutritonal quality index identifies consumer nutrient needs. Food Techn., 30:22.

WYSE, B.W., SORENSON, A.W., WITTWER, A.J. and HANSEN, R.G. 1976. Foods instead of drugs to offset diuretic potassium losses. Utah Sci., Sept. p. 86.

4

Nutritional Quality Index

APPLICATION OF NUTRIENT DENSITY TO CONSUMER DECISIONS

For general consumer applications of the Index of Nutritional Quality, the implementation of the U.S. RDAs in their present form was a necessary initial measure. Using this standard, we can for the first time specify to the family or institutional food buyer or meal planner more precisely the characteristics of a balanced diet. The U.S. RDAs are nutritional standards established for the purpose of guiding food selection of the population as a whole—not for specific individuals. Thus, they are an appropriate yardstick for general purposes of expressing food quality and guiding selection of appropriate food combinations.

Though each person has his/her own energy requirements just as he/she has individual needs for the other nutrients, the U.S. RDAs and an arbitrary 2300 kcal can be used in illustrative calculations as the reasonable intake goal of an average adult. Obviously an active young male will require more than 2300 kcal to maintain weight while a relatively sedentary middle-aged female will require fewer kcal.

Index values therefore represent the quality of a food or combination of foods relative to the standard U.S. RDAs. An index of "1" or more for a particular nutrient indicates that 2300 kcal of the food being evaluated will supply the U.S. RDA of that nutrient. (Hansen 1973).

For general illustrative purposes, the following nutrients and their U.S. RDAs are considered in this chapter: energy, 2300 kcal[1]; protein, 65 g[2]; calcium, 1,000 mg; iron, 18 mg; vitamin A, 5,000 I.U.; thiamin, 1.5 mg; riboflavin, 1.7 mg; niacin, 20 mg; and vitamin C, 60 mg.

An important assumption of the Index of Nutritional Quality is that if all kcal are derived from a single food or food combination, this would

---

(1) There is no established U.S. RDA for kcal.
(2) Assuming the Protein Efficiency Ration (PER) is less than that of casein.

give the consumer a general idea of the potential of such foods to contribute to a balanced diet. However, it is impractical and undesirable to use a single food source to supply dietary needs; a more meaningful food profile is based on the usual contribution of a particular food to a total diet. The base parameter in such a case is the number of calories contained in an estimated average adult portion.

The profile of a one-cup serving of milk that contains 160 kcal is presented in Figure 4.1. A one-cup serving provides 7% or 160 kcal of the daily adult energy standard. The base line in Figure 4.1 represents a food index of "1," or the nutrient allowance for the day. Each index value can be read directly from a bar graph of the type below. The length of the bar now becomes the percent of the daily allowance represented by one serving of the food under consideration.

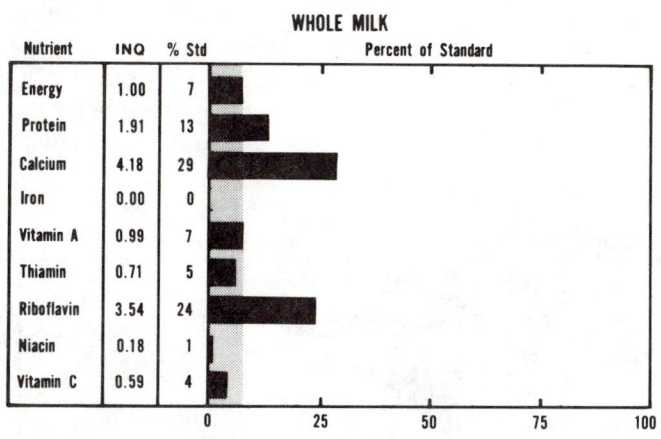

FIG. 4.1. CONTRIBUTION TO THE DAILY NUTRIENT ALLOWANCES BY ONE CUP OF WHOLE COW'S MILK

Obviously foods of high nutritional quality will have some nutrient values proportionately exceeding their energy content. Conversely, foods of lesser quality would provide most nutrients in adequate amounts only in conjunction with excess calories. The INQ profiles, therefore, convey two important concepts: the overall quality of the food as judged by the Index of Nutritional Quality and the contribution of a portion of that food to the total daily diet. Serving size information in this paper has been drawn in major part from Church and Church (1970).

FOOD COMPLEMENTATION

To balance a diet, nutrients that are in low amounts in one food need to be provided by other foods. The Index of Nutritional Quality Profiles make it easy to devise such food complementation. All that is required is an ability to offset the "short-bar" nutrients in a food profile with complementary food having "long-bars" for those nutrients. If a standard format is used for all food graphs, wherever and whenever they are presented, complementation could be understood by anyone. Familiarity with an Index of Nutritional Quality would permit individuals to readily see that a balanced diet can be achieved by choosing a variety of foods where the combined nutrient contents satisfy the U.S. RDAs. To meet nutritional goals, specific food combinations are immaterial so long as the additive result is adequate amounts of the needed nutrients.

To illustrate the concept of complementation, consider milk as shown in Figure 4.1, combined with other foods, including a pork chop, whose profile appears in Figure 4.2. The pork chop provides 19, 63, and 23% of the daily allowances, respectively, of iron, thiamin, and niacin. A pork chop is also a good source of high quality protein since one serving can yield 37% of the daily need by only 17% of the daily calories, yielding an INQ of 37% ÷ 17% = 2.24 for protein. The nutrients in a pork chop complement some of the nutrients less plentiful in a cup of milk.

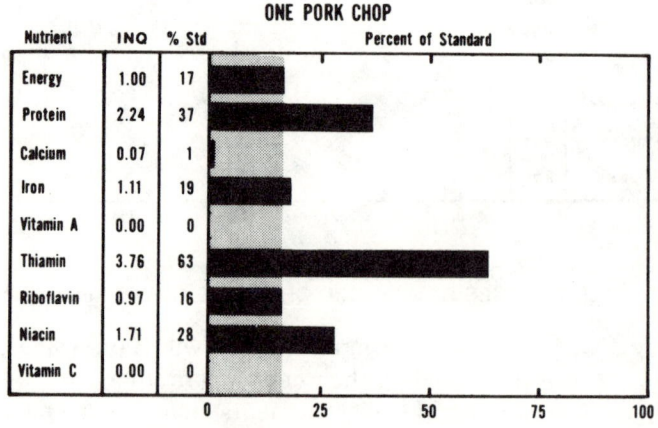

FIG. 4.2. CONTRIBUTION OF ONE PORK CHOP (3.5 OUNCES)
TO THE DAILY NUTRIENT ALLOWANCES

Raisins are a good source of iron in relation to calories (INQ = 1.55) as illustrated in Figure 4.3. A desirable iron level per calorie is probably the most difficult of all nutrient ratios to achieve. Unfortunately, serving sizes for raisins tend to be too small to help solve the problem. One-fourth cup of carrots (see Figure 4.4) contributes only 11 of the 2300 kcal but a large amount of vitamin A. Next, one-half cup of cauliflower (see Figure

4.5) yields 55% of the daily vitamin C allowance while adding only 13 kcal to the daily intake.

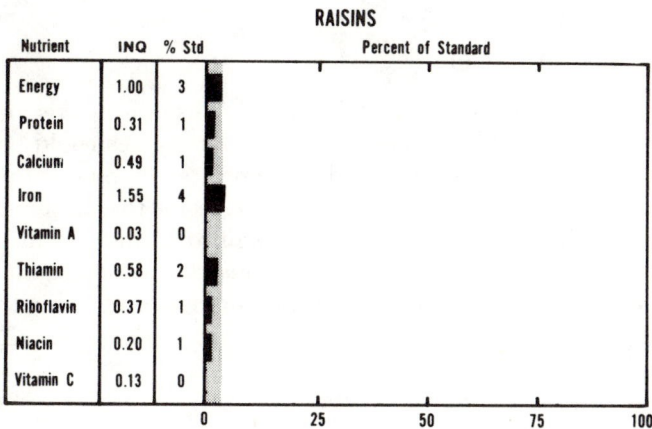

FIG. 4.3. CONTRIBUTION OF ONE SERVING (2 TABLESPOONS)
OF RAISINS TO THE DAILY NUTRIENT ALLOWANCES

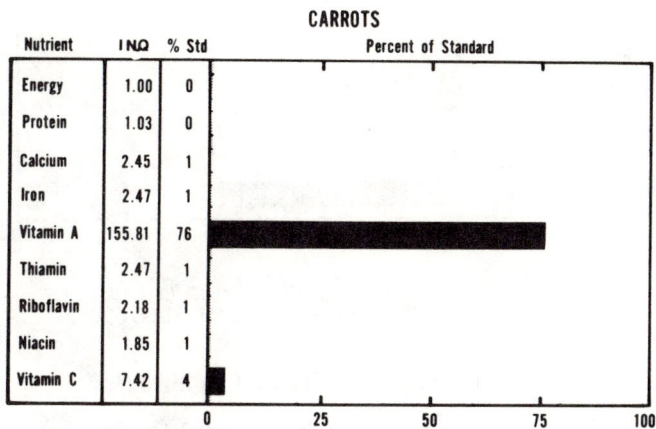

FIG. 4.4. CONTRIBUTION OF ONE SERVING (1½ CUP) OF
CARROTS TO THE DAILY NUTRIENT ALLOWANCES

The sum or composite of the individual foods mentioned above is illustrated in Figure 4.6. The composite represents a well-balanced meal. Every nutrient bar is longer than the energy line—-except iron which is only slightly low—indicating adequate or excess quantities. The foods combined in this meal provide 621 kcal, 27% of the 2300 kcal standard, leaving 73% for other meals and snacks. Its relatively low calorie and high nutrient content would make the meal an example for inclusion in a weight reduction program.

OTHER USES OF INQ

Nutrient density profiles included in cookbooks or other recipe sources could aid consumers in meal planning. Popular recipes could be supplemented with easily determined and appropriate complementary foods. For example, a one-cup portion of a standard recipe for chicken casserole provides proportionately high amounts of protein and niacin and adequate amounts of iron (see Figure 4.7). To insure a balanced meal, foods high in calcium, riboflavin, thiamin, and vitamins A and C should be used to complement the casserole.

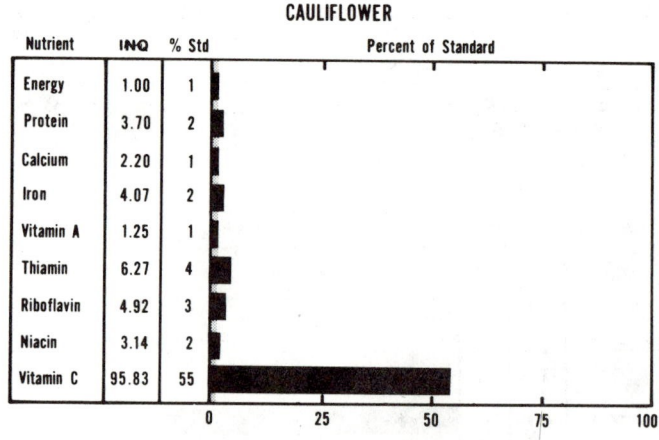

FIG. 4.5. CONTRIBUTION OF ONE SERVING (1½ CUP) OF CAULIFLOWER TO THE DAILY NUTRIENT ALLOWANCE

INDEX OF NUTRITIONAL QUALITY PROFILES

The potential value of the Index of Nutritional Quality as a nutrition education tool for the public will be realized only when food profiles are readily available. Toward this end, we have converted many of the foods in USDA Handbook No. 8 (Watt and Merril 1963), the major source of food composition data, to profile form by means of a computerized program. Amino acid composition data on proteins and some information on trace elements (including zinc) are also in computer storage for use in INQ calculations. As new information on food composition or nutrient standards becomes available, it is a simple matter to update the computer file. The resultant printout is the prototype for the figures in this chapter.

The dearth of information on trace elements content of foods and some vitamins such as B_6 and folacin limits the number of nutrients which can currently be included in INQ profiles. The limitations posed by incomplete food composition data in calculating INQ profiles emphasize the need to revise and add to the nutrient information currently available. Printouts obtained from the computer program can be collected into handbook form by direct offset printing, eliminating the need for costly and time consuming type setting. The handbook has been included at the end of the book as Part II. In addition, the handbook includes a supplement in which foods are grouped under a nutrient category, if they have an INQ of 1.5 and if they contain 15% (or more) of the U.S. RDA of that nutrient per serving. These lists make food complementation rapid and simple.

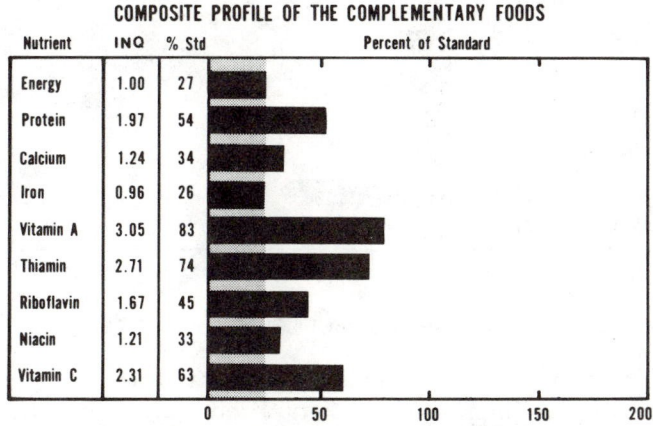

COMPOSITE PROFILE OF THE COMPLEMENTARY FOODS

Nutrient	INQ	% Std	Percent of Standard
Energy	1.00	27	
Protein	1.97	54	
Calcium	1.24	34	
Iron	0.96	26	
Vitamin A	3.05	83	
Thiamin	2.71	74	
Riboflavin	1.67	45	
Niacin	1.21	33	
Vitamin C	2.31	63	

FIG. 4.6. AGGREGATE CONTRIBUTION OF THE FOODS TO THE DAILY NUTRITIONAL NEEDS. THIS AMOUNT OF FOOD IN AGGREGATE CONTAINS 621 CALORIES.

To aid dietitians and other professionals who must know the quantities of nutrients contained in meals (or total diets), a plastic overlay is available for use with the Index of Nutritional Quality handbook. A printed outline of a food graph on the overlay enables one to mark off the length of the nutrient bars for each food used during a day's time. The resultant summation for each nutrient is seen as a typical profile (as drawn in the figures in this chapter) for any meal or diet under consideration.

Food profiles using the Index of Nutritional Quality concept could be used to amplify the value of information on the food labels and allow the consumer to practice broad complementation while making food selections in the supermarket.

The Index of Nutritional Quality is proposed for general use as a nutrition education tool. It provides a simple and reliable way to evaluate and balance individual diets in terms of the ratio of nutrients consumed in foods to allowances. The nutrient content of foods is expressed in proportion to the amount of energy they provide. For educational purposes, the expectation is that when individuals see for themselves whether their diets supply adequate amounts of nutrients within the framework of their energy needs, they will be less susceptible to misinformation.

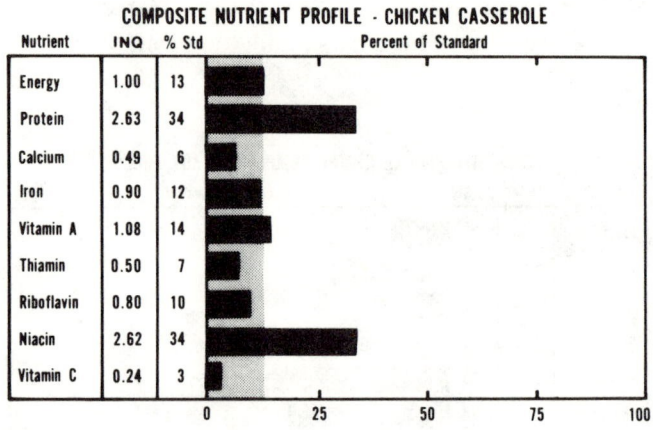

COMPOSITE NUTRIENT PROFILE · CHICKEN CASSEROLE

Nutrient	INQ	% Std
Energy	1.00	13
Protein	2.63	34
Calcium	0.49	6
Iron	0.90	12
Vitamin A	1.08	14
Thiamin	0.50	7
Riboflavin	0.80	10
Niacin	2.62	34
Vitamin C	0.24	3

FIG. 4.7. NUTRIENT PROFILE OF A FOOD ITEM

A basic problem of modern nutrition education is to motivate individuals to want to improve their diets. Food profiles and the Index of Nutritional Quality may not equate with motivation, but they will make it easier for people to visualize their dietary needs and deficiencies. Changes occur when an easily understood method to aid change with a minimum departure from present dietary practices is available.

NUTRITION EDUCATION FOR CHILDREN

Studies have shown that there is no instinct to guide man in the proper selection of his diet; therefore nutrition education is a universal need. Dietary and eating practices are established at a very early age and may often be the result of environmental and attitudinal influences. In addition, today's child is exposed to eating practices which reflect the tempo of a society involved in food fads, preparation shortcuts, packaged food machine products and diverse family interests which may interrupt traditional meal patterns. Broader exposure to nutritional value in food alternatives at the earliest possible age is an educational need which could help offset poor eating habits and provide stronger motivation for young children to seek a balanced diet from a diverse selection of food. Unfortunately much of the nutrition education in schools has been less than successful in establishing good eating habits in American school children, yet because of decrease in parental contact, every member of the family, especially young people, should be able to identify and be motivated to eat a balanced diet. However, few teachers are trained in the fundamentals of nutrition, and at present no state requires any nutrition courses for licensing or certification of teachers. (From Proposed Nutritional Bill S-3864, 1972).

A nutrition education program was developed at Utah State University between the years of 1974-1978. The purpose was to show that an Index of Nutritional Quality (INQ) could effectively be used as a tool to assist school children in making independent choices of appropriate food which will aid the children in selecting an adequate diet and aid in maintaining or advancing their general health and nutritional status. New tools and methods for promoting desired behavioral changes of the child in modern society were developed while incorporating existing nutrition teaching concepts into a workable continuing nutrition curriculum.

A number of supporting activities were included which integrated nutrition into other existing educational units. These activities were designed to use the applied skills and knowledge from other academic areas. They included projects within areas of mathematics, social studies, health science, art, music, and communication skills. These projects enriched the learning area and reinforced the nutrition concepts. Such integration into the curriculum made continuous nutrition education possible without overkill.

Student workbooks, teacher manuals, graphics and slide-tape teacher training modules are used to implement the program. The nutrition education program is a continuous sequence from kindergarten through grade 6. The concepts introduced at each grade level are predicated on the materials mastered in earlier grades, and become more sophisticated as the child matures. Sufficient material was developed to provide opportunities to reinforce the learning experiences of the slow learner as well as challenge the most gifted.

EDUCATIONAL APPROACH

All education involves a process of changing behavior in desirable directions. It has been found that the application of educational concepts is most likely to occur if they are related to the actual problems and interests of the student. (Eppright *et al.* 1970). Children do not change their food habits unless two prerequisites are satisfied. First, the individual must believe that such a change will help him toward some personally desired goal—whether that be weight loss, better health, a better physical appearance, or achieving peer acceptance. The goals will obviously differ for different groups based on age, sex and cultural background. Any successful nutrition program must respect family, ethnic, religious and traditional food patterns. It must be recognized that some students may already consume a nutritionally adequate diet which does not conform to traditional American tastes in either content or preparation. Second, the mechanics of the change process must be uncomplicated, easily activated and based on the previous experiences. Inductive or discovery teaching seemed to be a logical approach to achieve these goals in view of the nature of the material to be taught. Inductive learning occurs through personal experiences of the student. Through guided laboratory or classroom projects, the child assimilates and organizes the data he has examined and generalizes them into proper concepts.

The inductive learning approach should enable students to use academic skills to solve problems which have application and meaning for them. More precisely, meaningful education should prepare students to think for themselves; to retain facts, develop skills, and then use them to solve problems and finally evaluate the success of their efforts.

For nutrition education programs, it is customary to group foods according to the nutrient for which the foods are major sources. Guidelines are usually provided to illustrate how nutrient needs can be met by selecting from among relatively few groups of foods (Anon. NAS/NRC, 1974). A balanced diet is determined by daily selection of the appropriate number of servings from each group. Such food groupings are useful methods of dietary assessment as long as the usual diet consisted of traditional foods which are easily identified as a member of one of the food groups. However, modern supermarkets supply a phethora of analogs, processed and mixed foods, whose nutrient contents are unlike any food group. They also tend to encourage rigidity in teaching about food selection. It is important that such guides be adapted and modified imaginatively to meet the needs of individuals and families with different levels of income, cultural patterns, and life styles. Categorization of a food as being either good or bad is meaningless because individual foods must be considered to contribute to the balance of nutrients in a diet within caloric needs. A variety of food combinations can serve to meet recommended dietary allowances, provided the choice of foods is made with care.

The Index of Nutritional Quality used in this educational program

Hamburger

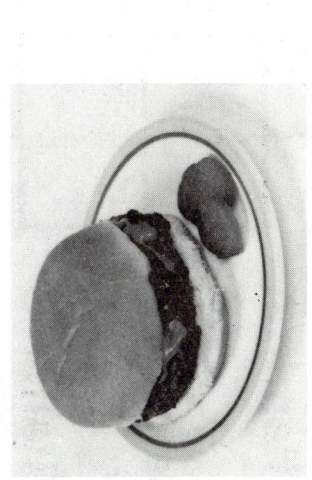

** HAMBURGER ON BUN, FAST FOOD CHAIN, FEG.
76 GRAMS WHICH SUPPLY 2CO CAL OF ENERGY

NUTRIENT	UNIT	AMOUNT	INQ	% STD
ENERGY	CAL	199.62	1.00	8
PROTEIN	G	12.76	4.26	35
VITAMIN A	IU	6.80	0.02	0
VITAMIN C	MG	0.00	0.00	0
THIAMIN	MG	0.15	1.48	12
RIBOFLAVN	MG	0.15	1.54	13
NIACIN	MG	2.96	2.23	19
CALCIUM	MG	35.16	0.53	4
IRON	MG	1.39	2.39	20

1 AVERAGE

0   25%   50%   75%   100%

FIG. 4.8. NUTRIENT PROFILE OF A HAMBURGER ON BUN WITH CATSUP, MUSTARD & PICKLE CHIPS, 3 OUNCE PATTY .164 GRAMS WHICH SUPPLY 329 KCAL OF ENERGY

Hamburger

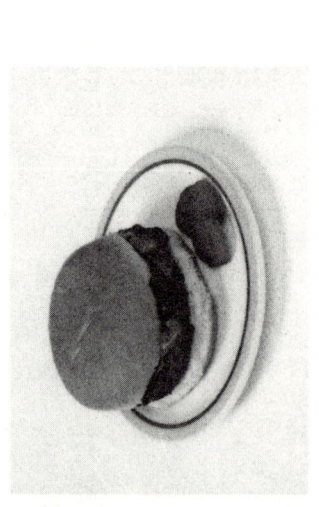

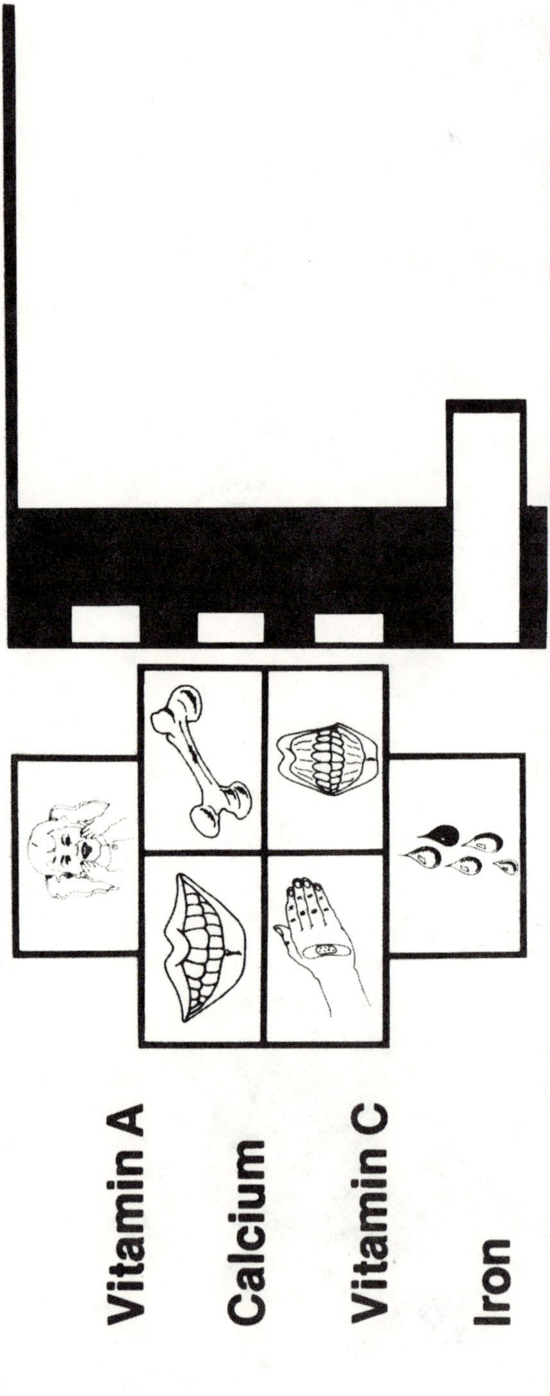

Vitamin A

Calcium

Vitamin C

Iron

expresses the nutrient potential of food in simple color coded graphs. The elementary school child's ability to relate to simple spatial relations and colors of the Index of Nutritional Quality food profiles has been effectively demonstrated in an elementary school setting. Figure 4.8 shows one of 128 nutrient density profile cards developed for the elementary grades. They are used to assist children to use food complementations as well as determine food quality.

After learning to assess the quality of foods by identifying good nutrient sources (long bars) and nutrients in short supply (absent or short bars) the children are taught to use food complementation to balance their diet by selecting food items which collectively have at least one long bar for each nutrient. For example, if a child selects milk for his lunch he must find foods with a long red (iron) bar and a long green (vitamin C) bar to complement the milk profile. Such choices may include beef stew, carrots, pizza, fruits, etc. Any combination of foods which pleases the child and meets the nutrient requirements is considered an acceptable meal. The child is not locked into traditional food choices or combinations. Atypical selections such as casseroles or tacos with a glass of milk or juice for breakfast, cannot only be condoned but encouraged if the child who does not like typical breakfast foods can get a balanced diet and reduce plate wastage. This program also allows for food choices of favorite but not so nutritious foods if they are placed in the proper frame of reference in combination with other higher nutrient density foods. The nutrient density approach to diet planning can also maximize the use of favorite and traditional foods. As long as a recipe or the ingredients for a complex food are known, the INQ profile can be produced automatically by computer, thus making special diets (alternative food patterns, vegetarianism, clinical prescriptions), and cultural foods (Kosher, Spanish, Oriental, dishes from developing countries, soul food, etc.) an integral part of the nutrition program.

EVALUATION

The determination of progress is an integral part of teaching. Evaluation of the success and failure of each aspect of the program must be made so that weak areas can be strengthened in the future. Students should be aware of their progress, reinforced in their success and encouraged to try additional learning experiences in areas where they lack confidence or expertise. The grade school program was evaluated by external reviewers chosen by the Food and Drug Administration as well as continuous internal evaluation by constant monitoring of the students ability to achieve the behavioral objectives.

Analysis of the nutrient density based nutrition education program indicated that elementary school children are not only capable of learning sophisticated nutrition concepts, but the program significantly improved participants' food attitudes and behaviors. For example the nutrient complementation concept was taught as a follow-up to nutrient addition. The behavioral objective for this concept involved adding the nutrients from two foods, and then selecting a third food from a large number of choices which would nutritionally complement the original two foods by supplying any lacking nutrients. Understanding of this concept was tested at the second and third grade levels. Eighty-seven percent of the students performed above the 80 percent accuracy level. There appeared to be a greater increase in knowledge concerning the nutritional quality of foods among the younger children than the older ones.

As part of the external review a letter was sent home to parents asking them to evaluate the impact of the nutrition education on their children. Even though the letter to parents did not mention that the program included learning to read nutritional information on food packages, 24 parents or 6 percent of those responding, stated their children showed an increased interest in food labels.

PRE-SCHOOL EDUCATION

A companion program for pre-school children is currently being developed through a grant from the Gerber Baby Products Company. The pre-school program is also based on a nutrient density concept and is designed to help children learn to make independent choices of groups of foods which provide both good nutrition and eating pleasure. The objectives of the program are to provide incentive for children to improve their eating habits, expand their experiences with foods and give them simple tools in the form of INQ food profiles with which they can evaluate the nutritional quality of individual foods and put them together in simple nutritionally adequate groups or meals. Figure 4.9 illustrates the modified food profile cards used with pre-school children. These profiles like the grade school graphics are flexible in all parameters and appropriate nutritional standards may be used for specific groups or U.S. RDA s used for the population as a whole.

Materials have been generated which reflect the actual dietary requirements of children four and five years of age, as well as materials which are based on the U.S. Recommended Daily Allowances developed for nutritional labeling by the Food and Drug Administration.

Fewer nutrients are appropriate for young children with budding cognitive abilities. Nutritional parameters include calcium, iron, vitamins

A and C because they have been identified as potential problems in the American diet (Anon 1978). They are also representative of essential nutrients, including a water soluble and a fat soluble vitamin, a mineral, and a micro-nutrient. The number of nutrients in the profile is increased for the older children as they become more sophisticated in nutrition theory.

The pre-school profiles are designed to eliminate the needs for any reading skills. Since "energy" is a rather abstract concept, the specific reference to an energy line has been replaced with a dark area whose length represents the reference line of caloric content. Therefore, nutrient bars which equal or fall above the black area represent nutrients which are supplied in adequate or excessive amounts in relation to calories. It should be noted that the length of the bar shows proportionally the amount of a nutrient in a food in relation to the calories it contains represented by the height of the black box.

Parent materials are also being developed. Parents are being instructed in the philosophy of the overall program and will be provided with the basic information that will enable them to support and reinforce the concepts the child learns in the laboratory. Exposure to the nutritional values reflected by nutrient density may also provide motivation for parents to provide appealing food choices of higher nutritional value which will advance the general health of the entire family.

SUMMARY

The implications of nutrition education based on nutrient density are numerous. It can provide ways of translating nutrition concepts into better shopping habits, food selection and food preparation for all members of the community, as well as improve the general quality of public education by teaching children to apply cognitive and social skills to the solution of relevant nutrition problems. It can also serve all segments of society, including minorities, by maximizing the use of foods which are the components of cultural and religious dietaries. Nutrient density has great potential for health education. It is an example of the broad perspective for preventive medicine and provides a method that health practioners can use in hospital or community settings for patient counseling.

Prior to 1970, categorical food guides were the almost exclusively used tools of nutrition education. Even today, relatively rigid delineations of acceptable types and amounts of foods are the standard approach. This food guide procedure has recently been criticized, however, and the need for a new teaching perspective has been suggested (see selected references).

A nutrient approach has been recommended as a way to effectively teach nutrition (see selected references). Since foods are vehicles for nutrients, food-based information is obviously still important. With nutrient sophistication, however, an individual has a more rational basis for making decisions about food, which is the ultimate goal of nutrition education.

A major purpose of the work reported here was to test whether a concept with such promising and diverse applications might also be an effective basis for nutrition education in elementary schools.

REFERENCES

ANON. 1968. Household Food Consumption Survey 1965-66. Dietary Levels of Households in the United States, Agricultural Research Service Report No. 16, U.S. Dept. of Agriculture, Washington, D.C.

ANON. 1969. Proposed criteria for food label information panel, Fed. Reg., *37*:6493.

ANON. 1974. Food and Nutrition Board, Recommended Dietary Allowances, 8th ed., National Academy of Sciences, Washington, D.C.

ANON. 1974b. U.S. RDA Comparison Cards. National Dairy Council, Chicago.

CHURCH, C.F. and CHURCH, H.N. 1970. Food Values of Portions Commonly Used—Bowes and Church, 11th ed., J.P. Lippincott Co., Philadelphia.

COWGILL, G.R. and ANDERSON, W.E. 1932. Laxative effects of wheat bran and washed bran in healthy men, J. Am. Med. Assn., *98*:1866.

EPPRIGHT, E., PATTERSON, M., and BARBOUR, H. 1970. Teaching Nutrition, 2nd Ed., Iowa State Univ. Press., Amer. p.345.

GOODHART, R.S. and SHILS, M.E. 1973. Modern Nutrition in Health and Disease, 5th ed., Lea and Febiger, Philadelphia.

GUNTHRIE, H.A. 1971. Introduction to Nutrition, 2nd ed., C.V. Mosby Co., St. Louis. p. 128.

HANSEN, R.G. 1973. An index of food quality, Nutr. Rev., *31*:1.

HENDERSON, L.M. 1972. Nutritional problems growing out of new patterns of food consumption, Am. J. Publ. Health, 62:1194.

LEVERTON, R.M. 1974. Fats in Food and Diet, Agricultural Research Service, Agr. Info. Bull. 361, U.S. Dept. of Agriculture, Washington, D.C.

PARRISH, J.B. 1971. Implications of changing food habits for nutrition educators, J. Nutr. Educ., 2:140.

ROBINSON, C.H. 1972. Normal and Therapeutic Nutrition, 14th ed., Macmillan Co., N. Y. 129, 548-549.

SORENSON, A.W., WYSE, B.W., WITTWER, A.J., and HANSEN, R.G. 1976. An Index of Nutritional Quality for a balanced diet, J. Amer. Dietet. Assn., 68:236.

STARE, F.J. 1972. Nutritional problems of affluent populations, S. African Med. J., *45*:1575.

WATT, B.K. and MERRIL, A.L. 1963. Composition of Foods-Raw, Processed, and Prepared. Agriculture Handbook No. 8, Rev. ed., U.S. Dept. of Agriculture, Washington, D.C.

WRETLIND, A. 1974. World Sugar Production and Usage in Europe, Sugars in Nutrition Ed., H.L. Sipple, and K.W. McNutt, Academic Press, New York, pp.88− 90.

USDA Agricultural Research Service, Progress Report of the Consumer and Food Economics Division, Marketing and Nutrition Research, Washington, D.C., Nov. 1971.

5

Current Nutritional
Problems of Consumers

Even though nutrition labeling has been in use for several years, many consumers still need to know how to apply the information that appears on the label when purchasing food in the grocery store or when planning menus at home. Whether or not consumers use labeling to make decisions, the food industry has opportunities to continue to improve the nutritional value of the products it produces. The education of the consumer is becoming a more critical factor and should be increasingly emphasized; at the same time, the food industry can concentrate on the problem of providing nutritious foods from which the consumer can make choices.

It is the purpose of this chapter to illustrate the problems of those at nutritional risk in today's society and to identify particular areas where the food industry can be of help in optimizing the nutritional health of consumers.

For the calculations which follow, Agricultural Handbook No. 8 has been used as the source of food composition data (Watt and Merrill 1963).

INFANTS DIETS ANALYZED

Figure 5.1a shows a computer-derived bar graph of the nutrients present in an evaporated milk formula representative of the diet for young infants. The length of the bars represents percentages of the Recommended Dietary Allowances (RDAs) for an infant one month of age. The profile shows a protein INQ of 2.18 (meaning that 2.18 times the protein standard is provided if the energy requirement of 535 kcal is satisfied). Other high INQ values are: riboflavin 2.70, calcium 2.21, and phosphorus 2.70. The calcium-to-phosphorus ratio of the formula can be derived from the tabular data in the INQ format (810 mg of Ca/660

a. Evaporated milk
Diet for child 1 mo of age
682 g which supply 535 kcal of energy

Nutrient	Amount		INQ	% of Std					
					0	50%	100%	150%	200%
Energy	535 000	kcal	1 00	102					
Protein	22 000	g	2 18	222					222 22 %
Vitamin A	1 050 000	IU	0 74	75					
Vitamin D	250 000	IU	0 61	63					
Vitamin C	5 000	mg	0 14	14					
Niacin	1 000	mg	0 20	20					
Riboflavin	1 100	mg	2 70	275					275 00 %
Thiamin	0 200	mg	0 66	67					
Calcium	810 000	mg	2 21	225					225 00 %
Phosphorus	660 000	mg	2 70	275					275 00 %
Iron	0 300	mg	0 03	3					

Nutrient standard

Nutrients as proportion of energy

b Proprietary formula

Suggested diet for child 1 mo of age
714 g which supply 514 kcal of energy

Nutrient	Amount	INQ	% of Std	0						
Energy	514 000 kcal	1 00	98							
Protein	14 800 g	1 53	149							
Vitamin A	3 257 000 IU	2 38	233							232 64%
Vitamin D	703 000 IU	1 80	176							
Vitamin C	97 000 mg	2 84	277							277 14%
Niacin	5 300 mg	1 08	106							
Riboflavin	0 310 mg	0 79	78							
Thiamin	0 400 mg	1 36	133							
Calcium	408 000 mg	1 16	137							
Phosphorus	329 000 mg	1 40	137							
Iron	10 500 mg	1 07	105							

Nutrients as proportion of energy

Nutrient standard

50%   100%   150%   200%

FIG. 5.1 NUTRIENT PROFILES OF INFANT FORMULAS

Based on U.S. RDAs for 0- to 6-month-old child. Fig. 1a = nutrient profile of evaporated milk formula (10 oz of evaporated milk, 12 oz of water, and 5 tsp of corn syrup). Fig. 1b = nutrient profile of proprietary formula (1:1 dilution of 25 oz of formula, 1 tbsp of fortified infant cereal, and 1 ml of dietary supplement including 2,000 IU of vitamin A, 400 IU of vitamin D, 60 mg of vitamin C, and fluoride.

mg of P=1.2 and approaches the desirable 1.5 set by the NAS/NRC in 1973.

Protein consumption in excess of requirement is characteristic of the national dietary. Until recently, this situation was not seriously considered, but now some have found that high protein consumption may interfere with utilization of other nutrients (Johnson et al., 1970; Waltker and Linkswiler 1972). This is of importance when making infant formula based on cow's milk, since, on an energy-equivalent basis, cow's milk contains about three times as much protein as breast milk. Manufacturers generally dilute the cow's milk with water and add sugar.

Figure 5.1a shows a well-known fact—that unless specifically fortified, evaporated milk formulas do not supply sufficient amounts of iron or vitamins A, D, and C (the INQs for these nutrients are less than 1.0). Tryptophan conversion to niacin from the excess protein (NAS/NRC 1973) meets a significant part of the niacin need.

Figure 5.1b is the profile of 25 oz of a proprietary iron-fortified baby formula currently being marketed, plus one tablespoon of fortified infant cereal and one ml of a common infant vitamin supplement (data obtained from labels). With the exception of riboflavin, the profile reflects a nutritious and calorically adequate diet for the one-month-old infant.

Obtaining an adequate amount of iron is a particular problem for infants and children. For its first few weeks of life, the infant may have sufficient iron stores if its mother consumed optimal iron during the prenatal period; this, however, is not always a valid assumption. Because the gastrointestinal tolerance of supplemented iron in the infant is controversial, the food industry has provided nutrient-supplemented formulas with and without iron. It remains for other groups to provide the needed guidance so that members of the medical profession and consumers alike can make wise selection based on nutrient balance and availability.

CHILDREN'S DIETS ANALYZED

Recognizing that a child must be well nourished if it is to learn efficiently, school lunch and, in some areas, school breakfast programs have been initiated. Such programs are especially important because, for many children, they may provide the only well-balanced meal of the day (Pyke 1970, Bralove 1972). The nutritional contributions of these programs to the health and development of children, assuming that the meals are consumed, may be seen by an analysis of the menus.

Table 5.1 is taken from the published week's menu for a school child in a metropolitan area of the United States. Designed to minimize waste and encourage appetites, the menu is varied and attractive, and caters to

TABLE 5.1. REPRESENTATIVE WEEK'S MENUS OF TYPE A SCHOOL LUNCH USED IN A METROPOLITAN AREA IN CALIFORNIA

Food	Serving size
Meal I	
Tacos (state recipe D-18)	2 oz
Mexican Corn (½ tsp)	¼ cup
Lettuce and tomato	¼ cup
Rosy applesauce	¼ cup
Rolled wheat pan bread	1 roll
Butter or margarine	½ tsp
Milk	½ pt
Meal II	
Diced turkey in gravy	1½ oz
Whipped Potatoes (½ tsp)	¼ cup
Cabbage confetti salad	¼ cup
Bulgur roll	1 roll
Butter or margarine	½ tsp
Chilled apricot halves	¼ cup
Peanut butter cookie	½ oz
Milk	½ pt
Meal III	
Italian spaghetti with meat and cheese	2 oz
Buttered (½ tsp) green beans	¼ cup
Lettuce-spinach salad	¼ cup
French bread	1 slice
Butter or margarine	½ tsp
Apple wedge and raisins	¼ cup
Milk	½ pt
Meal IV	
Barbecued beef	2 oz
Buttered (½ tsp) peas	¼ cup
Celery-carrot sticks	¼ cup
Buttered bun	½ tsp butter and 1 bun
Pineapple-grapefruit crisp	¼ cup
Milk	½ pt
Meal V	
Oven-browned fish sticks	1½ oz
Potatoes au gratin	⅜ cup
Tossed green salad	¼ cup
Cornbread	½ oz
Butter or margarine	½ tsp
Cherry gelatin with bananas	⅛ cup
Milk	½ pt

a. Based on RDAs for 7- to 10-year old children
693 g which supply 878 kcal of energy

Nutrient	Amount	INQ	% of Std
Energy	878.264 kcal	1.00	37
Protein	32.632 g	2.48	91
Calcium	569.438 mg	1.95	71
Iron	5.526 mg	1.51	55
Vitamin A	2,175.840 IU	1.80	66
Thiamin	0.445 mg	1.01	37
Riboflavin	0.898 mg	2.04	75
Niacin	5.198 mg	0.89	32
Vitamin C	21.792 mg	1.49	54

Nutrients as proportion of energy

Nutrient standard

b. Based on RDAs for 11- to 14-year old boys
632 g which supply 816 kcal of energy

Nutrient	Amount		INQ	% of Std	0 — 50% — 100%
Energy	815.846	kcal	1.00	29	LLLLLLLLLLLL
Protein	37.004	g	2.89	84	LLLLLLLLLLLLLLLLLLLLLLLLLLLLLLLLLL
Calcium	438.192	mg	1.25	37	LLLLLLLLLLLLLLL
Iron	4.291	mg	0.82	24	LLLLLLLLLL
Vitamin A	2,209.700	IU	1.52	44	LLLLLLLLLLLLLLLLLL
Thiamin	0.482	mg	1.18	34	LLLLLLLLLLLLLL
Riboflavin	0.806	mg	1.84	54	LLLLLLLLLLLLLLLLLLLLLL
Niacin	7.831	mg	1.49	44	LLLLLLLLLLLLLLLLL
Vitamin C	20.250	mg	1.54	45	LLLLLLLLLLLLLLLLLL

Nutrients as proportion of energy **Nutrient standard**

FIG. 5.2. PROFILES OF NUTRIENTS SUPPLIED BY TYPE A SCHOOL LUNCH MENU SHOWN IN TABLE 1

Fig. 2a = based on RDAs for children 7–10 years old. Fig. 2b = based on RDAs for boys 11–14 years old.

** GUM DROPS
   1-1/4 OUNCES

NUTRIENT	UNIT	AMOUNT	INQ	% STD	0	25%	50%	75%	100%
ENERGY	KCAL	123.2	1.00	4	XX				
PROTEIN	G	<0.1	0.02	<1	*				
VITAMIN A	IU	0.0	0.00	0	*				
VITAMIN C	MG	0.0	0.00	0	*				
THIAMIN	MG	0.0	0.00	0	*				
RIBOFLAVIN	MG	0.0	0.00	0	*				
NIACIN	MG	0.0	0.00	0	*				
CALCIUM	MG	2.1	0.05	<1	*				
IRON	MG	0.2	0.35	2	X*				

****

** SWEET CHOCOLATE BAR
   1-1/4 OUNCES

NUTRIENT	UNIT	AMOUNT	INQ	% STD	0	25%	50%	75%	100%
ENERGY	KCAL	187.4	1.00	8	XXXX				
PROTEIN	G	1.5	0.56	4	XX *				
VITAMIN A	IU	3.6	0.01	<1					
VITAMIN C	MG	0.0	0.00	0					
THIAMIN	MG	<0.1	0.08	1	X *				
RIBOFLAVIN	MG	<0.1	0.53	4	XX *				
NIACIN	MG	0.1	0.09	1	X *				
CALCIUM	MG	33.4	0.53	4	XX *				
IRON	MG	0.5	0.64	5	XXX*				

****

** MILK CHOCOLATE BAR
   1-1/4 OUNCES

NUTRIENT	UNIT	AMOUNT	INQ	% STD	0	25%	50%	75%	100%
ENERGY	KCAL	184.6	1.00	8	XXXX				
PROTEIN	G	2.7	0.00	8	XXX*				
VITAMIN A	IU	95.9	0.38	3	XX *				
VITAMIN C	MG	0.0	0.00	0	*				
THIAMIN	MG	<0.1	0.23	2	X *				
RIBOFLAVIN	MG	0.1	1.31	10	XXX*X				
NIACIN	MG	0.1	0.09	1	X *				
CALCIUM	MG	80.9	1.32	10	XXX*X				
IRON	MG	0.4	0.51	4	XX *				

****

** CHOCOLATE BAR WITH PEANUTS
   1-1/4 OUNCES

NUTRIENT	UNIT	AMOUNT	INQ	% STD	0	25%	50%	75%	100%
ENERGY	KCAL	192.8	1.00	8	XXXX				
PROTEIN	G	5.0	1.73	14	XXX*XXX				
VITAMIN A	IU	63.9	0.24	2	X *				
VITAMIN C	MG	0.0	0.00	0	*				
THIAMIN	MG	<0.1	0.92	7	XXX*				
RIBOFLAVIN	MG	10.0	0.96	8	XXX*				
NIACIN	MG	1.8	1.38	11	XXX*XX				
CALCIUM	MG	61.8	0.96	8	XXX*				
IRON	MG	9.5	0.62	5	XXX*				

****

FIG. 5.3. NUTRIENT PROFILES FOR 1¼ OZ OF VARIOUS
TYPES OF CANDY SOLD IN VENDING MACHINES

already-developed food preferences in many children, while conditioning food preferences for others.

As shown in Figure 5.2a, if a child consumed all the food provided, he would receive, on a daily basis, 37% of his energy requirement. He would also receive 91% of his vitamin A needs. All of the other common vitamins and minerals are in greater proportion to his needs than the energy (INQ$\geq$ 1.0), including niacin when considering the tryptophan conversion.

When evaluated against the RDAs for older preteenage children (Fig. 5.2b), the menu in Table 5.1 is even more appropriate because it provides 29% of the calories and 84% of the daily protein needs. The consumption of high-calorie, low-nutrient snacks would disproportionately lengthen the energy bar in Figure 5.2, thus reducing the nutrient density of the meal. A number of communities have specified the type of foods permitted in vending machines in schools. Considering some common candies, for example, INQs can provide a basis for selecting those with the highest nutrient density for sale in vending machines, as shown in Figure 5.3.

TEENAGE DIETS ANALYZED

The teenage girl has a particularly difficult problem. On the one hand, she is under peer pressures to consume a large number of her calories in the form of snack foods, while at the same time she is acutely aware that overweight will make her unattractive. This results in highly erratic food habits (Wyman 1972). She often times eliminates foods from her diet that have a high nutrient density, and she may thus lack nutrients that are important during a critical time of physiological development. Teenagers have tended to increase their consumption of snack foods over the past years (Parrish 1971).

Many snack items are refined forms of basically nutritious foods. The potato in various forms represents a good example of nutrient dilution. Figure 5.4a is a profile of a 150 kcal serving of potato (one medium-sized) baked in its skin. The standards are estimates from the literature and the RDAs for a female 15-18 years of age. The INQs indicate that the potato is a good source of protein, thiamin, niacin, vitamin C, pantothenic acid, vitamin B_6, carbohydrate, fiber, phosphorus, and potassium. Standards for nutrients for which RDAs have not been defined are discussed by Sorenson *et al.* (1975).

The isocaloric profile shown in Figure 5.4b of a 150 kcal protein of French-fried potatoes (11 pieces, 4 in. $\times$ ¼ in. $\times$ ¼ in.), however, shows graphically how the 65 kcal (9 kcal/g $\times$ 7.2 g) contributed by fat dilutes

a. Potatoes—baked in skin
161 g which supply 150 kcal of energy

Nutrient	Amount		INQ	% of Std
Energy	150.000	kcal	1.00	7
Protein	4.194	g	1.22	9
Calcium	14.516	mg	0.17	1
Iron	1.129	mg	0.88	6
Vitamin A	0.000	IU	0.00	0
Thiamin	0.161	mg	2.05	15
Riboflavin	0.065	mg	0.65	5
Niacin	2.742	mg	2.74	20
Vitamin C	32.258	mg	10.04	72
Pantothenic acid	0.613	mg	1.72	12
Vitamin B$_6$	0.165	mg	1.15	8
Vitamin B$_{12}$	0.000	µg	0.00	0
Fat	0.000	g	0.02	0
Saturated fatty acid	0.000	g	0.00	0
Unsaturated oleic	0.000	g	0.00	0
Unsaturated linoleic	0.000	g	0.00	0
Cholesterol	0.000	mg	0.00	0
Carbohydrate, total	34.032	g	1.76	13
Fiber	0.968	g	2.51	18
Phosphorus	104.839	mg	1.22	9
Sodium	6.452	mg	0.02	0
Potassium	811.290	mg	2.84	20

Nutrients as proportion of energy

(bar chart scale: 0   25%   50%   75%)

b. Potatoes—French-fried
55 g which supply 150 kcal of energy

Nutrient	Amount		INQ	% of Std	0 25%
Energy	150.000	kcal	1.00	7	
Protein	2.354	g	0.69	5	
Calcium	8.212	mg	0.10	1	
Iron	0.712	mg	0.55	4	
Vitamin A	0.000	IU	0.00	0	
Thiamin	0.071	mg	0.91	6	
Riboflavin	0.044	mg	0.44	3	
Niacin	1.697	mg	1.70	12	
Vitamin C	11.496	mg	3.58	28	
Pantothenic acid	0.208	mg	0.58	4	
Vitamin B6	0.056	mg	0.39	3	
Vitamin B12	0.000	µg	0.00	0	
Fat	7.226	g	1.10	8	
Saturated fatty acid	1.642	g	0.92	7	
Unsaturated oleic	1.642	g	0.70	5	
Unsaturated linoleic	3.832	g	2.15	15	
Cholesterol	0.000	mg	0.00	0	
Carbohydrate, total	19.708	g	1.02	7	
Fiber	0.547	g	1.42	10	
Phosphorus	60.766	mg	0.71	5	
Sodium	3.285	mg	0.01	0	
Potassium	466.971	mg	1.63	12	

Nutrients as proportion of energy

4c. Potato chips
26 g which supply 150 kcal of energy

Nutrient	Amount		INQ	% of Std	0 25%
Energy	150.000	kcal	1.00	7	
Protein	1.400	g	0.41	3	
Calcium	10.563	mg	0.12	1	
Iron	0.475	mg	0.37	3	
Vitamin A	0.000	IU	0.00	0	
Thiamin	0.055	mg	0.71	5	
Riboflavin	0.018	mg	0.18	1	
Niacin	1.268	mg	1.27	9	
Vitamin C	4.225	mg	1.31	9	
Pantothenic acid	0.100	mg	0.28	2	
Vitamin B6	0.048	mg	0.33	2	
Vitamin B12	0.000	µg	0.00	0	
Fat	10.511	g	1.60	11	
Saturated fatty acid	2.641	g	1.48	11	
Unsaturated oleic	2.113	g	0.90	6	
Unsaturated linoleic	5.282	g	2.96	21	
Cholesterol	0.000	mg	0.00	0	
Carbohydrate, total	13.204	g	0.68	5	
Fiber	0.423	g	1.10	8	
Phosphorus	36.708	mg	0.43	3	
Sodium	89.789	mg	0.31	2	
Potassium	298.415	mg	1.04	7	

Nutrients as proportion of energy

FIG. 5.4. NUTRIENT DILUTION BY FATS IS ILLUSTRATED BY ISOCALORIC PROFILES OF BAKED POTATOES, FRENCH-FRIED POTATOES, AND POTATO CHIPS

the proportions of other nutrients in the original food. In this form, the INQs of niacin and vitamin C have been reduced from 2.74 and 10.04 to 1.70 and 3.58, respectively. A further nutrient dilution is shown in the profile of 150 kcal of potato chips (about 13 chips) shown in Figure 5.4c. In this case, 95 kcal or 63% of the energy comes from fat. Niacin and vitamin C have been reduced to INQs of 1.27 and 1.31, respectively. Whereas the original potato contained significant extra quantities of vitamin C, the potato chip has barely enough to match the energy. There is nothing inherently wrong in consuming potato chips if the other food selections recognize the nutrient dilution caused by the added fat. One should note that since INQ profiles are independent of portion size the isocaloric representation makes an easy comparison by standardizing the energy baseline.

Because of insufficient food composition data in the literature for pantothenic acid and vitamins B_6 and B_{12}, these values should only be considered rough estimates. The food industry could be of service by providing reliable values for these nutrients, especially for canned and processed foods for which data are especially sparse. Watt and Murphy (1970) have suggested that these data be sent to the Consumer and Food Economics Research Division of the USDA's Agricultural Research Service.

Many processed foods cater to our liking for sugar. The share of total carbohydrate in the U.S. diet provided by sugars (predominantly sucrose) as compared to starch has risen from about 32% around the turn of the century to more than 50% (Page and Friend 1974). Concomitantly, intake of fat in the U.S. has risen from 35% of total calories to 45%, with a corresponding decrease in calories from complex carbohydrates (USDA 1972).

This trend is being modulated by preserving canned fruits in their own juices. Recently, high sugar prices have had a salutary nutritional consequence by encouraging the use of less sugar in food processing. The number of calories increases markedly between a 1-cup serving of juice-packed peaches (110 kcal) and an average 1-cup serving of canned peaches in heavy syrup (200 kcal). Figures 5.5a and b are isocaloric profiles of the two types of peaches. The dilution of vitamins A and C by the sugar is readily apparent—INQs for the respective nutrients go from 6.25 to 2.89 and 4.15 to 1.79, and iron and riboflavin are diluted below amounts necessary to meet RDAs (INQs because less than 1.0).

If a teenage girl makes her choices from soft drinks, snack foods, and highly sweetened foods which have been shown to constitute a significant number of calories of her energy requirement (Bauman and Ruch 1974), it becomes a difficult task to balance her diet. The recent move by some quick-service drive-in restaurants to have a self-service salad

Peaches, canned, solid and liquid, juice pack
333g which supply 150 kcal of energy

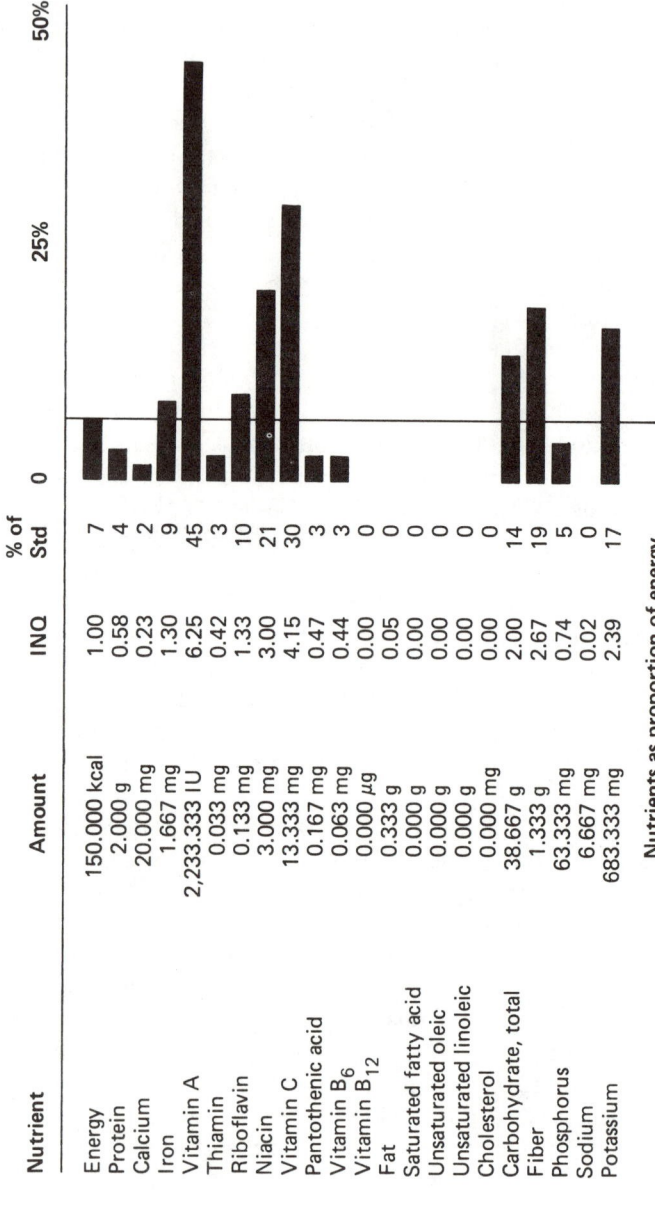

Nutrient	Amount	INQ	% of Std
Energy	150.000 kcal	1.00	7
Protein	2.000 g	0.58	4
Calcium	20.000 mg	0.23	2
Iron	1.667 mg	1.30	9
Vitamin A	2,233.333 IU	6.25	45
Thiamin	0.033 mg	0.42	3
Riboflavin	0.133 mg	1.33	10
Niacin	3.000 mg	3.00	21
Vitamin C	13.333 mg	4.15	30
Pantothenic acid	0.167 mg	0.47	3
Vitamin B$_6$	0.063 mg	0.44	3
Vitamin B$_{12}$	0.000 µg	0.00	0
Fat	0.333 g	0.05	0
Saturated fatty acid	0.000 g	0.00	0
Unsaturated oleic	0.000 g	0.00	0
Unsaturated linoleic	0.000 g	0.00	0
Cholesterol	0.000 mg	0.00	0
Carbohydrate, total	38.667 g	2.00	14
Fiber	1.333 g	2.67	19
Phosphorus	63.333 mg	0.74	5
Sodium	6.667 mg	0.02	0
Potassium	683.333 mg	2.39	17

Nutrients as proportion of energy

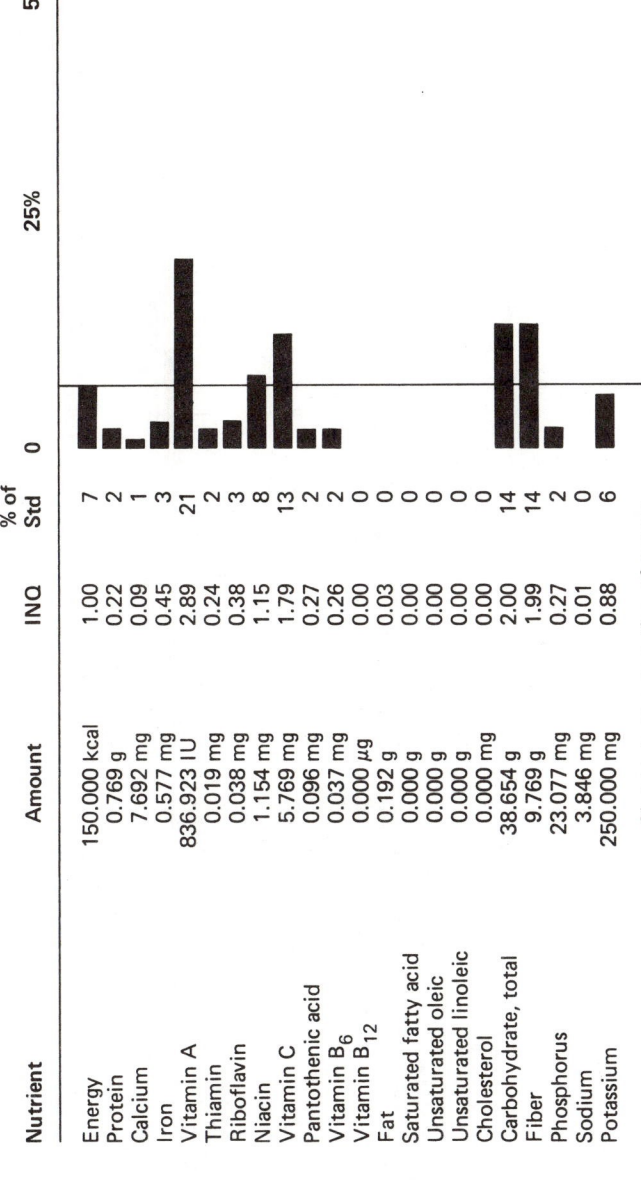

Peaches, canned, solid and liquid, syrup pack, heavy 192g which supply 150 kcal of energy

Nutrient	Amount	INQ	% of Std
Energy	150.000 kcal	1.00	7
Protein	0.769 g	0.22	2
Calcium	7.692 mg	0.09	1
Iron	0.577 mg	0.45	3
Vitamin A	836.923 IU	2.89	21
Thiamin	0.019 mg	0.24	2
Riboflavin	0.038 mg	0.38	3
Niacin	1.154 mg	1.15	8
Vitamin C	5.769 mg	1.79	13
Pantothenic acid	0.096 mg	0.27	2
Vitamin B$_6$	0.037 mg	0.26	2
Vitamin B$_{12}$	0.000 µg	0.00	0
Fat	0.192 g	0.03	0
Saturated fatty acid	0.000 g	0.00	0
Unsaturated oleic	0.000 g	0.00	0
Unsaturated linoleic	0.000 g	0.00	0
Cholesterol	0.000 mg	0.00	0
Carbohydrate, total	38.654 g	2.00	14
Fiber	9.769 g	1.99	14
Phosphorus	23.077 mg	0.27	2
Sodium	3.846 mg	0.01	0
Potassium	250.000 mg	0.88	6

Nutrients as proportion of energy

FIG. 5.5a & b. NUTRIENT DILUTION BY SUGAR IS ILLUSTRATED BY ISOCALORIC PROFILES OF PEACHES PACKED IN JUICE AND PEACHES PACKED IN HEAVY SYRUP

Hamburger, French fries, milk shake, and salad
917 g which supply 1,053 kcal of energy

Nutrient	Amount	INQ	% of Std			
				50%	100%	150%
Energy	1,052.660 kcal	1.00	50	HHHHFFFF MMMMMMS S S		
Protein	38.908 g	1.62	81	HHHHHHHHHHHF F MMMMMMMMMMMMS S		
Calcium	739.800 mg	1.23	62	HHF MMMMMMMMMMMMMMMMMS S		
Iron	5.720 mg	0.63	32	HHHHHFF MMS S S		
Vitamin A	2,966.400 IU	1.48	74	HFF F MMMMMMS S S S S S S S S S S		
Thiamin	0.597 mg	1.08	54	HHHHHFFF MMMMMMS S S S		
Riboflavin	1.291 mg	1.84	92	HHHHHF F MMMMMMMMMMMMMMMMMS S		
Niacin	7.568 mg	1.08	54	HHHHHHHHHHFFFFFF MS S S		
Vitamin C	63.630 mg	2.82	141	F MMMMS S S S S S S S S S S S S S S S S S S S S S S S S S S		

Nutrients as proportion of energy

Nutrient standard

FIG. 5.6. CONTRIBUTION MADE BY A HAMBURGER (H), FRENCH FRIES (F), MILK SHAKE (M), AND SALAD (S) TO THE NUTRITIONAL REQUIREMENTS (BASED ON RDAs) OF A GIRL 15–18 YEARS OLD

bar should be commended. The effect of the addition of a tossed salad to a typical meal of hamburger, French fries, and milk shake is shown in Figure 5.6. The difficulty of satisfying an individual's daily needs for nutrients without a meal that includes some fresh produce and milk products becomes obvious.

MIDDLE-AGE DIETS ANALYZED

Many men in middle age are faced with the problem of overweight. While their participation in physical activities has gradually decreased, their appetite is still geared to their earlier expenditures of energy. The basic problem of this age group is not usually a deficiency of particular nutrients, but rather an excess consumption of calories. Obesity, reinforced by other factors typical of this age group, makes such individuals good candidates for coronary heart disease (Stare 1972). To reduce the risk of coronary heart disease, some physicians recommend a modified diet that is low in overall fat and cholesterol and that increases the polyunsaturated fatty acid (P:S) ratio from the prevailing average of 1:3 (Guthrie 1971) to 1:1.

An individual would have a difficult time following such a prescription while selecting foods from the grocery shelf. The Food and Drug Administration had hoped that nutrition labeling would be useful to the 10-15% of the adult population on modified diets (Johnson 1974). The information on fatty acid content and amount of cholesterol in a food may or may not appear on the label. However, this information is invaluable to many who are on clinical diets. The food industry could provide a valuable service by giving fatty acid and cholesterol information on more foods, as allowed by current labeling standards. Some manufacturers are providing this information, and they are to be commended.

ELDERLY DIETS ANALYZED

The profile of the diet of a 69-year-old widow (Table 5.2 and Fig. 5.7) illustrates many of the nutritional problems of the elderly. Even though this individual is overconsuming her RDA for energy by 9%, the quality of her diet is poor for several nutrients. The nutrient profile shows the typical problem of many senior citizens, that of a limited calcium intake (authors' unpublished data). It is also obvious from Figure 5.7 that iron is a nutritional problem for women throughout their lifetime. The INQ for iron is 0.88, but because the woman's diet exceeded the energy standard selected (RDA for women over 51 years of age), she consumed 95% of her iron requirement.

24-hr dietary recall of a woman 69 years of age
1,444 g which supply 1,962 kcal of energy

Nutrient	Amount	INQ	% of Std	Nutrient profile (0–200%)
Energy	1,962.210 kcal	1.00	109	
Protein	49.748 g	0.99	108	
Calcium	531.540 mg	0.61	66	
Iron	9.549 mg	0.88	95	
Vitamin A	6,345.600 IU	1.46	159	
Thiamin	1.059 mg	0.97	106	
Riboflavin	1.073 mg	0.90	98	
Niacin	11.219 mg	0.86	93	
Vitamin C	215.060 mg	4.38	478	477.91%
Pantothenic acid	4.667 mg	0.43	47	
Vitamin B$_6$	0.796 mg	0.36	40	
Vitamin B$_{12}$	1.270 µg	0.19	21	
Fat	124.266 g	1.47	160	
Saturated fatty acid	38.220 g	1.67	182	
Unsaturated oleic	56.190 g	1.84	201	200.68%
Unsaturated linoleic	20.620 g	0.90	98	
Cholesterol	415.830 mg	0.64	69	
Carbohydrate, total	169.168 g	0.67	74	
Fiber	2.704 g	0.43	47	
Phosphorus	777.240 mg	0.89	97	
Sodium	3,049.880 mg	0.70	76	
Potassium	2,028.470 mg	0.47	51	

Nutrients as proportion of energy

FIG. 5.7. COMPOSITE NUTRIENT PROFILE OF THE DIET SHOWN IN TABLE 5.2 FOR A 69-YEAR-OLD WOMAN, SHOWING THE CONTRIBUTION OF EACH MEAL TO THE ENTIRE DAY'S DIET

B = breakfast, D = dinner, and S = a snack; lunch was not consumed.

TABLE 5.2.   24-HR DIETARY RECALL SHEET FOR AN
ELDERLY FEMALE*

Food	Serving size
Breakfast at 10:00 am	
Grapefruit	1 whole
Egg	1
Margarine	1 tbsp
Toast, white	2 slices
Margarine	2 tbsp
Postum coffee substitute	1 cup
Saccharin	2 tablets
Pream coffee whitener	1 tsp
Dinner at 6:00 pm	
Potatoes, creamed, with diced ham	1 cup medium white sauce
	1 medium potato
	½ cup diced ham
Bread, white	2 slices
Onion, steamed	1 whole
Margarine	1 tbsp
Snack at 9:00 pm	
Bread, white, with peanut butter and honey	1 tbsp peanut butter
	1 tbsp honey
	1 slice

*Lunch not consumed

The food industry could offer a real service by developing appetizing foods that would constitute good sources of these nutrients at reasonable cost. From our experience, vitamins A and C are also often in low supply in the diets of the elderly, and these deficiencies are correlated with seasons when fresh produce is neither plentiful nor inexpensive.

VEGETARIAN DIETS

Another nutritional concern which could become increasingly important is that of trace minerals in the dietary. These trace elements are known to be in abundant supply in whole grains (Fig. 5.8a). Meat is also a source of trace elements, and when it makes up a significant portion of the diet, it is unlikely that these nutrients will become marginal (Fig. 5.8c). For economic, nutritional, or other reasons, some people become essentially vegetarian. Also, with the current world food situation, many economists suggest that people in general will need to decrease their consumption of meat (Daly 1969). If refined wheat products are used in

Wheat flour, whole (from hard wheat)
45g which supply 150 kcal of energy

Nutrient	Amount	INQ	% of Std			
				0	25%	50%
Energy	150.00 kcal	1.00	7			
Calcium	18.47 mg	0.28	2			
Iron	1.49 mg	1.27	8			
Phosphorus	167.57 mg	2.57	17			
Sodium	1.35 mg	0.01	0			
Potassium	166.67 mg	0.64	4			
Magnesium	67.66 mg	2.59	17			
Chromium	2.25 µg	0.53	3			
Manganese	2,207.21 µg	5.64	37			
Cobalt	33.78 µg	1.73	11			
Copper	183.78 µg	1.41	9			
Zinc	1.40 mg	1.43	9			
Molybdenum	35.59 µg	5.46	36			

Nutrients as proportion of energy

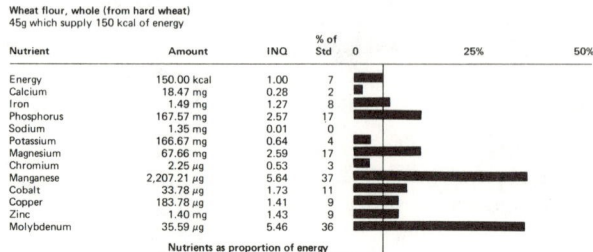

Wheat flour, patent, all-purpose flour, enriched
41 g which supply 150 kcal of energy

Nutrient	Amount	INQ	% of Std			
				0	25%	50%
Energy	150.00 kcal	1.00	7			
Calcium	6.59 mg	0.10	1			
Iron	1.19 mg	1.02	7			
Phosphorus	35.85 mg	0.55	4			
Sodium	0.82 mg	0.00	0			
Potassium	39.14 mg	0.15	1			
Magnesium	12.32 mg	0.47	3			
Chromium	1.23 µg	0.29	2			
Manganese	247.25 µg	0.63	4			
Cobalt	24.83 µg	0.76	5			
Copper	61.81 µg	0.47	3			
Zinc	0.37 mg	0.38	2			
Molybdenum	13.18 µg	2.02	13			

Nutrients as proportion of energy

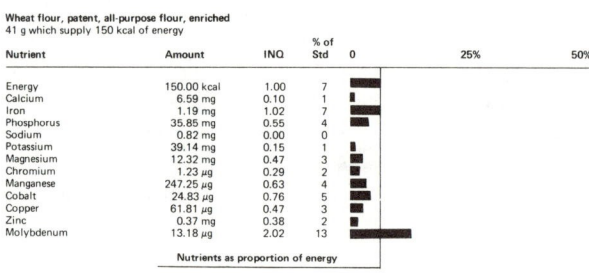

Average of equal portions of beef and pork
65g which supply 150 kcal of energy

Nutrients	Amount	INQ	% of Std		
				0	25%
Energy	150.00 kcal	1.00	7		
Calcium	8.50 mg	0.13	1		
Iron	2.48 mg	2.12	14		
Phosphorus	193.46 mg	2.97	19		
Sodium	40.86 mg	0.16	1		
Potassium	248.37 mg	0.95	6		
Magnesium	16.08 mg	0.62	4		
Chromium	5.88 µg	1.39	9		
Manganese	12.74 µg	0.03	0		
Cobalt	22.55 µg	1.15	8		
Copper	156.86 µg	1.20	8		
Zinc	2.48 mg	2.54	17		
Molybdenum	122.55 µg	18.79	123		

Nutrients as proportion of energy

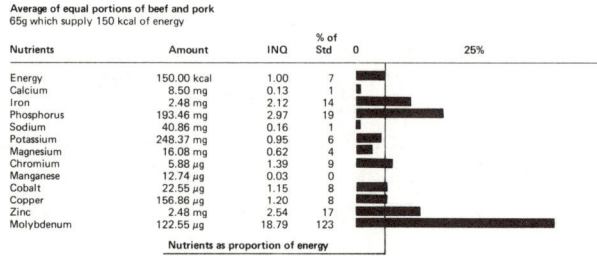

FIG. 5.8. ISOCALORIC PROFILES

Illustrating the wide range of mineral content in whole wheat flour, white enriched flour, and red meats (source: Schroeder, 1971). For nutrients with no U.S. RDA, a reasonable value has been assumed: energy 2,300.0 kcal, calcium 1,000.00 mg, iron 18.0 mg, phosphorus 1,000.0 mg, sodium 4,000.0 mg, potassium 4,000.0 mg, magnesium 400.0 mg, chromium 65.0 µg, manganese 6,000.0 µg, manganese 6,000.0 µg, cobalt 300.0 µg, copper 2,000.0 µg, zinc 15.0 mg, molybdenum 100.0 µg

the substitution for meat, it is possible that these individuals' diets may become limiting in the trace elements. (Fig 5.8b).

There may be other considerations, but for the most part, vegetarian diets can be nutritionally adequate. The food industry, if providing consumers with alternatives to meat, should be aware of the contribution that meat has made to the trace mineral content of the diet in the past.

CAN AID FOOD INDUSTRY

In addition to identifying nutritional needs in the population, the food industry can use the INQ for:

Planning and designing new foods for overall nutritional adequacy.

Evaluating current food fortification practices.

Determining enrichment and restoration policy in foods.

As a result of coordinated, long-term, intensive cooperation among food scientists, nutrition educators, and the food industry, consumers will be able to make adequate food choices within their personal food preference, economic, ethnic, religious, and social constraints. The nutritional quality of food products and complete nutrition labeling of food products are the variables which can be most influenced by the food industry.

LINOLEIC ACID

National food and nutrition policies are emerging in some countries in part because of the possible effects of diet on coronary heart disease, even though the evidence is controversial (Wretlind, 1974). Patients at risk of coronary heart disease are generally counseled to make dietary modifications. Reduction of calorie intake and total fat intake together with an increase in the ratio of polyunsaturated (linoleic acid) to saturated fatty acids in the diet are elements of diet modification for those at risk. Unfortunately in the U.S. over the last several decades, fat consumption from all sources has increased from 35% of an individual's calories up to 45%. This increased fat largely comes from soybean oil and other vegetable oils which, in many cases, are hydrogenated, making the linoleic acid content uncertain. (USDA-ARS, 1971).

Confronted by recommendations to modify fat intake, the patient may find implementation difficult. It is difficult to obtain fat information from most labels, according to current labeling practices. One solution would be to define a goal for linoleic acid consumption within a specified total fat intake and then examine each food's capacity to meet the specified goal. More informative labeling practices, based upon more detailed food composition data and better informed patients, would be required. The INQ approach could facilitate quantitating the recommendation and subsequent food choices to accomplish a prescribed goal.

Using a standard of 38% of the dietary energy as fat (Leverton, 1974), of which 30%, or 29 g, is linoleic acid, changes can be made in the average diet if a P:S ratio of 1 or greater is to be obtained (see Figure 5.9). The data used to generate Figure 5.9 indicate that vegetable fats and fat products, e.g., salad dressing, have INQs ≥ 1.64, while lard, olive oil, and butter have INQs equal to 0.88, 0.63 and 0.22, respectively. The 20% of the foods in the nut classification with INQs ≤ 0.16 for linoleic acid include extracted soybean products and coconut products. The 70% of the foods in the nut classification having INQs for linoleic acid ≥ 1 include walnuts, soybeans, Brazil nuts, peanuts and almonds, with INQs of 4.87, 2.31, 2.06, 1.01 and 1.52, respectively. Those foods that have INQs greater than 1.0 must be the predominant sources of polyunsaturated fats to ensure a P: S ratio of 1. The foods with the highest INQs become complementary sources of linoleic acid for foods low in polyunsaturates or high in saturated or animal fats.

LINOLEIC ACID

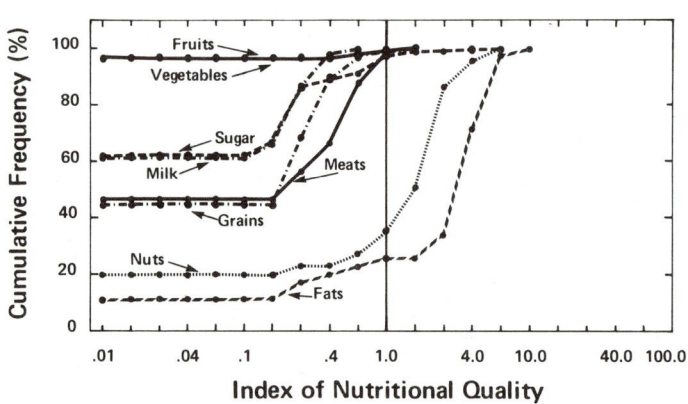

FIG. 5.9. LINOLEIC ACID IN FOODS IS IN RELATION TO ENERGY CONTENT

An INQ of 1 for linoleic acid is arbitrarily fixed at 29 g intake per day per 2300 kcal.

Foods in the rest of the food groups have INQs of less than 1.0 for linoleic acid. The data for the meat, poultry, fish and eggs category, however, are incomplete; Handbook No. 8 does not include linoleic acid values for most fish. Many kinds of fish are, however, considered to be good sources of linoleic acid. The supporting additional data would obviously modify Figure 5.9. This emphasizes the critical need for more food composition data if dietary recommendations for fat-modified diets are to be implemented.

Poultry is normally recommended for inclusion in a fat-modified diet. The linoleic acid INQs for chicken and turkey are 1.1 and 0.9, respectively. These products, therefore, are acceptable in such diets and hold their own in regard to nutrient density; however, they cannot be expected to raise the P: S ratio without other alterations in the diet. Unmodified vegetable fats and the foods in the nut categories, and probably fish, are the food groups which would need to be consumed in greater quantity to significantly increase P: S ratio.

The INQ approach, coupled with adequate compositional data, could materially ease professionals' efforts to help consumers learn how to make nutritionally advisable dietary modifications.

REFERENCES

AMA Council on Foods and Nutrition. 1973. Improvement of the nutritive quality of foods: General policies. J. Am. Med. Assn. 225(9):1118.

BAUMAN, H and RUCH, D. 1974. Problems of researching and marketing fortified foods and their implications for consumption trends. In *Nutrients in Processed Foods*, Ed. P.L. White and D.C. Fletcher, Publishing Sciences Group, Inc., Acton, Mass.

BRALOVE, M. 1972. We're eating ourselves to death. Medical Times *100*: 255.

CRAMPTON, E.W. 1964. Nutrient-to-calorie ratios in applied nutrition. J. Nutr. *82*:353.

DALY, R.F. 1969. Food enough for the U.S.? A crystal ball look ahead. In *Food for Us All,* Ed. E. Stefferud, U.S. Dept. of Agriculture, Washington, D.C.

FDA. 1972. Nutrition labeling: Proposed criteria for food label information panel. Food and Drug Administration. Fed. Reg. 37(62):6497, March 30.

GUTHRIE, H.A. 1971. *Introductory Nutrition*, 2nd ed. The C.V. Mosby Co., St. Louis, Mo.

HANSEN, R.G. 1973. An index of food quality. Nutr. Rev. *31*:1

JOHNSON, N.E., ALCANTARA, E.N., and LINKSWILER, H. 1970. Effect of level of protein intake on urinary and fecal calcium and calcium retention of young adult males. J. Nutr. *100*:1425.

JOHNSON, O.C. 1974. The FDA and labeling. J. Am. Dietet. Assn. 64:471.

LEVERTON, R.M. 1974. Fats in Food and Diet, USDA Agriculture Information Bulletin No. 361.

NAS/NRC. 1974. *Recommended Dietary Allowances,* 8th ed. Natl. Acad. of Sciences-Natl. Res. Council, Washington, D.C.

PAGE, L. and FRIEND, B. 1974. Levels of use of sugars in the United States. In *Sugars in Nutrition,* Ed. H. Sipple and J. McNutt, Nutrition Foundation Monograph Series, Academic Press, New York.

PARRISH, J.B. 1971. Implications of changing food habits for nutrition educators. J. Nutr. Educ. 2:140.

PYKE, M. 1970. Food technology and society. Nutr. Rev. 28:31.

ROSE, M.S., HESSLER, M.J., STIEBELING, H.K., and TAYLOR, C.N. 1928. Visualizing food values. J. Home Econ. 20:781.

SCHROEDER, H.A. 1971. Losses of vitamins and trace minerals resulting from processing and preservation of foods. Am. J. Clin. Nutr. 24:562.

SORENSON, A.W., WYSE, B.W., WITTWER, A.J., and HANSEN, R.G. 1975. A balanced diet—New help for an old problem in the form of the Index of Nutritional Quality. J. Am. Dietet. Assn. (In press).

STARE, F.J. 1972. Nutritional problems of affluent populations. S. Afr. Med. J. 46:1575.

USDA. 1971. Agricultural Research Service, Progress Report of the Consumer and Food Economics Division, Marking and Nutrition Research, July 1, 1971, Agricultural Research Service, Washington, D.C., Nov.

USDA. 1972. Food and nutrient intake of individuals in the United States, Spring 1965. Household Food Consumption Survey 1965-66 Report No. 11. U.S. Dept. of Agriculture-Agric. Res. Service, Washington, D.C.

WALKER, R.M. and LINKSWILER, H.M. 1972. Calcium retention in the adult human male as affected by protein intake. J. Nutr. 102:1297.

WATT, B.K. and MERRILL, A.L. 1963. *Composition of Foods—Raw, Processed, Prepared.* Agriculture Handbook No. 8. U.S. Dept. of Agriculture, Washington, D.C.

WATT, B.K. and MURPHY, E.W. 1970. Tables of food consumption: Scope and needed research. Food Technol. 24:50.

WRETLIND, A. 1974. World Sugar Production and Usage in Europe, Sugars in Nutrition Ed., H.L. Sipple and K.W. McNutt, Academic Press, New York, pp. 88-90.

WYMAN, J.R. 1972. Teenagers and food. Food and Nutr. 2(1):3.

6

Nutritional Quality of Snack Foods

Snack foods are contributing to an increasing percentage of the daily caloric intake in the American diet. Using nutrient density criteria, common snack foods are evaluated individually and in combination. Food fortification guidelines are discussed in relation to consumption of snack foods. A concept of intrinsic and extrinsic occurrence of nutrients in foods is presented below as a basis for comparison of nutritional quality of regular and fortified foods.

PLANNING FOR THE INEVITABLE SNACK FOODS IN THE DIET

For purposes of this discussion, "snack foods" are defined as items consumed between meals. In contrast "fast foods" are those prepared with minimum time, served in franchise restaurants, and consumed most often as meals but the group may include items that are also eaten as snacks. The choices offered by food vending machines continue to increase in variety and consumer appeal and currently may be either snacks or meal substitutes. In this chapter we are primarily concerned with snack foods, but some meal substitutes will inevitably be included, because as meal patterns blur or disappear, so do distinctions between meals and snacks (Breeling 1970).

For many individuals, between-meal consumption of foods provides up to 25 percent of their calories (Thomas and Call 1973). In a traditional sense, the only meal still taken by many is in the evening, with breakfast and lunch omitted or taken in haste under circumstances that do not allow for preparation of foods of a more traditional character.

Lee (1977) has suggested that urbanization and technological development have helped induce the increased popularity of nontraditional foods. Certainly food habits and customs are influenced by television and other forms of media, and changing food habits and food supplies may be partially responsible for the low levels of iron, calcium, and vitamin C identified in the population by nutrition surveys (Leverton 1968).

Whether as cause or effect, the fast food industry is enjoying an unparalleled, phenomenal growth. Most fast food chains are currently growing at a 12 percent plus per annum substantially above the 8 percent to 10 percent of the rest of the food service industry.

One result of these phenomena is that the average consumer finds it more and more difficult to make nutritionally sound snack selections. When 374 high school students in Indiana were surveyed, 73 percent of the students reported consuming foods from the vending machines either two or three times per week or every day (Hruban 1973). When confronted by a list of snack foods available from the vending machine which contained an equal number of snacks rated by the authors as "excellent", "fair" and "poor", the students did not select snack foods rated as excellent, favoring instead soda pop, gum, sweet roll, candy bars and mints.

NUTRITIONAL COMPARISON OF FOODS

If snack foods were generally equivalent in nutrient density to those common in more traditional diets, there would be little cause for concern. However, some are mainly a source of energy with little else, while others do contain significant quantities of nutrients.

The Index of Nutritional Quality (INQ) is an effective way to evaluate the nutritional equivalencies of foods. The INQ method is a quantitative and qualitative measure of nutrient-to-calorie density that provides a profile of ratios which may be represented graphically. An INQ value of 1.0 for a given nutrient in a food indicates that 2000 kcal of that food would supply the U.S. RDA of that nutrient. Conversely, a nutrient value less than 1.0 for a given food (or in graphical format, a bar shorter than the energy or kcal bar) means that an excess of calories must be eaten to fulfill the U.S. RDAs for that nutrient if only that food were eaten.

The nutrient density profiles of six common beverages illustrate various concepts (Figures 6.1—6.6). Empty calories are obvious in the carbonated beverage profile (Figure 6.1). Coffee, (Figure 6.2) in contrast, provides small amounts of niacin and iron (3 percent and 1 percent, respectively) and no calories. This nutrient source becomes significant for individuals who drink eight to ten cups of coffee per day.

The three profiles for milk (Figures 6.3, 6.4 and 6.5) illustrate how removing the calories provided by milk fat would affect the proportion of other nutrients relative to calories. Whole milk contains three nutrients in excess of calories, i.e. protein, riboflavin and calcium with INQs of 1.66, 3.08 and 3.63 respectively. In 2 percent lowfat milk the INQs for these three nutrients are 2.19, 4.19 and 4.05 respectively. While in skim milk they become 3.08, 5.88 and 6.72, respectively. Orange juice with break-

COLA CARBONATED BEVERAGE*

Nutrient	Amount		INQ	% STD	0	25%
Energy	95.94	KCAL	1.00	5	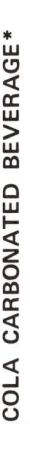	
Protein	0.00	G	0.00	0		
Vitamin A	0.00	IU	0.00	0		
Vitamin C	0.00	MG	0.00	0		
Thiamin	0.00	MG	0.00	0		
Riboflavin	0.00	MG	0.00	0		
Niacin	0.00	MG	0.00	0		
Calcium	0.00	MG	0.00	0		
Iron	0.00	MG	0.00	0		

*(8 ounces)

FIG. 6.1. NUTRIENT PROFILE FOR THE CONTRIBUTION OF EIGHT OUNCES OF CARBONATED BEVERAGE ILLUSTRATING ENERGY AND NUTRIENT CONTRIBUTION USING 2,000 KCAL AND U.S. RDAs FOR STANDARDS

COFFEE*

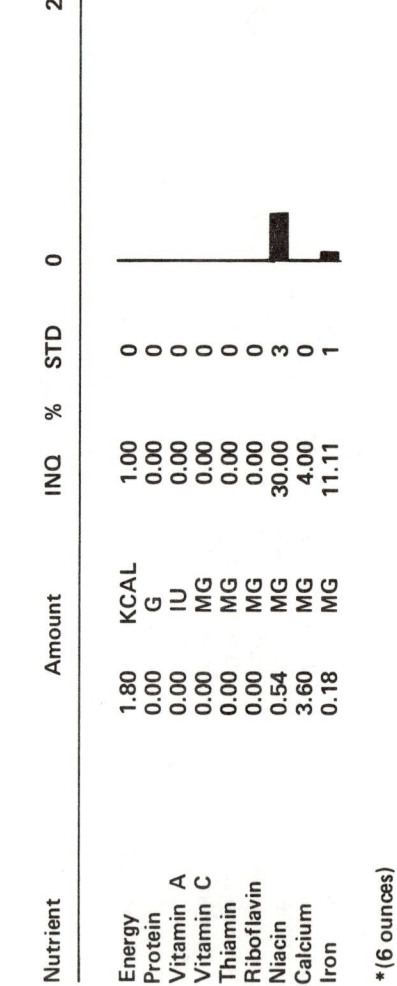

Nutrient	Amount		INQ	% STD	0		25%
Energy	1.80	KCAL	1.00	0			
Protein	0.00	G	0.00	0			
Vitamin A	0.00	IU	0.00	0			
Vitamin C	0.00	MG	0.00	0			
Thiamin	0.00	MG	0.00	0			
Riboflavin	0.00	MG	0.00	0			
Niacin	0.54	MG	30.00	3			
Calcium	3.60	MG	4.00	0			
Iron	0.18	MG	11.11	1			

*(6 ounces)

FIG. 6.2. NUTRIENT PROFILE FOR COFFEE INDICATING INSIGNIFICANT AMOUNTS OF CALORIES WHILE CONTRIBUTING SMALL AMOUNTS OF NIACIN AND IRON TO DAILY NUTRITIONAL NEEDS

WHOLE MILK *

Nutrient	Amount		INQ	% STD	0	25%
Energy	158.60	KCAL	1.00	8		
Protein	8.54	G	1.66	13		
Vitamin A	341.60	IU	0.86	7		
Vitamin C	2.44	MG	0.51	4		
Thiamin	0.07	MG	0.62	5		
Riboflavin	0.42	MG	3.08	24		
Niacin	0.24	MG	0.15	1		
Calcium	287.92	MG	3.63	29		
Iron	0.00	MG	0.00	0		

*(8 ounces)

FIG. 6.3. NUTRIENT PROFILE FOR WHOLE MILK

2% LOWFAT MILK *

Nutrient	Amount		INQ	% STD	
Energy	145.14	KCAL	1.00	7	
Protein	10.33	G	2.19	16	
Vitamin A	196.80	IU	0.54	4	
Vitamin C	2.46	MG	0.56	4	
Thiamin	0.10	MG	0.90	7	
Riboflavin	0.52	MG	4.19	30	
Niacin	0.25	MG	0.17	1	
Calcium	351.78	MG	4.85	35	
Iron	0.25	MG	0.19	1	

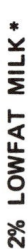

*(8 ounces)

FIG. 6.4. NUTRIENT PROFILE FOR 2% LOWFAT MILK

SKIM MILK*

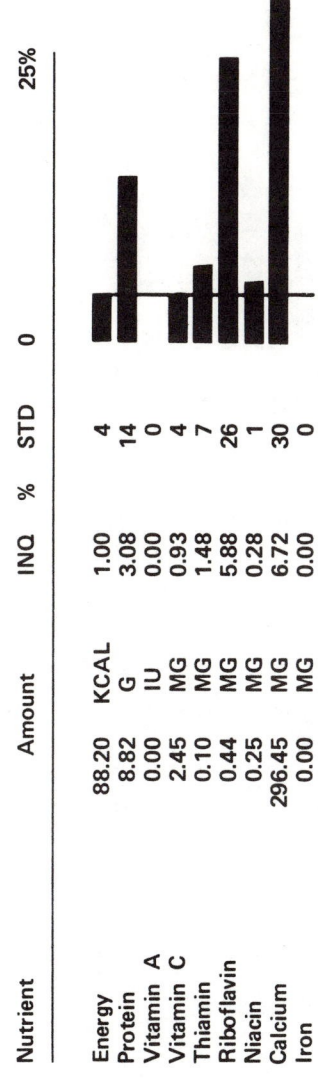

Nutrient	Amount		INQ	% STD	0	25%
Energy	88.20	KCAL	1.00	4		
Protein	8.82	G	3.08	14		
Vitamin A	0.00	IU	0.00	0		
Vitamin C	2.45	MG	0.93	4		
Thiamin	0.10	MG	1.48	7		
Riboflavin	0.44	MG	5.88	26		
Niacin	0.25	MG	0.28	1		
Calcium	296.45	MG	6.72	30		
Iron	0.00	MG	0.00	0		

*(8 ounces)

FIG. 6.5. NUTRIENT PROFILES FOR SKIM MILK ILLUSTRATING
THE EFFECT OF REMOVAL OF MILK FAT CALORIES ON THE
NUTRITIONAL CONTRIBUTION FOR THESE FOODS

ORANGE JUICE *

Nutrient	Amount		ING	% STD	0	25%
Energy	112.05	KCAL	1.00	6		
Protein	1.74	G	0.48	3		
Vitamin A	498.00	IU	1.78	10		
Vitamin C	112.05	MG	33.33	187		187%
Thiamin	0.22	MG	2.67	15		
Riboflavin	0.03	MG	0.26	1		
Niacin	0.75	MG	0.67	4		
Calcium	22.41	MG	0.40	2		
Iron	0.25	MG	0.25	1		

*(8 ounces)

FIG. 6.6. ORANGE JUICE PROFILE GRAPHICALLY
ILLUSTRATES THAT RELATIVE TO CALORIES THIS
BEVERAGE IS AN EXCELLENT DAILY SOURCE OF VITAMIN C

fast or as a snack is an excellent source of vitamin C with an INQ of 33.33 (Figure 6.6).

Snack foods can greatly contribute to satisfy daily nutritional needs. For example, the sweet roll in Figure 6.7 contains the same number of calories as the combination of fresh fruits, cheese and crackers illustrated in Figure 6.8. Relative to calories, however, the sweet roll is low in all of the nutrients shown, while the foods illustrated in Figure 6.8 are significantly short only in niacin (INQ = 0.54) relative to calories. With two cups of coffee, however, the latter snack becomes nearly adequate in niacin.

If one evaluates various meal substitutes using this methodology, interesting data emerge. The hamburger and carbonated beverage (Figure 6.9) is less nutritious than the same hamburger consumed with a milkshake (Figure 6.10). In the former profile, no nutrient has an INQ $\geq$ 1.0 while in the latter protein, riboflavin and calcium INQs exceed 1.0. The pizza profile (Figure 6.11) indicates that this favorite food is fairly well-balanced with vitamins A, C and thiamin (INQs = 0.82, 0.81, 0.83, respectively) being provided in "fair" amounts, while all other nutrients are in "adequate" supply except for protein (INQ = 1.91) which is provided in "good" quantity (Wittwer *et al* 1977).

NUTRIENT FORTIFICATION

Since most people choose foods on the basis of convenience and palatability, with minimum consideration given to nutrient content, the question of fortifying snack foods with nutrients arises.

The fortification of milk with vitamin D to prevent rickets, and salt with iodine to prevent goiter, along with the enrichment of flour with iron, thiamin, riboflavin, and niacin, have become widely accepted public health practices. Under consideration, therefore, is the extension of fortification practices to include other foods and a broader spectrum of nutrients. It is important to note that, in the milk and salt examples, the food is being used as a vehicle to provide nutrients to prevent deficiency diseases, namely, rickets and goiter. In the case of flour enrichment, some of the nutrients (thiamin, riboflavin, niacin and iron) discarded in the milling process are simply being added back to the flour. Changing dietary patterns may now necessitate adding other vitamins and minerals to flour and cereal products, since they also are concentrated in the discarded portion.

In 1974 the Food and Nutrition Board of the National Academy of Sciences proposed a fortification policy for cereal grain products (Anon 1974). Since 26 percent of the calories consumed by the general U.S. population are derived from cereals (on a flour equivalent about 17

SWEET ROLL*

Nutrient	Amount		INQ %	STD	0	25%
Energy	436.08	KCAL	1.00	22		
Protein	11.73	G	0.83	18		
Vitamin A	96.60	IU	0.09	2		
Vitamin C	0.00	MG	0.00	0		
Thiamin	0.10	MG	0.30	6		
Riboflavin	0.21	MG	0.56	12		
Niacin	1.10	MG	0.25	6		
Calcium	117.30	MG	0.54	12		
Iron	1.10	MG	0.28	6		

*(4½ x 3¾ x 2")

FIG. 6.7. THE NUTRIENT PROFILE FOR SWEET ROLL
ILLUSTRATES THE SMALL AMOUNT OF OTHER NUTRIENTS
RELATIVE TO CALORIES PROVIDED BY THIS SNACK ITEM

FRESH FRUIT, CHEESE & CRACKERS *

Nutrient	Amount		INQ	% STD
Energy	432.61	KCAL	1.00	22
Protein	12.04	G	0.86	19
Vitamin A	966.90	IU	0.89	19
Vitamin C	182.69	MG	14.08	304
Thiamin	0.34	MG	1.05	23
Riboflavin	0.37	MG	1.01	22
Niacin	2.33	MG	0.54	12
Calcium	351.80	MG	1.63	35
Iron	3.68	MG	0.94	20

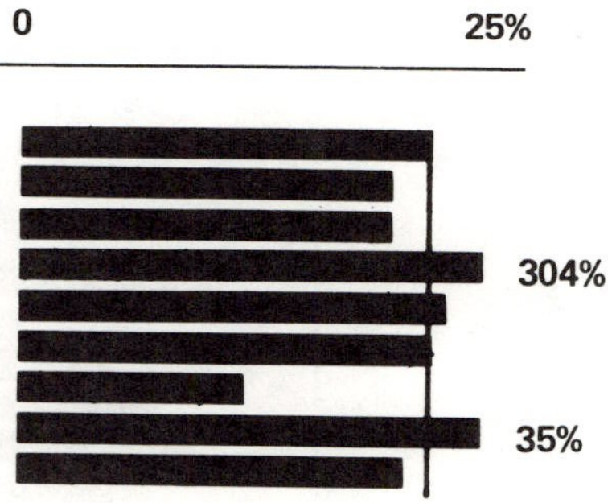

* (Same kilocalories as a sweet roll)

FIG. 6.8. ISOCALORIC PROFILE OF FRESH FRUIT, CHEESE AND CRACKERS COMBINATION WHEN COMPARED WITH A SWEET ROLL ILLUSTRATING THE NUTRITIONAL PREFERENCE OF THE FORMER OVER THE LATTER

HAMBURGER and CARBONATED BEVERAGE

Nutrient	Amount		INQ	% STD	0	25%	50%
Energy	432.36	KCAL	1.00	22			
Protein	13.66	G	0.97	21			
Vitamin A	433.70	IU	0.40	9			
Vitamin C	7.39	MG	0.57	12			
Thiamin	0.22	MG	0.68	15			
Riboflavin	0.20	MG	0.54	12			
Niacin	3.53	MG	0.82	18			
Calcium	52.99	MG	0.25	5			
Iron	2.45	MG	0.63	14			

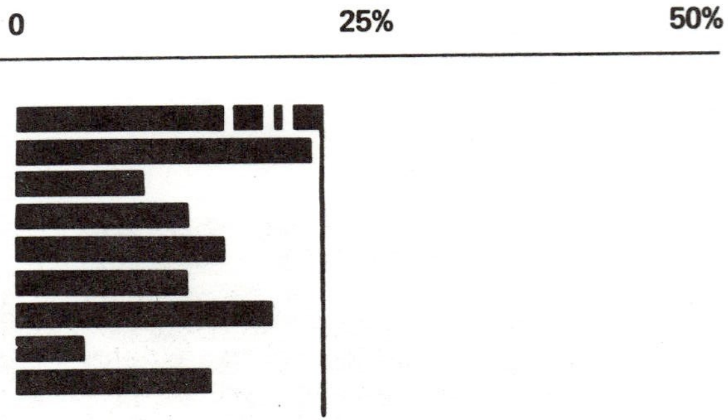

■ Hamburger with lettuce, tomato & catsup

▮▮▮ Carbonated Beverage (12 oz)

FIG. 6.9. NUTRIENT CONTRIBUTION OF A HAMBURGER AND
A CARBONATED BEVERAGE

HAMBURGER and MILKSHAKE

Nutrient	Amount		INQ	% STD
Energy	637.38	KCAL	1.00	32
Protein	24.44	G	1.18	38
Vitamin A	1218.30	IU	0.76	24
Vitamin C	10.08	MG	0.53	17
Thiamin	0.31	MG	0.66	21
Riboflavin	0.71	MG	1.31	42
Niacin	3.80	MG	0.60	19
Calcium	408.49	MG	1.28	41
Iron	2.59	MG	0.45	14

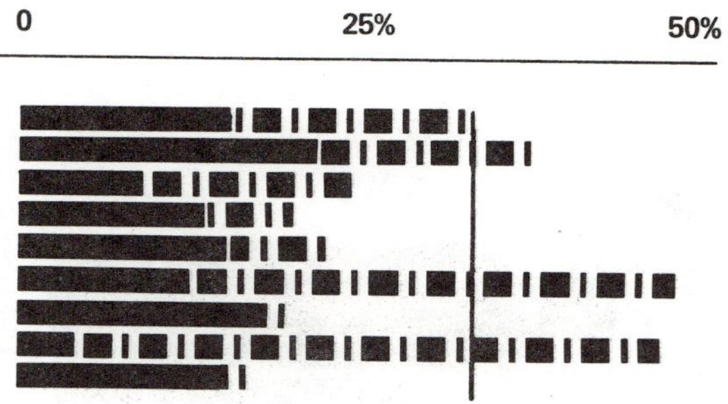

Hamburger with lettuce, tomato & catsup

Milkshake (12 oz)

FIG. 6.10. NUTRIENT PROFILE OF A HAMBURGER AND A MILKSHAKE ILLUSTRATING THAT COMBINATIONS OF FOOD CAN COMPLIMENT INDIVIDUAL STRENGTHS AND WEAKNESSES OF INDIVIDUAL FOODS

PIZZA—PEPPERONI, SAUSAGE, VEGETABLES *

Nutrient	Amount		INQ	% STD
Energy	599.05	KCAL	1.00	30
Protein	37.13	G	1.91	57
Vitamin A	1235.20	IU	0.82	25
Vitamin C	14.49	MG	0.81	24
Thiamin	0.37	MG	0.83	25
Riboflavin	0.53	MG	1.03	31
Niacin	7.06	MG	1.18	35
Calcium	337.66	MG	1.13	34
Iron	5.34	MG	0.99	30

* (¼ of 14″ pie)

FIG. 6.11. PIZZA PROFILE GRAPHICALLY ILLUSTRATING
NUTRITIONAL CONTRIBUTION OF THIS FAVORITE FAMILY
FOOD

percent), proper fortification could be nutritionally advisable. In addition to those nutrients now added to flour (thiamin, riboflavin, niacin and iron), the Food and Nutrition Board recommended that vitamin A, pyridoxine (vitamin B_6), folic acid, calcium, magnesium, and zinc be considered. These nutrients were selected primarily on the basis that significant segments of the population are consuming inadequate amounts of one or more of them.

The technical feasibility of adding the nutrients was not a principal factor in the recommendations. It was expected that adverse product acceptance by the consumer, or any color or flavor problems could be overcome. The questions of needs and public policy were (and are) the important issues.

REASONS AND CRITERIA FOR FORTIFICATION

Some reasons accepted in the past for fortifying foods with nutrients are (Anon. 1974):

(1) A significant number of people have intakes of the nutrient(s) below the desirable level.

(2) The food(s) to be fortified is/are likely to be consumed by the population in need of quantities sufficient to offset the problem without producing dietary imbalances.

(3) The added nutrient(s) is/are stable under usual storage and use conditions.

(4) The nutrient(s) is/are bioavailable from the food.

(5) There is reasonable assurance that toxicity will not occur even with excessive intakes.

(6) The cost involved in fortifying is reasonable relative to the anticipated benefit.

General purpose flour in the United States and in England is milled to about 70 to 75 percent extraction, which means that in the milling process 25 to 30 percent of the wheat kernel is discarded as animal feed —bran and middlings— and 70 to 75 percent is retained in the flour. Unfortunately, many of the important nutrients are concentrated in the discarded portion (Figure 6.12).

In England, Sir Rudolph Peters has suggested that consideration be given to returning to a wartime 85 percent extraction rate, since higher levels of the vitamins and trace minerals in proportion to energy would be retained with the flour. Since it has been shown that low income segments of the population, especially, consume a higher proportion of their calories from breads and cereals, this could have significant consequences if practiced in the United States (Anon. 1974).

Perhaps the best case for fortification or enrichment of foods can be

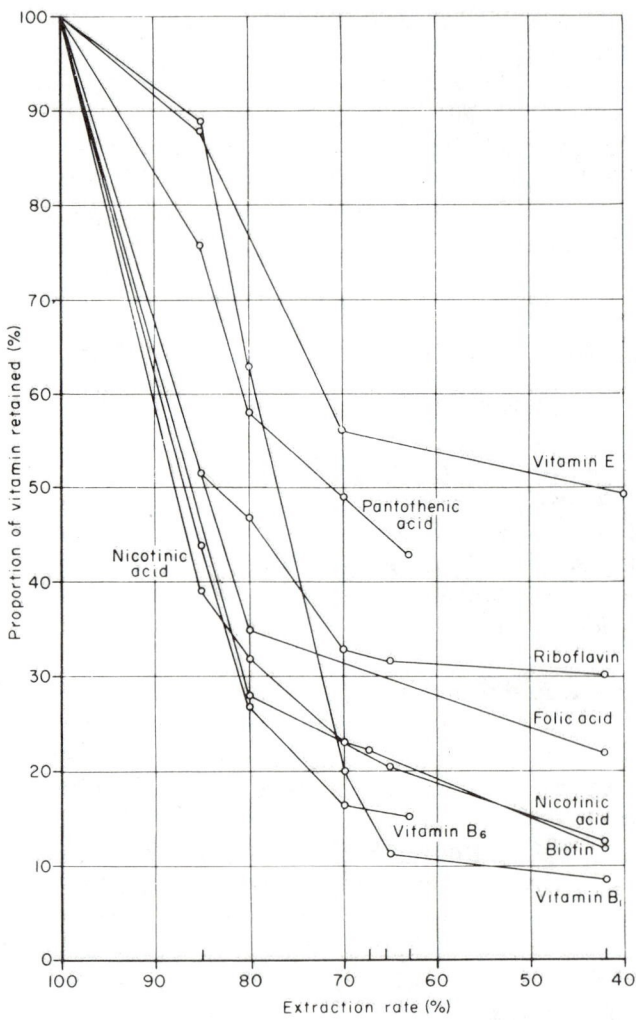

FIG. 6.12. RELATION BETWEEN EXTRACTION RATE AND
PROPORTION OF TOTAL VITAMINS OF THE GRAIN RETAINED
IN FLOUR

made for iron under item 1) above, that is, the intake of nutrient(s) is below the desirable level in the diets of a significant number of people. Iron deficiency anemia is commonly present in the population and current food preparation practices tend to reduce iron intake. Whereas cast iron cookware, especially with acid foods, was a significant source of iron, the change to stainless steel, aluminum, teflon, and even copper cooking utensils has reduced iron in food. Much of the iron in cereals lost in the milling process is added back to the flour, but there is no nationwide enrichment requirement.

To further increase iron content of food as consumed beyond current enrichment practice is neither universally accepted as being desirable nor technically has the best form of iron and vehicle for fortification been identified. The recognition of iron deficiency anemia in the population has, however, stimulated consideration of iron enrichment of foods generally, and upward adjustments in the RDA for iron for some segments of the population. Appropriate vehicles for iron fortification are under investigation, cereal products being an important traditional vehicle. Additionally, potatoes, sugar, salt, and coffee have all been suggested to be appropriate food carriers for iron fortification.

Aside from the specific food to use to increase iron intake is the question of chemical form of supplementary iron. Iron EDTA complexes have been proposed for fortification for reasons of efficacy and stability. Under some circumstances, iron EDTA added to foods is about twice as effective as ferrous sulphate. Efficacy of the iron supplement must certainly depend upon other constituents of the diet. The stability of iron and other nutrients in fortified foods is a matter for continuous study. However, one of the important problems remains the efficacy of fortification of food with iron.

Since folic acid deficiency occurs in the U.S., it is of practical interest to us that in South Africa folic acid deficiency can be corrected by food fortification. Folic acid added to cereal products will survive baking and cooking procedures and increase the folic acid in body tissue of the consumers. The possibility of prevention or cure of megaloblastic anemia by fortification of food with folic acid is promising.

As our food supply is increasingly defined by manufacturing practice, more people are likely to risk dietary deficiencies. Fortification of many snack foods could help keep average diets nutritionally balanced.

If newly fabricated popular foods have low nutrient density ratings (small amounts of nutrients in proportion to calories), it may be expected that, sooner or later, some essential nutrients will become limiting in the food supply. This could especially affect individuals whose nutrient needs are most critical, e.g., growing youngsters, women during pregnancy and lactation, and sedentary elderly who need fewer calories but an average amount of other nutrients. Thus, even without substantial evidence that nutrient deficits currently exist, increasing proportions of the population can be expected to be at nutritional risk in the future unless dietary trends change.

If every food offered in the market place contained a balanced supply of all the nutrients known to be required (related to some universal standard such as recommended dietary allowance per 1,000 kcal), a balanced diet could be achieved even with nothing but fabricated foods. However unattractive this may seem at the present, it could happen, but only with the fortification of many snack foods.

At the other extreme, the process of nutrition education may persuade everyone to consume sufficient quantities of the traditional foods containing "intrinsically" all of the nutrient requirements. In view of current lifestyles and the way people usually select their foods (on the basis of convenience, cost and taste rather than nutritional values), this will be difficult.

INTRINSIC VERSUS EXTRINSIC NUTRIENTS

Nutrients may be present in foods because they have been added "extrinsically," or because they are "intrinsic" parts of the food. Intrinsic refers to genetically determined constituents of plant and animal tissues, while extrinsic means that a nutrient has been artificially added to the food material.

If the principal nutrients are in a food intrinsically, another thirty or so additional nutrients may be expected to be associated in reasonable proportions, related to the biological function of the plant or animal tissue from which the food is derived. If, on the other hand, some of the principal nutrients are largely in a food by addition (extrinsically), others can be expected to be lacking. Use of the word intrinsic would avoid reference to such terms as "natural," with all of the unfortunate connotations it has acquired. For purposes of nutrition education, and discussions of food fortification and new foods, intrinsic and extrinsic could become precisely descriptive.

NUTRITION EDUCATION

Without adequate nutrition education, wise decisions about foods become an impossibility. Food choices could include nutritional evaluations if usable information about nutrient contents were available at the site of selection. That implies understandable, legible labels. Vending machines could be stocked with clearly labeled foods having high nutrient density ratings. It would also be important to note if the nutrients were intrinsic or extrinsic to the food to reinforce and encourage wise food selection habits.

REINFORCEMENT OF NUTRITION INFORMATION BY EDUCATION, ADVERTISEMENT, USE OF FOOD AND LABELS

For all of us, but especially for young people without a nutrition education background, to make a wise decision when selecting foods in a vending machine has become an important public health issue. Food choices could be made with nutritional value as part of the selection process if usable information about nutrient contents were included at the site of selection. It has been suggested that to enlighten the selections from vending machines it would be most useful to provide alternative choices with a major proportion of foods having a high nutrient density. It would, of course, be important to differentiate if the nutrients labeled were in the food intrinsically rather than from addition to reinforce and encourage wise food selection habits. It has been suggested that some children meet most all of their energy needs either from snacks or fast food items. This may be even more so as we substitute fast foods for Type A school lunches, as is being done in some locations. In order to insure a balanced diet, fortification of the foods with a broad spectrum of nutrients should be a consideration. Intelligent food choices to compliment good health are becoming more and more complex.

The choices that young people are also reported to be making through school cafeterias in many areas show a preference for snack food type items—items sold normally in fast-food restaurants. If free choice in selection of options continues to become more prevalent, an increasing burden is placed on the food containing many trace nutrients intrinsically to supply the elements of a balanced diet, or a more extensive enrichment or fortification program is needed to ensure an adequate diet.

CONCLUSIONS

To insure the population a balanced diet, fortification of snack foods with a broad spectrum of nutrients should be considered. Until the public can be better prepared to evaluate nutritional values, a more extensive enrichment or fortification program of snack foods is needed.

REFERENCES

ANON. 1974. Council on Foods and Nutrition. Improvement of the nutritive quality of foods. Jour. Amer. Med. Assoc. 225.

ANON. 1974. National Academy of Sciences. Proposed Fortification Policy for Cereal-Grain Products. Washington, D.C.

BREELING, J.L. 1970. Are we snacking our way to malnutrition? Today's Health 48:48-50.

HANSEN, R.G. 1973. An Index of food quality. Nutr. Rev. *31*:1. 1-7.

HANSEN, R.G., WYSE, B.W., and BROWN, G. 1978. Nutrient needs and their expression. Food Technol. *32*:44-53.

HRUBAN, J.A. 1976. Selection of snack foods from vending machines by high school students. Jour. Sch. Health *47*:33-37.

LEE, E.E. 1977. Food fads, nutrition and teenage mothers. Childhood Education *53*:143-146.

LEVERTON, R.M. 1968. The paradox of teenage nutrition. Jour. Amer. Diet. Assoc. *53*:1, 116-123.

THOMAS, J.A. and CALL, D.L. 1973. Eating between meals. Nutr. Rev. *31*: 5, 137-139.

WITTWER, A.J., SORENSON, A.W., WYSE, B.W., and HANSEN, R.G. 1977. Nutrient density offers a basis for quantitative description of foods for normal and therapeutic diets. Jour. Nutr. Educ. *9*:1, 26-30.

7

Nutritional Labeling – What's That?

INTRODUCTION

For several years we and some of our colleagues at Utah State University have been lecturing to groups throughout Utah on methods for improving one's personal diet. These groups have included community and service organizations, women's clubs, senior citizen and minority groups as well as county nutrition agents, their aides and other semi-professionals. Whenever we discuss the food labels based on nutrient composition, the audience response has been discouragingly uniform. Most of the people didn't know these labels existed, and those who had noticed them had little or no idea of how to apply the nutritional information to their own diet. Such reactions to and comments about nutritional labeling have prompted this chapter.

HISTORY OF NUTRITIONAL LABELING

The last nutrition labeling laws that were published in the Federal Register (1973) went into effect in January 1975. They are the end product of a three-year study of food labeling initiated by the 1969 White House Conference. Charles C. Edwards, then Commissioner of the Food and Drugs Administration (1973) defined the new labeling guides as aids designed to furnish the consumer more information about the ingredients and nutritional qualities of foods in a uniform and easily understood manner. Any food to which a nutrient is added, or that makes a nutritional claim, must conform to the nutrition label requirements.

According to these requirements, the nutrition portion of a label must state: the number of calories in a reasonable serving size of the food, and (in grams) the amounts of protein, carbohydrate and fat in that size serving. The percentages of the USRDA's established for protein and seven vitamins and minerals that the serving provides must also be listed. The label *may* include information of a clinical nature—but no claims may be made special for properties of the food in preventing or treating diseases or disorders. Nor may the label suggest that conventional foods (as usually consumed) are inadequate to meet nutritional needs or that natural sources of vitamins are better or different than vitamins chemically produced (Food and Drug Administration, 1972).

The FDA's efforts, of course, are aimed at giving consumers easily understood, usable nutrition information. Before activating this new labeling program, the FDA surveyed professionals and groups in the food and nutrition "business," as well as 1500 consumers. The nutrition-label program was then designed to try to avoid most of the problems defined by the survey data. The method finally chosen is therefore at least applicable to nutrient density concepts. Nutrient-density is based on fundamental nutritional concepts and terms rather than on some contrived index of food composition which generally sacrifices accuracy for simplicity (Moore and Wendt, 1973). Therefore, although other types of labels might have been simpler to comprehend, they were also judged likely to be of less value as teaching aids and be more prone to obsolescence.

PRESENT LABELING RULES NOT ENTIRELY SUCCESSFUL

Unfortunately, while consumers need the quantitative information provided by the new labeling system, many find it relatively difficult to comprehend. They are unable to readily switch from the traditional way of assessing the quality of foods by categorizing them into food groups (the "basic four" or the "basic seven") to interpreting percentage composition tables based on the nutrients in the foods.

Those who have been able to relate the label information to food quality must also face the problem of adjusting the given nutrient values to the amount of food they actually consume, which is often not the same as the serving size listed on the label.

A WAY TO IMPROVE THE NUTRIENT DENSITY LABEL

The Index of Nutritional Quality (INQ), a method of nutrient analysis, offers the advantages of both nutrient density accuracy and graphical simplicity. The INQ provides a "picture" profile of the quality of a food in terms of its caloric content. Unlike the present labeling system, the quality of the food is not related to an arbitrarily defined serving size. The information required by the new labeling law is incorporated into the INQ approach by superimposing the food quality profile on a percent of nutrients needed (usually an RDA) scale. The resultant profile gives not only the nutrient contribution of a specified serving size to the total daily diet, but (more important) it provides a simple qualitative as well as quantitative indication of the food's quality—independent of serving size. Further, because the bars on the graph are much larger than the print commonly used on food packages and cans, the nutrient information is more noticeable and more easily perceived by those who would ordinarily have to find and don their spectacles to read present labels.

Specifically, the INQ is based on the ratio of nutrient to calorie contents. It is the relationship between the percent of the nutritional standard and the percent of calorie requirement satisfied by a specified quantity of a food. Since the ratio remains constant, the quantity of food is immaterial to any quality evaluation. In other words, the INQ remains the same whether the amount of food is varied to contain 1000 kcal, 2300 kcal, or 2800 kcal, or whether the amount cited is 10 grams or 100 grams.

In this chapter, nutrients are expressed as percentages of the U.S. Recommended Daily Allowance (USRDAs) while the caloric values are percentages of 2800 kcal, the unit selected by the FDA for labeling. It might be argued that a 2000 kcal base, an average adult requirement, would be more realistic since it would not overestimate the energy needs of the majority of the population. In a practical sense, however, no caloric value would be universally valid.

The INQ values for a food may be hand- or, more easily, computer-calculated from food composition data then converted into a bar graph. Since the nutrient density profile is a graphical statement of food quality based on the human need for energy,* foods with nutrient to calorie ratios greater than one (1.0) will have bars on their graphs longer than the energy line. Such foods are good sources of those nutrients. Values smaller than 1.0 (or bars shorter than the energy line) indicate that the nutrients are being supplied by that food in insufficient quantities compared to energy content. For example, a quantity of a food that supplied 20 percent of the daily calorie requirement, 25 percent of the RDA for protein, and 10 percent of the RDA for iron would have an INQ value of .25/.20 or 1.25 for protein and an INQ of .10/.20 or 0.5 for iron. The graph's horizontal scale presents the percent of USRDA supplied by a specific food portion. The average consumer can thus easily see the potential nutrient contribution to his total diet of the food being consid-

---

*Using this line of reasoning, all essential nutrients should be consumed in their recommended amounts by the time one has just met his calorie requirements which ideally maintains his optimum weight without gain or loss.

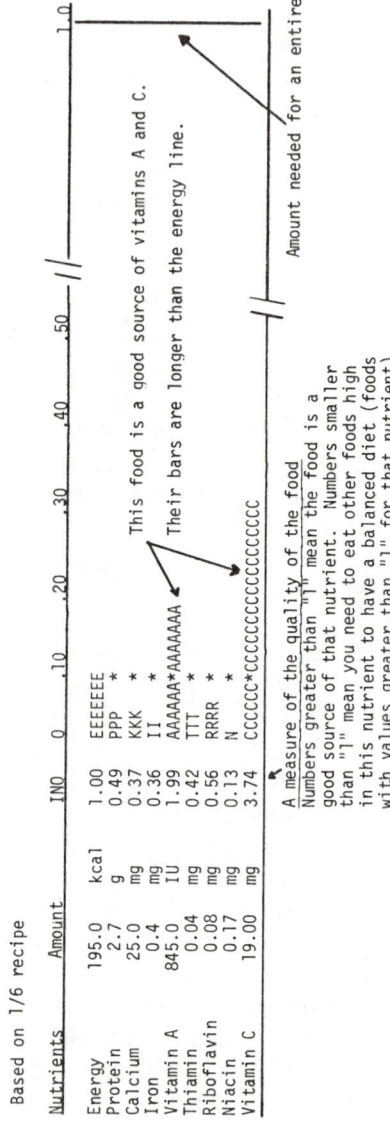

CREAM CHEESE SALAD

Blend the ingredients in the following order or:
Blend together in a blender.

In a large bowl, cream 1 large package (8 oz.) cream cheese
Add #2 can crushed pineapple, undrained
Add ½ cup heavy cream, whipped
Add 1 small can pimentos
Add mixture to
  2 packages (regular size) lemon or lime gelatin set in
  1 cup boiling water
Turn into mold and refrigerate. No salad dressing is required.

Based on 1/6 recipe

Nutrients	Amount		INQ	0	.10	.20	.30	.40	.50		1.0
Energy	195.0	kcal	1.00	EEEEEE							
Protein	2.7	g	0.49	PPP *							
Calcium	25.0	mg	0.37	KKK *							
Iron	0.4	mg	0.36	II *							
Vitamin A	845.0	IU	1.99	AAAAAA*AAAAAAA							
Thiamin	0.04	mg	0.42	TTT *							
Riboflavin	0.08	mg	0.56	RRRR *							
Niacin	0.17	mg	0.13	N *							
Vitamin C	19.00	mg	3.74	CCCCC*CCCCCCCCCCCCCCCC							

This food is a good source of vitamins A and C.

Their bars are longer than the energy line.

Amount needed for an entire day

A measure of the quality of the food
Numbers greater than "1" mean the food is a
good source of that nutrient. Numbers smaller
than "1" mean you need to eat other foods high
in this nutrient to have a balanced diet (foods
with values greater than "1" for that nutrient)

FIG. 7.1. THE NUTRITIONAL VALUE OF RECIPES CAN BE
REPRESENTED BY A NUTRIENT DENSITY PROFILE

The profile could be included in a cookbook to aid in food
complementation as seen in the example of a cream cheese salad. The profile components are pointed out in this illustration.

ered. A computer printout of a cream cheese salad (Fig. 7.1) illustrates a dual presentation of the INQ profile and the percent of RDA scale.

LABEL EXAMPLES

The INQ concept can be applied to food labeling requirements without significant modification of the computer format. Figure 7.2 is a stylized label of a serving of corn that satisfies the FDA regulations. The label format, which simply adds a graph to the usual tabular data, complies with the prescribed information and order of presentation (see Federal Register). The values in Figure 7.2 are based on USRDAs. If a different RDA or energy standard were to be adopted, the INQ profile could easily be recomputed accordingly.

The nutrient profile includes energy to show the percent of the recommended daily caloric intake represented by a serving of the food. The calorie "bår" also defines the base line for the INQ profile. Nutrient bars that are shorter than the calorie bar indicate a need to include other foods in the diet that contain supplementary amounts of these nutrients. In essence, then, with graphed INQ information, the individual can assess his dietary needs based on broadly conceived food complementation rather than in terms of food groups.

Figure 7.3 is a label format for a cereal that is usually consumed with a half-cup of milk. The nutrient contents of the cereal alone and of the cereal and milk combination are illustrated in the multicomponent profile; another feature of the computer program. Nutrients other than those legally required have been included in this label. Any nutrient that has been assayed and for which RDA's may or may not have been established, can be included in the profile, including cholesterol, total fat, and fatty acids. The label in Figure 7.3 also gives the nutrients and amounts that have been added to fortify the cereal product. Unfortunately, fortification with nutrients may tend to generate an overstatement of the quality of a food in INQ profiles and in present labels. Fortification or supplementation of a food with those nutrients required by labeling rules may make certain products appear to be nearly perfect foods when in reality they contain insufficient amounts of other essential nutrients not included on the label. One solution to the problem is to format profiles which show the intrinsic and added nutrients as segments of the bars on the graph.

By using labeling information of this type, the consumer can balance a diet using a variety of well-liked foods that may or may not be representative of the accepted four food groups. Since comprehension of the INQ profile does not require reading skills, labeling information could be used by children and non-English speaking persons. Most people will not regu-

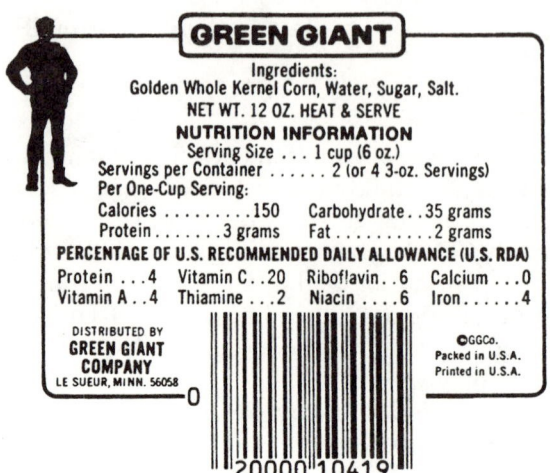

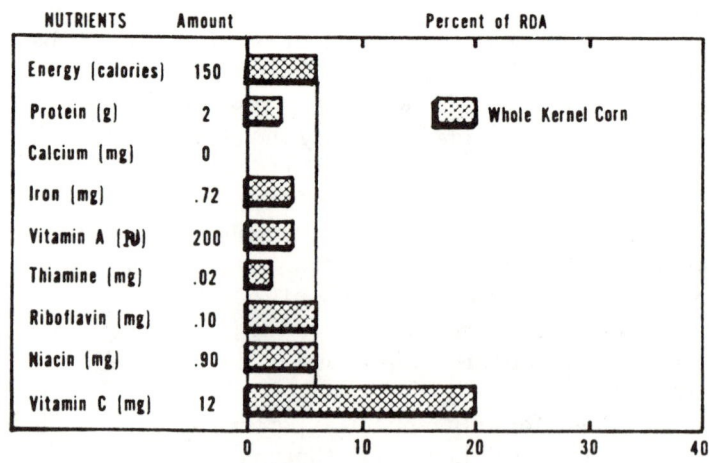

FIG. 7.2.   AN EXISTING AND A NUTRIENT DENSITY PROPOSED
LABEL FOR WHOLE KERNEL CORN

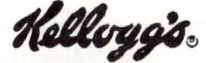

NUTRITION INFORMATION PER SERVING

SERVING SIZE: One ounce (1 cup) Sugar Pops alone and in combination with ½ cup vitamin D fortified whole milk.

SERVINGS PER CONTAINER: 13

	SUGAR POPS	
	1 oz.	with ½ cup whole milk
CALORIES	110	190
PROTEIN	1 gm	6 gm
CARBOHYDRATES	26 gm	32 gm
FAT	0 gm	5 gm

PERCENTAGE OF U.S. RECOMMENDED DAILY ALLOWANCE (U.S. RDA)

	SUGAR POPS	
	1 oz.	with ½ cup whole milk
PROTEIN	2	10
VITAMIN A	25	25
VITAMIN C	25	25
THIAMINE	25	25
RIBOFLAVIN	25	35
NIACIN	25	25
CALCIUM	*	15
IRON	10	10
VITAMIN D	10	25
VITAMIN B₆	25	25
FOLIC ACID	25	25
PHOSPHORUS	*	10
MAGNESIUM	*	4

*Contains less than 2 percent of the U.S. RDA of these nutrients.

Sugar Pops with ½ cup milk

Ingredients: Puffed corn, sugar, corn syrup, molasses, salt, hydrogenated veg. oil and certified colors. BHA and BHT added to preserve freshness. Net wt. 13 oz.

NUTRITION INFORMATION
servings per package: 13
one serving Sugar Pops; 110 kcal ≈ 28.4 grams ≈ 1 oz.
    with 1/2 cup milk; 190 kcal ≈ 150 grams.

	Sugar Pops	with 1/2 cup milk
Carbohydrate	26 g	32 g
Fat	0 g	5 g

Vit. A, Vit. C, Thiamine, riboflavin, niacin, Vit. D, Vit B₆, folic acid and iron added.

NUTRIENTS	Amount	
Energy (kcal)	110/190	
Protein (g)	1/6	
Calcium (mg)	0/120	
Iron (mg)	1.8/1.8	
Vitamin A (Iu)	1250/1250	
Thiamine (mg)	.3/.3	
Riboflavin (mg)	.4/.6	
Niacin (mg)	4/4	
Vitamin C (mg)	15/15	
Vitamin D (Iu)	40/100	
Vitamin B6 (mg)	.5/.5	
Folic Acid (mg)	.1/.1	
Phosphorus (mg)	0/80	
Magnesium (mg)	0/14	

Sugar Pops
1/2 cup Milk

0   10   20   30   40

FIG. 7.3. AN EXISTING AND A NUTRIENT DENSITY PROPOSED LABEL FOR A POPULAR CHILDREN'S BREAKFAST CEREAL

larly sum the nutrient contents of their daily diets to determine whether daily recommended allowances are met. Overall public nutrition would almost certainly improve, however, if the relative nutritional strengths and weaknesses of foods were made so unavoidably obvious that reasonable diet planning required minimal effort.

NEED FOR PUBLIC EDUCATION

As Johnson (1974) pointed out in a recent article, nutritional labeling should be given a fair chance. Present labeling rules and, in our opinion, especially nutrient density labeling, gives food manufacturers the opportunity for the first time to honestly state the nutritional quality of their product to the consumer.

Perhaps it is also time to give the public the chance to learn a new method of helping themselves to better health and nutrition. Certainly the concept of percentages is widely accepted and, with the added impetus of a standardized graphic, any time required to instruct the public on how to best use food label information would be well spent. Though certainly not everyone will capitalize on the availability of the new nutritional labeling, the potential interest seems high. Coupled with an educational effort, the nutritional labeling program should benefit substantial segments of the population.

REFERENCES

FDA. 1973. Nutrition labeling. Federal Register *38* (13):2124-2164.

JOHNSON, O.C. 1974. The Food and Drug Administration and labeling. The Journal of the American Dietetic Association. 64(5):471-475.

MOORE, J.L. and WENDT, P.F. 1973. Nutritional labeling—a summary and evaluation. Journal of Nutrition Education 5(2):121-124.

NATIONAL NUTRITION CONSORTIUM, INC. 1975. Nutritional Labeling how it can work for you. National Nutrition Consortium Inc., Bethesda Md. 134 p.

8

Nutritional Quality of Clinical Diets

The demands of modern society can increase the problems of obtaining a "balanced" diet. Despite new food regulations on fortification, additives, advertising, and labeling, many people are unaware of the nutritional quality of their diets. Assessment of nutritional intake is becoming ever more important because of the trend by the American public to consume more foods of relatively low nutritive value compared with the calories they provide. The average American citizen today, being more sedentary than his predecessor in previous generations, must consume fewer calories to maintain his weight (Anon. 1974); he, therefore, must obtain the nutrients necessary to maintain his health from less food. Thus, wiser food choices must be made by selecting combinations of foods that meet nutritive needs without providing excess calories.

Dietitians often find the demands of their jobs increasing, and regular detailed nutritional analysis of diets is sometimes so time consuming as to be impossible. Theoretical and technical advances have increased the quantitative information in the field of nutrition and though chemical analysis of foods are far from complete, a great deal of food composition data is available. However, the number and complexity of diets that can be evaluated by conventional methods for nutritional adequacy are limited by time and cost. Professionals need a method which can capitalize on available information to enable them to plan diets which provide sufficient quantities of all essential nutrients within energy requirements. Unfortunately, most clinical diets are calculated to meet the requirement of a few nutrients of immediate concern without regard for the total diet.

INDEX OF NUTRITIONAL QUALITY— AN EVALUATIVE TOOL

The Index of Nutritional Quality (INQ) is a readily understood means of nutrient analysis designed to take advantage of data processing techniques and to organize and clarify nutritional information. It can be used for menu and recipe analysis, dietary evaluation, assisting in the regulation of clinical diets, and determining nutritional trends, as well as providing a basis for public nutrition education. This concept provides (a) a quantitative analysis of the diet, using nutrient standards, e.g., percentage of the Recommended Dietary Allowances (RDAs), and also (b) a profile of nutritive quality based on a ratio of nutritive to caloric needs. For special dietary purposes, the INQ facilitates determination of the best food sources of nutrients. The purpose of this chapter is to demonstrate applications of the INQ, with examples illustrating its usefulness for evaluating and improving the nutritional quality of diets.

The standards usually used to calculate the INQ are the U.S. Recommended Daily Allowances (U.S. RDAs) of the Food and Drug Administration (FDA) for nutritional labeling (Anon. 1972); however, other values, such as the Recommended Dietary Allowances (RDAs) of the Food and Nutrition Board (Anon. 1974), may be used to describe more accurately the nutritional needs of an individual or group. When using either the RDAs or U.S. RDAs, the limitations of interpretation of nutritional requirements and the standards which ensue must be understood (Leverton 1975, Hegsted 1972). As a dietary evaluation, a profile of index numbers emerges which may be represented graphically. In graphic form, the INQ profile yields both qualitative and quantitative information. It can then be determined at a glance whether the RDAs or U.S. RDAs are met by observing whether the individual foods eaten additively give an INQ of "1" or greater (bars longer than the energy bar) for each nutrient. An INQ of "1" for a given nutrient in a food indicates that the amount of food just necessary to yield sufficient energy per day to maintain weight will also provide the appropriate allowance for that nutrient. Conversely, values less than "1" (bars shorter than the energy bar) identify nutrients in a food where an excess of calories must be eaten to fulfill the standards for those nutrients if only that food were eaten.

Because of variation in individual energy needs, it would be impossible to calculate INQs for foods for specific individuals; therefore, caloric levels are arbitrarily chosen to illustrate certain points.

A food can be examined as if it were the only source of energy in the diet and/or if consumed in normal quantities. A computer program has been developed which calculates the INQs and prints them in a tabular and graphic format. Figure 8.1 (top), taken from the computer printout, shows tomatoes as a total energy source for a 2,300 kcal requirement. The INQ for energy is "1" by definition (100 percent of the energy need). When considering the percentage of a nutrient standard, it can be redefined as:

Analysis of 11500 Grams Which Supply the Need for Energy (2300 Kcal)

NUTRIENT	UNIT	AMOUNT	INQ	% STD				
					0	1.0	2.0	3.0
ENERGY	kcal	2300.00	1.00	100	EEEEEEEEEEEEEEE*			
PROTEIN	g	115.00	1.77	177	PPPPPPPPPPPPPPPP*PPPPPPPPPPPPP			
CALCIUM	mg	1380.00	1.38	138	KKKKKKKKKKKKKKKK*KKKKKKKKK			
IRON	mg	51.75	2.88	288	IIIIIIIIIIIIIIIIII*IIIIIIIIIIIIIIIIIIIIIIIIIIIIIIIIII 288%			
VITAMIN A	IU	94300.00	18.86	1886	AAAAAAAAAAAAAAAAA*AAAAAAAAAAAAAAAAAAAAAAAAAAAAAAAAA 1886%			
THIAMIN	mg	6.33	4.22	422	TTTTTTTTTTTTTTTTT*TTTTTTTTTTTTTTTTTT 422%			
RIBOFLAVIN	mg	4.03	2.37	237	RRRRRRRRRRRRRRRRR*RRRRRRRRRRRRRRRRRRRRR			
NIACIN	mg	74.75	3.74	374	NNNNNNNNNNNNNNNNN*NNNNNNNNNNNNNNNNNNNN 374%			
VITAMIN C	mg	2415.00	40.25	4025	CCCCCCCCCCCCCCCCC*CCCCCCCCCCCCCCCCCCCCCCCCCCCCC 4025%			

Analysis of 1 Med. (3.5 oz) (100 Grams) Which Supplies 20 Kcal of Energy

NUTRIENT	UNIT	AMOUNT	INQ	% STD									
					0	10	20	30	40	50	60	70	80
ENERGY	kcal	20.00	1.00	1	E*								
PROTEIN	g	1.00	1.77	2	P*								
CALCIUM	mg	12.00	1.38	1	K*								
IRON	mg	0.45	2.88	3	I*								
VITAMIN A	IU	820.00	18.86	16	A*AAAAAAAAAA								
THIAMIN	mg	0.06	4.22	4	T*T								
RIBOFLAVIN	mg	0.04	2.37	2	M*								
NIACIN	mg	0.65	3.74	3	N*N								
VITAMIN C	mg	21.00	40.25	35	C*CCCCCCCCCCCCCCCCCCCCCCCCCCCCCCCCC								

FIG. 8.1. RAW, RIPE TOMATO

TOP: as a total source of food energy. BOTTOM: contribution of a 100-gm. serving to the total daily nutrient requirements.

$$INQ = \frac{\text{per cent of a standard or requirement of nutrient}}{\text{per cent of standard of energy}}$$

Using this as a basis of computation, when the energy requirement is met with a food, such as tomatoes, they would provide 177 per cent of the daily need for protein as recommended by the U.S. RDAs and have an INQ of 1.77 (177/100). The 177 per cent was calculated by dividing 115 gm. protein provided by the quantity of tomatoes supplying 2,300 kcal by 65 gm., the U.S. RDA for protein of low biologic value. The INQ does not reflect protein quality. The tomato is a high nutrient density food, each nutrient bar being far in excess of that for energy, indicating that each INQ is greater than "1". However, tomatoes are not a good choice as a single food to sustain life; an average adult would need to consume 11.5 kg. of the fruit daily to meet energy requirements.

In this case, a more useful calculation is one in which nutrients are described in terms of a portion size likely to be used in an average diet. Figure 8.1 (bottom) illustrates the contribution of a tomato of medium size weighing 100 gm. to the daily nutritive requirements. Since the proportion of nutritive content to energy content of a food remains constant, the INQ and, therefore, the relative profile of a food (relative lengths of the bars) remains the same, independent of serving size. The serving size graph (Figure 8.1, bottom) is, then, the INQ profile superimposed on a percentage of U.S. RDA scale. From the profile, it is seen that the energy supplied by a tomato is approximately 1 per cent of the daily need and that about 3 per cent of the U.S. RDA for iron is provided in a serving.

Many dietitians will recognize that Figure 8.1 (bottom) is similar in appearance to the share system popularized by Rose (See Taylor 1942). Representing the nutrient content of a food by a bar graph of the percentage of the daily requirements satisfied by a given portion is not a new concept. The most important aspect of Figure 8.1 (bottom) is the inclusion of the nutrient: calorie ratio (INQ) from which one may judge the true nutritional quality of the food.

For clinical and research purposes, the graphs can be programmed to include any number of nutrients, if adequate compositional data is available, such as vitamin B_6, pantothenic acid, and folacin. The eight presented in Figure 8.1 are only illustrative. They include a representative group of the best known and understood nutrients, which, if consumed in adequate amounts from a variety of traditional foods, are assumed also to meet the requirement for the other essential nutrients. However, this assumption may not be valid for fortified foods or food analogs. Fortification and supplementation programs can readily be evaluated by consideration of INQ.

SOME SELECTED APPLICATIONS OF THE INQ

Nutrient Analysis of Cycle Menus.—The INQ may be used in analyzing both meals and a diet, as well as evaluating individual foods. A composite of a meal, or a daily average of a diet, is calculated by adding the nutrient values of each food in the meal and printing the result in the standard profile form. A dietary evaluation is calculated in the same way and then divided by the number of days in the diet to yield a profile representative of a daily average of nutrient composition. Figure 8.2 is a seven-day institutional diet currently being served in the Intermountain area. Relative to the amount of energy, the figure shows that this diet supplies protein, calcium, vitamin A, riboflavin and ascorbic acid in adequate amounts by the U.S. RDA standard. If a maximum of 38 per cent of the 2,300 kcal is used for the fat standard (Leverton 1974), the diet meets this requirement. Assuming a constant proportion of nutrients to calories from foods in the diet, carbohydrate, sodium, and niacin reach the standards only because an excess of calories (136 per cent) is offered. The carbohydrate standard of 288 gm. (50 per cent of the 2,300 kcal energy standard) was determined by adding the energy values for the fat (Leverton 1974) and the protein specified by the U.S. RDA (Anon. 1972) and subtracting that sum from 2,300 kcal energy. The value of 4 gm. for sodium represents an average daily intake (Robinson 1972). For actual clinical analysis, the standards can be established to represent any dietary prescription. Generally, the pertinent standard is printed at the beginning of each analysis. Iron (84 per cent), thiamin (91 per cent), and fiber are low, even with the high energy content of the diet. A standard of 7 gm. fiber was arbitrarily set for this diet (Cowgill and Anderson 1932), assuming that 70 kg. represents an average adult weight. The authors have, of course, arbitrarily selected those standards for which RDAs (Anon. 1974) or U.S. RDAs (Anon. 1972) do not exist, and they do not necessarily represent a maximum or ideal intake; they are mainly presented for illustrative purposes.

The expanded number of nutrients included in this graph provide additional information for dietitians and physicians who must evaluate the nutritive intake of patients on modified-fat, -carbohydrate, or-electrolyte diets. The B, L and D components of the bars on the graph indicate the average contribution of each meal [B = breakfast, L = lunch (noon meal), D = dinner (evening meal)]. When the nutritive content of a profile exceeds the limits of the graph, the percentage of the standard is printed at the end of the bar, and the percentage contribution of each meal is shown on the next line. The sum of B, L, and D equals the total percentage of the standard. A profile for each day of the diet can be printed out by computer, as well as the week's composite shown here. As expected, daily evaluations usually show greater nutrient fluctuations

Calculations Based on The U.S.RDA 2300 Kcal, 38% Fat, 50% Carbo., 12% Protein:

Energy 2300.00 kcal   Protein 65.00 g   Fat 97.00 g   Carbo Tot 288.00 g   Fiber 7.00 g
Calcium 1000.00 mg   Iron 18.00 mg   Sodium 4000.00 mg   Potassium 4000.00 mg   Vitamin A 5000.00 IU
Thiamin 1.50 mg   Riboflavin 1.70 mg   Niacin 20.00 mg   Vitamin C 60.00 mg

NUTRIENT	UNIT	AMOUNT	INQ	%STD	0 50 100 150
ENERGY	kcal	3127.49	1.00	138	BBBBBBBBBBBBBBLLLLLLLLLLLLLLLLLLLLLLLLLLLLLLLDDDDDDD*DDDDDDDDDDDDDD/
PROTEIN	g	132.75	1.50	204	BBBBBBBBBBBBBBBBBBBLLLLLLLLLLLLLLLLLLLLLLLLLLLLLLLLL*LLDDDDDDDDDDDDDD/DDD 204%
					B* 40% L* 66% D* 98%
FAT	g	142.75	1.08	147	BBBBBBBBBBBBBBBLLLLLLLLLLLLLLLLLLLLLLLLLLLLLLDDDDDD*DDDDDDDDDDDDDD/DDD
CARBOHY	g	334.88	0.86	116	BBBBBBBBBBBBBBBBBBLLLLLLLLLLLLLLLLLLLLLLLLDDDDDDDDD*DDDDDD /
FIBER	g	4.05	0.43	58	BBBBLLLLLLLLDDDDDDDDD * /
CALCIUM	mg	1670.56	1.23	167	BBBBBBBBBBBBBBBBBBBLLLLLLLLLLLLLLLLLLLLLLLLLLLLLLLD*DDDDDDDDDDDDDD/DDD 167%
IRON	mg	15.05	0.61	84	BBBBBBBBLLLLLLLLLLLLLDDDDDDDD * /
SODIUM	mg	4568.92	0.84	114	BBBBBBBBBBBBLLLLLLLLLLLLLLLLLLLLLLLDDDDDDDDDDDD*DDDDD
POTASSIUM	mg	3957.09	0.73	99	BBBBBBBBBBLLLLLLLLLLLLLLLLLLLLLLDDDDDDDDDDD* /
VITAMIN A	IU	7717.21	1.14	154	BBBBBBBBBBBBBBLLLLLLLLLLLLLLLLLLLLLLLLLLLLLLDDDDDD* /
THIAMIN	mg	1.37	0.67	91	BBBBBBBBBLLLLLLLLLLLLLLDDDDDDDDD * /
RIBOFLAVIN	mg	2.98	1.29	175	BBBBBBBBBBBBBBBBBBLLLLLLLLLLLLLLLLLLLLLLLLLLLLLLLLLL*DDDDDDDDDDDDDDDD/DDD 175%
NIACIN	mg	22.20	0.82	111	BBBBBBBBBBBLLLLLLLLLLLLLLLLLLLLLLLDDDDDDDDDDDDDD*DDDD /
VITAMIN C	mg	96.38	1.18	161	BBBBBBBBBBBBBBBBLLLLLLLLLLLLLLLLLLLLLLLLLLLLLLLLLLDDDD*DDDDDDDDDDDDDDDD/DDD 161%

FIG. 8.2.   ASSESSMENT OF THE NUTRITIONAL QUALITY OF A SEVEN-DAY INSTITUTIONAL DIET COMPUTERIZED FOR AN ADULT BASED ON THE U.S. RDA AND AN ENERGY REQUIREMENT OF 2,300 kcal.

than the weekly average, emphasizing that analysis of long-term dietary intake is necessary for many types of nutritional assessments. In light of recent criticisms of institutional diets (Butterworth 1974, Enloe 1974), evaluations of this type would be helpful to administrative and clinical dietitians in determining the nutritional adequacy of menus they provide to their clients.

Clinical Application.—In addition to indicating the quality of the diet, the INQ can aid in evaluating or planning clinical menus to fit a patient's special nutritional requirements. In some cases, by prescription, nutrients are limited; in others, they are increased. Traditionally, dietitians have been concerned with planning diets which provide proper amounts of some of the nutrients of clinical significance, i.e., protein, sodium, potassium, carbohydrate, fat, cholesterol, or iron. The INQ can provide profiles which limit the nutrients under consideration and evaluate the nutritional quality of the diet with reference to other key nutrients.

Diabetes.—Diabetes mellitus is an example of a metabolic disease which requires special dietary care. Factors to be considered are age, sex, body weight, and activity. Calculation of such diets is often based on equivalents, in which foods have been grouped according to similar nutrient content, i.e., the Food Exchange lists (Caso 1950). This allows an individual to make choices according to personal preference, cost, and availability. A physician or clinical dietitian prescribes the diet and determines the number of daily Exchanges for each food group.

The Exchange lists have been evaluated for nutrient adequacy applying the INQ method. Figure 8.3 is based on a dietary prescription for 1,550 kcal, 150 gm. carbohydrate, 80 gm. protein and 70 gm. fat and for the following number of Exchanges for individual food groups: fruit—3; B vegetable—1; milk—2; bread—6; meat—7; and fat—3. The individual Exchange lists have been adjusted, so that each food could be chosen at least once.

The number of foods in each group made an eight-day diet convenient to calculate. For instance, there are twenty-four choices in the bread Exchange list, and six choices a day are intended from this group. Thus, there are enough foods to make a different choice for each Exchange item for four days. Doubling each serving of the foods in the bread Exchange list adjusts this group for an eight-day diet. Foods in each of the other Exchange lists were treated in the same way. The profile is the result of this compilation. Each nutrient examined, except iron (INQ—0.84), is adequately supplied, but when protein, fat, and carbohydrate values assigned to the different Exchange lists are used to calculate the content of these nutrients in the total diet, the index values are lower than if the

Calculations Based on the Requirements for a Diabetic Female 35 Years of Age (For Slow Weight Loss)

Energy 1550.00 kcal   Protein 80.00 g   Fat 70.00 g   Carbo-Tot 150.00 g   Fiber 5.00 g
Calcium 800.00 mg   Iron 18.00 mg   Vitamin A 4000.00 IU   Thiamin 1.00 mg   Riboflavin 1.20 mg
Niacin 13.00 mg   Vitamin C 45.00 mg

NUTRIENT	UNIT	AMOUNT	INQ	% STD	0 50 100 150
ENERGY	kcal	1893.61	1.00	122	DDDDDDDVVVFFFBBBBBBBBBBBBBBBMMMMMMM*MMMMOOOO/
PROTEIN	g	103.59	1.06	129	DDDDDDDDDVVVVVVFBBBBBBBBMMMMMMMMMMMM*MMMMMMM/MMMO
FAT	g	85.44	1.00	122	DDDDDDDDVBBBBBMMMMMMMMMMMMMMMMMM*00000000/0
CARBOHYDRATE	g	189.18	1.03	126	DDDDDVVVVVVFFFFFFBBBBBBBBBBBBB*BBBBBBBM/0
FIBER	g	10.51	1.72	210	VVVVVVVVVVVVVVVVVVVVVVVVVVVVV*VVVVVFF/FFFFFFFFFF D* 0% V*115% F* 32% B* 51% M* 6% 0* 7%
CALCIUM	mg	1442.47	1.48	180	DDDDDDDDDDDDDDDDDDDDDDDDDDVVVVVVVV*VVVVVVV/FFFBBBBBM 180%
IRON	mg	18.55	0.84	103	VVVVVVVVVVVVVFFFBBBBBBBBMMMMMMMMMM*0 /
VITAMIN A	IU	26136.16	5.35	653	DDDDDVVVVVVVVVVVVVVVVVVVFFFBBBBBBBBBB*VVVVVVV/VVVVVVVVV 653% D* 14% V* 406% F* 50% B* 39% M* 138% 0* 7%
THIAMIN	mg	1.46	1.20	146	DDDDDVVVVVVVVVVVVVVVVFFFFFBBBBBBBBBBB*BBBMMMM/MMMMMMMO
RIBOFLAVIN	mg	3.13	2.13	261	DDDDDDDDDDDDDDDDDDDDDDDDVVVVVVVVVVVV*VVVVVVV/VFFFBBBBBB 261% D* 71% V* 55% F* 9% B* 27% M* 95% 0* 4%
NIACIN	mg	22.55	1.42	173	DVVVVVVVVVVVVVVVVVVVFFFBBBBBBMMMMMMMMM*MMMMMMMMMM/MMMMMMMMM 173%
VITAMIN C	mg	245.13	4.46	545	DDDDVVVVVVVVVVVVVVVVVVVVVVVVV*VVVVVVV/VVVVVVVV 545% D* 9% V* 363% F* 114% B* 44% M* 12% 0* 2%

FIG. 8.3. NUTRITIVE PROFILE OF THE DIABETIC EXCHANGE LISTS

The letter component of the bars represents the contribution
of each food category of the Exchange list as follows: D = milk;
V = vegetable; F = fruit; B = bread; M = meat; O = fat.

analysis were based on data in Agriculture Handbook No. 8 (Watt and Merrill 1963).

If one considers that all of the foods in the Exchange lists could be used with equal probability (Caso defends the calculations for the food groupings on the basis that all foods would not be used equally as we have assumed in our analysis), then an additional 22 per cent of the energy (344 kcal), 29 per cent of protein (24 gm.), 22 per cent of fat (15 gm.), and 26 per cent of carbohydrate (39 gm.) are consumed. The INQs in this profile indicate that, if only 1,550 kcal are consumed, protein, fat, and carbohydrate in the diet would be near the prescribed optimum. On the assumption that 1,900 kcal are required to maintain weight, the prescription for this diet should result in a weight loss, but in actuality, the diet would maintain weight.

The profile in Figure 8.4 evaluates a dietary intake for a patient using the menus shown in Table 8.1. The Exchange lists were used to plan the menus in accordance with the prescription (Table 8.2). With the Exchange lists and the amounts of protein, fat and carbohydrate assigned to each list, the index values, as expected, are lower than if the composition of the food were taken from a table. Thus, carbohydrate actually exceeded the prescription by 16 per cent, protein by 13 per cent, and fat by 32 per cent. For other nutrients, the diet is low in calcium (INQ= 0.55), iron (INQ= 0.72), thiamin (INQ= 0.77), riboflavin (INQ= 0.78), and niacin (INQ= 0.91). If consumed, the diet would be adequate in niacin (108 per cent of U.S. RDA) only because of the additional energy provided (119 per cent of 1,750 kcal). Values below the standard for niacin are not cause for concern when tryptophan in the dietary protein exceeds the amino acid requirement.

Other conditions requiring modified diets. Diet Analysis.—If composite profiles of various popular reducing diets were available, interested persons could evaluate each total diet in terms of its nutrient-energy relationships and judge its intrinsic merit for themselves. For example, Figure 8.6 is the profile of a locally popular grapefruit and egg diet. This diet has some obvious serious nutritional inadequacies. One would most certainly lose weight with an energy intake drastically curtailed to 44% of the standard, and the diet's fruit and vegetables provide large quantities of vitamins A and C. However, lack of dairy products and whole grains and cereals means low intake levels of calcium and the B vitamins, especially thiamin. Iron levels are low as well, making this particular weight-loss diet a poor choice in terms of maintaining adequate amounts of nutrients as well as its inadvisably low energy value.

The composition of the fatty acids provided by the food shown in Tables 8.1 and 8.2 is also given in Figure 8.4. Using an arbitrary standard of 30 per cent of the fat being provided by both saturated and polyun-

Energy 1750.00 kcal   Protein 75.00 g   Fat 80.00 g   Carbo-Tot 185.00 g   Fiber 7.00 g
Calcium 1000.00 mg   Iron 18.00 mg   Vitamin A 5000.00 IU   Thiamin 1.50 mg   Riboflavin 1.70 mg
Niacin 20.00 mg   Vitamin C 60.00 mg   Sat Fat A 24.00 g   Uns Oleic 32.00 g   Uns Linol 24.00 g
Cholest 600.00 mg

NUTRIENT	UNIT	AMOUNT	INQ	% STD	0	50	100	150
ENERGY	kcal	2083.42	1.00	119	BBBBBBBBBBBLLLLLLLLLLLDDDDDDDDDDDDDDS*SSSSSSSS/			
PROTEIN	g	85.04	0.95	113	BBBBBBBBBBBLLLLLLLLLLLLLLDDDDDDDDDDDDDDDSS*SSSS /			
FAT	g	105.26	1.11	132	BBBBBBBBBBBLLLLLLLLLLLLLLLLLLLLDDDDDDDDDD*SSSSSSSS/SSSS			
CARBO-TOT	g	214.51	0.97	116	BBBBBBBBBBBLLLLLLLLLLLLLLLLLLLLLDDDDDDDDDDDDS*SSSS			
FIBER	g	11.92	1.43	170	BBBBBBBBBBBLLLLLLLLLLLLLLLLLLLLLLLLLL*LLLLLLLL/LDDDDDDD 170%			
CALCIUM	mg	658.25	0.55	66	BBBBBBBBBBBLLLLLLLDDDDSSSSS * /			
IRON	mg	15.46	0.72	86	BBBBBBBBBBBLLLLLLLLLLDDDDDDDDDSS * /			
VITAMIN A	IU	20381.90	3.42	408	BBBBBBBBBBBLLLLLLLLLDDDDDDDDDDDDDDDDD*DDDDDDD/DDDDDDDD 408% B* 30% L* 20% D* 351% S* 7%			
THIAMIN	mg	1.37	0.77	91	BBBBBBBBBBBLLLLLLLLLLLLLLLDDDDDDDDDSSS * /			
RIBOFLAVIN	mg	1.58	0.78	93	BBBBBBBBBBBLLLLLLLLLLLLLLLDDDDDDDSSSSS * /			
NIACIN	mg	21.55	0.91	108	BBBBBBBBBBBLLLLLLLLLLLLLLDDDDDDDDDSSSS*SSSS /			
VITAMIN C	mg	184.28	2.58	307	BBBBBBBBBBBLLLLLLLLLLLLLLLLLLLLLLLLLLL*LLLLLLLL/LLLLLLLLL 307% B* 102% L* 64% D* 137% S* 5%			
SAT FAT A	g	41.60	1.46	173	BBBBBBBBBBBLLLLLLLLLLLLLLLLLLLLLLLLLL*DDDDDDD/DDDDDDDSSS 173%			
UNS OLEIC	g	41.40	1.09	129	BBBBBBBBBBBLLLLLLLLLLLLLLLLLLLLDDDDDDDDSS*SSSSSSS/SS			
UNS LINOL	g	10.60	0.37	44	BLLLLLLLDSSSSSSS * /			
CHOLEST	mg	538.45	0.75	90	BBBBBBBBBBBLLLLLLLLDDDDDDSS * /			

FIG. 8.4.   ANALYSIS OF THE PRESCRIPTION FOR THE DIET IN TABLE 8.2

TABLE 8.1. ONE DAY'S SAMPLE MENUS TO
MEET DIETARY PRESCRIPTION IN TABLE 8.2.

food	serving size	
	measure	grams
Breakfast		
banana	1 small	100
egg, poached	1	50
whole wheat toast	1 slice	25
wheat flakes	¾ c.	20
milk	½ c.	120
butter	2 tsp.	10
coffee (no sugar)	—	—
Noon meal		
luncheon meat	2 slices	60
rye bread	2 slices	50
butter	2 tsp.	10
lettuce salad	¼ head	113
French dressing	1 Tbsp.	13
fresh blackberries	1 c.	150
Evening meal		
chopped round steak	3 oz.	90
potatoes, mashed	½ c.	100
carrots	½ c.	100
roll	1(2-in. diameter)	30
butter	1 tsp.	5
cantaloupe	½ of 6-in.	400
Evening snack		
milk	½ c.	120
saltines	5	20
peanut butter	2 Tbsp.	30
butter	1 tsp.	5
apple	1 small	80

TABLE 8.2. DIETARY PRESCRIPTION AND MEAL
PATTERN FOR A PATIENT WITH DIABETES

PRESCRIPTION: 1,750 kcal (185 gm. carbohydrate, 75 gm. protein, 80 gm. fat)

MEAL PATTERN

Exchange List	number of Exchanges
milk	1
vegetable, group B	1
fruit	6
bread	7
meat	7
fat	7

Calculations Based on The RDA for a Female Over 50 Years of Age:

```
Energy 1800.00 kcal   Protein 46.00 g    Fat 75.00 g       Carbo-Tot 235.00 g    Fiber 7.00 g
Ash 25.00 g           Calcium 800.00 mg  Phosphorus 800.00 mg  Iron 10.00 mg     Sodium 4000.00 mg
Potassium 4000.00 mg  Vitamin A 4000.00 IU  Thiamin 1.00 mg   Riboflavin 1.10 mg  Niacin 12.00 mg
Vitamin C 45.00 mg    Sat Fat A 22.50 g  Uns Oleic 30.00 g  Uns Linol 22.50 g    Cholest 600.00 mg
```

Composite Nutrient Profile - For Total Week of July 19-25 1974

```
NUTRIENT    UNIT  AMOUNT    INQ   %STD  0                       50                      100                     150

ENERGY      kcal  1262.16   1.00   70   BBBBBBLLLLLLLLDDDDDDDDDDDD/
PROTEIN     g       48.26   1.50  150   BBBBBBBBBBLLLLLLLLLLLLLLLDDDDDDD/DDDDDDDDDD*DD
FAT         g       69.97   1.33   93   BBBBBBBBBBBBBLLLLLLLLLLLLLDDDDDD/DDDDDDDD *
CARBO-TOT   g      109.04   0.66   46   BBBLLLLLDDDDDDDDDD *
FIBER       g        0.88   0.18   13   LDDDD /
ASH         g        8.08   0.46   32   BBLLLLDDDDDD /
CALCIUM     mg     462.39   0.82   58   BBBBBBBBBBBLLLLLLLDDDDDDV /
PHOSPHORUS  mg     687.94   1.23   86   BBBBBBBBBLLLLLDDDDDDDDDDDD/DDDD *
IRON        mg       5.70   0.81   57   BBLLLLLLLDDDDDDDDDDDDD /
SODIUM      mg    1526.73   0.54   38   BBLLLLLDDDDDDDDD *
POTASSIUM   mg    1384.93   0.49   35   BBBLLLDDDDDDD /
VITAMIN A   IU   12786.27   4.56  320   BBBBLLLLLLLLDDDDDDDDDDDDDDV/VVVVVVVVV*VVVVVVVVVVVVVVVVV 320%
                                        B*11% L*25%  D*33%  V*250%
THIAMIN     mg       5.48   7.82  548   BBLLLLLDDDDDDDDDDDVVVVVVVVV/VVVVVVV*VVVVVVVVVVVVVVVVV 548%
                                        B*6%  L*16%  D*26%  V*500%
RIBOFLAVIN  mg       5.99   7.77  545   BBBBBBBBBBBLLLLLLLLLLDDDDDD/DDDDDDDVV*VVVVVVVVVVVVVVVVV 545%
                                        B*30% L*23%  D*37%  V*455%
NIACIN      mg      50.79   6.04  423   BBBLLLLLLLLLLLDDDDDDDDDDDD/DDDDDDDVW*VVVVVVVVVVVVVVVVV 423%
                                        B*7%  L*33%  D*50%  V*333%
VITAMIN C   mg     123.78   3.92  275   BBLLLDDDDDDDDDDDDDDVVVVVVV/VVVVVVV*VVVVVVVVVVVVVVVV 275%
                                        B*5%  L*8%   D*40%  V*222%
SAT FAT A   g       27.15   1.72  121   BBBBBBBBBBBBBBBBBBBLLLLLLLLLLLL/LDDDDDDDD*DDDDDDD
UNS OLEIC   g       28.90   1.37   96   BBBBBBBBBBBBLLLLLLLLLLDDDDD/DDDDDDDD *
UNS LINOL   g        8.45   0.54   38   BBLLLLLLDDDDD /
CHOLEST     mg     191.80   0.46   32   BBBLLLDDDDDD *
```

FIG. 8.5. AN EXPANDED NUTRIENT PROFILE OF A SEVEN DAY DIETARY INTAKE FOR A WOMAN, BASED ON THE RECOMMENDED DIETARY ALLOWANCES

COMPOSITE PROFILE OF 2 WEEK WEIGHT REDUCTION DIET

Nutrient	INQ	% Std	Percent of Standard
Energy	1.00	44	
Protein	2.24	99	
Calcium	0.86	38	
Iron	1.62	72	
Vitamin A	7.35	326	
Thiamin	1.02	45	
Riboflavin	1.97	88	
Niacin	1.70	76	
Vitamin C	9.72	431	

0   50   100   150   200

FIG. 8.6. NUTRIENT PROFILE OF A WEIGHT REDUCTION DIET

The diet is consumed in various forms but essentially includes: Breakfast—one-half grapefruit, 1 or 2 eggs, and coffee; Lunch—salad (either fruit or vegetable), one egg, meat (3–4 oz of meat, fish, or poultry once during the week), and one-half grapefruit; Dinner—vegetable, meat (3–4 oz of meat, fish, or poultry), an egg on alternate days (bread on the other), one-half grapefruit, and coffee. The analysis presented is the average for 1 day calculated from food consumed for an entire week.

saturated fatty acids, the diet has an actual P:S ratio of 0.26. This information is sometimes useful in planning fat-modified diets.

When making a diagnosis and recommending treatment, it is often important for a physician to know the composition of the diet his patient has been consuming. However, unless the facilities of a large hospital and the service of a clinical dietitian are available, dietary evaluations are seldom made, and even those are sketchy, involving only a few nutrients.

A comprehensive dietary profile, such as shown in Figure 8.5, could be most helpful. Recommendations of a woman patient in her sixties with severe gastrointestinal problems resulting from radiotherapy and surgery for cancer are based on the RDAs. Thirty-eight per cent total calories from fat (40 per cent of fat calories from mono-unsaturated fatty acid and 30 per cent each from saturated and polyunsaturated fatty acids), 50 per cent carbohydrate, and 12 per cent protein were intended. From the recorded seven-day food intake, the computer was supplied with the corresponding food codes and amounts in grams, calories, or ounces, and with an identification of the meal at which the food was consumed. Figure 8.5 was the resulting analysis. It is apparent that foods high in roughage were avoided by this individual as shown by the low crude fiber INQ.

Anorexia reduced the energy content of the diet to 70 per cent of the RDA. By increasing portions to meet energy requirements, fat (INQ= 1.33) and phosphorus (INQ= 1.23) needs would then be met. Modification of the diet would be necessary to increase intakes of calcium, potassium, and iron, the latter being an important consideration since the patient is anemic. Evaluation of other nutrients, such as vitamins B_6 and B_{12} and copper, could be useful in patients with anemia of unknown etiology, but such food composition data are not available.

Sodium is below the average intake of 4 gm., but salt added to the food at the table has not been included in the calculations.

Vitamin A, thiamin, riboflavin, niacin, and ascorbic acid are supplied in excess of normal dietary needs. This imbalance occurs because a supplement was taken in the form of two multiple vitamin tablets a day. Note that this particular supplement contains no iron. The contribution to the diet of the supplement is shown by the "V" portion of the nutrient bars. Without supplementation, the diet supplies inadequate quantities of vitamin A (69 per cent), thiamin (48 per cent), riboflavin (90 per cent), and ascorbic acid (53 per cent).

Another consideration in the American diet is the source of fat. Standards for the above diet have been arbitrarily adjusted to reflect a 30 per cent allowance of the total dietary fat for both saturated and unsaturated fatty acids, or a P:S ratio of 1. The patient preferred butter to margarine and oils, even in cooking, which lowers the P:S ratio to 0.313 (8.5 gm. unsaturated fat, 27.1 gm. saturated fat). Mono-unsaturated fatty acids fall a little short of the standard of 40 per cent (30 gm.) of total fat. For this diet, cholesterol is well within the arbitrary 600-mg. standard.

After nutritional inadequacies in a diet have been identified, the dietitian must suggest foods to supply the deficient nutrients without excessive calories. Individual food profiles based on INQ are useful when made available to patients to aid them in selecting foods to ensure an adequate nutritive intake. Supplementary lists for eight common nutrients, given in Part II of this book, are also available to aid the patient to balance his diet. These lists are based on INQ numbers greater than "1.5," i.e., each portion provides at least one and a half times the requirement for that nutrient in comparison with the established energy standard of 2000 kcal. Food lists developed in this manner differ in that the foods included are not only good sources of individual nutrients, but they do not supply excessive calories per serving.

CONCLUSION AND SUMMARY

The INQ (Index of Nutritional Quality) has the potential for educational and clinical application in many areas of nutrition and food science. For foods, the INQ quantitatively evaluates nutrient composition in relation to energy. The concept has been computerized, and each parameter can be expanded or modified to fit a variety of purposes.

The INQ ratio printed by the computer in graphic form showing the composition of food compared with recommended standards for consumption. The standard format provides a rapid means of showing food composition while retaining specific quantitative information required for professional use. Individual foods and diets may be compared by determining their INQ values.

A graph with eight nutrients plus energy provides a workable means for general dietary purposes. This profile may be expanded to include other nutrients, depending on the purposes intended. Nutritional data are stored in the computer and readily retrieved, or specific data for a given study can be read from cards and then stored for subsequent use. Moreover, data banks can be easily updated as new information becomes available.

Data processing techniques can provide a rapid, accurate assessment of nutritional quality. Dietary analysis, which was prohibitive by hand calculation, is now possible.

REFERENCES

ANON. 1972. Federal Register 37: 6493 (No. 62), March 30, 1972.

ANON. 1974. National Academy of Science: Recommended Dietary Allowances. Eighth Revised Edition. Washington, D.C.

BUTTERWORTH, C.E., Jr. 1974. The skeleton in the hospital closet. Nutr. Today 9: 4 (Mar.-Apr.).

CASO, E.K. 1950. Calculation of diabetic diets. J. Am. Dietet. A. 26: 575.

COWGILL, G.R. and ANDERSON, W.E. 1932. Laxative effects of wheat bran and "washed bran" in healthy men. J. A.M.A. 98: 1866.

ENLOE, C.F., Jr. 1974. The view from the catbird's seat. Pts. 1 and 2. Food Nutr. News (Natl. Live Stock & Meat Bd.) 45: Mar.-Apr., May-June.

HANSEN, R.G. 1973. An index of food quality. Nutr. Rev. 31:1.

HEGSTED, D.M. 1972. Problems in the use and interpretation of the Recommended Dietary Allowances. Ecol. Food Nutr. 1:255.

LEVERTON, R.M. 1974. Fats in food and diet. USDA Agric. Info. Bull. No. 361.

LEVERTON, R.M. 1975. The RDAs are not for amateurs. J. Am. Dietet. A. 66:9.

ROBINSON, C.H. 1972. Normal and Therapeutic Nutrition, 14th Ed. Macmillan Book Co., N.Y.

TAYLOR, C.M. 1942. Food values in Shares and Weights in Common Servings. Macmillan Book Co., N.Y.

WATT, B.K. and MERRILL, A.L. 1963. Composition of Foods—Raw, Processed, Prepared. Rev. USDA Agric. Handbook No. 8.

9

Food Instead of Drugs

INTRODUCTION: EXAMPLE OF SPECIFIC APPLICATION

Besides general diet modification, nutrient density can be used to generalize specific clinical data for nutrition related diseases. For example, heart disease and hypertension have long been major health problems with nutritional ramification.

Potassium is one of the so-called electrolytes that are crucial to human health. Unfortunately, a wide variety of drugs and diseases can cause diverse electrolyte imbalances. In recent years, potassium loss has become a particularly common medical problem because of the increased use of diuretics.

Diuretics, which enhance the urinary excretion of sodium and water, are used to reduce the volume of extracellular fluid and to prevent or combat edema (excess retention of body water). They achieve that goal by accelerating urine formation or, more commonly, by depressing renal (kidney) reabsorption of water and sodium. Diuretics are often prescribed for patients with hypertension (high blood pressure), congestive heart failure, or hepatic (liver) abnormalities. Since each diuretic has its own mode of action and potential side effects, even a careful matching with the patient's particular situation cannot preclude the chance of problems.

The commonly used thiazide (diurel and hydroxydiurel) diuretics are called "potassium wasting." Other diuretics have little effect on potassium, while some actually conserve potassium at the expense of sodium. The more potent diuretics, however, tend to produce significant potassium loss.

Physicians currently deal with potassium deficiencies by combining potassium-sparing diuretics with supplemental potassium salts. Unfortunately, both of these classes of drugs incorporate certain disadvantages. For example, the potassium-sparing diuretics can produce elevated blood urea nitrogen, dizziness, vomiting, diarrhea, flaccid weakness, etc.

Potassium salts (especially the popular potassium chloride) can have side effects that generally include irritation of the upper small intestines. In addition, the supplements are not always well absorbed and can generate a false sense of security in patients who rely on them.

POTASSIUM FROM FOODS

As an alternative to the drug therapy side-effects merry-go-round, we propose a qualitative diet therapy. In other words, a proper choice of foods can effectively offset potassium depletion problems.

In general, of course, the diets of some individuals may not provide adequate potassium even before they encounter illnesses or drug therapy regimes. For example, some fully ambulatory geriatric patients have been found to have a potassium intake of only 50 milliequivalents (1950 mg) per day, when their estimated need was for 100 milliequivalents. But whether induced by low appetites, poor food choices, disease, or drugs, potassium deficiency can be more pleasantly cured by foods that provide adequate absorbable potassium than by drug supplements with their unpleasant side effects.

Patients are occasionally given food lists or counseled by physicians to consume foods high in potassium, but they are rarely given comprehensive instructions on the quantities that should be eaten. Many times, foods high in potassium are simply added to the patient's normal diet without being considered in terms of their caloric and other nutrient contributions.

SOME SPECIFICS

Admittedly, it has been difficult to determine the exact amount of potassium likely to be derived from food sources, but an effective, quantitative method for integrating high-potassium foods into the total diet is now available. The Index of Nutritional Quality (INQ) developed at Utah State University measures a food's nutrient to caloric density:

$$\frac{\text{Percent of Nutrient requirement in a quantity of Food}}{\text{Percent of energy requirement in a quantity of food}} = \text{INQ}$$

A computer program has been developed which can calculate the INQ for each nutrient of concern. The result is then summarized as a graphic profile of nutrient content. The ratio of the food's nutrient content to its energy content remains constant. The quantity of food in question is thus immaterial to calculations of the INQ. The USU research groups evaluated numerous foods to determine whether each has a high density of potassium relative to its kilocalorie and sodium contents. Sodium was included because patients on diuretic therapy are often on sodium-restricted intakes as well.

For illustrative purposes, the common prescription of 132 milliequivalents (5150 mg) of potassium and 87 milliequivalents (2000 mg) of sodium per day for patients on diuretic therapy has been used as a standard. The daily intake of potassium for most people averages 100 milliequivalents (3900 mg) per day, with a range of 40–153 milliequivalents (1560–5970 mg). The average potassium chloride supplementation level supplies 32 milliequivalents (1250 mg), which is believed to adequately offset the potassium lost during therapy. The sodium standard of 87 milliequivalents (2000 mg) represents the no-salt-added dietary prescription, which is given to many hypertensive patients.

An INQ above "1" for potassium in a food indicates that the amount of the food that would satisfy an individual's total energy requirement for a day (2300 kcal) should also supply the required amounts of potassium. Conversely, a food with an INQ lower than "1" would be a poor choice for the patient needing potassium repletion because it would not supply enough potassium relative to caloric contribution. To be appropriate for a patient on potassium-wasting diuretic therapy and a moderately sodium-restricted diet, a food would need to have an INQ above "1" for potassium and below "1" for sodium. The illustrations reflect standards that are appropriate for many patients. The computer program, however, can be easily modified to fit any sodium and potassium dietary requirements.

In the unlikely situation of fresh halibut being used as the sole source of a person's energy, a 2300 kilocalorie portion would supply 62 percent of the 87 milliequivalents (2000 mg) of sodium and 193 percent of the 132 milliequivalent (5150 mg) standard for potassium (Figure 9.1a). Most people, however, consume a variety of foods each day. Figure 9.1b shows the ratio of nutrients to energy (INQ), in a 3.5 ounce serving of halibut. Such a serving of halibut provides 100 kcal, which is 4 percent of our assumed 2300 kcal energy requirement per day for an average adult, and 8 percent of the daily potassium prescription. The same serving would also provide 3 percent of the sodium prescription.

A large baking potato has exceptionally high potassium, and low sodium contents (Figure 9.2). The potato would provide only 8 percent of a person's total energy requirement and less than one percent of the sodium prescription, but would contribute 19 percent of the dietary potassium prescription (INQ= 2.32).

Each one percent of the energy requirement satisfied by cooked asparagus (Figure 9.3) would provide 3.9 percent of the potassium requirement. Since the caloric content is so low, almost unlimited quantities can be consumed. One serving of asparagus provide 5 milliequivalents (195 mg) of potassium and only 20 kcal. A ⅝ cup serving of raisins, a more traditionally favored food supplement for dietary potassium, provides 20 milliequivalents (780 mg) of potassium but also contains 289 kcal(Figure 9.4). The raisins' potassium INQ is therefore only 1.13, or about one-third of asparagus. Thus, on a per calorie basis, asparagus contains approximately three times more potassium than raisins.

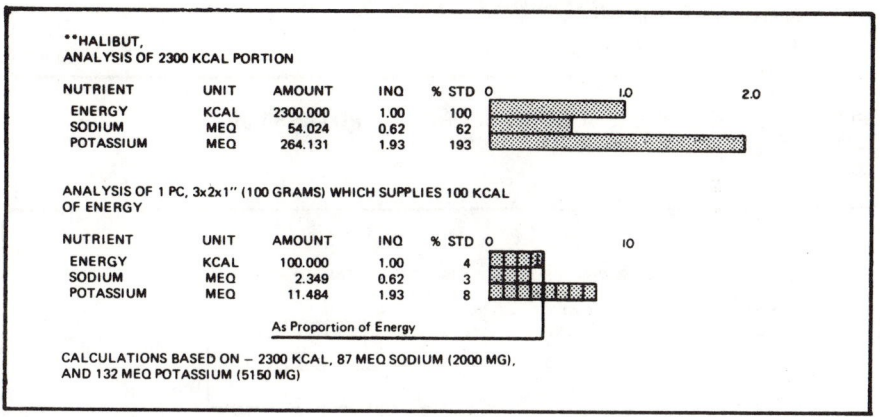

FIG. 9.1. POTASSIUM AND SODIUM PROFILE OF HALIBUT FOR: (a) A 2300 KCAL PORTION AND (b) A NORMAL SERVING SIZE

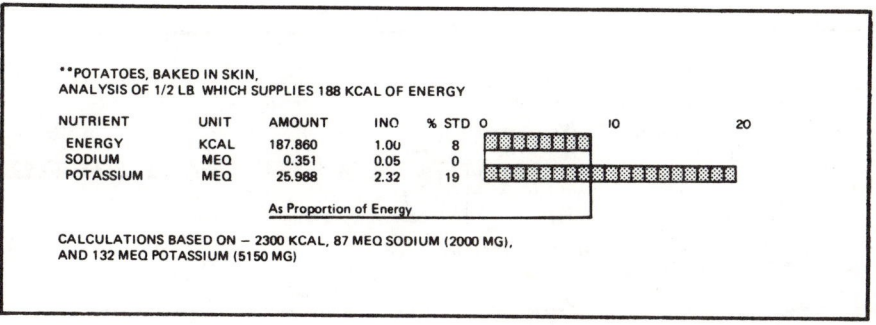

FIG. 9.2. POTATOES ARE A HIGH POTASSIUM, LOW SODIUM FOOD

Sauerkraut, as seen in Figure 9.5, has an excellent INQ for potassium (3.34), but would not be included on lists for potassium supplementation because of its inordinately high sodium content (INQ= 47.7).

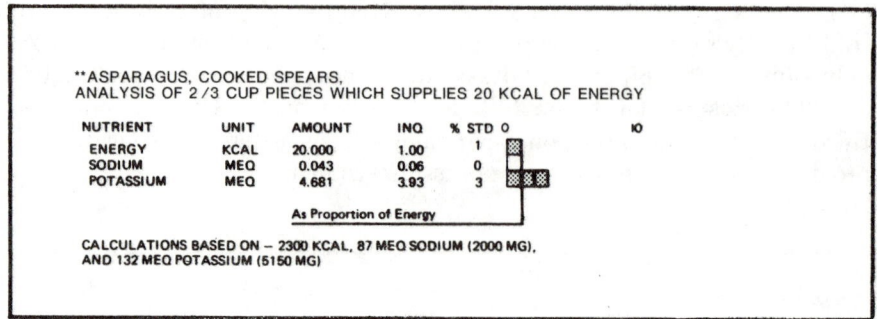

FIG. 9.3. ASPARAGUS IS A GOOD SOURCE OF POTASSIUM
COMPARED TO THE CALORIES PROVIDED

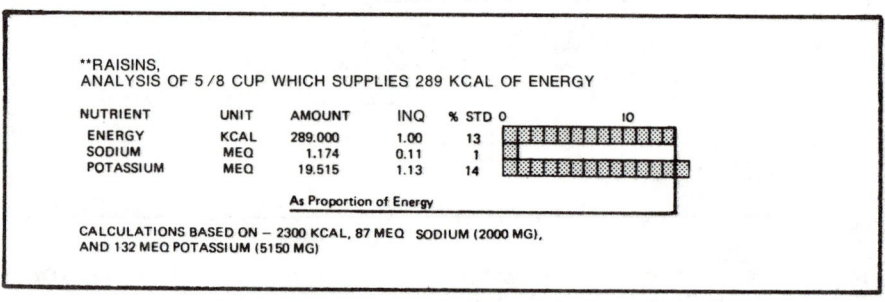

FIG. 9.4. RAISINS, A FOOD TRADITIONALLY USED FOR
POTASSIUM SUPPLEMENTATION, ONLY HAS A POTASSIUM
INQ OF 1.13

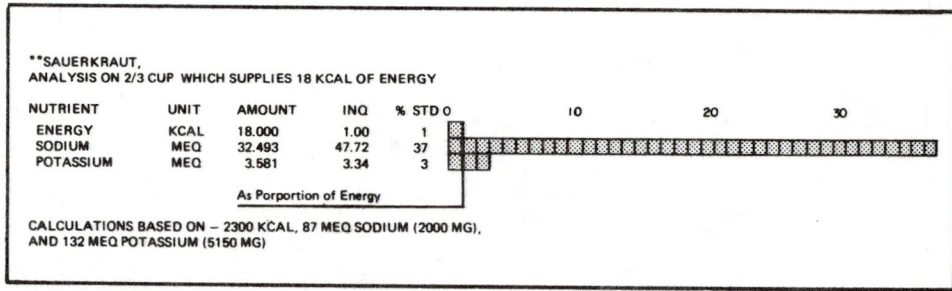

FIG. 9.5. SAUERKRAUT IS HIGH IN POTASSIUM (INQ = 3.34) AND SODIUM
(INQ = 47.72)

The USU research group has incorporated nutrient composition of over
2000 foods into their computer program (Table 9.1). To illustrate how
this data bank can be used to evaluate a food for its overall nutrient

TABLE 9.1. DIETARY POTASSIUM SUPPLEMENT LIST

	Dairy Products	Meat, Poultry, Fish	Dry Beans, Nuts	Vegetables (fresh)	Fruits	Grain Products	Misc. Items
Foods High in potassium (8.0 Meq/serving or more)	Milk, +Butter 　low fat 　2% 　skim +Yogurt from 　skim milk	+Abalone, canned Beef, ground 　oven roast 　pot roast 　pot pie 　sirloin steak 　vegetable stew Bluefish, baked Catfish Chicken 　+chow mein, 　　canned 　pot pie 　white & dark +Chili con carne 　with beans, 　　canned +Cod, canned +Flounder, baked Haddock, raw Halibut, baked Herring, raw Lamb chop Lake herring Mackerel, raw Perch, raw Pike, raw +Sardines, canned +Scallops, cooked Veal, roast	Almond meal Beans, navy 　red 　soy 　white	Avocado, raw Bamboo shoots, 　raw Beans, lima, 　boiled Mushrooms, raw Parsnips, cooked Potato, baked 　French fried 　salad +Swiss chard Winter squash, 　baked	Apricots, dried 　uncooked Bananas Breadfruit, raw Fruit cocktail, 　canned Grapefruit juice Grapefruit- 　orange juice Melon 　casaba 　honeydew 　musk 　water Nectarine Orange, navel Orange juice Papaya Pears, canned Prunes, uncooked Raisins		

TABLE 9.1. (CONTINUED)

| Foods moderately high in potassium (2.6-7.9 Meq/serving) | +Cottage cheese
Ice cream | Bass, fresh
+Beef, chipped dried
Clams, raw
Lamb leg, roasted
Liver
Pork chop
+Tuna, canned | +Beans with pork & tomato sauce
+Peanut butter
+Peanuts roasted, salted | +Artichoke, boiled
Asparagus boiled
Beans, green boiled
Beans, green yellow
+Beets, canned
Broccoli, cooked
Brussels sprouts
Cabbage, raw cooked
+Carrots, cooked
Cauliflower
Corn, sweet
Eggplant, cooked
Lettuce
Onion
Peas, fresh
Peas & carrots cooked
+Pickle, dill
Potato, boiled mashed
+Sauerkraut
+Spinach
Summer squash
Succotash, cooked
Tomato, raw
+juice
Vegetable, mixed | Apricots, raw canned nectar
Blackberries raw
Boysenberries, frozen
Cherries sour sweet
Currants, raw
Figs, canned
Gooseberries, canned
Grapefruit raw
Kumquats, raw
Peaches raw canned
Pears, raw
Pineapple, raw juice
Plums, raw
Prune, juice
Raspberries, red, raw
Strawberries, raw
Tangerines | Cereals:
oatmeal, cooked
+Macaroni & cheese
Rice, cooked | +Beef broth
+Chicken broth
+Soup *minestrone +vegetable beef
Tea, instant |

TABLE 9.1. (*CONTINUED*)

Foods low in potassium (2.5 Meq/serving or less)	+Cheese, cheddar +Swiss Eggs, boiled Sherbet	+Anchovy, pickled +Bacon +Bologna, 3" diam. slices +Sausage, links	+Celery, raw Cucumber, raw	Bread, white whole wheat Chocolate chip cookie Cupcake Fig **Bar** Cereal, corn meal corn flakes farina puffed rice	Butter +Catsup Cocoa, dry powder +French dressing +Mayonnaise +Mustard Salad oil Sugar, white

Underlined foods are good sources of potassium in terms of caloric content, i.e., INQ's greater than "1"

+High sodium foods, i.e., INQ > 1:00

value, Figure 9.6 presents a profile of eighteen of the essential nutrients in a medium banana. From this profile it can be seen that bananas are a good source of potassium (INQ= 1.87), and an even better source of ascorbic acid (INQ= 4.51). Bananas also contain adequate amounts of iron (the most difficult nutrient to supply in adequate amounts in American diets), and close to the required amounts of vitamin A, thiamin, riboflavin, and niacin.

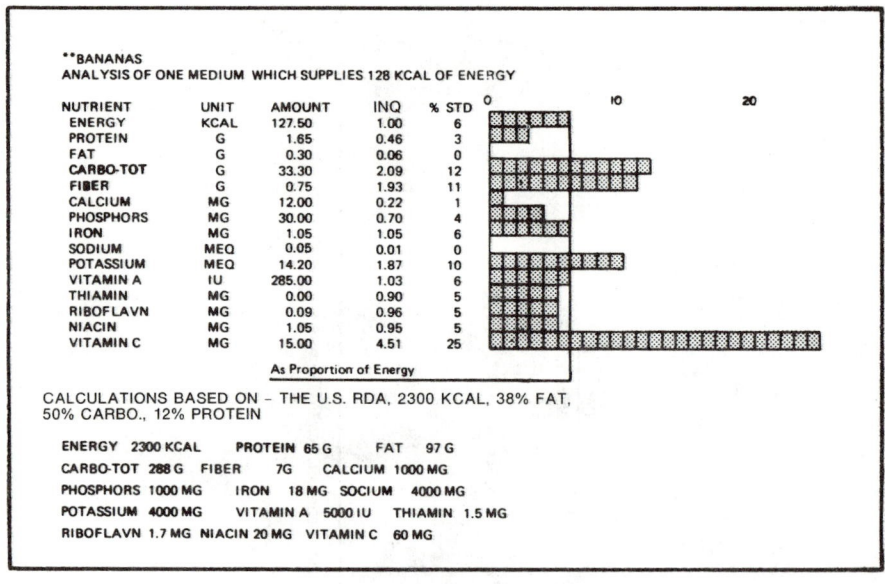

FIG. 9.6. THE PROFILE FOR A BANANA ILLUSTRATES A RANGE OF NUTRIENTS OR WHICH INQs CAN BE CALCULATED

In Table 9.1, individual foods have been grouped into classes that emphasize their potassium contents. Foods listed in regular type contain potassium in amounts relatively less than their calorie contents, i.e., they have potassium/caloric INQs less than "1." These foods would have to be consumed in excess of energy needs to meet the potassium supplementation requirement. In contrast, the foods underlined have high potassium/calorie INQs and should constitute most of the potassium-seeking individual's diet.

Foods high in sodium content have been marked with a "+," i.e. INQ greater than one. People on sodium-restricted diets should be aware of these foods except on rare occasions and in small amounts.

Obviously, foods can provide a practical alternative to drugs as a source of potassium. The computerized USU food data bank is also finding increasing use by physicians, dietitians and nutritionists as a basis for counseling individuals with diverse dietary problems. In essence, by devising and computerizing the INQ concept, the USU researchers have facilitated sensible food choices by anyone interested in optimizing their nutritional status.

POTASSIUM

The classes of foods that are high in potassium are clearly indicated by INQ analysis (see Figure 9.7). Setting an arbitrary potassium standard of 100 milliequivalents/2300 kcal, it can be seen that vegetables are the most substantial source. Those with an INQ of 10.0 would meet the total potassium standard with a 230 kcal portion. Nearly half of the vegetables have a potassium INQ of between 4.0 and 10.0, and they constitute the principal dietary sources of supplementary potassium.

POTASSIUM

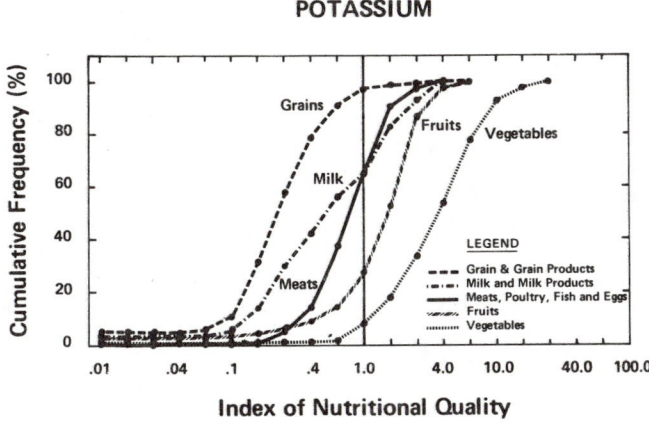

Index of Nutritional Quality

FIG. 9.7. POTASSIUM DISTRIBUTION IN FOODS IS IN
RELATION TO ENERGY CONTENT

Vegetables, fruits and nuts have the greatest potassium:energy ratio of any of the food categories. The standard of intake for potassium is 103 Meq per 2300 kcal.

Foods that are at the high end of the potassium INQ curve are listed in Table 9.2 in decreasing order of potassium content. The INQ suggests the potential of the food for supplementing a low potassium intake.

When a normal serving size is considered, certain practicalities become evident. A goal to meet a particular potassium intake can be set, and to realize the goal, the INQ can be an important informational item. Sodium content of the foods would, in practice, also be an important consideration.

TABLE 9.2. POTASSIUM CONTENT OF SELECTED FOODS

Food	Serving Size	Kcal	MEq Potassium	INQ
Spinach	3½ oz.	19	20.4	24.1
Beet greens	½ cup	24	14.6	13.7
Swiss chard	⅗ cup	25	14.1	12.6
Celery	1 sm. stalk	3	1.7	11.5
Lettuce	3½ oz.	14	6.8	10.8
Dill pickle	1 lg.	11	5.1	10.5
Artichokes	1 lg.	56	22.0	8.8
Mushrooms	4 lg.	28	10.6	8.5
Asparagus	1 oz.	3	1.0	7.3
Tomato juice	½ cup	19	5.8	6.9
Broccoli	1 stalk	32	9.8	6.9
Summer squash	1 cup	22	6.7	6.9
Cauliflower	⅞ cup	18	5.3	6.6
Cucumber	½ med.	7	2.0	6.6
Tomato	1 small	22	6.3	6.4
Cabbage	1 cup shredded	24	6.0	5.6
Sweet pepper	1 lg.	22	5.5	5.6
Musk melon	1 wedge	66	15.7	5.4
Brussels sprouts	10 oz.	102	23.9	5.2
Winter squash	8 oz.	122	28.3	5.2
Snap beans	1 cup	27	6.2	5.2
Orange juice	1 cup	98	13.1	3.0
Banana	½ med.	64	7.1	2.5
Dried apricots	10 halves	125	12.1	2.2
Dried prunes	5 med.	119	8.4	1.6
Raisins	⅝ cup	289	19.6	1.5

REFERENCES

FOOD AND NUTRITION BOARD. 1974. Recommended Dietary Allowances, 8th Ed., National Academy of Sciences, Washington, D.C.

MENEELY, G.R. and BATTARBEE, H.D. 1976. Sodium and potassium. Nutr. Rev., 34:225.

POTASSIUM therapy and gastrointestinal lesions. 1970. Missouri Med., 67: 310.

WYSE, B.W., SORENSON, A.W., WITTWER A.J., and HANSEN, R.G. 1976. Foods instead of drugs to offset diuretic potassium losses. Utah Sci., Sept., p. 86.

10

Dietitians: Contributing Members of the Health Care Team

Ten years have passed since the popularization of the problem-oriented record introduced by Lawrence Weed and much has been said—pro and con—about this method of recording patient information. Problem orientation has been hailed as the wave of the future, a method of making it possible for patient data to be stored, transmitted, and retrieved using computer technology.

Problem orientation is in reality an explicit declaration of a commitment to provide comprehensive care as it is recorded in the patient's chart. It is an acknowledgment that virtually any patient can, and frequently does, present more than the relatively limited scope of problems which may have directly resulted in hospitalization or the seeking of medical care. Through the development of a problem list and the representation of explicit data and conclusions within the patient's chart, a mechanism is provided whereby each member of the patient care team may enter or have access to that data which is pertinent to the identification of treatment for patient problems.

All too often, the health care team focuses narrowly on physicians and to a lesser extent nurses. Other members, such as clinical pharmacists, dietitians or social workers are relegated to peripheral positions in which their input is so obscured as to make it difficult for them to positively affect patient outcome. As new technology and knowledge are acquired, each member of the health care team is ready to assume an ever-expanding role in the identification and treatment of patient problems. That the extent of the abilities of the members of the team is not understood does not diminish the potential which they have for making a significant contribution. Too often the role that diet may have, not only in terms of history but also in its interaction with therapeutic regimen and possible long-term effects on patient outcome, is ignored or poorly understood.

THE CHANGING ROLE OF THE DIETITIAN

Traditionally, dietitians have instructed patients according to physicians' orders. These instructions and the impressions dietitians may have about the patients' dietary needs are often not recorded on the medical chart. Nurses have acted as intermediaries, transmitting orders and diet prescriptions made by physicians to the dietitians. There has been little dialogue between physicians and dietitians, and dietitians have been reticent to initiate dietary intervention for the patients.

Need for More Involvement in Patient Care.—The science of nutrition has become vastly more complicated in recent years and diet manuals have become so extensive that most other health professionals are unable to keep up with current theory. In order to provide the best patient care possible, the dietitian must become an integral part of the patient care team. There must be increased communication between the dietitian and the physician and delegation of clinical nutrition responsibility to the dietitian including the writing of nutritional notes and dietary orders in the patient's chart.

Increased Nutrition Responsibility.—The basic nutritional assessment tool for the dietitian is the dietary history with all of its inherent problems. This information must often be used to make assessments and recommendations without precise nutritional biochemical data. Because of the difficulty of calculating nutrient content from diet histories, only a few nutrients of clinical significance are monitored. One of the problems with diet therapy is that changing one or two nutrients from the normal eating pattern will often skew the overall nutritional intake, necessitating the assessment of indicator nutrients to preserve proper nutritional balance.

Although the energy content of diets should be evaluated in terms of patient energy balance (i.e., is weight changing on present diet), dietary history frequently reflects a lower energy content than is actually consumed. When energy content is inadequate all other nutrients may be proportionally low. For example, a nutrient may appear to be in insufficient quantities in a diet history, but if calories were adjusted to reflect a weight maintenance intake by a proportionally increased serving size of all dietary items, the nutrient may be found in adequate amounts. Conversely, a patient overconsuming calories may not receive adequate amounts of nutrients if calories are restricted to a maintenance level. In other words, a method of assessing a dietary potential is necessary in order for dietitians to do an adequate job of modifying patient diets to meet clinical and general health requirements; therefore, a nutrient density approach is preferred.

Clearly, the variability of individual needs for nutrients, our lack of detailed information about food composition and diverse food processing factors preclude absolute precision in the index. Nevertheless, using the concept of nutrient density, the index provides a useful means of monitoring the adequacy of specialty diets, individual meals and menu series. Nutrient density can be calculated by computer for any number of nutrients based on any nutritional standards desired, including the Food and Nutrition Board's RDAs, the USRDA, clinical diet prescriptions, or research standards. The resultant profile of nutrient density ratios is printed in a bar graph.

Dietary assessment using this nutrient density approach fits well into the problem-oriented medical record (POMR) system. The following case histories illustrate how the dietitian may act as a member of the health care team utilizing these techniques.

NUTRIENT DENSITY TECHNIQUE—TWO CASE HISTORIES

Case 1. A 59-year-old woman was admitted to the hospital for treatment of a third-degree burn to the arm caused by grease splashed from an overheated skillet. The wound became infected and failed to heal after treatment with a topical aerosol. She also complained of polydypsia and increasing nocturia and sweating. Chlorothiazide was prescribed for the patient in treatment of hypertension. Her blood pressure was recorded as 215/180 when hypertension was diagnosed six months earlier. Though she complained of a general malaise, she reported no other illness or disease.

The social history noted that the patient was married, and had two teenage sons (ages 14 and 16), a high school education and average intelligence. Her interests were limited to keeping house, participation in church functions and the PTA.

This case had several dietary considerations. As the procedure of the POMR was followed, the input of the dietitian as well as others on the health care team was necessary for maximum care of the patient.

Data Base and Problem List—Table 10.1 is an unstructured data base, derived from the medical history, physical examination and laboratory data. The problem list is derived from the information in the data base. (See Table 10.2). In some situations, the physician may take the responsibility for identifying the major problems, while in other cases, several members of the health care team develop the master list. Whenever practical, the latter is the recommended procedure.

PROGRESS NOTES

Next, the progress notes were recorded for specific problems using the subjective, objective, assessment and plan (SOAP) format. The initial progress notes were written in the "plan" for problems such as diabetes, hypertension and obesity. Dietary intervention was complicated by the interrelationships between the medical problems. A dietary evaluation was made using a dietary recall and an INQ profile.

TABLE 10.1. CASE I: DATA CASE OF POMR

Medical History
Slow-healing infected wound on right forearm.
History of hypertension BP 215/180 (date).
Intermittent use of chlorothiazide (does not follow
    prescription regularly).
Polydepsia.
Nocturea.
General malaise.

Physical Examination
Height 5'3".
Weight (obese) 230 lbs (10.1 kilo).
Respiration 20.
Pulse 95.
BP 160/90.
Mild (+) edema of extremities.

Laboratory Data
Flat plate indicates borderline enlarged (edematous)
    lung.
Hematocrit 42%.
BUN 10 mg%.
FBS 155 mg% (Folin—WU).
Glucose tolerance 4+ 300 to 400 mg% peak.
Cholesterol 230 mg%.
Calcium 9 mg%.
Potassium 3.3 mg%.
Sodium 355 mg %.
WBC 11,500.

TABLE 10.2. CASE I: PROBLEM LIST OF POMR

Date Entered	No.	Active	Inactive
	1	Infected wound	
	2	Adult onset diabetes mellitus	
	3	Hypertension	
	4	Obesity	

A computerized graph, or a specialized flow chart, was used in conjunction with POMR. New graphs were added as the progress of the nutrient was audited. Reference to the graph saved time and space in documenting dietary parameters. Table 10.3 shows the patient's average daily

TABLE 10.3. CASE I: NUTRIENT DENSITY PROFILE

Nutrient	Unit[2]	Amount	Inq	%Std	Profile (0 — 50% — 100% — 150% — 200%)
ENERGY	Kcal	2397.220	1.00	133	BBBB…LLLL…DDDDDDD
PROTEIN	g	80.897	1.10	147	BBBB…LLLL…DD·DDDDDDD DDDD
CALCIUM	mg	1155.370	1.08	144	BBBB…LLLL…DDDDDDDD LDD
IRON	mg	14.680	1.10	147	BBBB…LLLL…DDDDDDD·DDDDDDD DDDD
VITAMIN A	IU	4451.600	0.84	111	BBBB…LLLL…DDD
THIAMIN	mg	1.006	0.76	101	BBBB…LLLL…D
RIBOFLAVIN	mg	2.114	1.44	192	BBBB…·LLLLLLL LLLLDDDDDDDDDDDD
NIACIN	mg	14.228	0.89	119	BBBB…LLLL…DDDDD
VITAMIN C	mg	46.220	0.77	103	BBLLLL…DDDDD·D
PANTOTHENIC ACID	mg	4.195	0.63	84	BBLLLLDDDDDDD
VITAMIN B6	mg	0.734	0.28	37	BBBB…·DDDDD·DDDDDDD
VITAMIN B12	µg	3.628	0.91	121	BBBB…·LLLLLLL
FAT	g	109.069	1.82	242	D* 77.74 … DDDD242.38
···BREAKDOWN:	B* 50.71	L*	113.92	D* 77.74	
SATURATED FAT A	g	41.250	2.29	306	D* 119.78 … LLLLLLLLLLLLLL305.56
···BREAKDOWN:	B* 64.00	L*	121.78	D* 119.78	
UNSATURATED OLEIC	g	48.520	2.70	359	D* 102.15 … LLLLLLLLLLLLLL359.41
···BREAKDOWN:	B* 79.70	L*	177.56	D* 102.15	
UNSATURATED LINOL	g	9.930	0.55	74	BBBB…LLLLLLDD
CHOLESTEROL	mg	316.650	0.48	63	BBBB…DDDDDDDD
CARBOHYDRATE TOTAL	g	278.231	1.49	199	BBBB…·LLLLLLL LLLLLLLDDDDDDDDD
FIBER	g	4.062	0.51	68	BLLLLLDDDDDDDDD
PHOSPHOROUS	mg	1363.070	1.28	170	BBBB…·LLLLLLD DDDDDDDDDD
SODIUM	mg	3918.900	1.47	196	BBBB…·LLLLLLL LLLLLLDDDDDDDDD
POTASSIUM	mg	2363.430	0.44	59	BBBB…LLLLLL → + ++

[1] Calculations based on RDAs for 59-year-old woman with protein, fat and carbohydrate adjusted for a diabetic patient. Estimated nutritional requirements have been assumed to be: energy 1800 Kcal. protein 55 gm, calcium 800 mg, iron 10 mg, vitamin A 4000 IU, thiamin 1 mg, riboflavin 1.1 mg, niacin 12 mg, vitamin C 45 mg, pantothenic acid 5 mg, vitamin B6 2 mg, vitamin B12 3 mg, fat 45 g, saturated fat A 13.5 g, unsaturated oleic 13.5 g, unsaturated linoleic 13.5 g, cholesterol 500 mg, carbohydrate total 140 g, fiber 6 g, phosphorus 800 mg, sodium 2000 mg, potassium 4000 mg.

[2] 1662 grams supply 2397 Kcal of energy.

+ = USRDA.   ++ = As proportion of energy.   B = Contribution of breakfasts.   L = Contribution of lunches.   D = Contribution of dinners.   S = Contribution of snacks.

nutrient intake calculated from a three-day dietary recall recorded by the dietitian. The information on the graph enabled the health team to determine the potential of the diet as well as the actual patient intake.

Modifying the Diet.—In considering the patient's chart, the dietary standards were programmed to conform to a diabetic diet (problem 2) with a mild salt restriction and an 1800-calorie base and RDAs nutrients as recommended by the National Research Council for a 59-year-old female. (See Table 10.3). The patient consumed one-third more calories than her estimated needs, indicating her obese condition was probably due to overconsumption. A reduction in calories to 1200 kcal should have resulted in a one-pound-per-week loss without jeopardizing the patient's ability to maintain an adequate nutrient intake. A reduction in weight would have beneficial effects in the treatment of both hypertension and insulin-resistant diabetes (adult onset).

The admission diet information showed dietary intakes when compared to arbitrary standards for pantothenic acid (84 percent of RDA), fiber (68 percent of standard) and potassium (59 percent of standard). A low serum potassium corresponded with the low dietary intake. In addition, the patient had been taking a thiazide diuretic which produces urinary potassium loss and causes increased need for this nutrient. Unsaturated fat intake was below the standard and when compared to the value for saturated fat yielded a P/S ratio of 0.25. The high carbohydrate value with a low fiber intake often reflects the patient's preference for sugar and highly refined carbohydrate foods.

The sodium intake was about average (400 mg), but had to be reduced to 200 mg as part of the usual hypertension therapy. Adequate amounts of vitamins A, C, B_{12}, thiamin and niacin were acheived only because of the excess calories consumed. If the calories were adjusted to 1800, these nutrients would be deficient as shown by the INQ values below 1.0. When calories were reduced to 1200, even more care had to be given to the choice of high-nutrient density foods. (See Table 10.4 for the dietitian's progress notes.)

Case II. Mrs. L. is a 71-year-old female, status post-fracture of the hip, who has been the resident of a licensed nursing home for three months. She suffers mild rheumatoid arthritis and anorexia though no organic reason has been identified for her lack of appetite. She has suffered a weight loss of 15 pounds from her admission weight of 132 pounds. She is fond of fresh fruit but is disinterested in most other foods.

Mrs. L., a widow of two years from rural background some 300 miles away, is ambulatory with the aid of a walker but is unable to care for herself without help. She is considered mildly senile. The patient is shy, but generally friendly and cooperative with the staff. However, she has not made many friends among the other patients who, for the most part, have dissimilar interests. She looks forward to weekly visits from her son and daughter-in-law, who make a 100-mile trip to see her.

TABLE 10.4. *CASE I*: PROGRESS NOTES

Date	Progress Notes

Problem 2: Diabetes

S. Cooks and prepares large meals for her family. Especially fond of pastry, hot breads and fried foods. Frequently skips breakfast, takes a light lunch of a sandwich, tea and dessert and a heavy dinner. Not fond of vegetables, except potatoes, snacks on her home-baked products. Has very little exercise.

O. Diet high in total fat, saturated fat, refined carbohydrate, and INQs below 1.0 for vitamins A and C and fiber.

A. Inadequate diabetic diet.

P. Instruct patient as to the use of the ADA Diabetic Exchange List. Use a diet Rx: CHO 140 gm, fat 45 gm, protein 55 gm. Signature of RD.

Problem 3: Hypertension

S. Fond of many high-sodium foods such as lunch meat and cheese.

O. Diet is average in sodium content (approximately 4000 mg) and low in potassium content. Patient is receiving chlorothiazide, a potassium-losing diuretic.

A. Hypertension possibly aggravated by sodium intake with low dietary potassium implications.

P. Reduce patient sodium intake to 2000 mg and increase potassium intake to 135 meq[8,9] to help replace potassium loss from diet therapy. Give patient a list of low-salt foods (INQ ≤ .5) and potassium-containing foods with INQs of 1.5 or greater.[10] These lists are to be used in conjunction with the diabetic exchange list. Signature of RD.

Problem 4: Obesity

S. "Loves to eat" especially when watching television.

O. The patient's calorie intake is 133 percent above the estimated energy requirement.

A. Obesity due to overconsumption.

P. Reduce the calorie intake to 1200 Kcal as part of the diabetic Rx in the calculation of exchanges. Counsel the patient using some behavior modification techniques to include reducing the home baking, changing the television routine and increasing the physical activity. Signature of RD.

*See chap. 9

TABLE 10.5. *CASE II:* DATA BASE OF POMR

Sex:	female
Age:	71
Height:	63 inches
Weight:	117 lbs.
BP:	138/76
Hbg.:	15.3 g/100 ml
Hematocrit:	45%
Calcium:	8.1 mg/100 ml
T. Protein:	6.5 g/100 ml
Cholesterol:	170 mg/100 ml
Serum Iron:	107 mg/100 ml

The consultant dietitian for the convalescent center was one of several health professionals called together to assess the patient's problems and make recommendations for the management of her case. In addition to the personal history, the items in Table 10.5 were also available in the patient's POMR data base.

After reviewing the records, the dietitian interviewed the patient about past eating habits, foods liked and disliked, and problems which the patient felt influenced her attitude or ability to eat. The diet the patient had been offered was evaluated by a three-day plate waste study. The menu as served was found to be nutritionally adequate, but the actual intake during the study period showed nutritional deficiencies in several areas. An INQ profile of the average daily intake of the patient is presented in Table 10.6.

Using the RDAs for a female over 50, the data shows the patient was consuming only two-thirds of her estimated 1800 kcal requirement. Her actual requirement may be less because of immobility during convalescence, but her continual weight loss confirmed she was not receiving adequate calories to maintain weight. The actual diet is inadequate in all respects except protein, saturated fat and vitamin C (reflecting her acceptance of fresh fruit). If adequate calories were consumed, all nutrients with INQs of 1.0 or above would be adequate, leaving calcium (INQ= .73), vitamin B_6 (INQ= .77), unsaturated fat (INQ= .48), cholesterol (INQ= .81), carbohydrate (INQ= .72), fiber (INQ= .66), sodium (INQ= .37) and potassium (INQ= .79) in deficit of the programmed nutrient standards. The low bone density correlates with the low serum calcium. Insufficient calcium is a common problem of old age and the patient may have had chronic intake because of her dislike of milk and all but processed cheese. The initial immobility resulting from the fracture may have compounded the calcium loss from bone stores. The dietary considerations of the patient were added to the progress notes (See Table 10.7).

TABLE 10.6. CASE II: NUTRIENT DENSITY PROFILE[1]

Nutrient	Unit	Amount	Inq	Std %	Profile (50% — 100% — 150% — 200%)
ENERGY	Kcal	1185.117	1.00	66	BBLLLLLLLLLDDDDDDDSSS
PROTEIN	g	47.023	1.55	102	BBBLLLLLLLLLLLLLDDDD|DDDDDDDDDDDDSS
CALCIUM	mg	383.243	0.73	48	BBBLLLDDDDDDDDSSS
IRON	mg	8.059	1.22	81	BBBBLLLLLLLLLDDDDDDDDD DDDDDSSS
VITAMIN A	IU	3014.067	1.14	75	BBBBLLLLLLLLLDDDDDDDDD DDSSS
THIAMIN	mg	0.763	1.16	76	BBBLLLLLLLLLLLLDDDDDDDDD SSSS
RIBOFLAVIN	mg	0.905	1.25	82	BBLLLLLLLLLLLLLLDDDDDD DDDSSSS
NIACIN	mg	9.960	1.26	83	BBBBLLLLLLLLLLLLLLDDDDD DDDDDSSS
VITAMIN C	mg	105.773	3.57	235	BBBBBBBBBBBBBBBBB BBBLLLLLLLLLLLLLLLLLLLLLLLDDDDDDDDDDDDDDSSSS 235.05
***BREAKDOWN:		69.93	B* L* 43.15		D* 41.85 S* 80.12
PANT ACID	mg	3.226	0.98	65	BBBLLLLLLLLLDDDDDDDSS
VITAMIN B6	mg	1.020	0.77	51	BLLLLLLLDDDDDDSSSSSSS
VITAMIN B12	µg	2.140	1.08	71	BLLLLLLLLDDDDDDDDDD DDDD
FAT	g	64.631	1.27	84	BLLLLLLLLLLLLLDDDDDD DDDDDSS
SATURATED FAT A	g	24.307	1.60	105	BLLLLLLLLLLLLLLLLDD DDDDDDDDDDDDDSSS
UNSATURATED OLEIC	g	26.133	1.29	85	BLLLLLLLLLLLLLLLDDDDD DDDDDDDSSS
UNSATURATED LINOL	g	7.303	0.48	32	LLLLLDDDDD
CHOLESTEROL	mg	320.257	0.81	53	LLLLDDDDDDDDDDSSS
CARBOHYDRATE TOTAL	g	109.910	0.72	48	BBBLLLDDDDDSSSS
FIBER	g	3.039	0.66	43	BBBLLLLLDDDDSSSS
PHOSPHORS	mg	685.123	1.30	86	BBBLLLLLLLLDDDDDDDDD DDDDDSSS
SODIUM	mg	975.960	0.37	24	BLLDDDDD
POTASSIUM	mg	2067.787	0.79	52	BBBLLLLLDDDDDSSSS → ++

[1] Calculations based on RDAs for a female 51+ years of age, 38 percent Kcal total fat: P/S ratio = 1. cholesterol 600 mg. fiber 5 mg. phosphorus 800 mg. sodium 4000 mg. potassium 4000 mg.

+ = USRDA.   ++ = As proportion of energy.

TABLE 10.7. *CASE II*: PROGRESS NOTES

Date	Progress Notes
	S. ... *O.* ... *A.* ...

P. Use more fat, especially unsaturated fats like margarire in sauces, gravies, dressings and spreads. Egg nogs, milk shakes,ice cream, etc. should be offered. (Note: sugar and fat add palatability to the diet as well as calories.) Foods containing dairy prducts will help increase calcium intake and an increase in unsaturated fat will improve the P/S ratio. Change the time of medication. Try to have the patient interact with other patients or when possible have a staff member talk with her during meals. Encourage snacking on food from supplementary food lists (foods high in nutrients found lacking in the diet, i.e., foods which have INQ of 1.5 or greater for each limiting nutrient).

Problem 3: Anorexia

S. Likes fruit that is easily chewed; dislikes milk, vegetables and tough meats. Finds institution food "tasteless" and misses the family favorites she used to cook. Also misses having friends around. Medication upsets her stomach.

O. Missing teeth and uncomfortable dental plate makes chewing difficult. ASA for arthritis is often administered 20 to 30 minutes before a meal. Spends much time alone. Diet assessment indicates deficit in energy intake and insufficient quantities of several nutrients. (See Table 6.)

P. Consult dental personnel for evaluation of teeth. With the patient, consult INQ food lists as supplementary sources of foods which would be accpetable to her. Increase the use of eggs in the diet—omelets, souffles, casseroles. (Note: since dietary cholesterol is low, eggs are an easily chewed source of protein, vitamin A, riboflavin, vitamin B12 and iron.). Increase the use of seasonings including: moderate amounts of salt, MSG and vegetables salts. (Note: the salt content of the diet is only one-third of an acceptable adult intake and can materially increase the palatability of food.). Increase the vegetable intake. Using diet preferences of patient in dietary planning is an important psychological factor in food preference.

THE POMR AND NUTRITIONAL EVALUATION

The POMR makes it possible to correlate the medical care provided by each of the health professionals. By including a quantitative assessment of the patient's dietary needs, the dietitian becomes a bonafide member of the health care team. The INQ nutrient density computerized diet profile is a specialized flow sheet that fits logically into the POMR. The progress notes allow dietary information to be added to the charts used in the total assessment of the patient's progress. The graphical nature of the INQ profile illustrates nutrition data so that a minimum amount of discussion is necessary in the progress notes. The INQ is a concept which can be interpreted by professional personnel and administrators alike. When coupled with the POMR, nutritional evaluation becomes accessible to anyone who may find it useful.

REFERENCES

ANON. 1972. Federal Register 37:62 March 30, p. 6493.

ANON. 1974. Foods and Nutrition Board "Recommended Dietary Allowances." 8th Ed. Rev. National Academy of Sciences, Washington, D.C.

BIERMAN, E.L. *et al.* 1976. Committee on Food and Nutrition, American Dietetic Association Special Report: Principals of Nutrition and Dietary Recommendations for Patients with Diabetes Mellitus. Diabetes 20:9 p. 633-634.

EDMUNDS, C.J. 1973. Total Body Potassium Changes with Prolonged Diuretic Therapy. American Heart Journal 85:4 p. 569-571.

LUTWAK, L. 1974. Continuing Need for Dietary Calcium Throughout Life. Geriatrics 29:5 p.171-178.

MACFARLANE, J.P.R., *et al.* 1973. Clinical Experience with Ameloride in the Elderly. ACTA Cardiology (Brux) 28:1 p. 365-374.

MACK. P.B. *et al.* 1967. Effect of Recombency and Space Flight on Bone Density. American Journal of Clinical Nutrition 20:11 p. 1194-1205.

MERRIL, J.P. 1970. Hypertensive Vascular Disease in Principals of Internal Medicine, M.M. Wintrobe *et al.*, Eds. (New York) p. 1258.

SORENSON, A.W. *et al.* 1976. An Index of Nutritional Quality for a Balanced Diet. Journal of the American Diabetic Association 68:3 p.236-242.

WATKIN, D.M. 1973. Nutrition for the Aging and the Aged in Modern Nutrition in Health and Disease. R.S. Goodhart *et al.*, Eds. (Philadelphia: Lea and Febiger) p. 681.

WYSE, B.W. *et al.* 1976. Foods Instead of Drugs—To Offset Potassium Losses. Utah Science 37:4 (September) p. 86-91.

WYSE, B.W. *et al.* Nutritional Quality Index Identifies Consumer Nutrient Needs. Food Technol. 30:1 p. 22-40.

11

International Nutrition Examined With the Aid of Index of Nutritional Quality

The index of nutritional quality methodology can easily be applied to diets in third world countries because it is not geared to a specific food supply. Before discussing specific examples, however, it is thought necessary to review the "protein issue" which has pervaded nutritional thought in developing countries and consequently, until recently, mitigated against seeking creative and innovative solutions to complex nutritional problems.

PROTEIN–CALORIE MALNUTRITION ISSUE

The interest in protein nutritional status was heightened when, in tropical Africa, Cecily Williams discovered that, in populations consuming large quantities of starchy root crops, protein malnutrition resulted. "Kwashiorkor" was the term assigned to the protein deficiency disease which Dr. Williams described in post-weaning infants. With the observations that followed, there was little doubt that protein deficit plays a major role in the development of Kwashiorkor. It is faulty, however, as understood by Dr. Williams to assume that protein deficiency is the major nutritional problem of today's society. In tropical regions such as Africa where root crops high in starch and low in protein constitute the bulk of the food, children are particularly susceptible. Under these circumstances the amount of both the food and the protein in food are often inadequate, and marasmus and kwashiorkor are the result.

The total per capita protein intake in various countries ranges from 45 to 100 grams daily. At the higher intake of protein, animal sources usually constitute at least 50 percent of the total, and cereals predominate when dietary proteins fall below 50 grams a day. In the U.S. about two-thirds of the protein may come from animal sources such as meat, milk, and eggs.

141

Protein and energy requirements can most easily be understood as a ratio. By expressing protein needs in grams per kilocalories of food per kilogram of body weight per day, a direct comparison with energy is possible.

A minimum physiological level of protein in the food to which humans can adapt appears to be 5 percent of calories. Protein content in the diet may be directly stated as percent of calories. Between 6.5 and 8.5 percent of calories as protein in the diet seems to be adequate for normal development of children provided calorie intake is adequate to meet physiological needs. When caloric intake is reduced, protein intake is proportionately lowered and eventually reaches a point where protein becomes limiting.

Increasing the energy intake has produced catch-up growth in undernourished children. In India where extra calories were given to school children, the increase in weight in a six-month period was from 1.1 to 1.5 kilograms, with a height increase of about 4 inches. Alternately, a faster rate of catch-up growth in previously deprived young children is possible when the dietary protein level is raised to 15 percent of energy. However, attempts to produce and merchandise protein supplements to those who presumably are protein deprived have also not been highly successful. These have suggested that Western technology and marketing methods are not directly exportable, without modification, to meet the real nutritional needs of developing nations.

Considering the limited facilities available for transport and storage of foods in developing countries, processed foods and food concentrates cannot provide an adequate base for hunger prevention programs. When yield, disease, and drought resistance, or even milling qualities of a cereal, are compromised to produce more protein in cereals, the results are questionable. Seeking simple and effective interim expedients to improve protein supplies has limited value for society. Food supplements which cost more than the corn meal they replace most often use up too much of a daily wage. Obviously, such practices should receive attention for emergency feeding, but have limited application to the general population. The most likely effect of marketing protein supplements is to distract attention from the need for a broad-based attack on agricultural development. For most it may still be the best practice to supplement a cereal with indigenous legumes to meet the nutritional needs for protein and other nutrients. It should not be necessary to consume an excessive concentration of calories in order to include enough of the essential nutrients.

Overstatement of the protein requirement by some nutritional scientists has reinforced the notion that there is a major protein deficiency in the food supply of the world. As protein requirements have been better understood and allowances adjusted downward accordingly, we have unwittingly solved much of the problem of "protein deficit" in the food supply. Hence, the real problem for most deprived people is in obtaining adequate quantities of food. Man has learned through the centuries to cultivate and develop foods which generally provide adequate nourishment. With minimal disturbance of traditional patterns, improvement can take place when the technology of western society is applied to indigenous food supplies in developing countries with due caution.

The requirement for protein in food can be understood as a requirement for amino acids in reasonable balance. Foods complement each other, hence, cereal grains tend to have too little lysine and sometimes trytophane for normal human development, but they have plentiful amounts of the amino acids containing sulfur. Beans and peas have more than enough lysine, but are insufficient in the sulfur containing amino acid methionine. Hence, legumes such as beans and peas and cereal grains have a synergistic effect when consumed together. This can be shown graphically as follows:

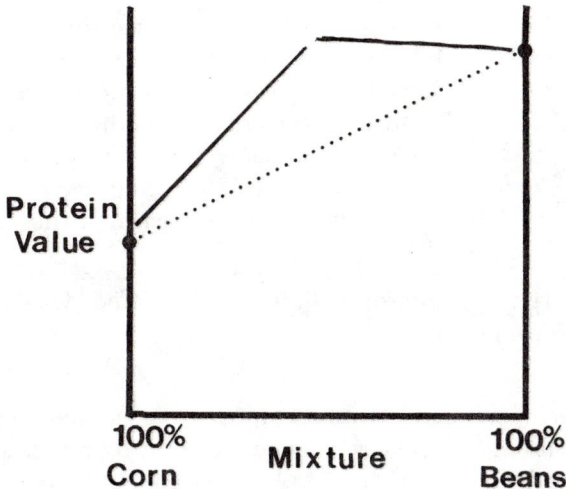

The protein value of an all corn diet is on the left and that of a bean diet on the right. When mixed in various proportions, the predicted value would follow the dotted line. Instead what is found is a reinforcing effect of the two foods upon each other in various combinations. This can best be understood as the corn and beans in combination having an amino acid content more nearly matching that of the human requirement. In a similar way, milk and cereal are complementary.

The syngergisms of the cereal and the pulses extend beyond the amino acids they supply. The legumes tend to have, in addition to more protein as a higher basic level of protein, more of some of the B vitamins and iron. The grains, on the other hand, are an important source of fiber and the complex polysaccharides, plus thiamin and some of the trace minerals if they are not removed by processing.

The general superiority of an equivalent amount of protein from meat, milk, or eggs over foods from plant origin in meeting the protein needs of humans again can be understood on two bases. First, the balanced supply of amino acids more nearly matches the human food requirement. Second, the proteins from animal sources are generally more digestible.

Emphasis on the protein problem has led governments to imagine that nutritional status and health could be significantly improved by such interim measures as the commercial and government sponsored production of protein rich foods, by fortification of staples with protein or amino acids, and on the agricultural side by the introduction of high protein varieties of cereals and by raising the ratio of legume to cereal production. Both of the latter could, in many instances, result in a lowering of total food supply.

The various recommending bodies have changed the suggested protein intake in recent decades generally trending downward but also reflecting some uncertainty in estimates of the actual requirement. In recent years the recommended dietary protein intake has been decreased so that it is now about where it was nearly 70 years ago.

The apparent nutritional quality of food is improved by reducing the recommended allowance for intake since, basically, the two considerations are related as follows:

$$\frac{\text{Nutrition composition of food}}{\text{Recommended allowances}} = \begin{array}{c} \text{Food Quality} \\ \text{or} \\ \text{Adequacy} \end{array}$$

Since the recommended allowance appears in the denominator in the above calculation, the quality or adequacy of a food improves as allowance is reduced. Even though overall a reduced and somewhat more realistic goal for protein consumption is appropriate, some note of caution should be interjected. That is, it is possible for the pendulum to swing too far, and we fail to consider that an adequate intake may be affected by environment. For resistance to and recovery from disease, optimum growth and development in a stressful situation, a precise statement of human requirements for protein suitable for all people may not be possible. Lower and upper limits of recommended intake may be important for health care professionals, and a reasonable median as a suggested guideline for consumers.

FOOD COMPLEMENTATION TO
REPAIR DIETARY INADEQUACIES

Availability of indigenous food in adequate quantity seems to be the prime prerequisite for improving the diet for many of the world's malnourished. For educational and also planning purposes, it may now be useful to concentrate on the need for a balanced intake of nutrients with an adequate supply of energy for all people. After a deficiency of energy has been met, other nutrients, including vitamin A, vitamin C, and the B vitamins, calcium, the trace elements and protein, must be considered for that balance.

The recognition of the deficiency diseases, such as scurvy, goiter, pellagra, and kwashiorkor, and the development of corrective measures rank among the most notable and dramatic achievements of man. The consequences of malnutrition, important to today's society, may be less dramatic and more difficult to characterize, but equally important. The results are inability to perform work efficiently, both thoughtful and physical, reduced resistance to infectious diseases, limited physical development of the young, and even impaired mental capacity.

Nevertheless to the extent that too much emphasis on protein obscures critical food energy and other nutrient shortages, efforts to improve food quality and quantity are less effective. In some areas of the world, vitamin A deficiency is a more significant problem. From the ICNND nutrition surveys as exemplified in Table 11.1, it has been deduced that many of the populations studied in South America consume more than 45 grams of protein each day, and furthermore, on the average more than 40 percent of this protein is derived from animal sources. A 45-gram daily standard with 40 percent from animal sources should meet the protein needs of practically all the population.

On the other hand, vitamin A availability in many diets in South America is far below an acceptable standard. Food quality analysis, using nutrient profiles of the ICNND study in Brazil, graphically depicts the situation (Figures 11.1 and 11.2). The vital question is, does this apparent deficit have clinical meaning? Keeping in mind that the analytical inputs for assessing dietary quality are chemical composition of food and an estimate of human requirement for nutrients, the question becomes, are there observable physical consequences of consuming diets containing too little vitamin A? Increasingly evident are eye difficulties, often correctable by supplementary vitamin A, but in the extreme result in irreversible blindness.

Food quality assessments by INQ method of analysis display graphically and understandably the strengths and weaknesses of the food supply. With the aid of the computer data bank, (preferably containing food composition values for indigenous food) recommendations can be made

TABLE 11.1. VITAMIN A AND PROTEIN COMPOSITION OF SOUTH AMERICAN DIETS

| | Vitamin A | | * Protein | |
	Units	% FAO**	gms	% FAO**
Brazil	152	4	44	105
Southern Zona de Mata	101	3	30	71
Agua Pieta	222	6	55	130
Catende	132	4	47	112
Primavora	160	5	51	121
Equador	1315	38	58	138
Chile	2094	60	70	166
Colombia	117	3	31	74
Bolivia	801	23	57	135
Venezuela	589	17	66	157
Paraguay	810	23	63	150

*Animal protein constitutes 50% or more of total
**FAO standard is 42 gms protein and 3500 IU Vitamin A

NUTRIENT	UNIT	AMOUNT	INQ	STD %	0 25% 50% 75% 100%
ENERGY	KCAL	1472.0	1.00	67	XXXXXXXXXXXXXXXXXXXXXXXXXXXXXXXXXXX
PROTEIN	G	51.4	2.64	177	XXXXXXXXXXXXXXXXXXXXXXXXXXXXXXXXXXXXXXX*XXXXXXXXXXXXXXXXXXX * 177%
VITAMIN A	IU	266.7	0.16	11	XXXXXX *
VITAMIN C	MG	26.0	1.30	87	XXXXXXXXXXXXXXXXXXXXXXXXXXXXXXXXXXXXXXXXX*XXXXXXXXXX
THIAMIN	MG	0.7	1.19	80	XXXXXXXXXXXXXXXXXXXXXXXXXXXXXXXXXXXXXXX*XXXXXX
RIBOFLAVIN	MG	0.54	0.63	42	XXXXXXXXXXXXXXXXXXXXXXX *
NIACIN	MG	12.4	1.28	86	XXXXXXXXXXXXXXXXXXXXXXXXXXXXXXXXXXXXXXXX*XXXXXXXX
CALCIUM	MG	471.0	1.57	105	XXXXXXXXXXXXXXXXXXXXXXXXXXXXXXXXXXXXXXXXXX*XXXXXXXXXXX * 105%
IRON	MG	17.4	1.85	124	XXXXXXXXXXXXXXXXXXXXXXXXXXXXXXXXXXXXXXXX*XXXXXXXXXXXXXX * 124%

****

FIG. 11.1. NORTHEAST BRAZILIAN AVERAGE*

*Using FAO standards for a woman with an energy base of 2200 kilocalories

NUTRIENT	UNIT	AMOUNT	INQ	STD %	0	25%	50%	75%	100%
ENERGY	KCAL	1729.0	1.00	79	XXXXXXXXXXXXXXXXXXXXXXXXXXXXXXXXXXXXXXXXXX				
PROTEIN	G	75.7	3.30	261	XXXXXXXXXXXXXXXXXXXXXXXXXXXXXXXXXXXXXXXXXXXXX*XXXXXXXXXXX * 261%				
VITAMIN A	IU	348.3	0.18	14	XXXXXXXXX				
VITAMIN C	MG	54.0	2.28	180	XXXXXXXXXXXXXXXXXXXXXXXXXXXXXXXXXXXXXX*XXXXXXXXXXX * 180%				
THIAMIN	MG	0.8	1.16	92	XXXXXXXXXXXXXXXXXXXXXXXXXXXXXXXXXXXXX*XXXXXXX				
RIBOFLAVIN	MG	0.7	0.65	51	XXXXXXXXXXXXXXXXXXXXXXXXXXX				
NIACIN	MG	17.9	1.56	123	XXXXXXXXXXXXXXXXXXXXXXXXXXXXXXXXXXX*XXXXXXXXXX * 123%				
CALCIUM	MG	625.0	1.76	139	XXXXXXXXXXXXXXXXXXXXXXXXXXXXXXXXXXX*XXXXXXXXXX * 139%				
IRON	MG	22.6	2.04	161	XXXXXXXXXXXXXXXXXXXXXXXXXXXXXX*XXXXXXXXXXX * 161%				

****

FIG. 11.2. SANTA RITA

incorporating local foods to correct nutritional deficiencies. The more accurate and complete the data bank containing the analytical values for the important nutrients, the more useful the resulting information is for intelligent food planning. Also, with increasing nutrition research, the nutrition community will be better able to circumscribe the human requirements for nutrients.

Use of the INQ method to improve dietaries can more easily be applied in third world countries because there are fewer food choices and more limited complementary foods to repair nutritional deficits. Under circumstances where most of the calorie needs of a group are supplied by as few as two dozen foods such as the situation in Hebron, Jordan when the ICNND survey was made, it would be relatively easy to provide adequate food quality to the consumers. But when the number of food selection choices is over 10,000 or more as in a modern U.S. supermarket, the educational task becomes vastly more complex.

The Hebron, Jordan nutrition survey as a case study is nevertheless informative since with relatively few foods, the quality differences and the unique and complementary value of each in the diet may be assessed.

KINGDOM OF JORDAN NUTRITION STUDY—A CASE STUDY

The Jordanian diet has been compared to the FAO standards for a woman using an energy base of 2200 kilocalories. The composite food index (Figure 11.3) shows that energy is consumed at almost double the 2200 kcal standard. Obviously, the population analyzed in Hebron was considerably more physically active than the average person in the U.S. since at that caloric intake general obesity would be the result. Even so, vitamin A, riboflavin, and calcium intake just barely meet the FAO standards. If the USRDAs standards are applied, the diet would be limiting vitamins A and C, calcium and iron.

The following figures depict the specific contribution of individual foods to the diet. The INQ values, assuming a 2200 kcal consumption, show the potential of a food to supply critical nutrients to the diet if all the calories come from this single food source. According to the survey, 1176 kcal, 420 gr of Arabic bread, is the average daily intake (Figure 11.4). Half of our FAO energy standard is met by bread which provides no vitamins A or C and because it was made from milled flour only limited quantities of riboflavin and other B vitamins and iron.

In 1962, rice (Figure 11.5) was an important calorie source in Hebron, Jordan, with 1195 kcal being derived from that source. Rice contains some protein and limited quantities of all of the other nutrients except vitamins A and C. Bread and rice are largely good energy sources but the diet needs improvement to bring intake of other nutrients into balance.

NUTRIENT	UNIT	AMOUNT	INQ	STD %
ENERGY	KCAL	4128.4	1.00	188
PROTEIN	G	108.4	1.99	374
VITAMIN A	IU	2552.0	0.54	102
VITAMIN C	MG	58.1	1.03	194
THIAMIN	MG	1.7	0.99	186
RIBOFLAVIN	MG	1.4	0.58	108
NIACIN	MG	25.5	0.94	176
CALCIUM	MG	554.7	0.66	123
IRON	MG	14.5	0.55	104

```
        0        25%       50%       75%      100%
ENERGY     XXXXXXXXXXXXXXXXXXXXXXXXXXXXXXXXXXXXXXXXXXXXXXX * 188%
PROTEIN    XXXXXXXXXXXXXXXXXXXXXXXXXXXXXXXXXXXXXXXXXXXXXXX * 374%
VITAMIN A  XXXXXXXXXXXXXXXXXXXXXXXXXXXXXXXXXXXXXXXXXXXXXXX * 102%
VITAMIN C  XXXXXXXXXXXXXXXXXXXXXXXXXXXXXXXXXXXXXXXXXXXXXXX * 194%
THIAMIN    XXXXXXXXXXXXXXXXXXXXXXXXXXXXXXXXXXXXXXXXXXXXXXX * 186%
RIBOFLAVIN XXXXXXXXXXXXXXXXXXXXXXXXXXXXXXXXXXXXXXXXXXXXXXX * 108%
NIACIN     XXXXXXXXXXXXXXXXXXXXXXXXXXXXXXXXXXXXXXXXXXXXXXX * 176%
CALCIUM    XXXXXXXXXXXXXXXXXXXXXXXXXXXXXXXXXXXXXXXXXXXXXXX * 123%
IRON       XXXXXXXXXXXXXXXXXXXXXXXXXXXXXXXXXXXXXXXXXXXXXXX * 104%
```

****

FIG. 11.3. JORDAN DIET

NUTRIENT	UNIT	AMOUNT	INQ	STD %	0 25% 50% 75% 100%
ENERGY	KCAL	1176.0	1.00	53	XXXXXXXXXXXXXXXXXXXXXXXXXXX
PROTEIN	G	37.8	2.44	130	XXXXXXXXXXXXXXXXXXXXXXXXXXXX*XXXXXXXXXXXXXXXXXXXXXX * 130%
VITAMIN A	IU	0.0	0.00	0	*
VITAMIN C	MG	0.0	0.00	0	*
THIAMIN	MG	0.8	1.57	84	XXXXXXXXXXXXXXXXXXXXXXXXXXXXXXXX*XXXXXXXXXXXXXXX
RIBOFLAVIN	MG	0.3	0.48	26	XXXXXXXXXXXX*
NIACIN	MG	8.0	1.03	55	XXXXXXXXXXXXXXXXXXXXXXXXXX*X
CALCIUM	MG	126.0	0.52	28	XXXXXXXXXXXXX*
IRON	MG	3.4	0.45	24	XXXXXXXXXXX*

****

FIG. 11.4. ARABIC BREAD 420 GRAMS

NUTRIENT	UNIT	AMOUNT	INQ	STD %	0	25%	50%	75%	100%
ENERGY	KCAL	1194.6	1.00	54	XXXXXXXXXXXXXXXXXXXXXXXXXXXX				
PROTEIN	G	25.1	1.59	86	XXXXXXXXXXXXXXXXXXXXXXXXXXXXX*XXXXXXXXXXXXXXXXXX				
VITAMIN A	IU	0.0	0.00	0			*		
VITAMIN C	MG	0.0	0.00	0			*		
THIAMIN	MG	0.2	0.47	26	XXXXXXXXXXXXX		*		
RIBOFLAVIN	MG	0.1	0.14	8	XXXX		*		
NIACIN	MG	5.3	0.67	36	XXXXXXXXXXXXXXXXXX		*		
CALCIUM	MG	79.2	0.32	18	XXXXXXXXX		*		
IRON	MG	2.6	0.35	19	XXXXXXXXXX		*		

FIG. 11.5. RICE 330 GRAMS

The potential of whole milk (Figure 11.6) to contribute substantial amounts of riboflavin and calcium and high quality protein is obviously not being realized because of limited intake of milk (41 kcal). A fermented milk, leben (Figure 11.7) is consumed in slightly larger quantitiy (63 kcal), and would improve the diet if more were consumed. Cheese (Figure 11.8) is consumed in even more limited quantities—7 kcals. The nutritional benefits of cheese, leben, and milk to the diet of the Jordanians are obvious, but to be effective, they should be consumed in larger quantities.

So much for the breads and cereals and milk and milk products. From the vegetable category of foods at the time of this survey the onion (Figure 11.9) was consumed in quantities that are insufficient to contribute a substantial amount of nutrients in the diet with the exception of vitamin C.

Potatoes (Figure 11.10), on the other hand, furnished important amounts of nutrients to the Hebron, Jordan diet. Their contribution of only 124 kcals, supplied more than three-fourths of the vitamin C and appreciable quantities of many of the other nutrients (except vitamin A) in proportion to their energy which they supply.

From only 134 g intake daily (27 kcal), tomatoes (Figure 11.11) were the other major source of vitamin C in the diet in Hebron. Futhermore, tomatoes provide a substantial amount of vitamin A—well in excess of the energy supplied.

This nutrient density system of describing food quality appears to amplify the contribution of the fruits and vegetables, since they generally satisfy only a small portion of the daily caloric needs. Even so, in Hebron, Jordan 60 percent of the vitamin A and twice the recommended amount of vitamin C is derived from vegetable sources, illustrating the importance of consuming foods from various categories.

Eggs (Figure 11.12) have the potential to contribute a substantial quantity of nutrients to any diet, but they were consumed in Hebron in such small quantities that the potential benefit was not realized.

The principal meat source was lamb (Figure 11.13) (653 kcal) which provides high quality protein, abundant amounts of niacin, iron, thiamin and riboflavin and not shown are significant amounts of trace minerals. Lamb thus is an important component of the food supply and parellels what beef, pork and chicken provide in the U.S. diet.

Foods such as olives (Figure 11.14) that were consumed in a limited quantity contribute more to aesthetic pleasure or taste than they do to meeting substantial nutrient needs. About 57 kcals daily were derived from butter in Hebron (Figure 11.15), which carries in addition to energy, a noticeable amount of vitamin A. Vegetable oil (Figure 11.16) was consumed in much more substantive quantities (486 kcal). Vegetable oils were probably an important source of vitamin E but available analyt-

NUTRIENT	UNIT	AMOUNT	INQ	STD %	0	25%	50%	75%	100%
ENERGY	KCAL	40.8	1.00	2	X				
PROTEIN	G	2.1	3.90	7	*XXX				
VITAMIN A	IU	96.0	2.07	4	*X				
VITAMIN C	MG	0.6	1.08	2	*				
THIAMIN	MG	<0.1	1.44	3	*X				
RIBOFLAVIN	MG	0.1	4.23	8	*XXX				
NIACIN	MG	0.1	0.22	<1					
CALCIUM	MG	70.8	8.48	16	*XXXXX				
IRON	MG	0.1	0.23	<1					

****

FIG. 11.6. WHOLE MILK 60 GRAMS

NUTRIENT	UNIT	AMOUNT	INQ	STD %	0	25%	50%	75%	100%
ENERGY	KCAL	63.3	1.00	3	XX				
PROTEIN	G	3.5	4.14	12	X*XXXX				
VITAMIN A	IU	379.5	5.28	15	X*XXXXXX				
VITAMIN C	MG	0.0	0.00	0	*				
THIAMIN	MG	0.1	4.00	12	X*XXXX				
RIBOFLAVIN	MG	0.2	6.46	19	X*XXXXXXXX				
NIACIN	MG	0.2	0.55	2	X*				
CALCIUM	MG	161.0	12.44	36	X*XXXXXXXXXXXXXXXXX				
IRON	MG	0.1	0.29	1	X*				

****

FIG. 11.7. LEBEN 115 GRAMS

NUTRIENT	UNIT	AMOUNT	INQ	STD %	0	25%	50%	75%	100%
ENERGY	KCAL	6.9	1.00	<1					
PROTEIN	G	0.5	5.61	2	X				
VITAMIN A	IU	48.0	6.12	2	X				
VITAMIN C	MG	0.0	0.00	0					
THIAMIN	MG	<0.1	1.06	<1					
RIBOFLAVIN	MG	<0.1	3.16	1	X				
NIACIN	MG	<0.1	0.07	<1					
CALCIUM	MG	3.2	2.23	1	X				
IRON	MG	<0.1	0.27	<1					

****

FIG. 11.8. CHEESE 3 GRAMS

NUTRIENT	UNIT	AMOUNT	INQ	STD %	0	25%	50%	75%	100%
ENERGY	KCAL	6.8	1.00	<1					
PROTEIN	G	0.2	2.36	1	X				
VITAMIN A	IU	7.5	0.98	<1					
VITAMIN C	MG	1.4	14.67	4	XX				
THIAMIN	MG	<0.1	1.63	<1					
RIBOFLAVIN	MG	<0.1	1.50	<1					
NIACIN	MG	<0.1	0.67	<1					
CALCIUM	MG	4.8	3.48	1	X				
IRON	MG	0.8	1.75	1	X				

****

FIG. 11.9. MATURE ONION 15 GRAMS

NUTRIENT	UNIT	AMOUNT	INQ	STD %	0	25%	50%	75%	100%
ENERGY	KCAL	123.7	1.00	6	XXX				
PROTEIN	G	3.0	1.83	10	XX*XX				
VITAMIN A	IU	29.8	0.21	1	X *				
VITAMIN C	MG	25.3	15.02	84	XX*XXXXXXXXXXXXXXXXXXXXXXXXXXXXXXXXXXXXXXXXXXX				
THIAMIN	MG	0.2	3.24	18	XX*XXXXXX				
RIBOFLAVIN	MG	0.1	0.82	5	XX*				
NIACIN	MG	1.8	2.19	12	XX*XXX				
CALCIUM	MG	16.4	0.65	4	XX*				
IRON	MG	1.0	1.33	7	XX*X				

****

FIG. 11.10. POTATOES 149 GRAMS

NUTRIENT	UNIT	AMOUNT	INQ	STD %	0	25%	50%	75%	100%
ENERGY	KCAL	26.8	1.00	1	X				
PROTEIN	G	1.3	3.79	5	*XX				
VITAMIN A	IU	1474.0	48.40	59	*XXXXXXXXXXXXXXXXXXXXXXXXXXX				
VITAMIN C	MG	30.8	84.33	103	*XXXXXXXXXXXXXXXXXXXXXXXXXXXXXXXXXXXXXXXXXXXXXXX * 103%				
THIAMIN	MG	0.1	7.33	9	*XXXX				
RIBOFLAVIN	MG	0.1	3.38	4	*X				
NIACIN	MG	0.7	3.79	5	*XX				
CALCIUM	MG	14.7	2.69	3	*X				
IRON	MG	0.8	4.71	6	*XXXXX				

****

FIG. 11.11. TOMATOES 134 GRAMS

NUTRIENT	UNIT	AMOUNT	INQ	STD %	0	25%	50%	75%	100%
ENERGY	KCAL	29.2	1.00	1	X				
PROTEIN	G	2.3	5.99	8	*XXX				
VITAMIN A	IU	205.2	6.19	8	*XXX				
VITAMIN C	MG	0.0	0.00	0	-				
THIAMIN	MG	<0.1	1.51	2	*				
RIBOFLAVIN	MG	<0.1	3.03	4	*X				
NIACIN	MG	<0.1	0.09	<1					
CALCIUM	MG	9.7	1.63	2	*				
IRON	MG	0.5	2.62	3	*X				

****

FIG. 11.12. EGGS 18 GRAMS

NUTRIENT	UNIT	AMOUNT	INQ	STD %	0	25%	50%	75%	100%
ENERGY	KCAL	653.0	1.00	30	XXXXXXXXXXXXXXXX				
PROTEIN	G	32.3	3.76	112	XXXXXXXXXXXXXXX*XXXXXXXXXXXXXXXXXXXXXXXXXXXXXXXXXX			*	112%
VITAMIN A	IU	0.0	0.00	0	*				
VITAMIN C	MG	0.0	0.00	0	*				
THIAMIN	MG	0.3	1.08	32	XXXXXXXXXXXXXXXX*X				
RIBOFLAVIN	MG	0.4	1.07	32	XXXXXXXXXXXXXXXX*X				
NIACIN	MG	9.3	2.15	64	XXXXXXXXXXXXXXX*XXXXXXXXXXXXXXXXXX				
CALCIUM	MG	18.6	0.14	4	XX *				
IRON	MG	4.9	1.19	35	XXXXXXXXXXXXXXX*XXXXXXXXXXXXXXXXXXXXXX				

****

FIG. 11.13. LAMB 206 GRAMS

NUTRIENT	UNIT	AMOUNT	INQ	STD %	0	25%	50%	75%	100%
ENERGY	KCAL	21.1	1.00	1	X				
PROTEIN	G	0.2	0.86	1	*				
VITAMIN A	IU	48.0	2.00	2	*				
VITAMIN C	MG	0.0	0.00	0	*				
THIAMIN	MG	<0.1	0.37	<1					
RIBOFLAVIN	MG	<0.1	2.31	2	*				
NIACIN	MG	0.1	0.80	1	*				
CALCIUM	MG	13.9	3.22	3	*X				
IRON	MG	0.3	1.90	2	*				

****

FIG. 11.14. OLIVES 16 GRAMS

NUTRIENT	UNIT	AMOUNT	INQ	STD %	0	25%	50%	75%	100%
ENERGY	KCAL	57.3	1.00	3	XX				
PROTEIN	G	<0.1	0.06	<1	*				
VITAMIN A	IU	264.0	4.06	11	X*XXXX				
VITAMIN C	MG	0.0	0.00	0	*				
THIAMIN	MG	0.0	0.00	0	*				
RIBOFLAVIN	MG	<0.1	0.02	<1	*				
NIACIN	MG	<0.1	0.02	<1	*				
CALCIUM	MG	1.6	0.14	<1	*				
IRON	MG	0.0	0.00	0	*				

****

FIG. 11.15. BUTTER 8 GRAMS

NUTRIENT	UNIT	AMOUNT	INQ	STD %	0	25%	50%	75%	100%
ENERGY	KCAL	485.7	1.00	22	XXXXXXXXXX				
PROTEIN	G	0.0	0.00	0	*				
VITAMIN A	IU	0.0	0.00	0	*				
VITAMIN C	MG	0.0	0.00	0	*				
THIAMIN	MG	0.0	0.00	0	*				
RIBOFLAVIN	MG	0.0	0.00	0	*				
NIACIN	MG	0.0	0.00	0	*				
CALCIUM	MG	0.0	0.00	0	*				
IRON	MG	0.0	0.00	0	*				

****

FIG. 11.16. VEGETABLE OIL 55 GRAMS

ical data with respect to vitamin E are too limited to permit a nutrient density analysis. Molasses (Figure 11.17) was consumed in a small quantity (28 kcals) and, in addition to energy, yields a small amount of calcium and iron. Molasses, which is largely sugar, contains calcium and iron as a consequence of processing techniques used. Sugar (Figure 11.18) constituted about 10 percent of calories, somewhat modest in comparison with diets in Europe or the U.S. and obviously the only nutrient derived from sugar is energy.

In summary, the nutritional index for the Hebron, Jordan diet is arrived at by adding all the individual food profiles for each food consumed in the amount given. For those whose intake of food is in the 2,000 to 3,000 kcal range, if the observed food consumption pattern persisted for any length of time a deficit in intake of some of the nutrients should be expected to result as shown by nutrients whose INQs are less than 1.0 (vitamin A, riboflavin, calcium and iron).

CONCLUSION

Until recently, dietary factors generally have been treated as of second line of order of importance, and only in the last year or two have we seen attempts to find ways to *include nutrition in policy planning* at the national and international levels.

REFERENCES

INTERDEPARTMENTAL COMMITTEE ON NUTRITION FOR NATIONAL DEFENSE. 1963. The Hashemite Kingdom of Jordan Nutrition Survey April—June 1962. Washington, D.C.

INTERDEPARTMENTAL COMMITTEE ON NUTRITION FOR NATIONAL DEFENSE. 1965. Northeast Brazil—Nutrition Survey March-May 1963. Washington, D.C.

VARELA, R.M., TEIXEIRA, S.G. and BATISTA, M.   1972. Hypovitaminosis A in the sugar cane zone of Southern Pernambuco State, Northeast Brazil. Amer. J. Clin. Nutr. 25: 800.

NUTRIENT	UNIT	AMOUNT	INQ	STD %	0	25%	50%	75%	100%
ENERGY	KCAL	27.8	1.00	1	X				
PROTEIN	G	0.0	0.00	0					
VITAMIN A	IU	0.0	0.00	0					
VITAMIN C	MG	0.0	0.00	0					
THIAMIN	MG	0.0	0.00	0					
RIBOFLAVIN	MG	0.0	0.00	0					
NIACIN	MG	0.0	0.00	0					
CALCIUM	MG	34.8	6.11	8	*XXX				
IRON	MG	0.7	4.06	5	*XX				

****

FIG. 11.17. MOLASSES 12 GRAMS

NUTRIENT	UNIT	AMOUNT	INQ	STD %	0	25%	50%	75%	100%
ENERGY	KCAL	215.6	1.00	10	XXXXX				
PROTEIN	G	0.0	0.00	0	*				
VITAMIN A	IU	0.0	0.00	0	*				
VITAMIN C	MG	0.0	0.00	0	*				
THIAMIN	MG	0.0	0.00	0	*				
RIBOFLAVIN	MG	0.0	0.00	0	*				
NIACIN	MG	0.0	0.00	0	*				
CALCIUM	MG	0.0	0.00	0	*				
IRON	MG	0.0	0.00	0	*				

****

FIG. 11.18. SUGAR 56 GRAMS

PART II
Index of Nutritional Quality
Food Profiles

12

Index of Nutritional Quality – Food Profiles

INTRODUCTION

The nutritional quality of any food or diet is a function of its nutrient components such as protein, vitamins and minerals as related to the specific nutrient needs of an individual. In the next section a concept called the Index of Nutritional Quality (INQ) is used to illustrate the nutritional content of foods. The Index of Nutritional Quality examines the nutritional quality of foods by relating the nutrients in foods to the kilocalories they contain. By using the INQ, an individual can simultaneously derive qualitative and quantitive evaluations of foods and food combinations such as menus and diets.

The food composition nutrient data in this manual were drawn from the Home and Garden Bulletin No. 72 of the U.S. Department of Agriculture. The calculations for the food profile graphs were based on the values shown on page 176 and a 2000 kcal requirement. The nutrient standards were derived from the Recommended Dietary Allowances of the Food and Nutrition Board of the National Academy of Sciences, expressed per 1000 kilocalories. The values cited are largely based on the allowances established for individuals whose nutrient-to-energy needs were greatest.These values were multiplied by two to obtain allowances per 2000 kilocalories. The potassium standard was calculated to provide a 1 to 1 molecular weight ratio when compared with sodium with the latter standard arbitrarily set at 3000 mg per 2000 kilocalories. This represents a sodium chloride intake of 7.5 g. The fat standard was established at 35 percent of 2000 kilocalories or 78 g. The P/S ratio was set at 0.7 with oleic fatty acids providing 11 percent of kilocalories, linoleic fatty acid providing 9 percent of kilocalories and saturated fatty acids providing 12.8 percent of kilocalories.

Nutritionists often use the terms "energy," "calories," and "kilocalories" (kcal) interchangeably. Energy comes from the assimilation of foods and is measured in terms of calories which are more correctly called kilocalories. To provide energy, foods must contain kilocalories. In the following section, we use energy to express the kilocalories provided by foods.

Examples: On page 201 you will find the nutrient profile for 1 cup of fluid whole milk (Item 50). The line beginning with the word "ENERGY" indicates that one cup of milk contains 150 kilocalories of energy or 8% of an adult's daily need (2000 kilocalories). The cup of milk also provides 8 grams of protein, which is 16% of the standard for protein.

To transform this information into an Index of Nutritional Quality or INQ for protein in milk, we divide the milk's percent of the standard for protein, i.e., 16%, by its percent of the standard for energy, i.e., 8%.This would equal 2. This means that a glass of milk provides twice as much of the protein required by an adult as of the required energy.

$$INQ = \frac{\% \text{ standard of nutrient}}{\% \text{ standard of energy}}$$

If we evaluate the other nutrients in milk using the same process, we find: vitamin A (INQ= 1.03), thiamin (INQ= 1.2), riboflavin (INQ= 4.44), phosphorus (INQ= 3.38), and calcium (INQ= 4.31). The other nutrients vitamin C (INQ= 0.44), niacin (INQ= 0.19), iron (INQ= 0.0810), and potassium (INQ= 0.99) have INQs less than 1.0.

An INQ of 1.0 or greater for any of these nutrients in a specified food indicates that the food supplies adequate amounts of that nutrient in comparison to the number of kilocalories it provides. If that food supplies a substantial number of nutrients with INQs for these nutrients of 1.0 or greater, it is of good nutritional quality. The nutrients that have INQs of less than 1.0, would have to be supplemented by other foods during the day. The Complementary Foods List in Part III of this book identify foods relatively high in particular nutrients.

The last five nutrients in the profile cannot be evaluated in this manner. Carbohydrate supplies energy and is important in the diet for this reason. The amount of carbohydrate is determined after providing adequate amounts of protein and providing fat within the 35 percent limitation. Ideally at the end of the day one should have consumed a combination of foods which does not exceed the calorie standard—nor contribute a disproportionate amount of the calorie-providing nutrients, i.e., protein, carbohydrate and fat.

USES

This book can be used to plan menus or to evaluate either a menu or a day's intake of food. Line up the enclosed plastic overlay over the food you wish to evaluate. Place the word ENERGY on the plastic overlay over the word ENERGY of the food being evaluated. Then, with a water-soluble, non-permanent marking pencil fill in the length of the bar corresponding to nutrient provided by the food. Additional foods can then be evaluated as follows: line up each one as you did originally, but move the plastic overlay to the left until the end of the marked line on the overlay is at the beginning of the ENERGY line for the new food. Using the marking pencil extend the ENERGY line to indicate the amount contributed by the food. Proceed similarly for each nutrient in each food being considered. If all positive nutrient lines exceed the energy line when all the foods being considered have been tabulated, the meal would be well-balanced.

To be valid, a tabulation must include such items as spreads used on breads and potatoes, jellies, or jams, sugar in beverages, etc. As an example of how the overlay works, consider a meal consisting of 1 cup skimmed milk, 1 cup tomato soup, and a brownie (Table 12.1).

The nutritional quality of the meal is seen when the length of each nutrient bar is compared to the length of the energy bar. This meal is adequate (nutrient bars longer than energy bar) in vitamins A, C, and thiamin, riboflavin and calcium and phosphorus. But it is inadequate relative to niacin, iron and potassium (bars shorter than energy bar). Though providing more protein than the standard, the meal provides reasonable amounts of carbohydrate and fat. The P to S ratio appears to be at least 0.7 and probably a little higher since the linoleic acid line is slightly longer than the saturated fatty acid line. Other meals and snacks for the day of this lunch should include foods that would extend all nutrient bars to 100% of the day's requirement.

The length of the energy line should be geared to individual needs. Some individuals like inactive adult women and young children may not require 2000 kcal per day. Although nutrient lines need to reach the 100% mark each day, the energy line may need to be curtailed below 100% (2000 kcal) to prevent weight gain or promote weight loss. Conversely, for teenage boys and physically active men the energy line may have to exceed the 100% mark in order to maintain weight.

TABLE 12.1. Your plastic overlay would look like this after being filled in for the skimmed milk (with **XXX**'s substituting for a solid inked bar).

Nutrient	0	10	20	30	40	50	60	70	80	90	100
ENERGY	XXX										
VITAMIN A	XXXXXXXXXX										
VITAMIN C	XXX										
THIAMIN	XXXXXXX										
RIBOFLAVIN	XXXXXXXXXXXXXXXXXXXXXXXXXXX										
NIACIN	X										
IRON	X										
CALCIUM	XXXXXXXXXXXXXXXXXXXXXXXXXXXXXX										
PHOSPHORUS	XXXXXXXXXXXXXXXXXXXXXX										
POTASSIUM	XXXXXX										
PROTEIN	XXXXXXXXXXXXX										
CARBOHYDRATE	XXX										
FAT											
OLEIC A											
LINOL A											
SAT FAT A	X										

The tomato soup's nutrients indicated by (---'s) would make your overlay appear as below.

```
Nutrient      0    10    20    30    40    50    60    70    80    90    100

ENERGY        XXX----
VITAMIN A     XXXXXXXXXXXX------------------
VITAMIN C     XXX-------------
THIAMIN       XXXXXX----
RIBOFLAVIN    XXXXXXXXXXXXXXXXXXXXXXXXXXXXX----
NIACIN        X-------
IRON          X-----
CALCIUM       XXXXXXXXXXXXXXXXXXXXXXXXXXXXXXX-
PHOSPHORUS    XXXXXXXXXXXXXXXXXXXXXXXXX---
POTASSIUM     XXXXXX----
PROTEIN       XXXXXXXXXXXX----
CARBOHYDRATE  XXX----
FAT           --
OLEIC A       --
LINOL A       --
SAT FAT A     X-
```

After adding the nutrients in a brownie (000's), your overlay would look like this:

```
Nutrient      0    10    20    30    40    50    60    70    80    90   100

ENERGY        XXX----0000
VITAMIN A     XXXXXXXXXXXX-----------------0
VITAMIN C     XXX-------------
THIAMIN       XXXXXX----000
RIBOFLAVIN    XXXXXXXXXXXXXXXXXXXXXXXXXX----00
NIACIN        X------0
IRON          X----00
CALCIUM       XXXXXXXXXXXXXXXXXXXXXXXXXXXXX-0
PHOSPHORUS    XXXXXXXXXXXXXXXXXXXXXXXXXX---000
POTASSIUM     XXXXXX---0
PROTEIN       XXXXXXXXXXXX---00
CARBOHYDRATE  XXX-----000
FAT           --000000
OLEIC A       --0000000000
LINOL A       ---00000
SAT FAT A     X-0000
```

TABLE OF FOOD PROFILES*

*See page 625 for alphabetical list of all food by name for reading location in text.

****

NUTRIENT PROFILE ANALYSIS OF FOODS FROM

THE HOME AND GARDEN BULLETIN NO.72-1

****

SOURCE: NUTRITIVE VALUE OF FOODS; HOME & GARDEN BULLETIN NO.72-1 REVISED 1977

CALCULATIONS BASED ON -- THE FOLLOWING VALUES

ENERGY	2000.00KCAL	VITAMIN A	4000.00 IU	VITAMIN C	60.00 MG	THIAMIN	1.00 MG	RIBOFLAVN	1.20 MG
NIACIN	14.00 MG	IRON	16.00 MG	CALCIUM	900.00 MG	PHOSPHRUS	900.00 MG	PUTASSIUM	5000.00 MG
PROTEIN	50.00 G	CARBOHYDT	275.00 G	FAT	78.00 G	OLEIC A	24.50 G	LINOL A	20.00 G
SAT FAT A	28.50 G								

1 BLUE CHEESE
ANALYSIS OF 28 GRAMS WHICH IS 1 OZ

NUTRIENT	UNIT	AMOUNT	INQ	% STD	0 10 20 30 40 50 60 70 80 90 100
ENERGY	KCAL	100.00	1.00	5	EEEE
VITAMIN A	IU	200.00	1.00	5	AAAA
VITAMIN C	MG	0.00	0.00	0	-
THIAMIN	MG	0.01	0.20	1	T	
RIBOFLAVN	MG	0.11	1.83	9	RRR|RRR
NIACIN	MG	0.30	0.43	2	NN	
IRON	MG	0.10	0.13	1	I	
CALCIUM	MG	150.00	3.33	17	KKK|KKKKKKKK
PHOSPHRUS	MG	110.00	2.44	12	XXX|XXXXX
POTASSIUM	MG	73.00	0.29	1	Y	
PROTEIN	G	6.00	2.40	12	PPP|PPPPP
CARBOHYDT	G	1.00	0.07	0	-
FAT	G	8.00	2.05	10	FFF|FFFF
OLEIC A	G	1.90	1.55	8	OOO|OO
LINOL A	G	0.20	0.20	1	L	
SAT FAT A	G	5.30	3.72	19	SSS|SSSSSSSSSS

****

2 CAMEMBERT CHEESE
ANALYSIS OF 38 GRAMS WHICH IS 1 WEDGE

NUTRIENT	UNIT	AMOUNT	INQ	% STD	0 10 20 30 40 50 60 70 80 90 100
ENERGY	KCAL	115.00	1.00	6	EEEEE
VITAMIN A	IU	350.00	1.52	9	AAAA|AA
VITAMIN C	MG	0.00	0.00	0	-
THIAMIN	MG	0.01	0.17	1	T	
RIBOFLAVN	MG	0.19	2.75	16	RRRR|RRRRRRR
NIACIN	MG	0.20	0.25	1	N	
IRON	MG	0.10	0.11	1	I	
CALCIUM	MG	147.00	2.84	16	KKKK|KKKKKKK
PHOSPHRUS	MG	132.00	2.55	15	XXXX|XXXXXX
POTASSIUM	MG	71.00	0.25	1	Y	
PROTEIN	G	8.00	2.78	16	PPPP|PPPPPPP
CARBOHYDT	G	0.00	0.00	0	-
FAT	G	9.00	2.01	12	FFFF|FFFF
OLEIC A	G	2.20	1.56	9	OOOO|OO
LINOL A	G	0.17	0.17	1	L	
SAT FAT A	G	5.80	3.54	20	SSSS|SSSSSSSSS

****

3   CHEDDAR CHEESE
ANALYSIS OF 28 GRAMS WHICH IS 1 OZ

NUTRIENT	UNIT	AMOUNT	INQ	% STD	0	10	20
ENERGY	KCAL	115.00	1.00	6	EEEEE		
VITAMIN A	IU	300.00	1.30	8	AAAIA		
VITAMIN C	MG	0.00	0.00	0	-		
THIAMIN	MG	0.01	0.17	1	T		
RIBOFLAVN	MG	0.11	1.59	9	RRRIRR		
NIACIN	MG	0.00	0.00	0	-		
IRON	MG	0.20	0.22	1	I		
CALCIUM	MG	204.00	3.94	23	KKKKIKKKKKKKKKKKK		
PHOSPHRUS	MG	145.00	2.80	16	XXXXIXXXXXXXX		
POTASSIUM	MG	28.00	0.10	1	-		
PROTEIN	G	7.00	2.43	14	PPPPIPPPPP		
CARBOHYDT	G	0.00	0.00	0	-		
FAT	G	9.00	2.01	12	FFFFIFFFF		
OLEIC A	G	2.10	1.49	9	OOOOIOO		
LINOL A	G	0.20	0.17	1	L		
SAT FAT A	G	6.10	3.72	21	SSSSISSSSSSSSSSSS		

4   CHEDDAR CHEESE
ANALYSIS OF 17 GRAMS WHICH IS 1 CUBIC INCH

NUTRIENT	UNIT	AMOUNT	INQ	% STD	0	10	20
ENERGY	KCAL	70.00	1.00	4	EEE		
VITAMIN A	IU	180.00	1.29	5	AAIA		
VITAMIN C	MG	0.00	0.00	0	-		
THIAMIN	MG	0.00	0.00	0	-		
RIBOFLAVN	MG	0.06	1.43	5	RRIR		
NIACIN	MG	0.00	0.00	0	-		
IRON	MG	0.10	0.18	1	I		
CALCIUM	MG	124.00	3.94	14	KKIKKKKKKK		
PHOSPHRUS	MG	88.00	2.79	10	XXIXXXXX		
POTASSIUM	MG	17.00	0.10	0	-		
PROTEIN	G	4.00	2.29	8	PPIPPP		
CARBOHYDT	G	0.00	0.00	0	-		
FAT	G	6.00	2.20	8	FFIFFF		
OLEIC A	G	1.30	1.52	5	OOIO		
LINOL A	G	0.10	0.14	1	-		
SAT FAT A	G	3.70	3.71	13	SSISSSSSS		

5 CHEDDAR CHEESE
ANALYSIS OF 113 GRAMS WHICH IS 1 CUP SHREDDED

```
                                0        10        20        30        40        50        60        70        80        90       100
                                *         *         *         *         *         *         *         *         *         *         *
NUTRIENT   UNIT  AMOUNT   INQ  %STD
ENERGY     KCAL  455.00   1.00   23   EEEEEEEEEEEEEEE
VITAMIN A  IU   1200.00   1.32   30   AAAAAAAAAAAAAAAAAAAIAAAAA
VITAMIN C  MG      0.00   0.00    0
THIAMIN    MG      0.03   0.13    3   TT
RIBOFLAVN  MG      0.42   1.54   35   RRRRRRRRRRRRRRRRIRRRRRRRR
NIACIN     MG      0.10   0.03    1   N
IRON       MG      0.80   0.22    5   IIII
CALCIUM    MG    815.00   3.98   91   KKKKKKKKKKKKKKKKKIKKKKKKKKKKKKKKKKKKKKKKKKKKKKKKK
PHOSPHRUS  MG    579.00   2.83   64   XXXXXXXXXXXXXXXXXIXXXXXXXXXXXXXXXXXX
POTASSIUM  MG    111.00   0.10    2   YY
PROTEIN    G      28.00   2.46   56   PPPPPPPPPPPPPPPPPIPPPPPPPPPPPPP
CARBOHYDT  G       1.00   0.02    0   -
FAT        G      37.00   2.09   47   FFFFFFFFFFFFFFFFFIFFFFFFFFFF
OLEIC A    G       8.50   1.53   35   OOOOOOOOOOOOOOOOIOOOOOOOO
LINOL A    G       0.70   0.15    4   LLL
SAT FAT A  G      24.20   3.73   85   SSSSSSSSSSSSSSSSSISSSSSSSSSSSSSSSSSSSSSSSSSSSS
*******************************************
```

6 COTTAGE CHEESE, CREAMED (4% FAT), LG CURD
ANALYSIS OF 225 GRAMS WHICH IS 1 CUP

```
                                0        10        20        30        40        50        60        70        80        90       100
                                *         *         *         *         *         *         *         *         *         *         *
NUTRIENT   UNIT  AMOUNT   INQ  %STD
ENERGY     KCAL  235.00   1.00   12   EEEEEEEE
VITAMIN A  IU    370.00   0.79    9   AAAAAAA
VITAMIN C  MG      0.00   0.00    0
THIAMIN    MG      0.05   0.43    5   TTTT
RIBOFLAVN  MG      0.37   2.62   31   RRRRRRRRIRRRRRRRRRRRRRRRRRR
NIACIN     MG      0.30   0.18    2   NN
IRON       MG      0.30   0.16    2   II
CALCIUM    MG    135.00   1.28   15   KKKKKKKIKKK
PHOSPHRUS  MG    297.00   2.81   33   XXXXXXXXIXXXXXXXXXXXXXXXX
POTASSIUM  MG    190.00   0.32    4   YYY
PROTEIN    G      28.00   4.77   56   PPPPPPPIPPPPPPPPPPPPPPPPPPPPPPPPPPPPPPPPPPPPPP
CARBOHYDT  G       6.00   0.19    2   HH
FAT        G      10.00   1.09   13   FFFFFFFFF
OLEIC A    G       2.40   0.83   10   OOOOOOOO
LINOL A    G       0.20   0.09    1   L
SAT FAT A  G       6.40   1.91   22   SSSSSSSSISSSSSSSS
*******************************************
```

7 COTTAGE CHEESE, CREAMED (4% FAT), SM CURD
ANALYSIS OF 210 GRAMS WHICH IS 1 CUP

NUTRIENT	UNIT	AMOUNT	INQ	% STD
ENERGY	KCAL	220.00	1.00	11
VITAMIN A	IU	340.00	0.77	9
VITAMIN C	MG	0.00	0.00	0
THIAMIN	MG	0.04	0.36	4
RIBOFLAVN	MG	0.34	2.58	28
NIACIN	MG	0.30	0.19	2
IRON	MG	0.30	0.17	2
CALCIUM	MG	126.00	1.27	14
PHOSPHRUS	MG	277.00	2.80	31
POTASSIUM	MG	177.00	0.32	4
PROTEIN	G	26.00	4.73	52
CARBOHYDT	G	6.00	0.20	2
FAT	G	9.00	1.05	12
OLEIC A	G	2.20	0.82	9
LINOL A	G	0.20	0.09	1
SAT FAT A	G	6.00	1.91	21

8 COTTAGE CHEESE, 2% FAT
ANALYSIS OF 226 GRAMS WHICH IS 1 CUP

NUTRIENT	UNIT	AMOUNT	INQ	% STD
ENERGY	KCAL	205.00	1.00	10
VITAMIN A	IU	160.00	0.39	4
VITAMIN C	MG	0.00	0.00	0
THIAMIN	MG	0.05	0.49	5
RIBOFLAVN	MG	0.42	3.41	35
NIACIN	MG	0.30	0.21	2
IRON	MG	0.40	0.24	3
CALCIUM	MG	155.00	1.68	17
PHOSPHRUS	MG	340.00	3.69	38
POTASSIUM	MG	217.00	0.42	4
PROTEIN	G	31.00	6.05	62
CARBOHYDT	G	8.00	0.28	3
FAT	G	4.00	0.50	5
OLEIC A	G	1.00	0.10	4
LINOL A	G	0.10	0.05	1
SAT FAT A	G	2.80	0.96	10

9 COTTAGE CHEESE, 1% FAT
ANALYSIS OF 226 GRAMS WHICH IS 1 CUP

NUTRIENT	UNIT	AMOUNT	INQ	% STD	0 10 20 30 40 50 60 70 80 90 100
ENERGY	KCAL	165.00	1.00	8	EEEEEEE
VITAMIN A	IU	80.00	0.24	2	AA
VITAMIN C	MG	0.00	0.00	0	-
THIAMIN	MG	0.05	0.61	5	TTTT
RIBOFLAVN	MG	0.37	3.74	31	RRRRRRRRRRRRRRRRRRRRR
NIACIN	MG	0.30	0.26	2	NN
IRON	MG	0.30	0.23	2	II
CALCIUM	MG	138.00	1.86	15	KKKKKK
PHOSPHRUS	MG	302.00	4.07	34	XXXXXXXXXXXXXXXXXXXXXXXX
POTASSIUM	MG	193.00	0.47	4	YYY
PROTEIN	G	28.00	6.79	56	PPPPPPPPPPPPPPPPPPPPPPPPPPPPPPPPPPPPPPPP
CARBOHYDT	G	6.00	0.26	2	HH
FAT	G	2.00	0.31	3	FF
OLEIC A	G	0.50	0.25	2	OO
LINOL A	G	0.10	0.06	1	-
SAT FAT A	G	1.50	0.64	5	SSSS

10 COTTAGE CHEESE, UNCREAMED (LESS THAN 0.5% FAT)
ANALYSIS OF 145 GRAMS WHICH IS 1 CUP

NUTRIENT	UNIT	AMOUNT	INQ	% STD	0 10 20 30 40 50 60 70 80 90 100
ENERGY	KCAL	125.00	1.00	6	EEEEE
VITAMIN A	IU	40.00	0.16	1	A
VITAMIN C	MG	0.00	0.00	0	-
THIAMIN	MG	0.04	0.64	4	TTT
RIBOFLAVN	MG	0.21	2.80	17	RRRRRRRRRR
NIACIN	MG	0.20	0.23	1	N
IRON	MG	0.30	0.30	2	II
CALCIUM	MG	46.00	0.82	5	KKKK
PHOSPHRUS	MG	151.00	2.68	17	XXXXXXXXX
POTASSIUM	MG	47.00	0.15	1	Y
PROTEIN	G	25.00	8.00	50	PPPPPPPPPPPPPPPPPPPPPPPPPPPPPPPPPPPPP
CARBOHYDT	G	3.00	0.17	1	H
FAT	G	1.00	0.21	1	F
OLEIC A	G	0.10	0.07	0	-
LINOL A	G	0.00	0.00	0	-
SAT FAT A	G	0.40	0.22	1	S

11 CREAM CHEESE
ANALYSIS OF 28 GRAMS WHICH IS 1 OZ

NUTRIENT	UNIT	AMOUNT	INQ	% STD	Profile (0 — 100)
ENERGY	KCAL	100.00	1.00	5	EEEE
VITAMIN A	IU	400.00	2.00	10	AAAIAAAA
VITAMIN C	MG	0.00	0.00	0	-
THIAMIN	MG	0.00	0.00	0	-
RIBOFLAVN	MG	0.06	1.00	5	RRRR
NIACIN	MG	0.30	0.38	2	II
IRON	MG	0.30	0.38	2	II
CALCIUM	MG	23.00	0.51	3	KKI
PHOSPHRUS	MG	30.00	0.67	3	XXXI
POTASSIUM	MG	34.00	0.14	1	Y
PROTEIN	G	2.00	0.80	4	PPPI
CARBOHYDT	G	1.00	0.07	0	-
FAT	G	10.00	2.56	13	FFFIFFFFF
OLEIC A	G	2.40	1.96	10	OOOIOOOO
LINOL A	G	0.20	0.20	1	L
SAT FAT A	G	6.20	4.35	22	SSSISSSSSSSSSSS

12 MOZZARELLA CHEESE, MADE WITH WHOLE MILK
ANALYSIS OF 28 GRAMS WHICH IS 1 OZ

NUTRIENT	UNIT	AMOUNT	INQ	% STD	Profile (0 — 100)
ENERGY	KCAL	90.00	1.00	5	EEEE
VITAMIN A	IU	260.00	1.44	7	AAAIA
VITAMIN C	MG	0.00	0.00	0	-
THIAMIN	MG	0.00	0.00	0	-
RIBOFLAVN	MG	0.08	1.48	7	RRRIR
NIACIN	MG	0.00	0.00	0	-
IRON	MG	0.10	0.14	1	I-
CALCIUM	MG	163.00	4.02	18	KKKIKKKKKKKK
PHOSPHRUS	MG	117.00	2.89	13	XXXIXXXXX
POTASSIUM	MG	21.00	0.09	0	-
PROTEIN	G	6.00	2.67	12	PPPIPPPPP
CARBOHYDT	G	1.00	0.08	0	-
FAT	G	7.00	1.99	9	FFFIFFF
OLEIC A	G	1.70	1.54	7	OOOIOO
LINOL A	G	0.20	0.22	1	L
SAT FAT A	G	4.40	3.43	15	SSSISSSSSSSS

Scale axis: 0   10   20   30   40   50   60   70   80   90   100

13 MOZZARELLA CHEESE, MADE WITH SKIM MILK
ANALYSIS OF 28 GRAMS WHICH IS 1 OZ

NUTRIENT	UNIT	AMOUNT	INQ	% STD
ENERGY	KCAL	80.00	1.00	4
VITAMIN A	IU	180.00	1.13	5
VITAMIN C	MG	0.00	0.00	0
THIAMIN	MG	0.01	0.00	1
RIBOFLAVN	MG	0.10	2.08	8
NIACIN	MG	0.00	0.00	0
IRON	MG	0.10	0.16	1
CALCIUM	MG	207.00	5.75	23
PHOSPHRUS	MG	149.00	4.14	17
POTASSIUM	MG	27.00	0.14	1
PROTEIN	G	8.00	4.00	16
CARBOHYDT	G	1.00	0.09	0
FAT	G	5.00	1.60	6
OLEIC A	G	1.20	1.22	5
LINOL A	G	0.10	0.13	1
SAT FAT A	G	3.10	2.72	11

14 PARMESAN CHEESE, GRATED
ANALYSIS OF 100 GRAMS WHICH IS 1 CUP

NUTRIENT	UNIT	AMOUNT	INQ	% STD
ENERGY	KCAL	455.00	1.00	23
VITAMIN A	IU	700.00	0.77	17
VITAMIN C	MG	0.00	0.00	0
THIAMIN	MG	0.05	0.22	5
RIBOFLAVN	MG	0.39	1.43	33
NIACIN	MG	0.30	0.09	2
IRON	MG	1.00	0.27	6
CALCIUM	MG	1376.00	6.72	153
PHOSPHRUS	MG	807.00	3.94	90
POTASSIUM	MG	107.00	0.09	2
PROTEIN	G	42.00	3.63	84
CARBOHYDT	G	4.00	0.06	1
FAT	G	30.00	1.69	38
OLEIC A	G	7.70	1.38	31
LINOL A	G	0.30	0.07	2
SAT FAT A	G	19.10	2.95	67

15 PARMESAN CHEESE, GRATED
ANALYSIS OF 5 GRAMS WHICH IS 1 TBSP

NUTRIENT	UNIT	AMOUNT	INQ	% STD
ENERGY	KCAL	25.00	1.00	1
VITAMIN A	IU	40.00	0.80	1
VITAMIN C	MG	0.00	0.00	0
THIAMIN	MG	0.00	0.00	0
RIBOFLAVN	MG	0.02	1.33	2
NIACIN	MG	0.00	0.00	0
IRON	MG	0.00	0.00	0
CALCIUM	MG	69.00	6.13	8
PHOSPHRUS	MG	40.00	3.56	4
POTASSIUM	MG	5.00	0.08	0
PROTEIN	G	2.00	3.20	4
CARBOHYDT	G	0.00	0.00	3
FAT	G	2.00	2.05	3
OLEIC A	G	0.40	1.31	2
LINOL A	G	0.00	0.00	4
SAT FAT A	G	1.00	2.81	4

16 PARMESAN CHEESE, GRATED
ANALYSIS OF 28 GRAMS WHICH IS 1 OZ

NUTRIENT	UNIT	AMOUNT	INQ	% STD
ENERGY	KCAL	130.00	1.00	7
VITAMIN A	IU	200.00	0.77	5
VITAMIN C	MG	0.00	0.00	0
THIAMIN	MG	0.01	0.15	1
RIBOFLAVN	MG	0.11	1.41	9
NIACIN	MG	0.10	0.11	1
IRON	MG	0.30	0.29	2
CALCIUM	MG	390.00	6.67	43
PHOSPHRUS	MG	229.00	3.91	25
POTASSIUM	MG	30.00	0.09	0
PROTEIN	G	12.00	3.69	24
CARBOHYDT	G	1.00	0.06	0
FAT	G	9.00	1.78	12
OLEIC A	G	2.20	1.38	9
LINOL A	G	0.10	0.08	1
SAT FAT A	G	5.40	2.91	19

```
                                   0    10    20    30    40    50    60    70    80    90   100
                                   * *  * * * * * * * * * * * * * * * * * * *
17  PROVOLONE CHEESE
ANALYSIS OF 28 GRAMS WHICH IS 1 OZ

NUTRIENT   UNIT   AMOUNT   INQ    % STD    0    10    20    30    40    50    60    70    80    90   100
ENERGY     KCAL   100.00   1.00     5    EEEE
VITAMIN A  IU     230.00   1.15     6    AAA|A
VITAMIN C  MG       0.00   0.00     0    -|
THIAMIN    MG       0.01   0.20     1    T|
RIBOFLAVN  MG       0.09   1.50     8    RRR|RR
NIACIN     MG       0.00   0.00     0    -|
IRON       MG       0.10   0.13     1    I|
CALCIUM    MG     214.00   4.76    24    KKK|KKKKKKKKKKK
PHOSPHRUS  MG     141.00   3.13    16    XXX|XXXXXXXX
POTASSIUM  MG      39.00   0.16     1    Y|
PROTEIN    G        7.00   2.80    14    PPP|PPPPPP
CARBOHYDT  G        1.00   0.07     0    -|
FAT        G        8.00   2.05    10    FFF|FFFF
OLEIC A    G        1.70   1.39     7    OUO|OO
LINOL A    G        0.10   0.10     1    -|
SAT FAT A  G        4.80   3.37    17    SSS|SSSSSSSSS
*****************************************************

18  RICOTTA CHEESE, MADE WITH WHOLE MILK
ANALYSIS OF 246 GRAMS WHICH IS 1 CUP

NUTRIENT   UNIT   AMOUNT    INQ   % STD    0    10    20    30    40    50    60    70    80    90   100
ENERGY     KCAL    428.00   1.00    21   EEEEEEEEEEEEEEEE
VITAMIN A  IU     1210.00   1.41    30   AAAAAAAAAAAAAAA|AAAAAA
VITAMIN C  MG        0.00   0.00     0   -|
THIAMIN    MG        0.03   0.14     3   TT|
RIBOFLAVN  MG        0.48   1.87    40   RRRRRRRRRRRRRRRR|RRRRRRRRRRRRR
NIACIN     MG        0.30   0.10     2   NN|
IRON       MG        0.90   0.26     6   IIIII|
CALCIUM    MG      509.00   2.64    57   KKKKKKKKKKKKKKKK|KKKKKKXXXXXXXXXXXXX
PHOSPHRUS  MG      389.00   2.02    43   XXXXXXXXXXXXXXXX|XXXXXXXXXXXXXXX
POTASSIUM  MG      257.00   0.24     5   YYYY|
PROTEIN    G        28.00   2.62    56   PPPPPPPPPPPPPPPP|PPPPPPPPPPPPPPPPPPPPPP
CARBOHYDT  G         7.00   0.12     3   HH|
FAT        G        32.00   1.92    41   FFFFFFFFFFFFFFFF|FFFFFFFFFFFFFFF
OLEIC A    G         7.10   1.35    29   OOOOOOOOOOOOOOO|OOOOO
LINOL A    G         0.70   0.16     4   LLL|
SAT FAT A  G        20.40   3.34    72   SSSSSSSSSSSSSSSS|SSSSSSSSSSSSSSSSSSSSSSSSSSSSSSSSSSSSSSSSSSSSSSSSSSSSSSS
*****************************************************
```

19 RICOTTA CHEESE, MADE WITH PART SKIM MILK
ANALYSIS OF 246 GRAMS WHICH IS 1 CUP

NUTRIENT	UNIT	AMOUNT	INQ	% STD
ENERGY	KCAL	340.00	1.00	17
VITAMIN A	IU	1060.00	1.56	27
VITAMIN C	MG	0.00	0.00	0
THIAMIN	MG	0.05	0.29	5
RIBOFLAVN	MG	0.46	2.25	38
NIACIN	MG	0.20	0.08	1
IRON	MG	1.10	0.40	7
CALCIUM	MG	669.00	4.37	74
PHOSPHRUS	MG	449.00	2.93	50
POTASSIUM	MG	308.00	0.36	6
PROTEIN	G	28.00	3.29	56
CARBOHYDT	G	13.00	0.28	5
FAT	G	19.00	1.43	24
OLEIC A	G	4.70	1.13	19
LINOL A	G	0.50	0.15	3
SAT FAT A	G	12.10	2.50	42

20 ROMANO CHEESE
ANALYSIS OF 28 GRAMS WHICH IS 1 OZ

NUTRIENT	UNIT	AMOUNT	INQ	% STD
ENERGY	KCAL	110.00	1.00	6
VITAMIN A	IU	160.00	0.73	4
VITAMIN C	MG	0.00	0.00	0
THIAMIN	MG	0.00	0.00	0
RIBOFLAVN	MG	0.11	1.67	9
NIACIN	MG	0.00	0.00	0
IRON	MG	0.10	0.11	1
CALCIUM	MG	302.00	6.10	34
PHOSPHRUS	MG	215.00	4.34	24
POTASSIUM	MG	30.00	0.11	1
PROTEIN	G	9.00	3.27	18
CARBOHYDT	G	0.00	0.07	0
FAT	G	8.00	1.86	10
OLEIC A	G	0.80	0.59	3
LINOL A	G	0.10	0.09	1
SAT FAT A	G	2.40	1.53	8

21 SWISS CHEESE
ANALYSIS OF 28 GRAMS WHICH IS 1 OZ

```
                              0        10        20        30        40        50        60        70        80        90       100
                                                                                                                                  *********************
```

NUTRIENT	UNIT	AMOUNT	INQ	% STD
ENERGY	KCAL	105.00	1.00	5	EEEE
VITAMIN A	IU	240.00	1.14	6	AAA|A
VITAMIN C	MG	0.00	0.00	0	—|
THIAMIN	MG	0.01	0.19	1	T|
RIBOFLAVN	MG	0.10	1.59	8	RRR|RRR
NIACIN	MG	0.00	0.00	0	—|
IRON	MG	0.00	0.00	0	—|
CALCIUM	MG	272.00	5.76	30	KKK|KKKKKKKKKKKKKKKKKK
PHOSPHRUS	MG	171.00	3.62	19	XXX|XXXXXXXXXXX
POTASSIUM	MG	31.00	0.12	1	—|
PROTEIN	G	8.00	3.05	16	PPP|PPPPPPPPP
CARBOHYDT	G	1.00	0.07	0	—|
FAT	G	8.00	1.95	10	FFF|FFFF
OLEIC A	G	1.70	1.32	7	OOO|OO
LINOL A	G	0.20	0.19	1	—|
SAT FAT A	G	5.00	3.34	18	SSS|SSSSSSSSS

22 AMERICAN PASTEURIZED PROCESS CHEESE
ANALYSIS OF 28 GRAMS WHICH IS 1 OZ

```
                              0        10        20        30        40        50        60        70        80        90       100
                                                                                                                                  *********************
```

NUTRIENT	UNIT	AMOUNT	INQ	% STD
ENERGY	KCAL	105.00	1.00	5	EEEE
VITAMIN A	IU	340.00	1.62	9	AAA|AAA
VITAMIN C	MG	0.00	0.00	0	—|
THIAMIN	MG	0.01	0.19	1	T|
RIBOFLAVN	MG	0.10	1.59	8	RRR|RRR
NIACIN	MG	0.00	0.00	0	—|
IRON	MG	0.10	0.12	1	I|
CALCIUM	MG	174.00	3.68	19	KKK|KKKKKKKK
PHOSPHRUS	MG	211.00	4.47	23	XXX|XXXXXXXXXXXXXX
POTASSIUM	MG	46.00	0.18	1	Y|
PROTEIN	G	6.00	2.29	12	PPP|PPPPP
CARBOHYDT	G	0.00	0.00	0	—|
FAT	G	9.00	2.20	12	FFF|FFFFF
OLEIC A	G	2.10	1.63	9	OOO|OOO
LINOL A	G	0.20	0.19	1	L|
SAT FAT A	G	5.60	3.74	20	SSS|SSSSSSSSSS

23 SWISS PASTEURIZED PROCESS CHEESE
ANALYSIS OF 28 GRAMS WHICH IS 1 OZ

NUTRIENT	UNIT	AMOUNT	INQ	% STD
ENERGY	KCAL	95.00	1.00	5
VITAMIN A	IU	230.00	1.21	6
VITAMIN C	MG	0.00	0.00	0
THIAMIN	MG	0.00	0.00	0
RIBOFLAVN	MG	0.08	1.40	7
NIACIN	MG	0.00	0.00	0
IRON	MG	0.20	0.26	1
CALCIUM	MG	219.00	5.12	24
PHOSPHRUS	MG	216.00	5.05	24
POTASSIUM	MG	61.00	0.26	1
PROTEIN	G	7.00	2.95	14
CARBOHYDT	G	1.00	0.08	0
FAT	G	7.00	1.89	9
OLEIC A	G	1.70	1.46	7
LINOL A	G	0.10	0.11	1
SAT FAT A	G	4.50	3.32	16

24 AMERICAN PASTEURIZED PROCESS CHEESE FOOD
ANALYSIS OF 28 GRAMS WHICH IS 1 OZ

NUTRIENT	UNIT	AMOUNT	INQ	% STD
ENERGY	KCAL	95.00	1.00	5
VITAMIN A	IU	260.00	1.37	7
VITAMIN C	MG	0.00	0.00	0
THIAMIN	MG	0.01	0.21	1
RIBOFLAVN	MG	0.13	2.28	11
NIACIN	MG	0.00	0.00	0
IRON	MG	0.20	0.26	1
CALCIUM	MG	163.00	3.81	18
PHOSPHRUS	MG	130.00	3.04	14
POTASSIUM	MG	79.00	0.33	2
PROTEIN	G	6.00	2.53	12
CARBOHYDT	G	2.00	0.15	1
FAT	G	7.00	1.89	9
OLEIC A	G	1.70	1.46	7
LINOL A	G	0.10	0.11	1
SAT FAT A	G	4.40	3.25	15

25 AMERICAN PASTEURIZED PROCESS CHEESE SPREAD
ANALYSIS OF 28 GRAMS WHICH IS 1 OZ

NUTRIENT	UNIT	AMOUNT	INQ	% STD	0 10 20 30 40 50 60 70 80 90 100
ENERGY	KCAL	82.00	1.00	4	EEE
VITAMIN A	IU	220.00	1.34	6	AA|A
VITAMIN C	MG	0.00	0.00	0	- |
THIAMIN	MG	0.01	0.24	1	T |
RIBOFLAVN	MG	0.12	2.44	10	RR|RRRR
NIACIN	MG	0.00	0.00	0	- |
IRON	MG	0.10	0.15	1	I |
CALCIUM	MG	159.00	4.31	18	KK|KKKKKKKK
PHOSPHRUS	MG	202.00	5.47	22	XX|XXXXXXXXXXXXXX
POTASSIUM	MG	69.00	0.34	1	Y |
PROTEIN	G	5.00	2.44	10	PP|PPPP
CARBOHYDT	G	2.00	0.18	1	H |
FAT	G	6.00	1.88	8	FF|FFF
OLEIC A	G	1.50	1.49	6	OO|OO
LINOL A	G	0.10	0.12	1	- |
SAT FAT A	G	3.80	3.25	13	SS|SSSSSSS

26 HALF AND HALF SWEET CREAM
ANALYSIS OF 242 GRAMS WHICH IS 1 CUP

NUTRIENT	UNIT	AMOUNT	INQ	% STD	0 10 20 30 40 50 60 70 80 90 100
ENERGY	KCAL	315.00	1.00	16	EEEEEEEEEE
VITAMIN A	IU	260.00	0.41	7	AAAAA
VITAMIN C	MG	2.00	0.21	3	CCC
THIAMIN	MG	0.08	0.51	8	TTTTTT
RIBOFLAVN	MG	0.36	1.90	30	RRRRRRRRRRR|RRRRRRRRRR
NIACIN	MG	0.20	0.09	1	N
IRON	MG	0.20	0.08	1	I
CALCIUM	MG	254.00	1.79	28	KKKKKKKKKK|KKKKKKKK
PHOSPHRUS	MG	230.00	1.62	26	XXXXXXXXXXX|XXXXXXX
POTASSIUM	MG	314.00	0.40	6	YYYY
PROTEIN	G	7.00	0.89	14	PPPPPPPPPP
CARBOHYDT	G	10.00	0.23	4	HHH
FAT	G	28.00	2.28	36	FFFFFFFFFF|FFFFFFFFFFFFFFFFF
OLEIC A	G	7.00	1.81	29	OOOOOOOOOO|OOOOOOOOO
LINOL A	G	0.60	0.19	3	LL
SAT FAT A	G	17.30	3.85	61	SSSSSSSSSS|SSSSSSSSSSSSSSSSSSSSSSSSSSSSSSSSSSSSSSSSSSSSSSSS

27 HALF AND HALF SWEET CREAM
ANALYSIS OF 15 GRAMS WHICH IS 1 TBSP

NUTRIENT	UNIT	AMOUNT	INQ	% STD
ENERGY	KCAL	20.00	1.00	1
VITAMIN A	IU	20.00	0.50	1
VITAMIN C	MG	0.00	0.00	0
THIAMIN	MG	0.01	1.00	1
RIBOFLAVN	MG	0.02	1.67	2
NIACIN	MG	0.00	0.00	0
IRON	MG	0.00	0.00	0
CALCIUM	MG	16.00	1.78	2
PHOSPHRUS	MG	14.00	1.56	2
POTASSIUM	MG	19.00	0.38	0
PROTEIN	G	0.00	0.00	0
CARBOHYDT	G	1.00	0.36	0
FAT	G	2.00	2.56	3
OLEIC A	G	0.40	1.63	2
LINOL A	G	0.00	0.00	0
SAT FAT A	G	1.10	3.86	4

28 LIGHT CREAM, 19% FAT
ANALYSIS OF 240 GRAMS WHICH IS 1 CUP

NUTRIENT	UNIT	AMOUNT	INQ	% STD
ENERGY	KCAL	470.00	1.00	24
VITAMIN A	IU	1730.00	1.84	43
VITAMIN C	MG	2.00	0.14	3
THIAMIN	MG	0.08	0.34	8
RIBOFLAVN	MG	0.36	1.28	30
NIACIN	MG	0.10	0.03	1
IRON	MG	0.10	0.03	1
CALCIUM	MG	231.00	1.09	26
PHOSPHRUS	MG	192.00	0.91	21
POTASSIUM	MG	292.00	0.25	6
PROTEIN	G	6.00	0.51	12
CARBOHYDT	G	9.00	0.14	3
FAT	G	46.00	2.51	59
OLEIC A	G	11.70	2.03	48
LINOL A	G	1.00	0.21	5
SAT FAT A	G	26.80	4.50	101

29 LIGHT CREAM, 19% FAT
ANALYSIS OF 15 GRAMS WHICH IS 1 TBSP

NUTRIENT	UNIT	AMOUNT	INQ	% STD	0	10	20	30	40	50	60	70	80	90	100
ENERGY	KCAL	30.00	1.00	2	E										*
VITAMIN A	IU	110.00	1.83	3	IA										*
VITAMIN C	MG	0.00	0.00	0	I										*
THIAMIN	MG	0.00	0.00	0	I										*
RIBOFLAVN	MG	0.02	1.11	2	X										*
NIACIN	MG	0.00	0.00	0	I										*
IRON	MG	0.00	0.00	2	K										*
CALCIUM	MG	14.00	1.04	2	K										*
PHOSPHRUS	MG	12.00	0.89	1	X										*
POTASSIUM	MG	18.00	0.24	0	I										*
PROTEIN	G	0.00	0.00	0	I										*
CARBOHYDT	G	1.00	0.24	0	I										*
FAT	G	3.00	2.56	4	IFF										*
OLEIC A	G	0.70	1.90	3	IO										*
LINOL A	G	0.10	0.33	1	I										*
SAT FAT A	G	1.80	4.21	6	ISSSS										*

****

30 LIGHT WHIPPING CREAM, UNWHIPPED, 31% FAT
ANALYSIS OF 239 GRAMS WHICH IS 1 CUP

NUTRIENT	UNIT	AMOUNT	INQ	% STD	0	10	20	30	40	50	60	70	80	90	100
ENERGY	KCAL	700.00	1.00	35	EEEEEEEEEEEEEEEEEEEE										*
VITAMIN A	IU	2690.00	1.92	67	AAAAAAAAAAAAAAAAAAAAAAAAAAAAAAAAAAAAA									*
VITAMIN C	MG	1.00	0.05	2	C										*
THIAMIN	MG	0.06	0.17	6	TTTT										*
RIBOFLAVN	MG	0.30	0.71	25	RRRRRRRRRRRRRR										*
NIACIN	MG	0.10	0.02	1	N										*
IRON	MG	0.10	0.02	1	I										*
CALCIUM	MG	166.00	0.53	18	KKKKKKKKKK										*
PHOSPHRUS	MG	146.00	0.46	16	XXXXXXXXX										*
POTASSIUM	MG	231.00	0.13	5	YYYY										*
PROTEIN	G	5.00	0.29	10	PPPPPP										*
CARBOHYDT	G	7.00	0.07	3	HH										*
FAT	G	74.00	2.71	95	FFFFFFFFFFFFFFFFFFFFFFFFFFFFFFFFFFFFFFFFFFFFFFFF						*
OLEIC A	G	18.30	2.13	75	OOOOOOOOOOOOOOOOOOOOOOOOOOOOOOOOOOOOOO							*
LINOL A	G	1.50	0.21	8	LLLLL										*
SAT FAT A	G	46.20	4.63	162	SSSSSSSSSSSSSSSSSSSSSSSSSSSSSSSSSSSSSSSSSSSSSSSSSS						*162

****

31 LIGHT WHIPPING CREAM, UNWHIPPED, 31% FAT
ANALYSIS OF 15 GRAMS WHICH IS 1 TBSP

NUTRIENT	UNIT	AMOUNT	INQ	% STD
ENERGY	KCAL	45.00	1.00	2
VITAMIN A	IU	170.00	1.89	4
VITAMIN C	MG	0.00	0.00	0
THIAMIN	MG	0.00	0.00	0
RIBOFLAVN	MG	0.02	0.74	2
NIACIN	MG	0.00	0.00	0
IRON	MG	0.00	0.00	0
CALCIUM	MG	10.00	0.49	1
PHOSPHRUS	MG	9.00	0.44	1
POTASSIUM	MG	15.00	0.13	0
PROTEIN	G	0.00	0.00	0
CARBOHYDT	G	0.00	0.00	0
FAT	G	5.00	2.85	6
OLEIC A	G	1.10	2.00	4
LINOL A	G	0.10	0.22	1
SAT FAT A	G	2.90	4.52	10

32 HEAVY WHIPPING CREAM, UNWHIPPED, 37% FAT
ANALYSIS OF 238 GRAMS WHICH IS 1 CUP

NUTRIENT	UNIT	AMOUNT	INQ	% STD
ENERGY	KCAL	820.00	1.00	41
VITAMIN A	IU	3500.00	2.13	88
VITAMIN C	MG	1.00	0.04	2
THIAMIN	MG	0.05	0.12	5
RIBOFLAVN	MG	0.26	0.53	22
NIACIN	MG	0.10	0.02	1
IRON	MG	0.10	0.02	1
CALCIUM	MG	154.00	0.42	17
PHOSPHRUS	MG	149.00	0.40	17
POTASSIUM	MG	179.00	0.09	4
PROTEIN	G	5.00	0.24	3
CARBOHYDT	G	7.00	0.06	3
FAT	G	88.00	2.75	113
OLEIC A	G	22.20	2.21	91
LINOL A	G	2.00	0.24	10
SAT FAT A	G	54.80	4.69	192

33 HEAVY WHIPPING CREAM, UNWHIPPED, 37% FAT
ANALYSIS OF 15 GRAMS WHICH IS 1 TBSP

NUTRIENT	UNIT	AMOUNT	INQ	% STD	0	10	20	30	40	50	60	70	80	90	100
ENERGY	KCAL	52.00	1.00	3	EE										
VITAMIN A	IU	220.00	2.12	6	AIAA										
VITAMIN C	MG	0.00	0.00	0	I										
THIAMIN	MG	0.00	0.00	0	I										
RIBOFLAVN	MG	0.02	0.64	2	RI										
NIACIN	MG	0.00	0.00	0	I										
IRON	MG	0.00	0.00	0	I										
CALCIUM	MG	10.00	0.43	1	KI										
PHOSPHRUS	MG	9.00	0.38	1	XI										
POTASSIUM	MG	11.00	0.08	0	I										
PROTEIN	G	0.00	0.00	0	I										
CARBOHYDT	G	0.00	0.00	0	I										
FAT	G	6.00	2.96	8	FIFFFF										
OLEIC A	G	1.40	2.20	6	O1000										
LINOL A	G	0.10	0.19	1	I										
SAT FAT A	G	3.50	4.72	12	SISSSSSSS										

34 WHIPPED TOPPING, PRESSURIZED
ANALYSIS OF 60 GRAMS WHICH IS 1 CUP

NUTRIENT	UNIT	AMOUNT	INQ	% STD	0	10	20	30	40	50	60	70	80	90	100
ENERGY	KCAL	155.00	1.00	8	EEEEEE										
VITAMIN A	IU	550.00	1.77	14	AAAAAIAAAAA										
VITAMIN C	MG	0.00	0.00	0	I										
THIAMIN	MG	0.02	0.26	2	TT										
RIBOFLAVN	MG	0.04	0.43	3	RRR										
NIACIN	MG	0.00	0.00	0	I										
IRON	MG	0.00	0.00	0	I										
CALCIUM	MG	61.00	0.87	7	KKKKKI										
PHOSPHRUS	MG	54.00	0.77	6	XXXXXI										
POTASSIUM	MG	88.00	0.23	2	Y										
PROTEIN	G	2.00	0.52	4	PPP										
CARBOHYDT	G	7.00	0.33	3	HH										
FAT	G	13.00	2.15	17	FFFFFIFFFFFF										
OLEIC A	G	3.40	1.79	14	OOOOOIOOOOO										
LINOL A	G	0.30	0.19	2	L										
SAT FAT A	G	8.30	3.76	29	SSSSSISSSSSSSSSSSSSSSSSSSS										

35 WHIPPED TOPPING, PRESSURIZED
ANALYSIS OF 3 GRAMS WHICH IS 1 TBSP

NUTRIENT	UNIT	AMOUNT	INQ	%STD	0	10	20	30	40	50	60	70	80	90	100
ENERGY	KCAL	10.00	1.00	1											
VITAMIN A	IU	4.00	0.20	0											
VITAMIN C	MG	0.00	0.00	0											
THIAMIN	MG	0.30	60.00	30	TTTTTTTTTTTTTTTTTTTTTTTTTTTTTT										
RIBOFLAVN	MG	0.00	0.00	0											
NIACIN	MG	0.00	0.00	0											
IRON	MG	0.30	3.75	2	II										
CALCIUM	MG	3.00	0.67	0											
PHOSPHRUS	MG	3.00	0.67	0											
POTASSIUM	MG	0.00	0.00	0											
PROTEIN	G	0.00	0.00	0											
CARBOHYDT	G	0.00	0.00	0											
FAT	G	1.00	2.56	1	F										
OLEIC A	G	0.20	1.63	1	O										
LINOL A	G	0.00	0.00	0											
SAT FAT A	G	0.40	2.81	1	S										

36 SOUR CREAM
ANALYSIS OF 230 GRAMS WHICH IS 1 CUP

NUTRIENT	UNIT	AMOUNT	INQ	%STD	0	10	20	30	40	50	60	70	80	90	100
ENERGY	KCAL	495.00	1.00	25	EEEEEEEEEEEEEEEEEEEEEEEEE										
VITAMIN A	IU	1820.00	1.84	46	AAAAAAAAAAAAAAAAAAAAAIAAAAAAAAAAAAAAAAAAAAAA									
VITAMIN C	MG	2.00	0.13	3	CCC										
THIAMIN	MG	0.08	0.32	8	TTTTTT										
RIBOFLAVN	MG	0.34	1.14	28	RRRRRRRRRRRRRRRRRRRRRRRRRRIRRR									
NIACIN	MG	0.20	0.06	1	N										
IRON	MG	0.10	0.03	1	I										
CALCIUM	MG	268.00	1.20	30	KKKKKKKKKKKKKKKKKKKKKKKKKKKKIKKKK									
PHOSPHRUS	MG	195.00	0.88	22	XXXXXXXXXXXXXXXXXXXXXX										
POTASSIUM	MG	331.00	0.27	7	YYYYY										
PROTEIN	G	7.00	0.57	14	PPPPPPPPPPPPPP										
CARBOHYDT	G	10.00	0.15	4	HHH										
FAT	G	48.00	2.49	62	FFFFFFFFFFFFFFFFFFFIFFFFFFFFFFFFFFFFFFFFFFFFFFFFFFFFFFFFFFFFFF						
OLEIC A	G	12.10	2.00	49	OOOOOOOOOOOOOOOOOOOOOIOOOOOOOOOOOOOOOOOOOOOOOOOOO							
LINOL A	G	1.10	0.22	6	LLLL										
SAT FAT A	G	30.00	4.25	105	SSSSSSSSSSSSSSSSSSSSSISSSSSSSSSSSSSSSSSSSSSSSSSSSSSSSSSSSSSSSSSSSSSSSSSSSSSSSSSSSSSSSSSSSSSSSSSSSSSSSSSSSSSSS * 105

37 SOUR CREAM
ANALYSIS OF 12 GRAMS WHICH IS 1 TBSP

NUTRIENT	UNIT	AMOUNT	INQ	% STD	0	10	20	30	40	50	60	70	80	90	100
ENERGY	KCAL	25.00	1.00	1	E										*
VITAMIN A	IU	90.00	1.80	2	IA										*
VITAMIN C	MG	0.00	0.00	0	I										*
THIAMIN	MG	0.00	0.00	0	I										*
RIBOFLAVN	MG	0.02	1.33	2	IX										*
NIACIN	MG	0.00	0.00	0	I										*
IRON	MG	0.00	0.00	0	I										*
CALCIUM	MG	14.00	1.24	2	IK										*
PHOSPHRUS	MG	10.00	0.89	1	IX										*
POTASSIUM	MG	17.00	0.27	0	I										*
PROTEIN	G	0.00	0.00	0	I										*
CARBOHYDT	G	1.00	0.29	0	I										*
FAT	G	3.00	3.08	4	IFF										*
OLEIC A	G	0.60	1.96	2	IO										*
LINOL A	G	0.10	0.40	1	I										*
SAT FAT A	G	1.60	4.49	6	ISSS										*

38 NON-DAIRY LIQUID (FROZEN) CREAMER
ANALYSIS OF 245 GRAMS WHICH IS 1 CUP

NUTRIENT	UNIT	AMOUNT	INQ	% STD	0	10	20	30	40	50	60	70	80	90	100
ENERGY	KCAL	335.00	1.00	17	EEEEEEEEEE										*
VITAMIN A	IU	220.00	0.33	6	AAAA										*
VITAMIN C	MG	0.00	0.00	0	I										*
THIAMIN	MG	0.00	0.00	0	I										*
RIBOFLAVN	MG	0.00	0.00	0	I										*
NIACIN	MG	0.00	0.00	0	I										*
IRON	MG	0.10	0.04	1	I										*
CALCIUM	MG	23.00	0.15	3	KK										*
PHOSPHRUS	MG	157.00	1.04	17	XXXXXXXXXXX	X									*
POTASSIUM	MG	467.00	0.56	9	YYYYYY										*
PROTEIN	G	2.00	0.24	4	PPP										*
CARBOHYDT	G	28.00	0.61	10	HHHHHHHH										*
FAT	G	24.00	1.84	31	FFFFFFFFFF	IFFFFFFFFFF									*
OLEIC A	G	0.30	0.07	1	O										*
LINOL A	G	0.00	0.00	0	I										*
SAT FAT A	G	22.80	4.78	80	SSSSSSSSSSI	SSSSSSSSSSSSSSSSSSSSSSSSSSSSSSSSSSSSSSSSSSSSSSSSSSSSSSSSSSSSSSSS									*

39 NON-DAIRY LIQUID (FROZEN) CREAMER
ANALYSIS OF 15 GRAMS WHICH IS 1 TBSP

NUTRIENT	UNIT	AMOUNT	INQ	% STD
ENERGY	KCAL	20.00	1.00	1
VITAMIN A	IU	10.00	0.25	0
VITAMIN C	MG	0.00	0.00	0
THIAMIN	MG	0.00	0.00	0
RIBOFLAVN	MG	0.00	0.00	0
NIACIN	MG	0.00	0.00	0
IRON	MG	0.00	0.00	0
CALCIUM	MG	1.00	0.11	0
PHOSPHRUS	MG	10.00	1.11	1
POTASSIUM	MG	29.00	0.58	1
PROTEIN	G	0.00	0.00	0
CARBOHYDT	G	2.00	0.73	1
FAT	G	1.00	1.28	1
OLEIC A	G	0.00	0.00	0
LINOL A	G	0.00	0.00	0
SAT FAT A	G	1.40	4.91	5

40 NON-DAIRY POWDERED CREAMER
ANALYSIS OF 94 GRAMS WHICH IS 1 CUP

NUTRIENT	UNIT	AMOUNT	INQ	% STD
ENERGY	KCAL	515.00	1.00	26
VITAMIN A	IU	190.00	0.18	5
VITAMIN C	MG	0.00	0.00	0
THIAMIN	MG	0.00	0.00	0
RIBOFLAVN	MG	0.16	0.52	13
NIACIN	MG	0.00	0.00	0
IRON	MG	0.10	0.02	1
CALCIUM	MG	21.00	0.09	2
PHOSPHRUS	MG	397.00	1.71	44
POTASSIUM	MG	763.00	0.59	15
PROTEIN	G	5.00	0.39	10
CARBOHYDT	G	52.00	0.73	19
FAT	G	33.00	1.64	42
OLEIC A	G	0.90	0.14	4
LINOL A	G	0.00	0.00	0
SAT FAT A	G	30.60	4.17	107

41 NON-DAIRY POWDERED CREAMER
ANALYSIS OF 2 GRAMS WHICH IS 1 TSP

NUTRIENT	UNIT	AMOUNT	INQ	% STD
ENERGY	KCAL	10.00	1.00	1
VITAMIN A	IU	0.00	0.00	0
VITAMIN C	MG	0.00	0.00	0
THIAMIN	MG	0.00	0.00	0
RIBOFLAVN	MG	0.00	0.00	0
NIACIN	MG	0.00	0.00	0
IRON	MG	0.00	0.00	0
CALCIUM	MG	0.00	0.00	0
PHOSPHRUS	MG	0.00	1.78	1
POTASSIUM	MG	16.00	0.64	0
PROTEIN	G	0.00	0.00	0
CARBOHYDT	G	1.00	0.73	0
FAT	G	1.00	2.56	1
OLEIC A	G	0.00	0.00	0
LINOL A	G	0.00	0.00	0
SAT FAT A	G	0.70	4.91	2

42 NON-DAIRY FROZEN WHIPPED TOPPING
ANALYSIS OF 75 GRAMS WHICH IS 1 CUP

NUTRIENT	UNIT	AMOUNT	INQ	% STD
ENERGY	KCAL	240.00	1.00	12
VITAMIN A	IU	650.00	1.35	16
VITAMIN C	MG	0.00	0.00	0
THIAMIN	MG	0.00	0.00	0
RIBOFLAVN	MG	0.00	0.00	0
NIACIN	MG	0.00	0.05	0
IRON	MG	0.10	0.05	1
CALCIUM	MG	5.00	0.06	1
PHOSPHRUS	MG	6.00	0.06	1
POTASSIUM	MG	14.00	0.02	1
PROTEIN	G	1.00	0.17	2
CARBOHYDT	G	17.00	0.52	6
FAT	G	19.00	2.03	24
OLEIC A	G	1.00	0.34	4
LINOL A	G	0.20	0.08	1
SAT FAT A	G	16.30	4.77	57

43   NON-DAIRY FROZEN WHIPPED TOPPING
ANALYSIS OF 4 GRAMS WHICH IS 1 TBSP

NUTRIENT	UNIT	AMOUNT	INQ	% STD
ENERGY	KCAL	15.00	1.00	1
VITAMIN A	IU	30.00	1.00	1
VITAMIN C	MG	0.00	0.00	0
THIAMIN	MG	0.00	0.00	0
RIBOFLAVN	MG	0.00	0.00	0
NIACIN	MG	0.00	0.00	0
IRON	MG	0.00	0.00	0
CALCIUM	MG	0.00	0.00	0
PHOSPHRUS	MG	0.00	0.00	0
POTASSIUM	MG	1.00	0.03	0
PROTEIN	G	0.00	0.00	0
CARBOHYDT	G	1.00	0.48	0
FAT	G	1.00	1.71	0
OLEIC A	G	0.10	0.54	0
LINOL A	G	0.00	0.00	0
SAT FAT A	G	0.90	4.21	3

44   NON-DAIRY POWDERED WHIPPED TOPPING
ANALYSIS OF 80 GRAMS WHICH IS 1 CUP

NUTRIENT	UNIT	AMOUNT	INQ	% STD
ENERGY	KCAL	150.00	1.00	8
VITAMIN A	IU	290.00	0.97	7
VITAMIN C	MG	1.00	0.22	2
THIAMIN	MG	0.02	0.27	2
RIBOFLAVN	MG	0.09	1.00	8
NIACIN	MG	0.00	0.00	0
IRON	MG	0.00	0.00	0
CALCIUM	MG	72.00	1.07	8
PHOSPHRUS	MG	69.00	1.02	8
POTASSIUM	MG	121.00	0.32	2
PROTEIN	G	3.00	0.80	6
CARBOHYDT	G	13.00	0.63	5
FAT	G	10.00	1.71	13
OLEIC A	G	0.60	0.33	2
LINOL A	G	0.10	0.07	1
SAT FAT A	G	8.50	3.98	30

45 NON-DAIRY POWDERED WHIPPED TOPPING
ANALYSIS OF 4 GRAMS WHICH IS 1 TBSP

```
                                  0    10   20   30   40   50   60   70   80   90   100
```

NUTRIENT	UNIT	AMOUNT	INQ	% STD	
ENERGY	KCAL	10.00	1.00	1	-
VITAMIN A	IU	10.00	0.50	0	-
VITAMIN C	MG	0.00	0.00	0	-
THIAMIN	MG	0.00	0.00	0	-
RIBOFLAVN	MG	0.00	0.00	0	-
NIACIN	MG	0.00	0.00	0	-
IRON	MG	0.00	0.00	0	-
CALCIUM	MG	4.00	0.89	0	-
PHOSPHRUS	MG	3.00	0.67	0	-
POTASSIUM	MG	6.00	0.24	0	-
PROTEIN	G	0.00	0.73	0	-
CARBOHYDT	G	1.00	0.00	0	-
FAT	G	0.00	0.00	0	-
OLEIC A	G	0.00	0.00	0	-
LINOL A	G	0.00	0.00	0	-
SAT FAT A	G	0.40	2.81	1	S

46 NON-DAIRY PRESSURIZED WHIPPED TOPPING
ANALYSIS OF 70 GRAMS WHICH IS 1 CUP

```
                                  0    10   20   30   40   50   60   70   80   90   100
```

NUTRIENT	UNIT	AMOUNT	INQ	% STD	
ENERGY	KCAL	185.00	1.00	9	EEEEEE
VITAMIN A	IU	330.00	0.89	8	AAAAAA
VITAMIN C	MG	0.00	0.00	0	-
THIAMIN	MG	0.00	0.00	0	-
RIBOFLAVN	MG	0.00	0.00	0	-
NIACIN	MG	0.00	0.00	0	-
IRON	MG	0.00	0.00	0	-
CALCIUM	MG	4.00	0.05	0	-
PHOSPHRUS	MG	13.00	0.16	1	X
POTASSIUM	MG	13.00	0.03	0	-
PROTEIN	G	1.00	0.22	2	PP
CARBOHYDT	G	11.00	0.43	4	HHH
FAT	G	16.00	2.22	21	FFFFFF|FFFFFFFFF
OLEIC A	G	1.40	0.62	6	OOOOO
LINOL A	G	0.20	0.11	1	L
SAT FAT A	G	13.20	5.01	46	SSSSSS|SSSSSSSSSSSSSSSSSSSSSSSSSSSSSSSSSSSS

47 NON-DAIRY PRESSURIZED WHIPPED TOPPING
ANALYSIS OF 4 GRAMS WHICH IS 1 TBSP

NUTRIENT	UNIT	AMOUNT	INQ	% STD
ENERGY	KCAL	10.00	1.00	1
VITAMIN A	IU	20.00	1.00	1
VITAMIN C	MG	0.00	0.00	0
THIAMIN	MG	0.00	0.00	0
RIBOFLAVN	MG	0.00	0.00	0
NIACIN	MG	0.00	0.00	0
IRON	MG	0.00	0.00	0
CALCIUM	MG	0.00	0.00	0
PHOSPHRUS	MG	1.00	0.22	0
POTASSIUM	MG	1.00	0.04	0
PROTEIN	G	0.00	0.00	0
CARBOHYDT	G	1.00	0.73	1
FAT	G	1.00	2.56	1
OLEIC A	G	0.10	0.82	0
LINOL A	G	0.00	0.00	0
SAT FAT A	G	0.80	5.61	3

48 NON-DAIRY SOUR CREAM (MADE WITH NONFAT DRY MILK)
ANALYSIS OF 235 GRAMS WHICH IS 1 CUP

NUTRIENT	UNIT	AMOUNT	INQ	% STD
ENERGY	KCAL	415.00	1.00	21
VITAMIN A	IU	20.00	0.02	1
VITAMIN C	MG	2.00	0.16	3
THIAMIN	MG	0.09	0.43	9
RIBOFLAVN	MG	0.38	1.53	32
NIACIN	MG	0.20	0.07	1
IRON	MG	0.10	0.03	1
CALCIUM	MG	266.00	1.42	30
PHOSPHRUS	MG	205.00	1.10	23
POTASSIUM	MG	380.00	0.37	8
PROTEIN	G	8.00	0.77	16
CARBOHYDT	G	11.00	0.19	4
FAT	G	39.00	2.41	50
OLEIC A	G	4.40	0.87	18
LINOL A	G	1.10	0.27	6
SAT FAT A	G	31.20	5.28	109

49 NON-DAIRY SOUR CREAM (MADE WITH NONFAT DRY MILK)
ANALYSIS OF 12 GRAMS WHICH IS 1 TBSP

```
NUTRIENT   UNIT  AMOUNT   INQ   % STD  0        10        20        30        40        50        60        70        80        90       100
ENERGY     KCAL   20.00   1.00    1    E                                                                                                  *
VITAMIN A  IU      0.00   0.00    0    -                                                                                                  *
VITAMIN C  MG      0.00   0.00    0    -                                                                                                  *
THIAMIN    MG      0.01   1.00    1    T                                                                                                  *
RIBOFLAVN  MG      0.02   1.67    2    R                                                                                                  *
NIACIN     MG      0.00   0.00    0    -                                                                                                  *
IRON       MG      0.00   0.00    0    -                                                                                                  *
CALCIUM    MG     14.00   1.56    2    K                                                                                                  *
PHOSPHRUS  MG     10.00   1.11    1    X                                                                                                  *
POTASSIUM  MG     19.00   0.38    0    -                                                                                                  *
PROTEIN    G       0.00   0.00    0    -                                                                                                  *
CARBOHYDT  G       1.00   0.36    0    -                                                                                                  *
FAT        G       2.00   2.56    3    |F                                                                                                 *
OLEIC A    G       0.20   0.82    1    O                                                                                                  *
LINOL A    G       0.10   0.50    1    -                                                                                                  *
SAT FAT A  G       1.60   5.61    6    |SSS                                                                                               *
*******************************************************************************************************************************************
```

50 MILK, FLUID WHOLE (3.3% FAT)
ANALYSIS OF 244 GRAMS WHICH IS 1 CUP

```
NUTRIENT   UNIT  AMOUNT   INQ   % STD  0        10        20        30        40        50        60        70        80        90       100
ENERGY     KCAL  150.00   1.00    8    EEEEEE                                                                                             *
VITAMIN A  IU    310.00   1.03    8    AAAAAA                                                                                             *
VITAMIN C  MG      2.00   0.44    3    CCC                                                                                                *
THIAMIN    MG      0.09   1.20    9    TTTTTT                                                                                             *
RIBOFLAVN  MG      0.40   4.44   33    RRRR|RRRRRRRRRRRRRRRRRRRRRR                                                                         *
NIACIN     MG      0.20   0.19    1    N                                                                                                  *
IRON       MG      0.10   0.08    1    I                                                                                                  *
CALCIUM    MG    291.00   4.31   32    KKKKK|KKKKKKKKKKKKKKKKKKKK                                                                          *
PHOSPHRUS  MG    228.00   3.38   25    XXXXX|XXXXXXXXXXXXXXX                                                                               *
POTASSIUM  MG    370.00   0.99    7    YYYYY                                                                                              *
PROTEIN    G       8.00   2.13   16    PPPPP|PPPPPPP                                                                                       *
CARBOHYDT  G      11.00   0.53    4    MHH                                                                                                *
FAT        G       8.00   1.37   10    FFFFF|FF                                                                                           *
OLEIC A    G       2.10   1.14    9    OOOOO|O                                                                                            *
LINOL A    G       0.20   0.13    1    L                                                                                                  *
SAT FAT A  G       5.10   2.39   18    SSSSS|SSSSSSSS                                                                                      *
*******************************************************************************************************************************************
```

51 MILK, FLUID LOWFAT (2% FAT), NO MILK SOLIDS ADDED
ANALYSIS OF 244 GRAMS WHICH IS 1 CUP

| | 0 | 10 | 20 | 30 | 40 | 50 | 60 | 70 | 80 | 90 | 100 |

NUTRIENT	UNIT	AMOUNT	INQ	% STD	
ENERGY	KCAL	120.00	1.00	6	EEEEE
VITAMIN A	IU	500.00	2.08	13	AAAA|AAAAA
VITAMIN C	MG	2.00	0.56	3	CCC |
THIAMIN	MG	0.10	1.67	10	TTT|TTT
RIBOFLAVN	MG	0.40	5.56	33	RRRR|RRRRRRRRRRRRRRRRRRRR
NIACIN	MG	0.20	0.24	1	N |
IRON	MG	0.10	0.10	1	I |
CALCIUM	MG	297.00	5.50	33	KKK|KKKKKKKKKKKKKKK
PHOSPHRUS	MG	232.00	4.30	26	XXXX|XXXXXXXXXXXXXXX
POTASSIUM	MG	377.00	1.26	8	YYYY|Y
PROTEIN	G	8.00	2.67	16	PPP|PPPPPPPP
CARBOHYDT	G	12.00	0.73	4	HHH |
FAT	G	5.00	1.07	6	FFFFF
OLEIC A	G	1.20	0.82	5	OOOO|
LINOL A	G	0.10	0.08	1	- |
SAT FAT A	G	2.90	1.70	10	SSSS|SSS

52 MILK, FLUID LOWFAT (2% FAT), LESS THAN 10 GRAMS OF PROTEIN PER CUP
ANALYSIS OF 245 GRAMS WHICH IS 1 CUP

| | 0 | 10 | 20 | 30 | 40 | 50 | 60 | 70 | 80 | 90 | 100 |

NUTRIENT	UNIT	AMOUNT	INQ	% STD	
ENERGY	KCAL	125.00	1.00	6	EEEEE
VITAMIN A	IU	500.00	2.00	13	AAAA|AAAAA
VITAMIN C	MG	2.00	0.53	3	CCC |
THIAMIN	MG	0.10	1.60	10	TTT|TTT
RIBOFLAVN	MG	0.42	5.60	35	RRRR|RRRRRRRRRRRRRRRRRRRRR
NIACIN	MG	0.20	0.23	1	N |
IRON	MG	0.10	0.10	1	I |
CALCIUM	MG	313.00	5.56	35	KKK|KKKKKKKKKKKKKKKKK
PHOSPHRUS	MG	245.00	4.36	27	XXXX|XXXXXXXXXXXXXX
POTASSIUM	MG	397.00	1.27	8	YYYY|Y
PROTEIN	G	9.00	2.88	18	PPPP|PPPPPPPP
CARBOHYDT	G	12.00	0.70	4	HHH |
FAT	G	5.00	1.03	6	FFFFF
OLEIC A	G	1.20	0.78	5	OOOO|
LINOL A	G	0.10	0.08	1	- |
SAT FAT A	G	2.90	1.63	10	SSSS|SSS

53 MILK, FLUID LOWFAT (2% FAT), MORE THAN 10 GRAMS OF PROTEIN PER CUP
ANALYSIS OF 246 GRAMS WHICH IS 1 CUP

NUTRIENT	UNIT	AMOUNT	INQ	% STD	0 10 20 30 40 50 60 70 80 90 100
ENERGY	KCAL	135.00	1.00	7	EEEE
VITAMIN A	IU	500.00	1.85	13	AAAAIAAAAA
VITAMIN C	MG	3.00	0.74	5	CCCI
THIAMIN	MG	0.11	1.63	11	TTTITTTT
RIBOFLAVN	MG	0.48	5.93	40	RRRRIRRRRRRRRRRRRRRRRRRRR
NIACIN	MG	0.20	0.21	1	N I
IRON	MG	0.10	0.09	1	I I
CALCIUM	MG	352.00	5.79	39	KKKKIKKKKKKXXXXXXXXXXXXXXXX
PHOSPHRUS	MG	276.00	4.54	31	XXXXIXXXXXXXXXXXXXXXXX
POTASSIUM	MG	447.00	1.32	9	YYYYIYY
PROTEIN	G	10.00	2.96	20	PPPPIPPPPPPPPPP
CARBOHYDT	G	14.00	0.75	5	HHHHI
FAT	G	5.00	0.95	6	FFFFF
OLEIC A	G	1.20	0.73	5	OOOOI
LINOL A	G	0.10	0.07	1	- I
SAT FAT A	G	3.00	1.56	11	SSSSISSS

54 MILK, FLUID LOWFAT (1% FAT), NO MILK SOLIDS ADDED
ANALYSIS OF 244 GRAMS WHICH IS 1 CUP

NUTRIENT	UNIT	AMOUNT	INQ	% STD	0 10 20 30 40 50 60 70 80 90 100
ENERGY	KCAL	100.00	1.00	5	EEEE
VITAMIN A	IU	500.00	2.50	13	AAAIAAAAA
VITAMIN C	MG	2.00	0.67	3	CCCI
THIAMIN	MG	0.10	2.00	10	TTTITTTT
RIBOFLAVN	MG	0.41	6.83	34	RRRIRRRRRRRRRRRRRRRRRRR
NIACIN	MG	0.20	0.29	1	N I
IRON	MG	0.10	0.13	1	I I
CALCIUM	MG	300.00	6.67	33	KKKIKKKKKKKKKKXXXXXXX
PHOSPHRUS	MG	235.00	5.22	26	XXXIXXXXXXXXXXXXX
POTASSIUM	MG	381.00	1.52	8	YYYIYY
PROTEIN	G	8.00	3.20	16	PPPIPPPPPPPP
CARBOHYDT	G	12.00	0.87	4	HHHI
FAT	G	3.00	0.77	4	FFFI
OLEIC A	G	0.70	0.57	3	OO I
LINOL A	G	0.10	0.10	1	- I
SAT FAT A	G	1.60	1.12	6	SSSS

55 MILK, FLUID LOWFAT (1% FAT), LESS THAN 10 GRAMS OF PROTEIN PER CUP
ANALYSIS OF 245 GRAMS WHICH IS 1 CUP

NUTRIENT	UNIT	AMOUNT	INQ	% STD	0 10 20 30 40 50 60 70 80 90 100
ENERGY	KCAL	105.00	1.00	5	EEEE
VITAMIN A	IU	500.00	2.38	13	AAA|AAAAA
VITAMIN C	MG	2.00	0.63	3	CCC|
THIAMIN	MG	0.10	1.90	10	TTT|TTTT
RIBOFLAVN	MG	0.42	6.67	35	RRR|RRRRRRRRRRRRRRRRR
NIACIN	MG	0.20	0.27	1	N|
IRON	MG	0.10	0.12	1	I|
CALCIUM	MG	313.00	6.62	35	KKK|KKKKKKKKKKKXXXXXXXXXXX
PHOSPHRUS	MG	245.00	5.19	27	XXX|XXXXXXXXXXXX
POTASSIUM	MG	397.00	1.51	8	YYY|YY
PROTEIN	G	9.00	3.43	18	PPP|PPPPPPPP
CARBOHYDT	G	12.00	0.83	4	HHH|
FAT	G	2.00	0.49	3	FF|
OLEIC A	G	0.60	0.47	2	OO|
LINOL A	G	0.10	0.10	1	-|
SAT FAT A	G	1.50	1.00	5	SSSS

56 MILK, FLUID LOWFAT (1% FAT), MORE THAN 10 GRAMS OF PROTEIN PER CUP
ANALYSIS OF 246 GRAMS WHICH IS 1 CUP

NUTRIENT	UNIT	AMOUNT	INQ	% STD	0 10 20 30 40 50 60 70 80 90 100
ENERGY	KCAL	120.00	1.00	6	EEEEE
VITAMIN A	IU	500.00	2.08	13	AAAA|AAAA
VITAMIN C	MG	3.00	0.83	5	CCCC|
THIAMIN	MG	0.11	1.83	11	TTTT|TTTT
RIBOFLAVN	MG	0.47	6.53	39	RRRR|RRRRRRRRRRRRRRRRRRRR
NIACIN	MG	0.24	0.30	1	N|
IRON	MG	0.10	0.10	1	I|
CALCIUM	MG	349.00	6.46	39	KKKK|KKKKKKKKKKKXXXXXXXXXXXXX
PHOSPHRUS	MG	273.00	5.06	30	XXXX|XXXXXXXXXXXXXXX
POTASSIUM	MG	444.00	1.48	9	YYYY|YY
PROTEIN	G	10.00	3.33	20	PPPP|PPPPPPPPP
CARBOHYDT	G	14.00	0.85	5	HHHH|
FAT	G	3.00	0.64	4	FFF|
OLEIC A	G	0.70	0.48	3	OO|
LINOL A	G	0.10	0.08	1	-|
SAT FAT A	G	1.80	1.05	6	SSSS

57 MILK, FLUID NONFAT (SKIM), NO MILK SOLIDS ADDED
ANALYSIS OF 245 GRAMS WHICH IS 1 CUP

NUTRIENT	UNIT	AMOUNT	INQ	% STD	0	10	20	30	40	50	60	70	80	90	100
ENERGY	KCAL	85.00	1.00	4	EEE										*
VITAMIN A	IU	500.00	2.94	13	AA|AAAAAA										*
VITAMIN C	MG	2.00	0.78	3	CCC										*
THIAMIN	MG	0.09	2.12	9	TT|TTTT										*
RIBOFLAVN	MG	0.37	7.25	31	RR	RRRRRRRRRRRRRRRR									*
NIACIN	MG	0.20	0.34	1	N										*
IRON	MG	0.10	0.15	1	I										*
CALCIUM	MG	302.00	7.90	34	KK	KKKKKKKKKXXXXXXXXXKKKK									*
PHOSPHRUS	MG	247.00	6.46	27	XX|XXXXXXXXXXXXXXXXX										*
POTASSIUM	MG	406.00	1.91	8	YY|YYY										*
PROTEIN	G	8.00	3.76	16	PP|PPPPPPPP										*
CARBOHYDT	G	12.00	1.03	4	HHH										*
FAT	G	0.10	0.00	0	-										*
OLEIC A	G	0.10	0.00	0	-										*
LINOL A	G	0.00	0.00	0	-										*
SAT FAT A	G	0.30	0.25	1	S										*

****

58 MILK, FLUID NONFAT (SKIM), LESS THAN 10 GRAMS OF PROTEIN PER CUP
ANALYSIS OF 245 GRAMS WHICH IS 1 CUP

NUTRIENT	UNIT	AMOUNT	INQ	% STD	0	10	20	30	40	50	60	70	80	90	100
ENERGY	KCAL	90.00	1.00	5	EEEE										*
VITAMIN A	IU	500.00	2.78	13	AAA|AAAAA										*
VITAMIN C	MG	2.00	0.74	3	CCC|										*
THIAMIN	MG	0.10	2.22	10	TTT|TTTT										*
RIBOFLAVN	MG	0.43	7.96	36	RHR	RRRRRRRRRRRRRRRRRRR									*
NIACIN	MG	0.20	0.32	1	N											*
IRON	MG	0.10	0.14	1	I											*
CALCIUM	MG	316.00	7.80	35	KKK	KKKKKKKKKKKKKKKKKK									*
PHOSPHRUS	MG	255.00	6.30	28	XXX|XXXXXXXXXXXXXXXX										*
POTASSIUM	MG	418.00	1.86	8	YYY|YYY										*
PROTEIN	G	9.00	4.00	18	PPP|PPPPPPPP										*
CARBOHYDT	G	12.00	0.97	4	HHH|										*
FAT	G	1.00	0.28	1	F											*
OLEIC A	G	0.10	0.09	0	-											*
LINOL A	G	0.00	0.00	0	-											*
SAT FAT A	G	0.40	0.31	1	S											*

****

59 MILK, FLUID NONFAT (SKIM), MORE THAN 10 GRAMS OF PROTEIN PER CUP
ANALYSIS OF 246 GRAMS WHICH IS 1 CUP

NUTRIENT	UNIT	AMOUNT	INQ	% STD	
ENERGY	KCAL	100.00	1.00	5	EEEE
VITAMIN A	IU	500.00	2.50	13	AAAIAAAAAA
VITAMIN C	MG	3.00	1.00	5	CCCC
THIAMIN	MG	0.11	2.20	11	TTTITTTT
RIBOFLAVN	MG	0.48	8.00	40	RRRIRRRRRRRRRRRRRRRRRRRRRR
NIACIN	MG	0.20	0.29	1	N
IRON	MG	0.10	0.13	1	I
CALCIUM	MG	352.00	7.82	39	KKKIKKKKKKKKKKKKKKKKKKKKKKXXXXX
PHOSPHRUS	MG	275.00	6.11	31	XXXIXXXXXXXXXXXXXXXXXX
POTASSIUM	MG	446.00	1.78	9	YYYIYYY
PROTEIN	G	10.00	4.00	20	PPPIPPPPPPPPPP
CARBOHYDT	G	14.00	1.02	5	HHHH
FAT	G	1.00	0.26	1	F
OLEIC A	G	0.10	0.08	0	-
LINOL A	G	0.00	0.00	0	-
SAT FAT A	G	0.40	0.28	1	S

60 BUTTERMILK, FLUID
ANALYSIS OF 245 GRAMS WHICH IS 1 CUP

NUTRIENT	UNIT	AMOUNT	INQ	% STD	
ENERGY	KCAL	100.00	1.00	5	EEEE
VITAMIN A	IU	80.00	0.40	2	AA
VITAMIN C	MG	2.00	0.67	3	CCC
THIAMIN	MG	0.08	1.60	8	TTTITT
RIBOFLAVN	MG	0.38	6.33	32	RRRIRRRRRRRRRRRRRRRRRRRRRR
NIACIN	MG	0.10	0.14	1	N
IRON	MG	0.10	0.13	1	I
CALCIUM	MG	285.00	6.33	32	KKKIKKKKKKKKKKKKKKKKKKKKKK
PHUSPHRUS	MG	219.00	4.87	24	XXXIXXXXXXXXXXXXXXX
POTASSIUM	MG	371.00	1.48	7	YYYIYY
PROTEIN	G	8.00	3.20	16	PPPIPPPPPPPP
CARBOHYDT	G	12.00	0.87	4	HHHH
FAT	G	2.00	0.51	3	FF
OLEIC A	G	0.50	0.41	2	OO
LINOL A	G	0.00	0.00	0	-
SAT FAT A	G	1.30	0.91	5	SSSS

61 EVAPORATED CANNED WHOLE MILK
ANALYSIS OF 252 GRAMS WHICH IS 1 CUP

NUTRIENT	UNIT	AMOUNT	INQ	% STD	0 10 20 30 40 50 60 70 80 90 100
ENERGY	KCAL	340.00	1.00	17	EEEEEEEEEEE
VITAMIN A	IU	610.00	0.90	15	AAAAAAAAAA
VITAMIN C	MG	5.00	0.49	8	CCCCCC
THIAMIN	MG	0.12	0.71	12	TTTTTTTT
RIBOFLAVN	MG	0.80	3.92	67	RRRRRRRRRRRRRRRRRRRRRRRRRRRRRRRRR
NIACIN	MG	0.50	0.21	4	NNN
IRON	MG	0.50	0.18	3	III
CALCIUM	MG	657.00	4.29	73	KKKKKKKKKKKXXXXXXXXXXXXXXXXXXXXXXXXXXX
PHOSPHRUS	MG	510.00	3.33	57	XXXXXXXXXXXXXXXXXXXXXXXXXXXXX
POTASSIUM	MG	764.00	0.90	15	YYYYYYYYYY
PROTEIN	G	17.00	2.00	34	PPPPPPPPPPPPPPPPP
CARBOHYDT	G	25.00	0.53	9	HHHHHH
FAT	G	19.00	1.43	24	FFFFFFFFFFFF
OLEIC A	G	5.30	1.27	22	OOOOOOOOOOO
LINOL A	G	0.40	0.12	2	LL
SAT FAT A	G	11.60	2.39	41	SSSSSSSSSSSSSSSSSSSS

62 EVAPORATED CANNED SKIM MILK
ANALYSIS OF 255 GRAMS WHICH IS 1 CUP

NUTRIENT	UNIT	AMOUNT	INQ	% STD	0 10 20 30 40 50 60 70 80 90 100
ENERGY	KCAL	200.00	1.00	10	EEEEEEE
VITAMIN A	IU	1000.00	2.50	25	AAAAAAAAAAAAAAAAA
VITAMIN C	MG	3.00	0.50	5	CCCC
THIAMIN	MG	0.11	1.10	11	TTTTTTT
RIBOFLAVN	MG	0.79	6.58	66	RRRRRRRRRRRRRRRRRRRRRRRRRRRRRRRR
NIACIN	MG	0.40	0.29	3	NN
IRON	MG	0.70	0.44	4	IIII
CALCIUM	MG	738.00	8.20	82	KKKKKKKKKKKKKKKKKKKKKKKKKKKKKKKKKKKKKKKKK
PHOSPHRUS	MG	497.00	5.52	55	XXXXXXXXXXXXXXXXXXXXXXXXXXXX
POTASSIUM	MG	845.00	1.69	17	YYYYYYYY
PROTEIN	G	19.00	3.80	38	PPPPPPPPPPPPPPPPPPP
CARBOHYDT	G	29.00	1.05	11	HHHHHHH
FAT	G	1.00	0.13	1	F
OLEIC A	G	0.10	0.04	0	-
LINOL A	G	0.00	0.00	0	-
SAT FAT A	G	0.30	0.11	1	S

63 SWEETENED CONDENSED MILK
ANALYSIS OF 306 GRAMS WHICH IS 1 CUP

NUTRIENT	UNIT	AMOUNT	INQ	% STD
ENERGY	KCAL	980.00	1.00	49
VITAMIN A	IU	1000.00	0.51	25
VITAMIN C	MG	8.00	0.27	13
THIAMIN	MG	0.28	0.57	28
RIBOFLAVN	MG	1.27	2.16	106
NIACIN	MG	0.60	0.09	4
IRON	MG	0.60	0.08	4
CALCIUM	MG	868.00	1.97	96
PHOSPHRUS	MG	775.00	1.76	86
POTASSIUM	MG	1136.00	0.46	23
PROTEIN	G	24.00	0.98	48
CARBOHYDT	G	166.00	1.23	60
FAT	G	27.00	0.71	35
OLEIC A	G	6.70	0.56	27
LINOL A	G	0.70	0.07	4
SAT FAT A	G	16.80	1.20	59

64 BUTTERMILK, DRIED
ANALYSIS OF 120 GRAMS WHICH IS 1 CUP

NUTRIENT	UNIT	AMOUNT	INQ	% STD
ENERGY	KCAL	465.00	1.00	23
VITAMIN A	IU	260.00	0.28	7
VITAMIN C	MG	7.00	0.50	12
THIAMIN	MG	0.47	2.02	47
RIBOFLAVN	MG	1.90	6.81	158
NIACIN	MG	1.10	0.34	8
IRON	MG	0.40	0.11	3
CALCIUM	MG	1421.00	6.79	158
PHOSPHRUS	MG	1119.00	5.35	124
POTASSIUM	MG	1910.00	1.64	38
PROTEIN	G	41.00	3.53	82
CARBOHYDT	G	59.00	0.92	21
FAT	G	7.00	0.39	9
OLEIC A	G	1.70	0.30	7
LINOL A	G	0.20	0.04	1
SAT FAT A	G	4.30	0.65	15

65 NONFAT INSTANT DRIED MILK
ANALYSIS OF 91 GRAMS WHICH IS 1 ENVELOPE (3.2 OZ)

NUTRIENT	UNIT	AMOUNT	INQ	% STD	
ENERGY	KCAL	325.00	1.00	16	EEEEEEEEEE
VITAMIN A	IU	2160.00	3.32	54	AAAAAAAAAAAAAAAAAAAAAAAAAAAA
VITAMIN C	MG	5.00	0.51	8	CCCCCC
THIAMIN	MG	0.38	2.34	38	TTTTTTTTTTTTTTTTTTTT
RIBOFLAVN	MG	1.59	8.15	133	RRRRRRRRRRRRRRRRRRRRRRRRRRRRRRRRRRRRRRRRRRRRR *133
NIACIN	MG	0.80	0.35	6	NNNNN
IRON	MG	0.30	0.12	2	II
CALCIUM	MG	1120.00	7.66	124	KKKKKKKKKKKKKKKKKKKKKKKKKKKKKKKKKKKKKKKKKKKKKKKK *124
PHOSPHRUS	MG	896.00	6.13	100	XXXXXXXXXXXXXXXXXXXXXXXXXXXXXXXXXXXXXXXXXX
POTASSIUM	MG	1552.00	1.91	31	YYYYYYYYYYYYY
PROTEIN	G	32.00	3.94	64	PPPPPPPPPPPPPPPPPPPPPPPPPP
CARBOHYDT	G	47.00	1.05	17	HHHHHHHHH
FAT	G	1.00	0.08	1	F
OLEIC A	G	0.10	0.03	0	-
LINOL A	G	0.00	0.00	0	-
SAT FAT A	G	0.40	0.09	1	S

66 NONFAT INSTANT DRIED MILK
ANALYSIS OF 68 GRAMS WHICH IS 1 CUP

NUTRIENT	UNIT	AMOUNT	INQ	% STD	
ENERGY	KCAL	245.00	1.00	12	EEEEEEE
VITAMIN A	IU	1610.00	3.29	40	AAAAAAAAAAAAAAAAAAAAA
VITAMIN C	MG	4.00	0.54	7	CCCCC
THIAMIN	MG	0.28	2.29	28	TTTTTTTTTTTTTT
RIBOFLAVN	MG	1.19	8.10	99	RRRRRRRRRRRRRRRRRRRRRRRRRRRRRRRRRRRRRRRRRRRRRRRRRR
NIACIN	MG	0.60	0.35	4	NNN
IRON	MG	0.20	0.10	1	I
CALCIUM	MG	837.00	7.59	93	KKKKKKKKKKKKKKKKKKKKKKKKKKKKKKKKKKKKKKKKKKKKKKK
PHOSPHRUS	MG	670.00	6.06	74	XXXXXXXXXXXXXXXXXXXXXXXXXXXXXXXXXXXXX
POTASSIUM	MG	1160.00	1.89	23	YYYYYYYYY
PROTEIN	G	24.00	3.92	48	PPPPPPPPPPPPPPPPPPPPPPPP
CARBOHYDT	G	35.00	1.04	13	HHHHHHH
FAT	G	0.00	0.00	0	-
OLEIC A	G	0.10	0.03	0	-
LINOL A	G	0.00	0.00	0	-
SAT FAT A	G	0.30	0.09	1	S

67 CHOCOLATE MILK (COMMERCIAL)
ANALYSIS OF 250 GRAMS WHICH IS 1 CUP

NUTRIENT	UNIT	AMOUNT	INQ	% STD	GRAPH (0–100)
ENERGY	KCAL	210.00	1.00	11	EEEEEEE
VITAMIN A	IU	300.00	0.71	8	AAAAAA|
VITAMIN C	MG	2.00	0.32	3	CCC
THIAMIN	MG	0.09	0.86	9	TTTTTTT|
RIBOFLAVN	MG	0.41	3.25	34	RRRRRRR|RRRRRRRRRRRRRRRRR
NIACIN	MG	0.20	0.20	2	NN
IRON	MG	0.60	0.36	4	III|
CALCIUM	MG	280.00	2.96	31	KKKKKKK|KKKKKKKKKKKKKK
PHOSPHRUS	MG	251.00	2.66	28	XXXXXXX|XXXXXXXXXXXXX
POTASSIUM	MG	417.00	0.79	8	YYYYYYY|
PROTEIN	G	8.00	1.52	16	PPPPPPP|PPPP
CARBOHYDT	G	26.00	0.90	9	HHHHHHH
FAT	G	8.00	0.98	10	FFFFFFF
OLEIC A	G	2.20	0.86	9	OOOOOOO|
LINOL A	G	0.20	0.10	1	L
SAT FAT A	G	5.30	1.77	19	SSSSSSS|SSSSSSS

68 CHOCOLATE MILK, LOWFAT (2%)(COMMERCIAL)
ANALYSIS OF 250 GRAMS WHICH IS 1 CUP

NUTRIENT	UNIT	AMOUNT	INQ	% STD	GRAPH (0–100)
ENERGY	KCAL	180.00	1.00	9	EEEEEEE
VITAMIN A	IU	500.00	1.39	13	AAAAAAA|AAA
VITAMIN C	MG	2.00	0.37	3	CCC
THIAMIN	MG	0.10	1.11	10	TTTTTTT|T
RIBOFLAVN	MG	0.42	3.89	35	RRRRRRR|RRRRRRRRRRRRRRRRRR
NIACIN	MG	0.30	0.24	2	NN
IRON	MG	0.60	0.42	4	III|
CALCIUM	MG	284.00	3.51	32	KKKKKKK|KKKKKKKKKKKKKK
PHOSPHRUS	MG	254.00	3.14	28	XXXXXXX|XXXXXXXXXXXXX
POTASSIUM	MG	422.00	0.94	8	YYYYYYY|
PROTEIN	G	8.00	1.78	16	PPPPPPP|PPPP
CARBOHYDT	G	26.00	1.05	9	HHHHHHH|H
FAT	G	5.00	0.71	6	FFFFF
OLEIC A	G	1.30	0.59	5	OOOO
LINOL A	G	0.10	0.06	1	-
SAT FAT A	G	3.10	1.21	11	SSSSSSS|SS

```
69  CHOCOLATE MILK, LOWFAT (1%)(COMMERCIAL)
ANALYSIS OF 250 GRAMS WHICH IS 1 CUP

NUTRIENT   UNIT  AMOUNT   INQ   %STD   0        10        20        30        40        50        60        70        80        90       100
ENERGY     KCAL  160.00   1.00    8    EEEEE
VITAMIN A  IU    500.00   1.56   13    AAAAAIAAAA
VITAMIN C  MG      2.00   0.42    3    CCC
THIAMIN    MG      0.10   1.25   10    TITTTTT
RIBOFLAVN  MG      0.40   4.17   33    RRRRRIRRRRRRRRRRRRRRRRRRR
NIACIN     MG      0.20   0.18    1    N
IRON       MG      0.60   0.47    4    III
CALCIUM    MG    287.00   3.99   32    KKKKKIKKKKKKKKKKKKKKKKK
PHOSPHRUS  MG    257.00   3.57   29    XXXXXIXXXXXXXXXXXXXXXX
POTASSIUM  MG    426.00   1.07    9    YYYYYIY
PROTEIN    G       8.00   2.00   16    PPPPPIPPPPP
CARBOHYDT  G      26.00   1.18    9    HHHHHIHH
FAT        G       3.00   0.48    4    FFF
OLEIC A    G       0.70   0.36    3    OO
LINOL A    G       0.10   0.06    1    -
SAT FAT A  G       1.50   0.66    5    SSSS
**********************************************************
```

```
70  EGGNOG (COMMERCIAL)
ANALYSIS OF 254 GRAMS WHICH IS 1 CUP

NUTRIENT   UNIT  AMOUNT   INQ   %STD   0        10        20        30        40        50        60        70        80        90       100
ENERGY     KCAL  340.00   1.00   17    EEEEEEEEEEEE
VITAMIN A  IU    890.00   1.31   22    AAAAAAAAAAAIAAAA
VITAMIN C  MG      4.00   0.39    7    CCCCC
THIAMIN    MG      0.09   0.53    9    TITTTTT
RIBOFLAVN  MG      0.48   2.35   40    RRRRRRRRRRRRRIRRRRRRRRRRRRRRR
NIACIN     MG      0.30   0.13    2    NN
IRON       MG      0.50   0.18    3    III
CALCIUM    MG    330.00   2.16   37    KKKKKKKKKKKXXXXIKKKKKKKKKKXXXXXXX
PHOSPHRUS  MG    278.00   1.82   31    XXXXXXXXXXXIXXXXXXXXXX
POTASSIUM  MG    420.00   0.49    8    YYYYYYY
PROTEIN    G      10.00   1.18   20    PPPPPPPPPPIPP
CARBOHYDT  G      34.00   0.73   12    HHHHHHHHHH
FAT        G      19.00   1.43   24    FFFFFFFFFFFFIFFFF
OLEIC A    G       5.00   1.20   20    OOOOOOOOOOOOOOIOO
LINOL A    G       0.60   0.18    3    LL
SAT FAT A  G      11.30   2.33   40    SSSSSSSSSSSSSISSSSSSSSSSSSSSS
**********************************************************
```

71 CHOCOLATE MALTED MILK (1 CUP WHOLE MILK AND 3/4 OZ MALTED MILK POWDER)
ANALYSIS OF 265 GRAMS WHICH IS 1 CUP PLUS POWDER

NUTRIENT	UNIT	AMOUNT	INQ	% STD	0 10 20 30 40 50 60 70 80 90 100
ENERGY	KCAL	235.00	1.00	12	EEEEEEE
VITAMIN A	IU	330.00	0.70	8	AAAAAAA I
VITAMIN C	MG	2.00	0.28	3	CCC
THIAMIN	MG	0.14	1.19	14	TTTTTTTITTT
RIBOFLAVN	MG	0.43	3.05	36	RRRRRRRIRRRRRRRRRRRRRRRRRR
NIACIN	MG	0.70	0.43	5	NNNN
IRON	MG	0.50	0.27	3	III
CALCIUM	MG	304.00	2.87	34	KKKKKKKIKKKKKKKKKKKKKKKXX
PHOSPHRUS	MG	265.00	2.51	29	XXXXXXXIXXXXXXXXXXXXX
POTASSIUM	MG	500.00	0.85	10	YYYYYYYI
PROTEIN	G	9.00	1.53	18	PPPPPPPIPPPPP
CARBOHYDT	G	29.00	0.90	11	HHHHHHHI
FAT	G	9.00	0.98	12	FFFFFFFF
OLEIC A	G	2.30	0.80	9	OOOOOOOI
LINOL A	G	0.30	0.13	2	L
SAT FAT A	G	5.50	1.64	19	SSSSSSSISSSSSS

72 NATURAL MALTED MILK (1CUP WHOLE MILK AND 3/4 OZ MALTED MILK POWDER)
ANALYSIS OF 265 GRAMS WHICH IS 1 CUP PLUS POWDER

NUTRIENT	UNIT	AMOUNT	INQ	% STD	0 10 20 30 40 50 60 70 80 90 100
ENERGY	KCAL	235.00	1.00	12	EEEEEEE
VITAMIN A	IU	380.00	0.81	10	AAAAAAAI
VITAMIN C	MG	2.00	0.28	3	CCC
THIAMIN	MG	0.20	1.70	20	TTTTTTTITTTTTT
RIBOFLAVN	MG	0.54	3.83	45	RRRRRRRIRRRRRRRRRRRRRRRRRRRRRRRR
NIACIN	MG	1.30	0.79	9	NNNNNNN
IRON	MG	0.30	0.16	2	II
CALCIUM	MG	347.00	3.28	39	KKKKKKKIKKKKKKKKKKKKKKKKKKKK
PHOSPHRUS	MG	307.00	2.90	34	XXXXXXXIXXXXXXXXXXXXXXXX
POTASSIUM	MG	529.00	0.90	11	YYYYYYYI
PROTEIN	G	11.00	1.87	22	PPPPPPPIPPPPPPP
CARBOHYDT	G	27.00	0.84	10	HHHHHHHI
FAT	G	10.00	1.09	13	FFFFFFFIF
OLEIC A	G	6.30	2.19	26	OOOOOOOIOOOOOOOOOOOO
LINOL A	G	2.60	1.11	13	LLLLLLIL
SAT FAT A	G	6.00	1.79	21	SSSSSSSISSSSSS

73 CHOCOLATE MILK SHAKE
ANALYSIS OF 300 GRAMS WHICH IS 10.6 OZ, NET WT.

NUTRIENT	UNIT	AMOUNT	INQ	% STD	PROFILE (0–100)
ENERGY	KCAL	355.00	1.00	18	EEEEEEEEEEE
VITAMIN A	IU	0.00	0.37	7	AAAAA
VITAMIN C	MG	0.00	0.00	0	-
THIAMIN	MG	0.14	0.79	14	TTTTTTTT
RIBOFLAVN	MG	0.67	3.15	56	RRRRRRRRRRR|RRRRRRRRRRRRRRRRRRRRRRR
NIACIN	MG	0.40	0.16	3	NN
IRON	MG	0.90	0.32	6	IIIII
CALCIUM	MG	396.00	2.48	44	KKKKKKKKKKKK|KKKKKKKKKKK
PHOSPHRUS	MG	378.00	2.37	42	XXXXXXXXXXXX|XXXXXXXXXXXXXXXXXXX
POTASSIUM	MG	672.00	0.76	13	YYYYYYYYY
PROTEIN	G	9.00	1.01	18	PPPPPPPPPPPPP
CARBOHYDT	G	63.00	1.29	23	HHHHHHHHHHHHHHHH|HHHH
FAT	G	8.00	0.58	10	FFFFFFF
OLEIC A	G	2.00	0.46	8	OOOOOOO
LINOL A	G	0.20	0.06	1	L
SAT FAT A	G	5.00	0.99	18	SSSSSSSSSSSSSS

74 VANILLA MILK SHAKE
ANALYSIS OF 313 GRAMS WHICH IS 11 OZ, NET WT.

NUTRIENT	UNIT	AMOUNT	INQ	% STD	PROFILE (0–100)
ENERGY	KCAL	350.00	1.00	17	EEEEEEEEEEE
VITAMIN A	IU	360.00	0.51	9	AAAAAA
VITAMIN C	MG	0.00	0.00	0	-
THIAMIN	MG	0.09	0.51	9	TTTTTT
RIBOFLAVN	MG	0.61	2.90	51	RRRRRRRRRRR|RRRRRRRRRRRRRRRRRRRRR
NIACIN	MG	0.50	0.20	4	NNN
IRON	MG	0.30	0.11	2	II
CALCIUM	MG	457.00	2.90	51	KKKKKKKKKKKK|KKKKKKKKKKK
PHOSPHRUS	MG	361.00	2.29	40	XXXXXXXXXXX|XXXXXXXXXXXXXXXXXX
POTASSIUM	MG	572.00	0.65	11	YYYYYYYY
PROTEIN	G	12.00	1.37	24	PPPPPPPPPPPPP|PPPP
CARBOHYDT	G	56.00	1.16	20	HHHHHHHHHHHHHH|HH
FAT	G	9.00	0.66	12	FFFFFFFF
OLEIC A	G	2.40	0.56	10	OOOOOOO
LINOL A	G	0.20	0.06	1	L
SAT FAT A	G	5.90	1.18	21	SSSSSSSSSSSSS|SSS

75 ICE CREAM, REGULAR (11% FAT), HARDENED
ANALYSIS OF 1064 GRAMS WHICH IS 1/2 GAL

NUTRIENT	UNIT	AMOUNT	INQ	% STD	
ENERGY	KCAL	2155.00	1.00	108	* 108
VITAMIN A	IU	4340.00	1.01	109	* 109
VITAMIN C	MG	6.00	0.09	10	*
THIAMIN	MG	0.42	0.39	42	*
RIBOFLAVN	MG	2.63	2.03	219	* 219
NIACIN	MG	1.10	0.07	8	*
IRON	MG	1.00	0.06	6	*
CALCIUM	MG	1406.00	1.45	156	* 156
PHOSPHRUS	MG	1075.00	1.11	119	* 119
POTASSIUM	MG	2052.00	0.38	41	*
PROTEIN	G	38.00	0.71	76	*
CARBOHYDT	G	254.00	0.86	92	*
FAT	G	115.00	1.37	147	* 147
OLEIC A	G	28.80	1.09	118	* 118
LINOL A	G	2.60	0.12	13	*
SAT FAT A	G	71.30	2.32	250	* 250

76 ICE CREAM, REGULAR (11% FAT), HARDENED
ANALYSIS OF 133 GRAMS WHICH IS 1 CUP

NUTRIENT	UNIT	AMOUNT	INQ	% STD	
ENERGY	KCAL	270.00	1.00	14	*
VITAMIN A	IU	540.00	1.00	14	*
VITAMIN C	MG	1.00	0.12	2	*
THIAMIN	MG	0.05	0.37	5	*
RIBOFLAVN	MG	0.33	2.04	28	*
NIACIN	MG	0.10	0.05	1	*
IRON	MG	0.10	0.05	1	*
CALCIUM	MG	176.00	1.45	20	*
PHOSPHRUS	MG	134.00	1.10	15	*
POTASSIUM	MG	257.00	0.38	5	*
PROTEIN	G	5.00	0.74	10	*
CARBOHYDT	G	32.00	0.86	12	*
FAT	G	14.00	1.33	18	*
OLEIC A	G	3.60	1.09	15	*
LINOL A	G	0.30	0.11	2	*
SAT FAT A	G	8.90	2.31	31	*

77 ICE CREAM, REGULAR (11% FAT), HARDENED
ANALYSIS OF 50 GRAMS WHICH IS 3-FL OZ

NUTRIENT	UNIT	AMOUNT	INQ	% STD	0 10 20 30 40 50 60 70 80 90 100
ENERGY	KCAL	100.00	1.00	5	EEEE
VITAMIN A	IU	200.00	1.00	5	AAAA
VITAMIN C	MG	0.00	0.00	0	--I
THIAMIN	MG	0.02	0.40	2	TT I
RIBOFLAVN	MG	0.12	2.00	10	RRR|RRRR
NIACIN	MG	0.10	0.14	1	N I
IRON	MG	0.00	0.00	0	- I
CALCIUM	MG	66.00	1.47	7	KKK|KK
PHOSPHRUS	MG	51.00	1.13	6	XXX|X
POTASSIUM	MG	96.00	0.38	2	YY I
PROTEIN	G	2.00	0.80	4	PPP|
CARBOHYDT	G	12.00	0.87	4	HHH|
FAT	G	5.00	1.28	6	FFF|F
OLEIC A	G	1.40	1.14	6	OOO|O
LINOL A	G	0.10	0.14	1	- I
SAT FAT A	G	3.40	2.39	12	SSS|SSSSS

78 ICE CREAM, REGULAR (11% FAT), SOFT SERVE
ANALYSIS OF 173 GRAMS WHICH IS 1 CUP

NUTRIENT	UNIT	AMOUNT	INQ	% STD	0 10 20 30 40 50 60 70 80 90 100
ENERGY	KCAL	375.00	1.00	19	EEEEEEEEEEEE
VITAMIN A	IU	790.00	1.05	20	AAAAAAAAAAAA|A
VITAMIN C	MG	1.00	0.09	2	C
THIAMIN	MG	0.08	0.43	8	TTTTT
RIBOFLAVN	MG	0.45	2.00	38	RRRRRRRRRRRR|RRRRRRRRRRRR
NIACIN	MG	0.20	0.08	1	N
IRON	MG	0.40	0.13	3	II
CALCIUM	MG	236.00	1.40	26	KKKKKKKKKKKK|KKKK
PHOSPHRUS	MG	199.00	1.18	22	XXXXXXXXXXXX|XXX
POTASSIUM	MG	338.00	0.36	7	YYYY
PROTEIN	G	7.00	0.75	14	PPPPPPPPP
CARBOHYDT	G	38.00	0.74	14	HHHHHHHHH
FAT	G	23.00	1.57	29	FFFFFFFFFFFF|FFFFFFF
OLEIC A	G	5.90	1.28	24	OOOOOOOOOOOO|OOOO
LINOL A	G	0.60	0.16	3	LL
SAT FAT A	G	13.50	2.53	47	SSSSSSSSSSSS|SSSSSSSSSSSSSSSSSSSSSSS

79 ICE CREAM, RICH (16% FAT), HARDENED
ANALYSIS OF 1188 GRAMS WHICH IS 1/2 GAL

NUTRIENT	UNIT	AMOUNT	INQ	% STD
ENERGY	KCAL	2805.00	1.00	140
VITAMIN A	IU	7200.00	1.28	180
VITAMIN C	MG	5.00	0.06	8
THIAMIN	MG	0.36	0.26	36
RIBOFLAVN	MG	2.27	1.35	189
NIACIN	MG	0.90	0.05	6
IRON	MG	0.80	0.04	5
CALCIUM	MG	1213.00	0.96	135
PHOSPHRUS	MG	927.00	0.73	103
POTASSIUM	MG	1771.00	0.25	35
PROTEIN	G	33.00	0.47	66
CARBOHYDT	G	256.00	0.66	93
FAT	G	190.00	1.74	244
OLEIC A	G	47.80	1.39	195
LINOL A	G	4.30	0.15	22
SAT FAT A	G	11.80	0.30	41

80 ICE CREAM, RICH (16% FAT), HARDENED
ANALYSIS OF 148 GRAMS WHICH IS 1 CUP

NUTRIENT	UNIT	AMOUNT	INQ	% STD
ENERGY	KCAL	350.00	1.00	17
VITAMIN A	IU	900.00	1.29	23
VITAMIN C	MG	1.00	0.10	2
THIAMIN	MG	0.04	0.23	4
RIBOFLAVN	MG	0.28	1.33	23
NIACIN	MG	0.10	0.04	1
IRON	MG	0.10	0.04	1
CALCIUM	MG	151.00	0.96	17
PHOSPHRUS	MG	115.00	0.73	13
POTASSIUM	MG	221.00	0.25	4
PROTEIN	G	4.00	0.46	8
CARBOHYDT	G	32.00	0.66	12
FAT	G	24.00	1.76	31
OLEIC A	G	6.00	1.40	24
LINOL A	G	0.50	0.14	3
SAT FAT A	G	14.70	2.95	52

81 ICE MILK, HARDENED (4.3% FAT)
ANALYSIS OF 1048 GRAMS WHICH IS 1/2 GAL

```
NUTRIENT   UNIT   AMOUNT    INQ   % STD    0        10        20        30        40        50        60        70        80        90       100
ENERGY     KCAL   1470.00   1.00    74   EEEEEEEEEEEEEEEEEEEEEEEEEEEEEEEEEEEEEEEEEEEEEEEEEEEEEEEEEEEEEEEEEEEEEEEEEE                                    *
VITAMIN A  IU     1710.00   0.58    43   AAAAAAAAAAAAAAAAAAAAAAAAAAAAAAAAAAAAAAAAAAA                                                                 *
VITAMIN C  MG        6.00   0.14    10   CCCCCCCC                                                                                                   *
THIAMIN    MG        0.61   0.83    61   TTTTTTTTTTTTTTTTTTTTTTTTTTTTTTTTTTTTTTTTTTTTTTTTTTTTTTTTTTTTTT                                               *
RIBOFLAVN  MG        2.78   3.15   232   RRRRRRRRRRRRRRRRRRRRRRRRRRRRRRRRRRRRRRRRRRRRRRRRRRRRRRRRRRRRRRRRRRRRRR|RRRRRRRRRRRRRRRRR *232
NIACIN     MG        0.90   0.09     6   NNNNN                                                                                                      *
IRON       MG        1.50   0.13     9   IIIIIII                                                                                                    *
CALCIUM    MG     1409.00   2.13   157   KKKKKKKKKKKKKKKKKKKKKKKKKKKKKKKKKKKKKKKKKKKKKKKKKKKKKKKKKKKKKKKKKKKKKK|KKKKKKKKKKKK *157
PHOSPHRUS  MG     1035.00   1.56   115   XXXXXXXXXXXXXXXXXXXXXXXXXXXXXXXXXXXXXXXXXXXXXXXXXXXXXXXXXXXXXXXXXXXXXX|XXXXXXXXX *115
POTASSIUM  MG     2117.00   0.58    42   YYYYYYYYYYYYYYYYYYYYYYYYYYYYYYYYYYYYYY                                                                      *
PROTEIN    G        41.00   1.12    82   PPPPPPPPPPPPPPPPPPPPPPPPPPPPPPPPPPPPPPPPPPPPPPPPPPPPPPPPPPPPPPPPPPPPPPPPP                                    *
CARBOHYDT  G       232.00   1.15    84   HHHHHHHHHHHHHHHHHHHHHHHHHHHHHHHHHHHHHHHHHHHHHHHHHHHHHHHHHHHHHHHHHHHHHHHHHH                                   *
FAT        G        45.00   0.78    58   FFFFFFFFFFFFFFFFFFFFFFFFFFFFFFFFFFFFFFFFFFFFFFFFFFFFFFFFFF                                                   *
OLEIC A    G        11.30   0.63    46   OOOOOOOOOOOOOOOOOOOOOOOOOOOOOOOOOOOOOOOOOOOOOOOO                                                             *
LINOL A    G         1.00   0.07     5   LLLL                                                                                                       *
SAT FAT A  G        28.10   1.34    99   SSSSSSSSSSSSSSSSSSSSSSSSSSSSSSSSSSSSSSSSSSSSSSSSSSSSSSSSSSSSSSSSSSSSSSSSSSSSSSSSSSSSSSSSSSSSSSSSSSSS*
*************************************************************************************************************************
```

82 ICE MILK, HARDENED (4.3% FAT)
ANALYSIS OF 131 GRAMS WHICH IS 1 CUP

```
NUTRIENT   UNIT   AMOUNT   INQ   % STD     0        10        20        30        40        50        60        70        80        90       100
ENERGY     KCAL   185.00   1.00     9   EEEEEEE                                                                                                    *
VITAMIN A  IU     210.00   0.57     5   AAAA|                                                                                                      *
VITAMIN C  MG       1.00   0.18     2   C  |                                                                                                       *
THIAMIN    MG       0.08   0.86     8   TTTTTT|                                                                                                    *
RIBOFLAVN  MG       0.35   3.15    29   RRRRR|RRRRRRRRRRRRRRRRR                                                                                     *
NIACIN     MG       0.10   0.08     1   N  |                                                                                                       *
IRON       MG       0.10   0.07     1   I  |                                                                                                       *
CALCIUM    MG     176.00   2.11    20   KKKKKK|KKKKKKKK                                                                                             *
PHOSPHRUS  MG     129.00   1.55    14   XXXXXX|XXXX                                                                                                 *
POTASSIUM  MG     265.00   0.57     5   YYYY |                                                                                                     *
PROTEIN    G        5.00   1.08    10   PPPPPPP|P                                                                                                   *
CARBOHYDT  G       29.00   1.14    11   HHHHHHH|H                                                                                                   *
FAT        G        6.00   0.83     8   FFFFFF|                                                                                                     *
OLEIC A    G        1.40   0.62     6   OOOOO|                                                                                                      *
LINOL A    G        0.10   0.05     1   - |                                                                                                         *
SAT FAT A  G        3.50   1.33    12   SSSSSS|SSS                                                                                                  *
*************************************************************************************************************************
```

83 ICE MILK, SOFT SERVE (2.6% FAT)
NALYSIS OF 175 GRAMS WHICH IS 1 CUP

NUTRIENT	UNIT	AMOUNT	INQ	% STD	0 10 20 30 40 50 60 70 80 90 100
ENERGY	KCAL	225.00	1.00	11	EEEEEEEE
VITAMIN A	IU	180.00	0.40	5	AAAA
VITAMIN C	MG	1.00	0.15	2	C
THIAMIN	MG	0.12	1.07	12	TTTTTTTT|T
RIBOFLAVN	MG	0.54	4.00	45	RRRRRRRR|RRRRRRRRRRRRRRRRRRR
NIACIN	MG	0.20	0.13	1	N
IRON	MG	0.30	0.17	2	II
CALCIUM	MG	274.00	2.71	30	KKKKKKKK|KKKKKKKKKKKK
PHOSPHRUS	MG	202.00	2.00	22	XXXXXXXX|XXXXXXXX
POTASSIUM	MG	412.00	0.73	8	YYYYYY
PROTEIN	G	8.00	1.42	16	PPPPPPPP|PPPP
CARBOHYDT	G	38.00	1.23	14	HHHHHHHH|HH
FAT	G	5.00	0.57	6	FFFFF
OLEIC A	G	1.20	0.44	5	OOOO
LINOL A	G	0.10	0.04	1	-
SAT FAT A	G	2.90	0.90	10	SSSSSSSS|

84 SHERBET (2% FAT)
ANALYSIS OF 1542 GRAMS WHICH IS 1/2 GAL

NUTRIENT	UNIT	AMOUNT	INQ	% STD	0 10 20 30 40 50 60 70 80 90 100
ENERGY	KCAL	2160.00	1.00	108	EEEEEEEEEEEEEEEEEEEEEEEEEEEEEEEEEEEEEEEEEEEEEEEEEEEEEEEEEEEEEEEEEEEEEEEEEEEEEEEEEEEEEEEEEEEEEEEEEEEEEE *108
VITAMIN A	IU	1480.00	0.34	37	AAAAAAAAAAAAAAAAAAAAAAAAAAAAAAAAAAAAA
VITAMIN C	MG	31.00	0.48	52	CCCCCCCCCCCCCCCCCCCCCCCCCCCCCCCCCCCCCCCCCCCCCCCCCCCC
THIAMIN	MG	0.26	0.24	26	TTTTTTTTTTTTTTTTTTTTTTTTTT
RIBOFLAVN	MG	0.71	0.55	59	RRRRRRRRRRRRRRRRRRRRRRRRRRRRRRRRRRRRRRRRRRRRRRRRRRRRRRRRRRRRR
NIACIN	MG	1.00	0.07	7	NNNNN
IRON	MG	2.50	0.14	16	IIIIIIIIIIII
CALCIUM	MG	827.00	0.85	92	KKKKKKKKKKKKKKKKKKKKKKXXXXXXXXXXXXXXXXXXXXXXXXXXXXXXXXXXKKKKKKKKKKKKKKKKKKKKKKKKKKKKKKK
PHOSPHRUS	MG	594.00	0.61	66	XXXXXXXXXXXXXXXXXXXXXXXXXXXXXXXXXXXXXXXXXXXXXXXXXXXXXXXXXXXXXXXXXXXX
POTASSIUM	MG	1585.00	0.29	32	YYYYYYYYYYYYYYYYYYYYYYYYYYYYYYYY
PROTEIN	G	17.00	0.31	34	PPPPPPPPPPPPPPPPPPPPPPPPPPPPPPPPPP
CARBOHYDT	G	469.00	1.58	171	HHHHHHHHHHHHHHHHHHHHHHHHHHHHHHHHHHHHHHHHHHHHHHHHHHHHHHHHHHHHHHHHHHHHHHHHHHHHHHHHHHHHHHHHHHHHHHHHHHHHHHHHHHHHHHHHHHHHHHHHHHHHHHHHHHHHHHHHHHHHHHHHHHHHHHHHHHHHHHHHHHHHHHHHHHHHHH *171
FAT	G	31.00	0.37	40	FFFFFFFFFFFFFFFFFFFFFFFFFFFFFFFFFFFFFFFF
OLEIC A	G	7.70	0.29	31	OOOOOOOOOOOOOOOOOOOOOOOOOOOOOOO
LINOL A	G	0.70	0.03	4	LLL
SAT FAT A	G	19.00	0.62	67	SSSSSSSSSSSSSSSSSSSSSSSSSSSSSSSSSSSSSSSSSSSSSSSSSSSSSSSSSSSSSSSSSSSSSSS

85 SHERBET (2% FAT)
ANALYSIS OF 193 GRAMS WHICH IS 1 CUP

```
                                    0        10        20        30        40        50        60        70        80        90       100
NUTRIENT    UNIT   AMOUNT   INQ  % STD
ENERGY      KCAL   270.00   1.00   14   EEEEEEEEEE
VITAMIN A   IU     190.00   0.35    5   AAAA
VITAMIN C   MG       4.00   0.49    7   CCCCC
THIAMIN     MG       0.03   0.22    3   TT
RIBOFLAVN   MG       0.09   0.56    8   RRRRR
NIACIN      MG       0.10   0.05    1   N
IRON        MG       0.30   0.14    2   II
CALCIUM     MG     103.00   0.85   11   KKKKKKKK
PHOSPHRUS   MG      74.00   0.61    8   XXXXXXX
POTASSIUM   MG     198.00   0.29    4   YYY
PROTEIN     G        2.00   0.30    4   PPP
CARBOHYDT   G       59.00   1.59   21   HHHHHHHHHH|HHHHH
FAT         G        4.00   0.38    5   FFFF
OLEIC A     G        1.00   0.30    4   OOO
LINOL A     G        0.10   0.04    1   -
SAT FAT A   G        2.40   0.62    8   SSSSSS
*********************************************************
```

86 CUSTARD, BAKED
ANALYSIS OF 265 GRAMS WHICH IS 1 CUP

```
                                    0        10        20        30        40        50        60        70        80        90       100
NUTRIENT    UNIT   AMOUNT   INQ  % STD
ENERGY      KCAL   305.00   1.00   15   EEEEEEEEEE
VITAMIN A   IU     930.00   1.52   23   AAAAAAAAAA|AAAAAA
VITAMIN C   MG       1.00   0.11    2   C
THIAMIN     MG       0.11   0.72   11   TTTTTTT
RIBOFLAVN   MG       0.50   2.73   42   RRRRRRRRRR|RRRRRRRRRRRRRRRRRRRRRR
NIACIN      MG       0.30   0.14    2   NN
IRON        MG       1.10   0.45    7   IIIIII
CALCIUM     MG     297.00   2.16   33   KKKKKKKKKK|KKKKKKKKKKKKKKKKKKKKK
PHOSPHRUS   MG     310.00   2.26   34   XXXXXXXXXX|XXXXXXXXXXXXXXXXXXXXXXXX
POTASSIUM   MG     387.00   0.51    8   YYYYYY
PROTEIN     G       14.00   1.84   28   PPPPPPPPPP|PPPPPPPPP
CARBOHYDT   G       29.00   0.69   11   HHHHHHH
FAT         G       15.00   1.26   19   FFFFFFFFFF|FFF
OLEIC A     G        5.40   1.45   22   OOOOOOOOOO|OOOOOO
LINOL A     G        0.70   0.23    4   LLL
SAT FAT A   G        6.80   1.56   24   SSSSSSSSSS|SSSSSSSSSSSSSS
*********************************************************
```

87 CHOCOLATE PUDDING, HOME RECIPE, STARCH BASE
ANALYSIS OF 260 GRAMS WHICH IS 1 CUP

NUTRIENT	UNIT	AMOUNT	INQ	% STD
ENERGY	KCAL	385.00	1.00	19
VITAMIN A	IU	390.00	0.51	10
VITAMIN C	MG	1.00	0.09	2
THIAMIN	MG	0.05	0.26	5
RIBOFLAVN	MG	0.36	1.56	30
NIACIN	MG	0.11	0.11	2
IRON	MG	1.30	0.42	8
CALCIUM	MG	250.00	1.44	28
PHOSPHRUS	MG	255.00	1.47	28
POTASSIUM	MG	445.00	0.46	9
PROTEIN	G	8.00	0.83	16
CARBOHYDT	G	67.00	1.27	24
FAT	G	12.00	0.80	15
OLEIC A	G	3.30	0.70	13
LINOL A	G	0.30	0.08	2
SAT FAT A	G	7.60	1.39	27

88 VANILLA PUDDING (BLANCMANGE), HOME RECIPE, STARCH BASE
ANALYSIS OF 255 GRAMS WHICH IS 1 CUP

NUTRIENT	UNIT	AMOUNT	INQ	% STD
ENERGY	KCAL	285.00	1.00	14
VITAMIN A	IU	410.00	0.72	10
VITAMIN C	MG	2.00	0.23	3
THIAMIN	MG	0.08	0.56	8
RIBOFLAVN	MG	0.41	2.40	34
NIACIN	MG	0.30	0.15	2
IRON	MG	0.00	0.00	0
CALCIUM	MG	298.00	2.32	33
PHOSPHRUS	MG	232.00	1.81	26
POTASSIUM	MG	352.00	0.49	7
PROTEIN	G	9.00	1.26	18
CARBOHYDT	G	41.00	1.05	15
FAT	G	10.00	0.90	13
OLEIC A	G	2.50	0.72	10
LINOL A	G	0.20	0.07	1
SAT FAT A	G	6.20	1.53	22

89 TAPIOCA CREAM PUDDING, HOME RECIPE
ANALYSIS OF 165 GRAMS WHICH IS 1 CUP

```
                                    0        10        20        30        40        50        60        70        80        90       100
NUTRIENT   UNIT  AMOUNT   INQ  %STD
ENERGY     KCAL  220.00   1.00   11  EEEEEEEE
VITAMIN A  IU    480.00   1.09   12  AAAAAAA|A
VITAMIN C  MG      2.00   0.30    3  CCC
THIAMIN    MG      0.07   0.64    7  TTTTTT|
RIBOFLAVN  MG      0.30   2.27   25  RRRRRRRR|RRRRRRRRRR
NIACIN     MG      0.20   0.13    1  N
IRON       MG      0.70   0.40    4  IIII
CALCIUM    MG    173.00   1.75   19  KKKKKKKK|KKKKK
PHOSPHRUS  MG    180.00   1.82   20  XXXXXXXX|XXXXXXX
POTASSIUM  MG    223.00   0.41    4  YYYY
PROTEIN    G       8.00   1.45   16  PPPPPPP|PPPP
CARBOHYDT  G      28.00   0.93   10  HHHHHHHH|
FAT        G       8.00   0.93   10  FFFFFFF|
OLEIC A    G       2.50   0.93   10  OOOOOOOO|
LINOL A    G       0.50   0.23    3  LL
SAT FAT A  G       4.10   1.31   14  SSSSSSS|SSS
```

90 CHOCOLATE PUDDING, COOKED FROM A MIX
ANALYSIS OF 260 GRAMS WHICH IS 1 CUP

```
                                    0        10        20        30        40        50        60        70        80        90       100
NUTRIENT   UNIT  AMOUNT   INQ  %STD
ENERGY     KCAL  320.00   1.00   16  EEEEEEEEEE
VITAMIN A  IU    340.00   0.53    9  AAAAAAA
VITAMIN C  MG      2.00   0.21    3  CCC
THIAMIN    MG      0.05   0.31    5  TTTT
RIBOFLAVN  MG      0.39   2.03   33  RRRRRRRRRR|RRRRRRRRRRR
NIACIN     MG      0.30   0.13    2  NN
IRON       MG      0.80   0.31    5  IIII
CALCIUM    MG    265.00   1.84   29  KKKKKKKKKK|KKKKKKKKK
PHOSPHRUS  MG    247.00   1.72   27  XXXXXXXXXX|XXXXXXX
POTASSIUM  MG    354.00   0.44    7  YYYYY
PROTEIN    G       9.00   1.13   18  PPPPPPPPP|P
CARBOHYDT  G      59.00   1.34   21  HHHHHHHHHH|HHHH
FAT        G       8.00   0.64   10  FFFFFFF|
OLEIC A    G       2.60   0.66   11  OOOOOOOO
LINOL A    G       0.20   0.06    1  L
SAT FAT A  G       4.30   0.94   15  SSSSSSSSSS|S
```

91 CHOCOLATE PUDDING, INSTANT
ANALYSIS OF 260 GRAMS WHICH IS 1 CUP

NUTRIENT	UNIT	AMOUNT	INQ	%STD
ENERGY	KCAL	325.00	1.00	16
VITAMIN A	IU	340.00	0.52	9
VITAMIN C	MG	2.00	0.21	3
THIAMIN	MG	0.08	0.49	8
RIBOFLAVN	MG	0.39	2.00	33
NIACIN	MG	0.30	0.13	2
IRON	MG	1.30	0.50	8
CALCIUM	MG	374.00	2.56	42
PHOSPHRUS	MG	237.00	1.62	26
POTASSIUM	MG	335.00	0.41	7
PROTEIN	G	8.00	0.98	16
CARBOHYDT	G	63.00	1.41	23
FAT	G	7.00	0.55	9
OLEIC A	G	2.20	0.55	9
LINOL A	G	0.30	0.09	2
SAT FAT A	G	3.60	0.78	13

92 FRUIT-FLAVORED YOGURT MADE WITH LOWFAT MILK, WITH ADDED MILK SOLIDS
ANALYSIS OF 227 GRAMS WHICH IS 8 OZ, NET WT.

NUTRIENT	UNIT	AMOUNT	INQ	%STD
ENERGY	KCAL	230.00	1.00	12
VITAMIN A	IU	120.00	0.26	3
VITAMIN C	MG	1.00	0.14	2
THIAMIN	MG	0.08	0.70	8
RIBOFLAVN	MG	0.40	2.90	33
NIACIN	MG	0.20	0.12	1
IRON	MG	0.20	0.11	1
CALCIUM	MG	343.00	3.31	38
PHOSPHRUS	MG	269.00	2.60	30
POTASSIUM	MG	439.00	0.76	9
PROTEIN	G	10.00	1.74	20
CARBOHYDT	G	42.00	1.33	15
FAT	G	3.00	0.33	4
OLEIC A	G	0.60	0.21	2
LINOL A	G	0.10	0.04	2
SAT FAT A	G	1.80	0.55	6

93 PLAIN YOGURT MADE WITH LOWFAT MILK, WITH ADDED MILK SOLIDS
ANALYSIS OF 227 GRAMS WHICH IS 8 OZ, NET WT.

NUTRIENT	UNIT	AMOUNT	INQ	% STD	0	10	20	30	40	50	60	70	80	90	100
ENERGY	KCAL	145.00	1.00	7	EEEEEE										*
VITAMIN A	IU	150.00	0.52	4	AAA										*
VITAMIN C	MG	2.00	0.46	3	CCC										*
THIAMIN	MG	0.10	1.38	10	TTTTITTT										*
RIBOFLAVN	MG	0.49	5.63	41	RHRRIRRRRRRRRRRRRRRRRRR									*
NIACIN	MG	0.30	0.30	2	NN										*
IRON	MG	0.20	0.17	1	I										*
CALCIUM	MG	415.00	6.36	46	KKKKIKKKKKKKKKKKXXXXXXXXXXXXX									*
PHUSPHRUS	MG	326.00	5.00	36	XXXXXIXXXXXXXXXXXXXXXXX									*
POTASSIUM	MG	531.00	1.46	11	YYYYYIYY										*
PROTEIN	G	12.00	3.31	24	PPPPPIPPPPPPPPP										*
CARBOHYDT	G	16.00	0.80	6	HHHHHI										*
FAT	G	4.00	0.71	5	FFFF										*
OLEIC A	G	0.80	0.45	3	OOO										*
LINOL A	G	0.10	0.07	1	-										*
SAT FAT A	G	2.30	1.11	8	SSSSS										*

94 PLAIN YOGURT MADE WITH NONFAT MILK, WITH ADDED MILK SOLIDS
ANALYSIS OF 227 GRAMS WHICH IS 8 OZ, NET WT.

NUTRIENT	UNIT	AMOUNT	INQ	% STD	0	10	20	30	40	50	60	70	80	90	100
ENERGY	KCAL	125.00	1.00	6	EEEEE										*
VITAMIN A	IU	20.00	0.08	1	-										*
VITAMIN C	MG	2.00	0.53	3	CCC I										*
THIAMIN	MG	0.11	1.76	11	TTTTITTT										*
RIBOFLAVN	MG	0.53	7.07	44	RRRRIRRRRRRRRRRRRRRRRRRRR									*
NIACIN	MG	0.30	0.34	2	NN										*
IRON	MG	0.20	0.20	1	I										*
CALCIUM	MG	452.00	8.04	50	KKKKIKKKKKKKKKKKXXXXXXXXXXXXXXXXXX									*
PHUSPHRUS	MG	355.00	6.31	39	XXXXIXXXXXXXXXXXXXXXXXXX									*
POTASSIUM	MG	579.00	1.85	12	YYYYIYYYY										*
PROTEIN	G	13.00	4.16	26	PPPPIPPPPPPPPPPPPPPP										*
CARBOHYDT	G	17.00	0.99	6	HHHHH										*
FAT	G	0.00	0.00	0	-										*
OLEIC A	G	0.10	0.07	0	-										*
LINOL A	G	0.00	0.00	0	-										*
SAT FAT A	G	0.30	0.17	1	S										*

95 PLAIN YOGURT MADE WITH WHOLE MILK, WITHOUT ADDED MILK SOLIDS
ANALYSIS OF 227 GRAMS WHICH IS 8 OZ, NET WT.

```
                                      0    10        20        30        40   50   60   70   80   90   100
NUTRIENT   UNIT   AMOUNT   INQ   % STD
ENERGY     KCAL   140.00   1.00    7   EEEEE                                                              * * * * * * * * * * * * * * * * *
VITAMIN A  IU     280.00   1.00    7   AAAAA
VITAMIN C  MG       1.00   0.24    2   C   I
THIAMIN    MG       0.07   1.00    7   TTTTT
RIBOFLAVN  MG       0.32   3.81   27   RRRRIRRRRRRRRRRRRR
NIACIN     MG       0.20   0.20    1   N   I
IRON       MG       0.10   0.09    1   I   I
CALCIUM    MG     274.00   4.35   30   KKKKKIKKKKKKKKKKKKKKKKKK
PHOSPHRUS  MG     215.00   3.41   24   XXXXXIXXXXXXXXXXXXX
POTASSIUM  MG     351.00   1.00    7   YYYYY
PROTEIN    G        8.00   2.29   16   PPPPPIPPPPPP
CARBOHYDT  G       11.00   0.57    4   HHH
FAT        G        7.00   1.28    9   FFFFFIF
OLEIC A    G        1.70   0.99    7   OOOOOO
LINOL A    G        0.10   0.07    1   -   I
SAT FAT A  G        4.80   2.41   17   SSSSSISSSSSS
                                      *****************
```

96 EGG, WHOLE, RAW, LARGE, WITHOUT SHELL
ANALYSIS OF 50 GRAMS WHICH IS 1 EGG

```
                                      0    10        20        30        40   50   60   70   80   90   100
NUTRIENT   UNIT   AMOUNT   INQ   % STD
ENERGY     KCAL    80.00   1.00    4   EEE                                                                * * * * * * * * * * * * * * * * *
VITAMIN A  IU     260.00   1.63    7   AAIAA
VITAMIN C  MG       0.00   0.00    0   -   I
THIAMIN    MG       0.04   1.00    4   TTT
RIBOFLAVN  MG       0.15   3.13   13   RRIRRRRRR
NIACIN     MG       0.00   0.00    0   -   I
IRON       MG       1.00   1.56    6   IIjII
CALCIUM    MG      28.00   0.78    3   KKI
PHOSPHRUS  MG      90.00   2.50   10   XXIXXXXX
POTASSIUM  MG      65.00   0.33    1   Y   I
PROTEIN    G        6.00   3.00   12   PPIPPPPP
CARBOHYDT  G        1.00   0.09    0   -   I
FAT        G        6.00   1.92    8   FFIFFF
OLEIC A    G        2.00   2.04    8   OOIOOOO
LINOL A    G        0.60   0.75    3   LLI
SAT FAT A  G        1.70   1.49    6   SSISS
                                      *****************
```

```
                                    10      20      30      40      50      60      70      80      90      100
                                                                                                        ***************
```

97 EGG, WHITE, RAW
ANALYSIS OF 33 GRAMS WHICH IS 1 WHITE

NUTRIENT	UNIT	AMOUNT	INQ	% STD	0
ENERGY	KCAL	15.00	1.00	1	E
VITAMIN A	IU	0.00	0.00	0	-
VITAMIN C	MG	0.00	0.00	0	-
THIAMIN	MG	0.00	0.00	0	-
RIBOFLAVN	MG	0.09	10.00	8	IRRRRR
NIACIN	MG	0.00	0.00	0	-
IRON	MG	0.00	0.00	0	-
CALCIUM	MG	4.00	0.59	0	-
PHOSPHRUS	MG	4.00	0.59	0	-
POTASSIUM	MG	45.00	1.20	1	Y
PROTEIN	G	3.00	8.00	6	IPPPP
CARBOHYDT	G	0.00	0.00	0	-
FAT	G	0.00	0.00	0	-
OLEIC A	G	0.00	0.00	0	-
LINOL A	G	0.00	0.00	0	-
SAT FAT A	G	0.00	0.00	0	-

```
*********************************************
```

```
                                    10      20      30      40      50      60      70      80      90      100
                                                                                                        ***************
```

98 EGG, YOLK, RAW
ANALYSIS OF 17 GRAMS WHICH IS 1 YOLK

NUTRIENT	UNIT	AMOUNT	INQ	% STD	0
ENERGY	KCAL	65.00	1.00	3	EEE
VITAMIN A	IU	310.00	2.38	8	AAIAAA
VITAMIN C	MG	0.00	0.00	0	-I
THIAMIN	MG	0.04	1.23	4	TTT
RIBOFLAVN	MG	0.07	1.79	6	RRIRR
NIACIN	MG	0.00	0.00	0	-I
IRON	MG	0.90	1.73	6	IIIII
CALCIUM	MG	26.00	0.89	3	KKI
PHOSPHRUS	MG	86.00	2.94	10	XXIXXXXX
POTASSIUM	MG	15.00	0.09	0	-I
PROTEIN	G	3.00	1.85	6	PPIPP
CARBOHYDT	G	0.00	0.00	0	-I
FAT	G	6.00	2.37	8	FFIFFF
OLEIC A	G	2.10	2.64	9	OOIOOOO
LINOL A	G	0.60	0.92	3	LLI
SAT FAT A	G	1.70	1.84	6	SSISS

```
*********************************************
```

99 EGG, FRIED IN BUTTER (LARGE)
ANALYSIS OF 46 GRAMS WHICH IS 1 EGG

```
                               0        10   20   30   40   50   60   70   80   90   100
NUTRIENT   UNIT  AMOUNT  INQ   % STD                                                   **************
ENERGY     KCAL   85.00  1.00    4   EEE
VITAMIN A  IU    290.00  1.71    7   AAIAAA
VITAMIN C  MG      0.00  0.00    0   -I
THIAMIN    MG      0.03  0.71    3   TTI
RIBOFLAVN  MG      0.13  2.55   11   RRIRRRRR
NIACIN     MG      0.00  0.00    0   -I
IRON       MG      0.90  1.32    6   IIIII
CALCIUM    MG     26.00  0.68    3   KKI
PHOSPHRUS  MG     80.00  2.09    9   XXIXXXX
POTASSIUM  MG     58.00  0.27    1   YI
PROTEIN    G       5.00  2.35   10   PPIPPPPP
CARBOHYDT  G       1.00  0.09    0   FFIFFF
FAT        G       6.00  1.81    8   OOIOOOO
OLEIC A    G       2.20  2.11    9   LLI
LINOL A    G       0.60  0.71    3   SSISSSS
SAT FAT A  G       2.40  1.98    8
```

100 EGG, HARD-COOKED (LARGE), WITHOUT SHELL
ANALYSIS OF 50 GRAMS WHICH IS 1 EGG

```
                               0        10   20   30   40   50   60   70   80   90   100
NUTRIENT   UNIT  AMOUNT  INQ   % STD                                                   **************
ENERGY     KCAL   80.00  1.00    4   EEE
VITAMIN A  IU    260.00  1.63    7   AAIAA
VITAMIN C  MG      0.00  0.00    0   -I
THIAMIN    MG      0.04  1.00    4   TTT
RIBOFLAVN  MG      0.14  2.92   12   RRIRRRRR
NIACIN     MG      0.00  0.00    0   -I
IRON       MG      1.00  1.56    6   IIIII
CALCIUM    MG     28.00  0.78    3   KKI
PHOSPHRUS  MG     90.00  2.50   10   XXIXXXXX
POTASSIUM  MG     65.00  0.33    1   YI
PROTEIN    G       6.00  3.00   12   PPIPPPPPP
CARBOHYDT  G       1.00  0.09    0   -I
FAT        G       6.00  1.92    8   FFIFFF
OLEIC A    G       2.00  2.04    8   OOIOOOO
LINOL A    G       0.60  0.75    3   LLI
SAT FAT A  G       1.70  1.49    6   SSISS
```

101 EGG, POACHED (LARGE)
ANALYSIS OF 50 GRAMS WHICH IS 1 EGG

NUTRIENT	UNIT	AMOUNT	INQ	% STD	0 10
ENERGY	KCAL	80.00	1.00	4	EEE
VITAMIN A	IU	260.00	1.63	7	AAIAA
VITAMIN C	MG	0.00	0.00	0	– I
THIAMIN	MG	0.04	1.00	4	TTT
RIBOFLAVN	MG	0.13	2.71	11	RRIRRRRRR
NIACIN	MG	0.00	0.00	0	– I
IRON	MG	1.00	1.56	6	IIIII
CALCIUM	MG	28.00	0.78	3	KKI
PHOSPHRUS	MG	90.00	2.50	10	XXIXXXXX
POTASSIUM	MG	65.00	0.33	1	Y I
PROTEIN	G	6.00	3.00	12	PPIPPPPPP
CARBOHYDT	G	1.00	0.09	0	I
FAT	G	6.00	1.92	8	FFIFFF
OLEIC A	G	2.00	2.04	8	OOIOOOO
LINOL A	G	0.60	0.75	3	LLI
SAT FAT A	G	1.70	1.49	6	SSISS

****

102 EGG, SCRAMBLED (MILK ADDED) IN BUTTER (LARGE)
ANALYSIS OF 64 GRAMS WHICH IS 1 EGG

NUTRIENT	UNIT	AMOUNT	INQ	% STD	0 10
ENERGY	KCAL	95.00	1.00	5	EEEE
VITAMIN A	IU	310.00	1.63	8	AAAIAA
VITAMIN C	MG	0.00	0.00	0	– I
THIAMIN	MG	0.04	0.84	4	TTT
RIBOFLAVN	MG	0.16	2.81	13	RNRIRRRRRRR
NIACIN	MG	0.00	0.00	0	– I
IRON	MG	0.90	1.18	6	IIIII
CALCIUM	MG	47.00	1.10	5	KKKK
PHOSPHRUS	MG	97.00	2.27	11	XXXIXXXX
POTASSIUM	MG	85.00	0.36	2	Y I
PROTEIN	G	6.00	2.53	12	PPPIPPPPP
CARBOHYDT	G	1.00	0.08	0	I
FAT	G	7.00	1.89	9	FFFIFFF
OLEIC A	G	2.30	1.98	9	OOOIOOOO
LINOL A	G	0.60	0.63	3	LL I
SAT FAT A	G	2.80	2.07	10	SSSISSSS

****

103 BUTTER, REGULAR
ANALYSIS OF 113 GRAMS WHICH IS 1/2 CUP STICK

NUTRIENT	UNIT	AMOUNT	INQ	% STD
ENERGY	KCAL	815.00	1.00	41
VITAMIN A	IU	3470.00	2.13	87
VITAMIN C	MG	0.00	0.00	0
THIAMIN	MG	0.01	0.02	1
RIBOFLAVN	MG	0.04	0.08	3
NIACIN	MG	0.00	0.00	0
IRON	MG	0.20	0.03	1
CALCIUM	MG	27.00	0.07	3
PHOSPHRUS	MG	26.00	0.07	3
POTASSIUM	MG	29.00	0.01	1
PROTEIN	G	1.00	0.05	2
CARBOHYDT	G	0.00	0.00	0
FAT	G	92.00	2.89	118
OLEIC A	G	23.10	2.31	94
LINOL A	G	2.10	0.26	11
SAT FAT A	G	57.30	4.93	201

104 BUTTER, REGULAR
ANALYSIS OF 14 GRAMS WHICH IS 1 TBSP

NUTRIENT	UNIT	AMOUNT	INQ	% STD
ENERGY	KCAL	100.00	1.00	5
VITAMIN A	IU	430.00	2.15	11
VITAMIN C	MG	0.00	0.00	0
THIAMIN	MG	0.00	0.00	0
RIBOFLAVN	MG	0.00	0.00	0
NIACIN	MG	0.00	0.00	0
IRON	MG	0.00	0.00	0
CALCIUM	MG	3.00	0.07	0
PHOSPHRUS	MG	3.00	0.07	0
POTASSIUM	MG	4.00	0.02	0
PROTEIN	G	0.00	0.00	0
CARBOHYDT	G	0.00	0.00	0
FAT	G	12.00	3.08	15
OLEIC A	G	2.90	2.37	12
LINOL A	G	0.30	0.30	2
SAT FAT A	G	7.20	5.05	25

105 BUTTER, REGULAR
ANALYSIS OF 5 GRAMS WHICH IS 1 PAT (90 PER LB)

```
                                   0    10   20   30   40   50   60   70   80   90  100
NUTRIENT   UNIT  AMOUNT   INQ  % STD
ENERGY     KCAL   35.00  1.00    2  E
VITAMIN A  IU    150.00  2.14    4  IAA
VITAMIN C  MG      0.00  0.00    0  I
THIAMIN    MG      0.00  0.00    0  I
RIBOFLAVN  MG      0.00  0.00    0  I
NIACIN     MG      0.00  0.00    0  I
IRON       MG      0.00  0.00    0  I
CALCIUM    MG      1.00  0.06    0  I
PHOSPHRUS  MG      1.00  0.06    0  I
POTASSIUM  MG      1.00  0.01    0  I
PROTEIN    G       0.00  0.00    0  I
CARBOHYDT  G       0.00  0.00    0  I
FAT        G       4.00  2.93    5  IFFF
OLEIC A    G       1.00  2.33    4  I00
LINOL A    G       0.10  0.29    1  I
SAT FAT A  G       2.50  5.01    9  ISSSSSS
***************************************************
```

106 BUTTER, WHIPPED
ANALYSIS OF 76 GRAMS WHICH IS 1/2 CUP STICK

```
                                   0    10   20   30   40   50   60   70   80   90  100
NUTRIENT   UNIT  AMOUNT   INQ  % STD
ENERGY     KCAL  540.00  1.00   27  EEEEEEEEEEEEEEEEEEEEEEEEEE
VITAMIN A  IU   2310.00  2.14   58  AAAAAAAAAAAAAAAAAAAAAAAAAAAAAAAAAAAAAAAAAAAAAAAAAA
VITAMIN C  MG      0.00  0.00    0  I
THIAMIN    MG      0.00  0.00    0  I
RIBOFLAVN  MG      0.03  0.09    3  HR
NIACIN     MG      0.00  0.02    0  I
IRON       MG      0.10  0.02    1  I
CALCIUM    MG     18.00  0.07    2  KK
PHOSPHRUS  MG     17.00  0.07    2  XX
POTASSIUM  MG     20.00  0.01    2  I
PROTEIN    G       1.00  0.07    2  PP
CARBOHYDT  G       0.00  0.00    0  I
FAT        G      61.00  2.90   78  FFFFFFFFFFFFFFFFFFFFFFFFFFFFFFFFFFFFFFFFFFFFFFFFFFFFFFFFFFFFFFFFFFFFFFFFFF
OLEIC A    G      15.40  2.33   63  OOOOOOOOOOOOOOOOOOOOOOOOOOOOOOOOOOOOOOOOOOOOOOOOOOOOOOOOOOOOOOO
LINOL A    G       1.40  0.26    7  LLLLL
SAT FAT A  G      38.20  4.96  134  SSSSSSSSSSSSSSSSSSSSSSSSSSSSSSSSSSSSSSSSSSSSSSSSSSSSSSSSSSSSSSSSSSSSSSSSSSSSSSSSSSSSSSSSSSSS *134
***************************************************
```

107 BUTTER, WHIPPED
ANALYSIS OF 9 GRAMS WHICH IS 1 TBSP

NUTRIENT	UNIT	AMOUNT	INQ	% STD
ENERGY	KCAL	65.00	1.00	3
VITAMIN A	IU	290.00	2.23	7
VITAMIN C	MG	0.00	0.00	0
THIAMIN	MG	0.00	0.00	0
RIBOFLAVN	MG	0.00	0.00	0
NIACIN	MG	0.00	0.00	0
IRON	MG	0.00	0.00	0
CALCIUM	MG	2.00	0.07	0
PHOSPHRUS	MG	2.00	0.07	0
POTASSIUM	MG	2.00	0.01	0
PROTEIN	G	0.00	0.00	0
CARBOHYDT	G	0.00	0.00	0
FAT	G	8.00	3.16	10
OLEIC A	G	1.90	2.39	8
LINOL A	G	0.20	0.31	1
SAT FAT A	G	4.70	5.07	16

108 BUTTER, WHIPPED
ANALYSIS OF 4 GRAMS WHICH IS 1 PAT (120 PER LB)

NUTRIENT	UNIT	AMOUNT	INQ	% STD
ENERGY	KCAL	25.00	1.00	1
VITAMIN A	IU	120.00	2.40	3
VITAMIN C	MG	0.00	0.00	0
THIAMIN	MG	0.00	0.00	0
RIBOFLAVN	MG	0.00	0.00	0
NIACIN	MG	0.00	0.00	0
IRON	MG	0.00	0.00	0
CALCIUM	MG	1.00	0.09	0
PHOSPHRUS	MG	1.00	0.09	0
POTASSIUM	MG	1.00	0.02	0
PROTEIN	G	0.00	0.00	0
CARBOHYDT	G	0.00	0.00	0
FAT	G	3.00	3.08	4
OLEIC A	G	0.80	2.61	3
LINOL A	G	0.10	0.40	1
SAT FAT A	G	1.90	5.33	7

109 VEGETABLE SHORTENINGS
ANALYSIS OF 200 GRAMS WHICH IS 1 CUP

NUTRIENT	UNIT	AMOUNT	INQ	% STD
ENERGY	KCAL	1770.00	1.00	89
VITAMIN A	IU	0.00	0.00	0
VITAMIN C	MG	0.00	0.00	0
THIAMIN	MG	0.00	0.00	0
RIBOFLAVN	MG	0.00	0.00	0
NIACIN	MG	0.00	0.00	0
IRON	MG	0.00	0.00	0
CALCIUM	MG	0.00	0.00	0
PHOSPHRUS	MG	0.00	0.00	0
POTASSIUM	MG	0.00	0.00	0
PROTEIN	G	0.00	0.00	0
CARBOHYDT	G	0.00	0.00	0
FAT	G	200.00	2.90	256
OLEIC A	G	88.20	4.07	360
LINOL A	G	48.40	2.73	242
SAT FAT A	G	48.80	1.93	171

110 VEGETABLE SHORTENINGS
ANALYSIS OF 13 GRAMS WHICH IS 1 TBSP

NUTRIENT	UNIT	AMOUNT	INQ	% STD
ENERGY	KCAL	110.00	1.00	6
VITAMIN A	IU	0.00	0.00	0
VITAMIN C	MG	0.00	0.00	0
THIAMIN	MG	0.00	0.00	0
RIBOFLAVN	MG	0.00	0.00	0
NIACIN	MG	0.00	0.00	0
IRON	MG	0.00	0.00	0
CALCIUM	MG	0.00	0.00	0
PHOSPHRUS	MG	0.00	0.00	0
POTASSIUM	MG	0.00	0.00	0
PROTEIN	G	0.00	0.00	0
CARBOHYDT	G	0.00	0.00	0
FAT	G	13.00	3.03	17
OLEIC A	G	5.70	4.23	23
LINOL A	G	3.10	2.82	16
SAT FAT A	G	3.20	2.04	11

111 LARD
ANALYSIS OF 205 GRAMS WHICH IS 1 CUP

NUTRIENT	UNIT	AMOUNT	INQ	X STD
ENERGY	KCAL	1850.00	1.00	95
VITAMIN A	IU	0.00	0.00	0
VITAMIN C	MG	0.00	0.00	0
THIAMIN	MG	0.00	0.00	0
RIBOFLAVN	MG	0.00	0.00	0
NIACIN	MG	0.00	0.00	0
IRON	MG	0.00	0.00	0
CALCIUM	MG	0.00	0.00	0
PHOSPHRUS	MG	0.00	0.00	0
POTASSIUM	MG	0.00	0.00	0
PROTEIN	G	0.00	0.00	0
CARBOHYDT	G	0.00	0.00	0
FAT	G	205.00	2.84	263
OLEIC A	G	83.80	3.70	342
LINOL A	G	20.50	1.11	102
SAT FAT A	G	81.00	3.07	284

112 LARD
ANALYSIS OF 13 GRAMS WHICH IS 1 TBSP

NUTRIENT	UNIT	AMOUNT	INQ	X STD
ENERGY	KCAL	115.00	1.00	6
VITAMIN A	IU	0.00	0.00	0
VITAMIN C	MG	0.00	0.00	0
THIAMIN	MG	0.00	0.00	0
RIBOFLAVN	MG	0.00	0.00	0
NIACIN	MG	0.00	0.00	0
IRON	MG	0.00	0.00	0
CALCIUM	MG	0.00	0.00	0
PHOSPHRUS	MG	0.00	0.00	0
POTASSIUM	MG	0.00	0.00	0
PROTEIN	G	0.00	0.00	0
CARBOHYDT	G	0.00	0.00	0
FAT	G	13.00	2.90	17
OLEIC A	G	5.30	3.76	22
LINOL A	G	1.30	1.13	7
SAT FAT A	G	5.10	3.11	18

113 MARGARINE, REGULAR
ANALYSIS OF 113 GRAMS WHICH IS 1/2 CUP STICK

NUTRIENT	UNIT	AMOUNT	INQ	% STD	0 10 20 30 40 50 60 70 80 90 100
ENERGY	KCAL	815.00	1.00	41	EEEEEEEEEEEEEEEEEEEEEEEEEEEEEEEEEEEEEEEE
VITAMIN A	IU	3750.00	2.30	94	AAAAAAAAAAAAAAAAAAAAAAAAAAAAAAAAAAAAAAAAIAAAAAAAAAAAAAAAAAAAAAAAAAAAAAAAAAAAAAAAAAAAAA
VITAMIN C	MG	0.00	0.00	0	-
THIAMIN	MG	0.01	0.02	1	T
RIBOFLAVN	MG	0.04	0.08	3	RRR
NIACIN	MG	0.00	0.00	0	
IRON	MG	0.20	0.03	1	I
CALCIUM	MG	27.00	0.07	3	KK
PHOSPHRUS	MG	26.00	0.07	3	XX
POTASSIUM	MG	29.00	0.01	1	-
PROTEIN	G	1.00	0.05	2	PP
CARBOHYDT	G	0.00	0.00	0	
FAT	G	92.00	2.89	118	FFFFFFFFFFFFFFFFFFFFFFFFFFFFFFFFFFFFFFFFFIFFFFFFFFFFFFFFFFFFFFFFFFFFFFFFFFFFFFFFFFFFFFFFFFFFFFFFFFFFFFFFFF * 118
OLEIC A	G	42.90	4.30	175	OOOOOOOOOOOOOOOOOOOOOOOOOOOOOOOOOOOOOOOOIOOOOOOOOOOOOOOOOOOOOOOOOOOOOOOOOOOOOOOOOOOOOOOOOOOOOOOOOOOOO * 175
LINOL A	G	24.90	3.06	125	LLLLLLLLLLLLLLLLLLLLLLLLLLLLLLLLLLLLLLLLILLLLLLLLLLLLLLLLLLLLLLLLLLLLLLLLLLLLLLLLLLLLL * 125
SAT FAT A	G	16.70	1.44	59	SSSSSSSSSSSSSSSSSSSSSSSSSSSSSSSSSSSSSSSSSSSSSSSSSSSSSSSSSSS

****

114 MARGARINE, REGULAR
ANALYSIS OF 14 GRAMS WHICH IS 1 TBSP

NUTRIENT	UNIT	AMOUNT	INQ	% STD	0 10 20 30 40 50 60 70 80 90 100
ENERGY	KCAL	100.00	1.00	5	EEEE
VITAMIN A	IU	470.00	2.35	12	AAAIAAAA
VITAMIN C	MG	0.00	0.00	0	-
THIAMIN	MG	0.00	0.00	0	-
RIBOFLAVN	MG	0.00	0.00	0	-
NIACIN	MG	0.00	0.00	0	-
IRON	MG	0.00	0.00	0	-
CALCIUM	MG	3.00	0.07	0	-
PHOSPHRUS	MG	3.00	0.07	0	-
POTASSIUM	MG	4.00	0.02	0	-
PROTEIN	G	0.00	0.00	0	-
CARBOHYDT	G	0.00	0.00	0	-
FAT	G	12.00	3.08	15	FFFIFFFFFFF
OLEIC A	G	5.30	4.33	22	OOOIOOOOOOOOOOOO
LINOL A	G	3.10	3.10	16	LLLILLLLLLL
SAT FAT A	G	2.10	1.47	7	SSSISS

****

115 MARGARINE, REGULAR
ANALYSIS OF 5 GRAMS WHICH IS 1 PAT (90 PER LB)

NUTRIENT	UNIT	AMOUNT	INQ	% STD	0 10 20 30 40 50 60 70 80 90 100
ENERGY	KCAL	35.00	1.00	2	E
VITAMIN A	IU	170.00	2.43	4	IAA
VITAMIN C	MG	0.00	0.00	0	I
THIAMIN	MG	0.00	0.00	0	I
RIBOFLAVN	MG	0.00	0.00	0	I
NIACIN	MG	0.00	0.00	0	I
IRON	MG	0.00	0.00	0	I
CALCIUM	MG	1.00	0.06	0	I
PHOSPHRUS	MG	1.00	0.06	0	I
POTASSIUM	MG	1.00	0.01	0	I
PROTEIN	G	0.00	0.00	0	I
CARBOHYDT	G	0.00	0.00	0	I
FAT	G	4.00	2.93	5	IFFF
OLEIC A	G	1.90	4.43	8	IOOOOO
LINOL A	G	1.10	3.14	6	ILLL
SAT FAT A	G	0.70	1.40	2	IS

116 MARGARINE, SOFT
ANALYSIS OF 227 GRAMS WHICH IS 8 OZ CONTAINER

NUTRIENT	UNIT	AMOUNT	INQ	% STD	0 10 20 30 40 50 60 70 80 90 100
ENERGY	KCAL	1635.00	1.00	82	EEEEEEEEEEEEEEEEEEEEEEEEEEEEEEEEEEEEEEEEEEEEEEEEEEEEEEEEEEEEEEEEEEEEEEEEEEEEEEEEEE
VITAMIN A	IU	7500.00	2.29	188	AAAAAAAAAAAAAAAAAAAAAAAAAAAAAAAAAAAAAAAAAAAAAAAAAAAAAAAAAAAAAAAAAAAAAAAAAAAAAAAAAAAAAAAAAAAAAAAAAA *188
VITAMIN C	MG	0.00	0.00	0	-
THIAMIN	MG	0.01	0.01	1	T
RIBOFLAVN	MG	0.08	0.08	7	RRRR
NIACIN	MG	0.10	0.01	1	N
IRON	MG	0.40	0.03	3	II
CALCIUM	MG	53.00	0.07	6	KKKK
PHOSPHRUS	MG	52.00	0.07	6	XXXXX
POTASSIUM	MG	59.00	0.01	1	Y
PROTEIN	G	1.00	0.02	2	PP
CARBOHYDT	G	0.00	0.00	0	-
FAT	G	184.00	2.89	236	FFFFFFFFFFFFFFFFFFFFFFFFFFFFFFFFFFFFFFFFFFFFFFFFFFFFFFFFFFFFFFFFFFFFFFFFFFFFFFFFFF *236
OLEIC A	G	71.50	3.57	292	OOOOOOOOOOOOOOOOOOOOOOOOOOOOOOOOOOOOOOOOOOOOOOOOOOOOOOOOOOOOOOOOOOOOOOOOOOOOOOOOOO *292
LINOL A	G	65.40	4.00	327	LLLLLLLLLLLLLLLLLLLLLLLLLLLLLLLLLLLLLLLLLLLLLLLLLLLLLLLLLLLLLLLLLLLLLLLLLLLLLLLLLL *327
SAT FAT A	G	32.50	1.39	114	SSSSSSSSSSSSSSSSSSSSSSSSSSSSSSSSSSSSSSSSSSSSSSSSSSSSSSSSSSSSSSSSSSSSSSSSSSSSSSSSSS *114

117 MARGARINE, SOFT
ANALYSIS OF 14 GRAMS WHICH IS 1 TBSP

NUTRIENT	UNIT	AMOUNT	INQ	% STD	0	10	20	30	40	50	60	70	80	90	100
ENERGY	KCAL	100.00	1.00	5	EEEE										*
VITAMIN A	IU	470.00	2.35	12	AAA|AAAAA										*
VITAMIN C	MG	0.00	0.00	0	-										*
THIAMIN	MG	0.00	0.00	0	-										*
RIBOFLAVN	MG	0.00	0.00	0	-										*
NIACIN	MG	0.00	0.00	0	-										*
IRON	MG	0.00	0.00	0	-										*
CALCIUM	MG	3.00	0.07	0	-										*
PHOSPHRUS	MG	3.00	0.07	0	-										*
POTASSIUM	MG	4.00	0.02	0	-										*
PROTEIN	G	0.00	0.00	0	-										*
CARBOHYDT	G	0.00	0.00	0	-										*
FAT	G	12.00	3.08	15	FFF|FFFFFFFF										*
OLEIC A	G	4.50	3.67	18	OOO|OOOOOOOOOO										*
LINOL A	G	4.10	4.10	21	LLL|LLLLLLLLLL										*
SAT FAT A	G	2.00	1.40	7	SSS|SS										*

118 MARGARINE, WHIPPED
ANALYSIS OF 76 GRAMS WHICH IS 1/2 CUP STICK

NUTRIENT	UNIT	AMOUNT	INQ	% STD	0	10	20	30	40	50	60	70	80	90	100
ENERGY	KCAL	545.00	1.00	27	EEEEEEEEEEEEEEEEEEEEEEEEEE										*
VITAMIN A	IU	2500.00	2.29	63	AAAAAAAAAAAAAAAAAAAAAA	AAAAAAAAAAAAAAAAAAAAA								*
VITAMIN C	MG	0.00	0.00	0	-										*
THIAMIN	MG	0.00	0.00	0	-										*
RIBOFLAVN	MG	0.03	0.09	3	RR										*
NIACIN	MG	0.10	0.02	1	I										*
IRON	MG	0.10	0.07	2	KK										*
CALCIUM	MG	18.00	0.07	2	XX										*
PHOSPHRUS	MG	17.00	0.07	2	-										*
POTASSIUM	MG	20.00	0.01	0	-										*
PROTEIN	G	0.00	0.00	0	-										*
CARBOHYDT	G	0.00	0.00	0	FFFFFFFFFFFFFFFFFFFFFFFFFFFFFFFFFFFFFFFFFFFFFFFFFFFFFFFFFFFFFFFFFFFFFFFFFF										* 117
FAT	G	61.00	2.87	78	OOOOOOOOOOOOOOOOOOOOOOOOOOOOOOOOOOOOOOOOOOOOOOOOOOOOOOOOOOOOOOOOOOOOOOOOOOOOOOOOO								*
OLEIC A	G	28.70	4.30	117	LLLLLLLLLLLLLLLLLLLLLLLLLLLLLLLLLLLLLLLLLLLLLLLLLLLLLLLLLLLLLLLLLLLLL									*
LINOL A	G	16.70	3.06	84	SSSSSSSSSSSSSSSSSSSSSSSSSSSSSSSSSSSSSSS										*
SAT FAT A	G	11.20	1.44	39											*

119 MARGARINE, WHIPPED
ANALYSIS OF 9 GRAMS WHICH IS 1 TBSP

NUTRIENT	UNIT	AMOUNT	INQ	% STD
ENERGY	KCAL	70.00	1.00	4
VITAMIN A	IU	310.00	2.21	8
VITAMIN C	MG	0.00	0.00	0
THIAMIN	MG	0.00	0.00	0
RIBOFLAVN	MG	0.00	0.00	0
NIACIN	MG	0.00	0.00	0
IRON	MG	0.00	0.00	0
CALCIUM	MG	2.00	0.06	0
PHOSPHRUS	MG	2.00	0.06	0
POTASSIUM	MG	2.00	0.01	0
PROTEIN	G	0.00	0.00	0
CARBOHYDT	G	0.00	0.00	0
FAT	G	8.00	2.93	10
OLEIC A	G	3.60	4.20	15
LINOL A	G	2.10	3.00	11
SAT FAT A	G	1.40	1.40	5

120 CORN OIL
ANALYSIS OF 218 GRAMS WHICH IS 1 CUP

NUTRIENT	UNIT	AMOUNT	INQ	% STD
ENERGY	KCAL	1925.00	1.00	96
VITAMIN A	IU	0.00	0.00	0
VITAMIN C	MG	0.00	0.00	0
THIAMIN	MG	0.00	0.00	0
RIBOFLAVN	MG	0.00	0.00	0
NIACIN	MG	0.00	0.00	0
IRON	MG	0.00	0.00	0
CALCIUM	MG	0.00	0.00	0
PHOSPHRUS	MG	0.00	0.00	0
POTASSIUM	MG	0.00	0.00	0
PROTEIN	G	0.00	0.00	0
CARBOHYDT	G	0.00	0.00	0
FAT	G	218.00	2.90	279
OLEIC A	G	53.60	2.27	219
LINOL A	G	12.50	0.65	63
SAT FAT A	G	27.70	1.01	97

121 CORN OIL
ANALYSIS OF 14 GRAMS WHICH IS 1 TBSP

NUTRIENT	UNIT	AMOUNT	INQ	% STD
ENERGY	KCAL	120.00	1.00	6
VITAMIN A	IU	0.00	0.00	0
VITAMIN C	MG	0.00	0.00	0
THIAMIN	MG	0.00	0.00	0
RIBOFLAVN	MG	0.00	0.00	0
NIACIN	MG	0.00	0.00	0
IRON	MG	0.00	0.00	0
CALCIUM	MG	0.00	0.00	0
PHOSPHRUS	MG	0.00	0.00	0
POTASSIUM	MG	0.00	0.00	0
PROTEIN	G	0.00	0.00	0
CARBOHYDT	G	0.00	0.00	0
FAT	G	14.00	2.99	18
OLEIC A	G	3.30	2.24	13
LINOL A	G	7.80	6.50	39
SAT FAT A	G	1.70	0.99	6

122 OLIVE OIL
ANALYSIS OF 216 GRAMS WHICH IS 1 CUP

NUTRIENT	UNIT	AMOUNT	INQ	% STD
ENERGY	KCAL	1910.00	1.00	96
VITAMIN A	IU	0.00	0.00	0
VITAMIN C	MG	0.00	0.00	0
THIAMIN	MG	0.00	0.00	0
RIBOFLAVN	MG	0.00	0.00	0
NIACIN	MG	0.00	0.00	0
IRON	MG	0.00	0.00	0
CALCIUM	MG	0.00	0.00	0
PHOSPHRUS	MG	0.00	0.00	0
POTASSIUM	MG	0.00	0.00	0
PROTEIN	G	0.00	0.00	0
CARBOHYDT	G	0.00	0.00	0
FAT	G	216.00	2.90	277
OLEIC A	G	15.40	0.66	63
LINOL A	G	17.70	0.93	89
SAT FAT A	G	30.70	1.13	108

123 OLIVE OIL
ANALYSIS OF 14 GRAMS WHICH IS 1 TBSP

NUTRIENT	UNIT	AMOUNT	INQ	% STD
ENERGY	KCAL	120.00	1.00	6
VITAMIN A	IU	0.00	0.00	0
VITAMIN C	MG	0.00	0.00	0
THIAMIN	MG	0.00	0.00	0
RIBOFLAVN	MG	0.00	0.00	0
NIACIN	MG	0.00	0.00	0
IRON	MG	0.00	0.00	0
CALCIUM	MG	0.00	0.00	0
PHOSPHRUS	MG	0.00	0.00	0
POTASSIUM	MG	0.00	0.00	0
PROTEIN	G	0.00	0.00	0
CARBOHYDT	G	0.00	0.00	0
FAT	G	14.00	2.99	18
OLEIC A	G	9.70	6.60	40
LINOL A	G	1.10	0.92	6
SAT FAT A	G	1.90	1.11	7

124 PEANUT OIL
ANALYSIS OF 216 GRAMS WHICH IS 1 CUP

NUTRIENT	UNIT	AMOUNT	INQ	% STD
ENERGY	KCAL	1910.00	1.00	96
VITAMIN A	IU	0.00	0.00	0
VITAMIN C	MG	0.00	0.00	0
THIAMIN	MG	0.00	0.00	0
RIBOFLAVN	MG	0.00	0.00	0
NIACIN	MG	0.00	0.00	0
IRON	MG	0.00	0.00	0
CALCIUM	MG	0.00	0.00	0
PHOSPHRUS	MG	0.00	0.00	0
POTASSIUM	MG	0.00	0.00	0
PROTEIN	G	0.00	0.00	0
CARBOHYDT	G	0.00	0.00	0
FAT	G	216.00	2.90	277
OLEIC A	G	98.50	4.21	402
LINOL A	G	67.00	3.51	335
SAT FAT A	G	37.40	1.37	131

125 PEANUT OIL
ANALYSIS OF 14 GRAMS WHICH IS 1 TBSP

NUTRIENT	UNIT	AMOUNT	INQ	% STD	0	10	20	30	40	50	60	70	80	90	100
ENERGY	KCAL	120.00	1.00	6	EEEEE										
VITAMIN A	IU	0.00	0.00	0	-										
VITAMIN C	MG	0.00	0.00	0	-										
THIAMIN	MG	0.00	0.00	0	-										
RIBOFLAVN	MG	0.00	0.00	0	-										
NIACIN	MG	0.00	0.00	0	-										
IRON	MG	0.00	0.00	0	-										
CALCIUM	MG	0.00	0.00	0	-										
PHOSPHRUS	MG	0.00	0.00	0	-										
POTASSIUM	MG	0.00	0.00	0	-										
PROTEIN	G	0.00	0.00	0	-										
CARBOHYDT	G	0.00	0.00	0	-										
FAT	G	14.00	2.99	18	FFFFIFFFFFFFF										
OLEIC A	G	6.20	4.22	25	OOOOIOOOOOOOOOOOOOOO										
LINOL A	G	4.20	3.50	21	LLLLLLLLLLLLLLLL										
SAT FAT A	G	2.30	1.35	8	SSSSIS										

****

126 SAFFLOWER OIL
ANALYSIS OF 218 GRAMS WHICH IS 1 CUP

NUTRIENT	UNIT	AMOUNT	INQ	% STD	0	10	20	30	40	50	60	70	80	90	100
ENERGY	KCAL	1925.00	1.00	96	EEEEEEEEEEEEEEEEEEEEEEEEEEEEEEEEEEEEEEEEEEEEEEEEE										
VITAMIN A	IU	0.00	0.00	0	-										
VITAMIN C	MG	0.00	0.00	0	-										
THIAMIN	MG	0.00	0.00	0	-										
RIBOFLAVN	MG	0.00	0.00	0	-										
NIACIN	MG	0.00	0.00	0	-										
IRON	MG	0.00	0.00	0	-										
CALCIUM	MG	0.00	0.00	0	-										
PHOSPHRUS	MG	0.00	0.00	0	-										
POTASSIUM	MG	0.00	0.00	0	-										
PROTEIN	G	0.00	0.00	0	-										
CARBOHYDT	G	0.00	0.00	0	-										
FAT	G	218.00	2.90	279	FFFFFFFFFFFFFFFFFFFFFFFFFFFFFFFFFFFFFFFFFFFFFFFFFFFFFFFFFFFFFFFFFFFIFF * 279										
OLEIC A	G	25.90	1.10	106	OOOOOOOOOOOOOOOOOOOOOOOOOOOOOOOOOOOOOOOOOOOOOOOOOOOOOOOOI000 * 106										
LINOL A	G	15.90	0.83	80	LLLLLLLLLLLLLLLLLLLLLLLLLLLLLLLLLLLLLLLL										
SAT FAT A	G	20.50	0.75	72	SSSSSSSSSSSSSSSSSSSSSSSSSSSSSSSSSSSSS										

****

127 SAFFLOWER OIL
ANALYSIS OF 14 GRAMS WHICH IS 1 TBSP

NUTRIENT	UNIT	AMOUNT	INQ	% STD	0 10 20 30 40 50 60 70 80 90 100
ENERGY	KCAL	120.00	1.00	6	EEEE
VITAMIN A	IU	0.00	0.00	0	-
VITAMIN C	MG	0.00	0.00	0	I
THIAMIN	MG	0.00	0.00	0	I
RIBOFLAVN	MG	0.00	0.00	0	I
NIACIN	MG	0.00	0.00	0	I
IRON	MG	0.00	0.00	0	I
CALCIUM	MG	0.00	0.00	0	I
PHOSPHRUS	MG	0.00	0.00	0	I
POTASSIUM	MG	0.00	0.00	0	I
PROTEIN	G	0.00	0.00	0	I
CARBOHYDT	G	0.00	0.00	0	I
FAT	G	14.00	2.99	18	FFFFIFFFFFFF
OLEIC A	G	1.60	1.09	7	OOOOO
LINOL A	G	10.00	8.33	50	LLLLILLLLLLLLLLLLLLLLLLLLLLLLLLLLLLLLLLLLLLLLLLLL
SAT FAT A	G	1.30	0.76	5	SSSSI

128 SOYBEAN OIL, HYDROGENATED
ANALYSIS OF 218 GRAMS WHICH IS 1 CUP

NUTRIENT	UNIT	AMOUNT	INQ	% STD	0 10 20 30 40 50 60 70 80 90 100	
ENERGY	KCAL	1925.00	1.00	96	EEEEEEEEEEEEEEEEEEEEEEEEEEEEEEEEEEEEEEEEEEEEEEEE	
VITAMIN A	IU	0.00	0.00	0	I	
VITAMIN C	MG	0.00	0.00	0	I	
THIAMIN	MG	0.00	0.00	0	I	
RIBOFLAVN	MG	0.00	0.00	0	I	
NIACIN	MG	0.00	0.00	0	I	
IRON	MG	0.00	0.00	0	I	
CALCIUM	MG	0.00	0.00	0	I	
PHOSPHRUS	MG	0.00	0.00	0	I	
POTASSIUM	MG	0.00	0.00	0	I	
PROTEIN	G	0.00	0.00	0	I	
CARBOHYDT	G	0.00	0.00	0	I	
FAT	G	218.00	2.90	279	FFFFFFFFFFFFFFFFFFFFFFFFFFFFFFFFFFFFFFFFFFFFFFFFFFFFFFFFFFFFFFFFFFFFFFFFFFFFFFFIFFF	*279
OLEIC A	G	93.10	3.95	380	OOOOOOOOOOOOOOOOOOOOOOOOOOOOOOOOOOOOOOOOOOOOOOOOOOOOOOOOOOOOOOOOOOOOOOOOOOOOOOOOOI000	*380
LINOL A	G	75.60	3.93	378	LLLLLLLLLLLLLLLLLLLLLLLLLLLLLLLLLLLLLLLLLLLLLLLLLLLLLLLLLLLLLLLLLLLLLLLLLLLLLLLILLL	*378
SAT FAT A	G	31.80	1.16	112	SSSSSSSSSSSSSSSSSSSSSSSSSSSSSSSSSSSSSSSSSSSISSS	*112

129 SOYBEAN OIL, HYDROGENATED
ANALYSIS OF 14 GRAMS WHICH IS 1 TBSP

NUTRIENT	UNIT	AMOUNT	INQ	% STD
ENERGY	KCAL	120.00	1.00	6
VITAMIN A	IU	0.00	0.00	0
VITAMIN C	MG	0.00	0.00	0
THIAMIN	MG	0.00	0.00	0
RIBOFLAVN	MG	0.00	0.00	0
NIACIN	MG	0.00	0.00	0
IRON	MG	0.00	0.00	0
CALCIUM	MG	0.00	0.00	0
PHOSPHRUS	MG	0.00	0.00	0
POTASSIUM	MG	0.00	0.00	0
PROTEIN	G	0.00	0.00	0
CARBOHYDT	G	0.00	0.00	0
FAT	G	14.00	2.99	18
OLEIC A	G	5.80	3.95	24
LINOL A	G	4.70	3.92	24
SAT FAT A	G	2.00	1.17	7

130 SOYBEAN-COTTONSEED OIL BLEND, HYDROGENATED
ANALYSIS OF 218 GRAMS WHICH IS 1 CUP

NUTRIENT	UNIT	AMOUNT	INQ	% STD
ENERGY	KCAL	1925.00	1.00	96
VITAMIN A	IU	0.00	0.00	0
VITAMIN C	MG	0.00	0.00	0
THIAMIN	MG	0.00	0.00	0
RIBOFLAVN	MG	0.00	0.00	0
NIACIN	MG	0.00	0.00	0
IRON	MG	0.00	0.00	0
CALCIUM	MG	0.00	0.00	0
PHOSPHRUS	MG	0.00	0.00	0
POTASSIUM	MG	0.00	0.00	0
PROTEIN	G	0.00	0.00	0
CARBOHYDT	G	0.00	0.00	0
FAT	G	218.00	2.90	*279
OLEIC A	G	63.00	2.67	*257
LINOL A	G	99.60	5.17	*498
SAT FAT A	G	38.20	1.39	*134

131 SOYBEAN-COTTONSEED OIL BLEND, HYDROGENATED
ANALYSIS OF 14 GRAMS WHICH IS 1 TBSP

NUTRIENT	UNIT	AMOUNT	INQ	% STD
ENERGY	KCAL	120.00	1.00	6
VITAMIN A	IU	0.00	0.00	0
VITAMIN C	MG	0.00	0.00	0
THIAMIN	MG	0.00	0.00	0
RIBOFLAVN	MG	0.00	0.00	0
NIACIN	MG	0.00	0.00	0
IRON	MG	0.00	0.00	0
CALCIUM	MG	0.00	0.00	0
PHOSPHRUS	MG	0.00	0.00	0
POTASSIUM	MG	0.00	0.00	0
PROTEIN	G	0.00	0.00	0
CARBOHYDT	G	0.00	0.00	0
FAT	G	14.00	2.99	18
OLEIC A	G	3.90	2.65	16
LINOL A	G	6.20	5.17	31
SAT FAT A	G	2.40	1.40	8

132 BLUE CHEESE REGULAR SALAD DRESSING
ANALYSIS OF 15 GRAMS WHICH IS 1 TBSP

NUTRIENT	UNIT	AMOUNT	INQ	% STD
ENERGY	KCAL	75.00	1.00	4
VITAMIN A	IU	30.00	0.20	1
VITAMIN C	MG	0.00	0.00	0
THIAMIN	MG	0.00	0.00	0
RIBOFLAVN	MG	0.02	0.44	2
NIACIN	MG	0.00	0.00	0
IRON	MG	0.00	0.00	0
CALCIUM	MG	12.00	0.36	1
PHOSPHRUS	MG	11.00	0.33	1
POTASSIUM	MG	6.00	0.03	0
PROTEIN	G	1.00	0.53	2
CARBOHYDT	G	1.00	0.10	0
FAT	G	8.00	2.74	10
OLEIC A	G	1.70	1.85	7
LINOL A	G	3.80	5.07	19
SAT FAT A	G	1.60	1.50	6

133 BLUE CHEESE LOW CALORIE SALAD DRESSING
ANALYSIS OF 16 GRAMS WHICH IS 1 TBSP

NUTRIENT	UNIT	AMOUNT	INQ	% STD		10 20 30 40 50 60 70 80 90 100
ENERGY	KCAL	10.00	1.00	1	A	
VITAMIN A	IU	30.00	1.50	1	A	
VITAMIN C	MG	0.00	0.00	0	I	
THIAMIN	MG	0.00	0.00	0	I	
RIBOFLAVN	MG	0.01	1.67	1	R	
NIACIN	MG	0.00	0.00	0	I	
IRON	MG	0.00	0.00	0	I	
CALCIUM	MG	10.00	2.22	1	K	
PHOSPHRUS	MG	8.00	1.78	1	X	
POTASSIUM	MG	5.00	0.20	0	I	
PROTEIN	G	0.00	0.00	0	I	
CARBOHYDT	G	1.00	0.73	0	F	
FAT	G	1.00	2.56	1	O	
OLEIC A	G	0.30	2.45	1	O	
LINOL A	G	0.00	0.00	0	I	
SAT FAT A	G	0.50	3.51	2	S	

134 FRENCH REGULAR SALAD DRESSING
ANALYSIS OF 16 GRAMS WHICH IS 1 TBSP

NUTRIENT	UNIT	AMOUNT	INQ	% STD		10 20 30 40 50 60 70 80 90 100
ENERGY	KCAL	65.00	1.00	3	EEE	
VITAMIN A	IU	0.00	0.00	0	I	
VITAMIN C	MG	0.00	0.00	0	I	
THIAMIN	MG	0.00	0.00	0	I	
RIBOFLAVN	MG	0.00	0.00	0	I	
NIACIN	MG	0.00	0.00	0	I	
IRON	MG	0.10	0.19	1	I	
CALCIUM	MG	2.00	0.07	0	I	
PHOSPHRUS	MG	2.00	0.07	0	I	
POTASSIUM	MG	13.00	0.08	0	I	
PROTEIN	G	0.00	0.00	0	I	
CARBOHYDT	G	3.00	0.34	1	H	
FAT	G	6.00	2.37	8	FFIFFF	
OLEIC A	G	1.30	1.63	5	OOIO	
LINOL A	G	3.20	4.92	16	LLILLLLLLLLL	
SAT FAT A	G	1.10	1.19	4	SSS	

135 FRENCH LOW CALORIE SALAD DRESSING
ANALYSIS OF 16 GRAMS WHICH IS 1 TBSP

NUTRIENT	UNIT	AMOUNT	INQ	%STD	0	10	20	30	40	50	60	70	80	90	100
ENERGY	KCAL	15.00	1.00	1	E										
VITAMIN A	IU	0.00	0.00	0	-										
VITAMIN C	MG	0.00	0.00	0	-										
THIAMIN	MG	0.00	0.00	0	-										
RIBOFLAVN	MG	0.00	0.00	0	-										
NIACIN	MG	0.00	0.00	0	-										
IRON	MG	0.10	0.83	1	I										
CALCIUM	MG	2.00	0.30	0	-										
PHOSPHRUS	MG	2.00	0.30	0	-										
POTASSIUM	MG	13.00	0.35	0	-										
PROTEIN	G	0.00	0.00	0	-										
CARBOHYDT	G	2.00	0.97	1	H										
FAT	G	1.00	1.71	1	F										
OLEIC A	G	0.10	0.54	0	-										
LINOL A	G	0.40	2.67	2	IL										
SAT FAT A	G	0.10	0.47	0	-										

136 ITALIAN REGULAR SALAD DRESSING
ANALYSIS OF 15 GRAMS WHICH IS 1 TBSP

NUTRIENT	UNIT	AMOUNT	INQ	%STD	0	10	20	30	40	50	60	70	80	90	100
ENERGY	KCAL	85.00	1.00	4	EEE										
VITAMIN A	IU	0.00	0.00	0	-										
VITAMIN C	MG	0.00	0.00	0	-										
THIAMIN	MG	0.00	0.00	0	-										
RIBOFLAVN	MG	0.00	0.00	0	-										
NIACIN	MG	0.00	0.00	0	-										
IRON	MG	0.00	0.00	0	-										
CALCIUM	MG	2.00	0.05	0	-										
PHOSPHRUS	MG	1.00	0.03	0	-										
POTASSIUM	MG	2.00	0.01	0	-										
PROTEIN	G	0.00	0.00	0	-										
CARBOHYDT	G	1.00	0.09	0	-										
FAT	G	9.00	2.71	12	FFIFFFFFF										
OLEIC A	G	1.90	1.82	8	OOIOOO										
LINOL A	G	4.70	5.53	24	LLILLLLLLLLLLLLL										
SAT FAT A	G	1.60	1.32	6	SSIS										

137 ITALIAN LOW CALORIE SALAD DRESSING
ANALYSIS OF 15 GRAMS WHICH IS 1 TBSP

NUTRIENT	UNIT	AMOUNT	INQ	% STD
ENERGY	KCAL	10.00	1.00	1
VITAMIN A	IU	0.00	0.00	0
VITAMIN C	MG	0.00	0.00	0
THIAMIN	MG	0.00	0.00	0
RIBOFLAVN	MG	0.00	0.00	0
NIACIN	MG	0.00	0.00	0
IRON	MG	0.00	0.00	0
CALCIUM	MG	0.00	0.00	0
PHOSPHRUS	MG	1.00	0.22	0
POTASSIUM	MG	2.00	0.08	0
PROTEIN	G	0.00	0.00	0
CARBOHYDT	G	0.00	0.00	0
FAT	G	1.00	2.56	1
OLEIC A	G	0.10	0.82	0
LINOL A	G	0.40	4.00	2
SAT FAT A	G	0.10	0.70	0

138 MAYONNAISE
ANALYSIS OF 14 GRAMS WHICH IS 1 TBSP

NUTRIENT	UNIT	AMOUNT	INQ	% STD
ENERGY	KCAL	100.00	1.00	5
VITAMIN A	IU	40.00	0.20	1
VITAMIN C	MG	0.00	0.00	0
THIAMIN	MG	0.00	0.00	0
RIBOFLAVN	MG	0.01	0.17	1
NIACIN	MG	0.00	0.00	0
IRON	MG	0.10	0.13	1
CALCIUM	MG	3.00	0.07	0
PHOSPHRUS	MG	4.00	0.09	0
POTASSIUM	MG	5.00	0.02	0
PROTEIN	G	0.00	0.00	0
CARBOHYDT	G	0.00	0.00	0
FAT	G	11.00	2.82	14
OLEIC A	G	2.40	1.96	10
LINOL A	G	5.60	5.60	28
SAT FAT A	G	2.00	1.40	7

139 MAYONNAISE TYPE SALAD DRESSING
ANALYSIS OF 15 GRAMS WHICH IS 1 TBSP

NUTRIENT	UNIT	AMOUNT	INQ	% STD	0 ... 100
ENERGY	KCAL	65.00	1.00	3	E
VITAMIN A	IU	30.00	0.23	1	A
VITAMIN C	MG	0.00	0.00	0	I
THIAMIN	MG	0.00	0.00	0	I
RIBOFLAVN	MG	0.00	0.00	0	I
NIACIN	MG	0.00	0.00	0	I
IRON	MG	0.00	0.00	0	I
CALCIUM	MG	2.00	0.07	0	I
PHOSPHRUS	MG	4.00	0.14	0	I
POTASSIUM	MG	1.00	0.01	0	I
PROTEIN	G	0.00	0.00	0	I
CARBOHYDT	G	2.00	0.22	1	H
FAT	G	6.00	2.37	8	FF|FFF
OLEIC A	G	1.40	1.76	6	OO|OO
LINOL A	G	3.20	4.92	16	LL|LLLLLLLLL
SAT FAT A	G	1.10	1.19	4	SSS

140 MAYONNAISE TYPE LOW CALORIE SALAD DRESSING
ANALYSIS OF 16 GRAMS WHICH IS 1 TBSP

NUTRIENT	UNIT	AMOUNT	INQ	% STD	0 ... 100
ENERGY	KCAL	20.00	1.00	1	E
VITAMIN A	IU	40.00	1.00	1	A
VITAMIN C	MG	0.00	0.00	0	I
THIAMIN	MG	0.00	0.00	0	I
RIBOFLAVN	MG	0.00	0.00	0	I
NIACIN	MG	0.00	0.63	1	I
IRON	MG	0.10	0.33	0	I
CALCIUM	MG	3.00	0.44	0	I
PHOSPHRUS	MG	4.00	0.02	0	I
POTASSIUM	MG	1.00	0.00	0	I
PROTEIN	G	0.00	0.73	1	H
CARBOHYDT	G	2.00	2.56	3	IF
FAT	G	2.00	1.63	2	O
OLEIC A	G	0.40	5.00	5	ILLL
LINOL A	G	1.00	1.40	1	S

141 TARTAR SAUCE
ANALYSIS OF 14 GRAMS WHICH IS 1 TBSP

NUTRIENT	UNIT	AMOUNT	INQ	% STD	0	10	20	30	40	50	60	70	80	90	100
ENERGY	KCAL	75.00	1.00	4	EEE										
VITAMIN A	IU	30.00	0.20	1	A										
VITAMIN C	MG	0.00	0.00	0	-										
THIAMIN	MG	0.00	0.00	0	-										
RIBOFLAVN	MG	0.00	0.00	0	-										
NIACIN	MG	0.00	0.00	0	-										
IRON	MG	0.10	0.17	1	I										
CALCIUM	MG	3.00	0.09	0	-										
PHOSPHRUS	MG	4.00	0.12	0	-										
POTASSIUM	MG	11.00	0.06	0	-										
PROTEIN	G	0.00	0.10	0	-										
CARBOHYDT	G	1.00	0.10	0	-										
FAT	G	8.00	2.74	10	FFIFFFFF										
OLEIC A	G	1.80	1.96	7	OOIOOO										
LINOL A	G	4.10	5.47	21	LLILLLLLLLLLLLL										
SAT FAT A	G	1.50	1.40	5	SSIS										

142 THOUSAND ISLAND REGULAR SALAD DRESSING
ANALYSIS OF 16 GRAMS WHICH IS 1 TBSP

NUTRIENT	UNIT	AMOUNT	INQ	% STD	0	10	20	30	40	50	60	70	80	90	100
ENERGY	KCAL	80.00	1.00	4	EEE										
VITAMIN A	IU	50.00	0.31	1	A										
VITAMIN C	MG	0.00	0.00	0	-										
THIAMIN	MG	0.00	0.00	0	-										
RIBOFLAVN	MG	0.00	0.00	0	-										
NIACIN	MG	0.00	0.00	0	-										
IRON	MG	0.10	0.16	1	I										
CALCIUM	MG	2.00	0.06	0	-										
PHOSPHRUS	MG	3.00	0.08	0	-										
POTASSIUM	MG	18.00	0.09	0	-										
PROTEIN	G	0.00	0.00	0	-										
CARBOHYDT	G	2.00	0.18	1	H										
FAT	G	8.00	2.56	10	FFIFFFFF										
OLEIC A	G	1.70	1.73	7	OOIOOO										
LINOL A	G	4.00	5.00	20	LLILLLLLLLLLLLL										
SAT FAT A	G	1.40	1.23	5	SSIS										

143 THOUSAND ISLAND LOW CALORIE SALAD DRESSING
ANALYSIS OF 15 GRAMS WHICH IS 1 TBSP

NUTRIENT	UNIT	AMOUNT	INQ	% STD
ENERGY	KCAL	25.00	1.00	1
VITAMIN A	IU	50.00	1.00	1
VITAMIN C	MG	0.00	0.00	0
THIAMIN	MG	0.00	0.00	0
RIBOFLAVN	MG	0.00	0.00	0
NIACIN	MG	0.00	0.00	0
IRON	MG	0.10	0.50	1
CALCIUM	MG	2.00	0.18	0
PHOSPHRUS	MG	3.00	0.27	0
POTASSIUM	MG	17.00	0.27	0
PROTEIN	G	0.00	0.00	0
CARBOHYDT	G	2.00	0.58	1
FAT	G	2.00	2.05	3
OLEIC A	G	0.40	1.31	2
LINOL A	G	1.00	4.00	5
SAT FAT A	G	0.40	1.12	1

144 COOKED SALAD DRESSING, HOME RECIPE
ANALYSIS OF 16 GRAMS WHICH IS 1 TBSP

NUTRIENT	UNIT	AMOUNT	INQ	% STD
ENERGY	KCAL	25.00	1.00	1
VITAMIN A	IU	80.00	1.60	2
VITAMIN C	MG	0.00	0.00	0
THIAMIN	MG	0.01	0.80	1
RIBOFLAVN	MG	0.03	2.00	3
NIACIN	MG	0.00	0.00	0
IRON	MG	0.10	0.50	1
CALCIUM	MG	14.00	1.24	2
PHOSPHRUS	MG	15.00	1.33	2
POTASSIUM	MG	15.00	0.30	0
PROTEIN	G	1.00	1.60	2
CARBOHYDT	G	2.00	0.58	1
FAT	G	2.00	2.05	3
OLEIC A	G	0.60	1.96	2
LINOL A	G	0.30	1.20	2
SAT FAT A	G	0.50	1.40	2

145 BLUEFISH, BAKED WITH BUTTER OR MARGARINE
ANALYSIS OF 85 GRAMS WHICH IS 3 OZ

NUTRIENT	UNIT	AMOUNT	INQ	% STD	0	10	20	30	40	50	60	70	80	90	100
ENERGY	KCAL	135.00	1.00	7	EEEE										
VITAMIN A	IU	40.00	0.15	1	A										
VITAMIN C	MG	0.00	0.00	0	-										
THIAMIN	MG	0.09	1.33	9	TTTT TT										
RIBOFLAVN	MG	0.08	0.99	7	RRRR										
NIACIN	MG	1.60	1.69	11	NNNN NNNN										
IRON	MG	0.60	0.56	4	III										
CALCIUM	MG	25.00	0.41	3	KK										
PHOSPHRUS	MG	244.00	4.02	27	XXXX XXXXXXXXXXXXXXXX										
POTASSIUM	MG	357.00	1.06	7	YYYY Y										
PROTEIN	G	22.00	6.52	44	PPPP PPPPPPPPPPPPPPPPPPPPPPPPPPPPPPPPPPPP										
CARBOHYDT	G	0.00	0.00	0	-										
FAT	G	4.00	0.76	5	FFFF										
OLEIC A	G	0.00	0.00	0	-										
LINOL A	G	0.80	0.59	4	LLL										
SAT FAT A	G	0.80	0.42	3	SS										

146 CLAMS, RAW, MEAT ONLY
ANALYSIS OF 85 GRAMS WHICH IS 3 OZ

NUTRIENT	UNIT	AMOUNT	INQ	% STD	0	10	20	30	40	50	60	70	80	90	100
ENERGY	KCAL	65.00	1.00	3	EEE										
VITAMIN A	IU	90.00	0.69	2	AA										
VITAMIN C	MG	8.00	4.10	13	CC CCCCCCCC										
THIAMIN	MG	0.08	2.46	8	TT TTT										
RIBOFLAVN	MG	0.15	3.85	13	RR RRRRRRR										
NIACIN	MG	1.10	2.42	8	NN NNN										
IRON	MG	5.20	10.00	33	II IIIIIIIIIIIIIIIIIIIIIIIII										
CALCIUM	MG	59.00	2.02	7	KK KK										
PHOSPHRUS	MG	138.00	4.72	15	XX XXXXXXXXX										
POTASSIUM	MG	154.00	0.95	3	YY										
PROTEIN	G	11.00	6.77	22	PP PPPPPPPPPPPPPPP										
CARBOHYDT	G	2.00	0.22	1	H										
FAT	G	1.00	0.39	1	F										
OLEIC A	G	0.00	0.00	0	-										
LINOL A	G	0.00	0.00	0	-										
SAT FAT A	G	0.00	0.00	0	-										

147 CLAMS, CANNED, SOLIDS AND LIQUIDS
ANALYSIS OF 85 GRAMS WHICH IS 3 OZ

NUTRIENT	UNIT	AMOUNT	INQ	% STD	0	10	20	30	40	50	60	70	80	90	100
ENERGY	KCAL	45.00	1.00	2	EE										
VITAMIN A	IU	90.00	1.00	2	AA										
VITAMIN C	MG	0.00	0.00	0	-										
THIAMIN	MG	0.01	0.44	1	TI										
RIBOFLAVN	MG	0.09	3.33	8	RIRRRR										
NIACIN	MG	0.90	2.86	6	NINNN										
IRON	MG	3.50	9.72	22	IIIIIIIIIIIIIIIIIII										
CALCIUM	MG	47.00	2.32	5	KIKK										
PHOSPHRUS	MG	116.00	5.73	13	XIXXXXXXX										
POTASSIUM	MG	119.00	1.06	2	YY										
PROTEIN	G	7.00	6.22	14	PIPPPPPPPP										
CARBOHYDT	G	2.00	0.57	1	HI										
FAT	G	1.00	0.57	1	FI										
OLEIC A	G	0.00	0.00	0	-I										
LINOL A	G	0.00	0.00	0	-I										
SAT FAT A	G	0.20	0.31	1	SI										

148 CRABMEAT, CANNED
ANALYSIS OF 135 GRAMS WHICH IS 1 CUP

NUTRIENT	UNIT	AMOUNT	INQ	% STD	0	10	20	30	40	50	60	70	80	90	100
ENERGY	KCAL	135.00	1.00	7	EEEEE										
VITAMIN A	IU	150.00	0.56	4	AAA										
VITAMIN C	MG	0.00	0.00	0	-										
THIAMIN	MG	0.11	1.63	11	TTTITTT										
RIBOFLAVN	MG	0.11	1.36	9	RRRHIRR										
NIACIN	MG	2.60	2.75	19	NNNNINNNNNNNNNN										
IRON	MG	1.10	1.02	7	IIIIII										
CALCIUM	MG	61.00	1.00	7	KKKKK										
PHOSPHRUS	MG	246.00	4.05	27	XXXXIXXXXXXXXXXXXXXXXXXX										
POTASSIUM	MG	149.00	0.44	3	YY										
PROTEIN	G	24.00	7.11	48	PPPPIPPPPPPPPPPPPPPPPPPPPPPPPPPPPPPPPPPPPPPPP										
CARBOHYDT	G	1.00	0.05	0	-										
FAT	G	3.00	0.57	4	FFF										
OLEIC A	G	0.40	0.24	2	O										
LINOL A	G	0.10	0.07	0	-										
SAT FAT A	G	0.60	0.31	2	SS										

149 FISH STICKS, BREADED, COOKED
ANALYSIS OF 28 GRAMS WHICH IS 1(4 BY 1 BY 1/2 IN) STICK OR 1 OZ

NUTRIENT	UNIT	AMOUNT	INQ	% STD	0 10 20 30 40 50 60 70 80 90 100
ENERGY	KCAL	50.00	1.00	3	EE
VITAMIN A	IU	0.00	0.00	0	-
VITAMIN C	MG	0.00	0.00	0	-
THIAMIN	MG	0.01	0.40	1	T
RIBOFLAVN	MG	0.02	0.67	2	R
NIACIN	MG	0.50	1.43	4	NIN
IRON	MG	0.10	0.25	0	I
CALCIUM	MG	3.00	0.13	0	I
PHOSPHRUS	MG	47.00	2.09	5	XIxx
POTASSIUM	MG	99.00	0.79	2	YY
PROTEIN	G	5.00	4.00	10	PIPPPPPP
CARBOHYDT	G	2.00	0.29	1	HI
FAT	G	3.00	1.54	4	FIF
OLEIC A	G	0.80	1.31	3	OIO
LINOL A	G	0.60	1.20	3	LL
SAT FAT A	G	0.80	1.12	3	SS

150 HADDOCK, BREADED, FRIED
ANALYSIS OF 85 GRAMS WHICH IS 3 OZ

NUTRIENT	UNIT	AMOUNT	INQ	% STD	0 10 20 30 40 50 60 70 80 90 100
ENERGY	KCAL	140.00	1.00	7	EEEEEE
VITAMIN A	IU	0.00	0.00	0	-
VITAMIN C	MG	2.00	0.48	3	CCC
THIAMIN	MG	0.03	0.43	3	TT
RIBOFLAVN	MG	0.06	0.71	5	RRRR
NIACIN	MG	2.70	2.76	19	NNNNINNNNNNNN
IRON	MG	1.00	0.89	6	IIIII
CALCIUM	MG	34.00	0.54	4	KKK
PHOSPHRUS	MG	210.00	3.33	23	XXXXXIxxxxxxxxxx
POTASSIUM	MG	296.00	0.85	6	YYYYYI
PROTEIN	G	17.00	4.86	34	PPPPPIPPPPPPPPPPPPPPPPPP
CARBOHYDT	G	5.00	0.26	2	H
FAT	G	5.00	0.92	6	FFFFI
OLEIC A	G	2.20	1.28	9	OOOOOIO
LINOL A	G	1.20	0.86	6	LLLLLI
SAT FAT A	G	1.40	0.70	5	SSSS

151 OCEAN PERCH, BREADED, FRIED
ANALYSIS OF 85 GRAMS WHICH IS 1 FILLET

NUTRIENT	UNIT	AMOUNT	INQ	% STD											
					0	10	20	30	40	50	60	70	80	90	100
ENERGY	KCAL	195.00	1.00	10	EEEEEEE										
VITAMIN A	IU	0.00	0.00	0	-										
VITAMIN C	MG	0.00	0.00	0	-										
THIAMIN	MG	0.10	1.03	10	TTTTTTT										
RIBOFLAVN	MG	0.10	0.85	8	RRRRRRR										
NIACIN	MG	1.60	1.17	11	NNNNNNNN										
IRON	MG	1.10	0.71	7	IIIIII										
CALCIUM	MG	28.00	0.32	3	KK										
PHOSPHRUS	MG	192.00	2.19	21	XXXXXXXXXXXXXXXXX										
POTASSIUM	MG	242.00	0.50	5	YYYY										
PROTEIN	G	16.00	3.28	32	PPPPPPPPPPPPPPPPPPPPPPPPPP										
CARBOHYDT	G	6.00	0.22	2	HH										
FAT	G	11.00	1.45	14	FFFFFFFFF										
OLEIC A	G	4.40	1.84	18	OOOOOOOOOOOO										
LINOL A	G	2.30	1.18	12	LLLLLLLL										
SAT FAT A	G	2.70	0.97	9	SSSSSSS										

152 OYSTERS, RAW, MEAT ONLY
ANALYSIS OF 240 GRAMS WHICH IS 1 CUP, 13-19 MEDIUM SELECTS

NUTRIENT	UNIT	AMOUNT	INQ	% STD											
					0	10	20	30	40	50	60	70	80	90	100
ENERGY	KCAL	160.00	1.00	8	EEEEEE										
VITAMIN A	IU	740.00	2.31	19	AAAAAIAAAAAAAA										
VITAMIN C	MG	72.00	15.00	120	CCCCCICCCCCCCCCCCCCCCCCCCCCCCCCCCCCCCCCCCCCCCCCCCCCCCCCCCCCCCCC							*120
THIAMIN	MG	0.34	4.25	34	TTTTTITTTTTTTTTTTTTTTTTTTT										
RIBOFLAVN	MG	0.43	4.48	36	RRRRIRRRRRRRRRRRRRRRRRRRRRRR										
NIACIN	MG	6.00	5.36	43	NNNNNINNNNNNNNNNNNNNNNNNNNNNNNNNN										
IRON	MG	13.20	10.31	83	IIIIIIIIIIIIIIIIIIIIIIIIIIIIIIIIIIIIIIIIIIIIIIIIIIIIIIIIIIII								
CALCIUM	MG	226.00	3.14	25	KKKKKIKKKKKKKKKKKKKKKK										
PHOSPHRUS	MG	343.00	4.76	38	XXXXXIXXXXXXXXXXXXXXXXXXXXXXXXX										
POTASSIUM	MG	290.00	0.73	6	YYYYYI										
PROTEIN	G	20.00	5.00	40	PPPPPIPPPPPPPPPPPPPPPPPPPPPPPPPPP										
CARBOHYDT	G	8.00	0.36	3	HH										
FAT	G	4.00	0.64	5	FFFF										
OLEIC A	G	0.20	0.10	1	O										
LINOL A	G	0.10	0.06	1	-										
SAT FAT A	G	1.30	0.57	5	SSSS										

153 SALMON, PINK, CANNED, SOLIDS AND LIQUIDS
ANALYSIS OF 85 GRAMS WHICH IS 3 OZ

NUTRIENT	UNIT	AMOUNT	INQ	% STD	
ENERGY	KCAL	120.00	1.00	6	EEEEE
VITAMIN A	IU	60.00	0.25	2	A
VITAMIN C	MG	0.00	0.00	0	-
THIAMIN	MG	0.03	0.50	3	TT
RIBOFLAVN	MG	0.16	2.22	13	RRRRIRRRRR
NIACIN	MG	6.80	8.10	49	NNNNINNNNNNNNNNNNNNNNNNNNNNNN
IRON	MG	0.70	0.73	4	IIIII
CALCIUM	MG	167.00	3.09	19	KKKKIKKKKKKKK
PHOSPHRUS	MG	243.00	4.50	27	XXXXIXXXXXXXXXXXXXXX
POTASSIUM	MG	307.00	1.02	6	YYYYY
PROTEIN	G	17.00	5.67	34	PPPPIPPPPPPPPPPPPPPPPP
CARBOHYDT	G	0.00	0.00	0	-
FAT	G	5.00	1.07	6	FFFFF
OLEIC A	G	0.80	0.54	3	OOO
LINOL A	G	0.10	0.08	1	-
SAT FAT A	G	0.90	0.53	3	SSS

154 SARDINES, ATLANTIC, CANNED IN OIL, DRAINED SOLIDS
ANALYSIS OF 85 GRAMS WHICH IS 3 OZ

NUTRIENT	UNIT	AMOUNT	INQ	% STD	
ENERGY	KCAL	175.00	1.00	9	EEEEEE
VITAMIN A	IU	190.00	0.54	5	AAAA
VITAMIN C	MG	0.00	0.00	0	-
THIAMIN	MG	0.02	0.23	2	TT
RIBOFLAVN	MG	0.17	1.62	14	RRRRRIRRRR
NIACIN	MG	4.60	3.76	33	NNNNNNINNNNNNNNNNNNNNNNN
IRON	MG	2.50	1.79	16	IIIIIIIIIIIII
CALCIUM	MG	372.00	4.72	41	KKKKKIKKKKKKKKKKKKKKKKKKKK
PHOSPHRUS	MG	424.00	5.38	47	XXXXXIXXXXXXXXXXXXXXXXXXXXXXXXXX
POTASSIUM	MG	502.00	1.15	10	YYYYYIY
PROTEIN	G	20.00	4.57	40	PPPPPIPPPPPPPPPPPPPPPPPPPP
CARBOHYDT	G	0.00	0.00	0	-
FAT	G	9.00	1.32	12	FFFFFFFIFF
OLEIC A	G	2.50	1.17	10	OOOOOOIO
LINOL A	G	0.50	0.29	3	LL
SAT FAT A	G	3.00	1.20	11	SSSSSIS

155 SCALLOPS, FROZEN, BREADED, FRIED, REHEATED
ANALYSIS OF 90 GRAMS WHICH IS 6 SCALLOPS

NUTRIENT	UNIT	AMOUNT	INQ	% STD
ENERGY	KCAL	175.00	1.00	9
VITAMIN A	IU	100.00	0.29	3
VITAMIN C	MG	0.00	0.00	0
THIAMIN	MG	0.03	0.34	3
RIBOFLAVN	MG	0.11	1.05	9
NIACIN	MG	0.80	0.65	6
IRON	MG	3.20	2.29	20
CALCIUM	MG	68.00	0.86	8
PHOSPHRUS	MG	176.00	2.23	20
POTASSIUM	MG	132.00	0.30	3
PROTEIN	G	16.00	3.66	32
CARBOHYDT	G	9.00	0.37	3
FAT	G	8.00	1.17	10
OLEIC A	G	4.50	2.10	18
LINOL A	G	0.80	0.46	4
SAT FAT A	G	1.80	0.72	6

156 SHAD, BAKED WITH FAT
ANALYSIS OF 85 GRAMS WHICH IS 3 OZ

NUTRIENT	UNIT	AMOUNT	INQ	% STD
ENERGY	KCAL	170.00	1.00	9
VITAMIN A	IU	30.00	0.09	1
VITAMIN C	MG	0.00	0.00	0
THIAMIN	MG	0.11	1.29	11
RIBOFLAVN	MG	0.22	2.16	18
NIACIN	MG	7.30	6.13	52
IRON	MG	0.50	0.37	3
CALCIUM	MG	20.00	0.26	2
PHOSPHRUS	MG	266.00	3.48	30
POTASSIUM	MG	320.00	0.75	6
PROTEIN	G	20.00	4.71	40
CARBOHYDT	G	0.00	0.00	0
FAT	G	10.00	1.51	13
OLEIC A	G	3.40	1.63	14
LINOL A	G	0.80	0.47	4
SAT FAT A	G	3.40	1.40	12

157 SHRIMP, CANNED
ANALYSIS OF 85 GRAMS WHICH IS 3 OZ

NUTRIENT	UNIT	AMOUNT	INQ	% STD	0 10 20 30 40 50 60 70 80 90 100
ENERGY	KCAL	100.00	1.00	5	EEEE
VITAMIN A	IU	50.00	0.25	1	A
VITAMIN C	MG	0.00	0.00	0	-
THIAMIN	MG	0.01	0.20	1	T
RIBOFLAVN	MG	0.03	0.50	3	RR
NIACIN	MG	1.50	2.14	11	NNNINNNNN
IRON	MG	2.60	3.25	16	IIIIIIIIIIIII
CALCIUM	MG	98.00	2.18	11	KKKIKKKKK
PHOSPHRUS	MG	224.00	4.98	25	XXXIXXXXXXXXXXXXXX
POTASSIUM	MG	104.00	0.42	2	YY
PROTEIN	G	21.00	8.40	42	PPPIPPPPPPPPPPPPPPPPPPPPPPPPPPPP
CARBOHYDT	G	1.00	0.07	0	F
FAT	G	1.00	0.26	1	-
OLEIC A	G	0.10	0.08	0	-
LINOL A	G	0.00	0.00	0	-
SAT FAT A	G	0.10	0.07	0	-

158 SHRIMP, FRENCH FRIED
ANALYSIS OF 85 GRAMS WHICH IS 3 OZ

NUTRIENT	UNIT	AMOUNT	INQ	% STD	0 10 20 30 40 50 60 70 80 90 100
ENERGY	KCAL	190.00	1.00	10	EEEEEEE
VITAMIN A	IU	0.00	0.00	0	-
VITAMIN C	MG	0.00	0.00	0	-
THIAMIN	MG	0.03	0.32	3	TT
RIBOFLAVN	MG	0.07	0.61	6	RRRR
NIACIN	MG	2.30	1.73	16	NNNNNNNINNNNN
IRON	MG	1.70	1.12	11	IIIIIIIII
CALCIUM	MG	61.00	0.71	7	KKKKK
PHOSPHRUS	MG	162.00	1.89	18	XXXXXXXIXXXXXX
POTASSIUM	MG	195.00	0.41	4	YYY
PROTEIN	G	17.00	3.58	34	PPPPPIPPPPPPPPPPPPPPPPPPPPPP
CARBOHYDT	G	9.00	0.34	3	HHH
FAT	G	9.00	1.21	12	FFFFFFFIF
OLEIC A	G	3.70	1.59	15	OOOOOOOIOOOO
LINOL A	G	2.00	1.05	10	LLLLLLL
SAT FAT A	G	2.30	0.85	8	SSSSSS

159 TUNA, CANNED IN OIL, DRAINED SOLIDS
ANALYSIS OF 85 GRAMS WHICH IS 3 OZ

NUTRIENT	UNIT	AMOUNT	INQ	% STD
ENERGY	KCAL	170.00	1.00	9
VITAMIN A	IU	70.00	0.21	2
VITAMIN C	MG	0.00	0.00	0
THIAMIN	MG	0.04	0.47	4
RIBOFLAVN	MG	0.10	0.98	8
NIACIN	MG	10.10	8.49	72
IRON	MG	1.60	1.18	10
CALCIUM	MG	7.00	0.09	1
PHOSPHRUS	MG	199.00	2.60	22
POTASSIUM	MG	256.00	0.60	5
PROTEIN	G	24.00	5.65	48
CARBOHYDT	G	0.00	0.00	0
FAT	G	7.00	1.06	9
OLEIC A	G	1.70	0.82	7
LINOL A	G	0.70	0.41	4
SAT FAT A	G	1.70	0.70	6

160 TUNA SALAD(WITH CELERY, MAYONNAISE TYPE DRESSING, PICKLE, ONION, EGG)
ANALYSIS OF 205 GRAMS WHICH IS 1 CUP

NUTRIENT	UNIT	AMOUNT	INQ	% STD
ENERGY	KCAL	350.00	1.00	17
VITAMIN A	IU	590.00	0.84	15
VITAMIN C	MG	2.00	0.19	3
THIAMIN	MG	0.08	0.46	8
RIBOFLAVN	MG	0.23	1.10	19
NIACIN	MG	10.30	4.20	74
IRON	MG	2.70	0.96	17
CALCIUM	MG	41.00	0.26	5
PHOSPHRUS	MG	291.00	1.85	32
POTASSIUM	MG	494.00	0.56	10
PROTEIN	G	30.00	3.43	60
CARBOHYDT	G	7.00	0.15	3
FAT	G	22.00	1.61	28
OLEIC A	G	6.30	1.47	26
LINOL A	G	6.70	1.91	33
SAT FAT A	G	4.30	0.86	15

161 BACON, CRISP
ANALYSIS OF 15 GRAMS WHICH IS 2 SLICES

Scale: 0 ── 10 ── 20 ── 30 ── 40 ── 50 ── 60 ── 70 ── 80 ── 90 ── 100

NUTRIENT	UNIT	AMOUNT	INQ	% STD	PROFILE
ENERGY	KCAL	85.00	1.00	4	EEE
VITAMIN A	IU	0.00	0.00	0	-
VITAMIN C	MG	0.00	0.00	0	-
THIAMIN	MG	0.08	1.88	8	TT|TTT
RIBOFLAVN	MG	0.05	0.98	6	RRR
NIACIN	MG	0.50	1.34	3	NN|NN
IRON	MG	0.50	0.74	3	III
CALCIUM	MG	2.00	0.05	0	-
PHOSPHRUS	MG	34.00	0.89	4	XXX
POTASSIUM	MG	35.00	0.16	1	Y|
PROTEIN	G	4.00	1.88	8	PP|PPP
CARBOHYDT	G	0.00	0.00	0	-
FAT	G	8.00	2.41	10	FF|FFFFF
OLEIC A	G	3.70	3.55	15	00|000000000
LINOL A	G	0.70	0.82	4	LLL
SAT FAT A	G	2.50	2.06	9	SS|SSSS

162 BEEF CUTS COOKED, LEAN AND FAT
ANALYSIS OF 85 GRAMS WHICH IS 3 OZ - 2 1/2 BY 2 1/2 BY 3/4 IN

Scale: 0 ── 10 ── 20 ── 30 ── 40 ── 50 ── 60 ── 70 ── 80 ── 90 ── 100

NUTRIENT	UNIT	AMOUNT	INQ	% STD	PROFILE
ENERGY	KCAL	245.00	1.00	12	EEEEEEEE
VITAMIN A	IU	30.00	0.06	1	A|
VITAMIN C	MG	0.00	0.00	0	-
THIAMIN	MG	0.04	0.33	4	TTT
RIBOFLAVN	MG	0.18	1.22	15	RRRRRRRR|RR
NIACIN	MG	3.60	2.10	26	NNNNNNNNN|NNNNNNNNN
IRON	MG	2.90	1.48	18	IIIIIIIII|IIIII
CALCIUM	MG	10.00	0.09	1	K|
PHOSPHRUS	MG	114.00	1.03	13	XXXXXXXXX|
POTASSIUM	MG	184.00	0.30	4	YYY|
PROTEIN	G	23.00	3.76	46	PPPPPPPP|PPPPPPPPPPPPPPPPPPPPPPPPPPPPPPPPPP
CARBOHYDT	G	0.00	0.00	0	-
FAT	G	16.00	1.67	21	FFFFFFFF|FFFFF
OLEIC A	G	6.50	2.17	27	000000000|00000000000
LINOL A	G	0.40	0.16	2	LL|
SAT FAT A	G	6.80	1.95	24	SSSSSSSSS|SSSSSSSSS

163 BEEF CUTS COOKED, LEAN ONLY
ANALYSIS OF 72 GRAMS WHICH IS 2.5 OZ

NUTRIENT	UNIT	AMOUNT	INQ	% STD
ENERGY	KCAL	140.00	1.00	7
VITAMIN A	IU	10.00	0.04	0
VITAMIN C	MG	0.00	0.00	0
THIAMIN	MG	0.04	0.57	4
RIBOFLAVN	MG	0.17	2.02	14
NIACIN	MG	3.30	3.37	24
IRON	MG	2.70	2.41	17
CALCIUM	MG	10.00	0.16	1
PHOSPHRUS	MG	108.00	1.71	12
POTASSIUM	MG	176.00	0.50	4
PROTEIN	G	22.00	6.29	44
CARBOHYDT	G	0.00	0.00	0
FAT	G	5.00	0.92	6
OLEIC A	G	1.80	1.05	7
LINOL A	G	0.20	0.14	1
SAT FAT A	G	2.10	1.05	7

164 GROUND BEEF, BROILED, LEAN WITH 10% FAT
ANALYSIS OF 85 GRAMS WHICH IS 3 OZ OR 3 BY 5/8 IN PATTY

NUTRIENT	UNIT	AMOUNT	INQ	% STD
ENERGY	KCAL	185.00	1.00	9
VITAMIN A	IU	20.00	0.05	1
VITAMIN C	MG	0.00	0.00	0
THIAMIN	MG	0.08	0.86	8
RIBOFLAVN	MG	0.20	1.80	17
NIACIN	MG	5.10	3.94	36
IRON	MG	3.00	2.03	19
CALCIUM	MG	10.00	0.12	1
PHOSPHRUS	MG	196.00	2.35	22
POTASSIUM	MG	261.00	0.56	5
PROTEIN	G	23.00	4.97	46
CARBOHYDT	G	0.00	0.00	0
FAT	G	10.00	1.39	13
OLEIC A	G	3.90	1.72	16
LINOL A	G	0.50	0.16	2
SAT FAT A	G	4.00	1.52	14

165 GROUND BEEF, BROILED, LEAN WITH 21% FAT
ANALYSIS OF 82 GRAMS WHICH IS 2.9 OZ OR 3 BY 5/8 IN PATTY

NUTRIENT	UNIT	AMOUNT	INQ	% STD	0 10 20 30 40 50 60 70 80 90 100
ENERGY	KCAL	235.00	1.00	12	EEEEEEEE
VITAMIN A	IU	30.00	0.06	1	A
VITAMIN C	MG	0.00	0.00	0	-
THIAMIN	MG	0.07	0.60	7	TTTTT
RIBOFLAVN	MG	0.17	1.21	14	RRRRRRRRIRR
NIACIN	MG	4.40	2.67	31	NNNNNNNNINNNNNNNNNNNNN
IRON	MG	2.60	1.38	16	IIIIIIIIIIIII
CALCIUM	MG	9.00	0.09	1	K
PHOSPHRUS	MG	159.00	1.50	18	XXXXXXXIXXXX
POTASSIUM	MG	221.00	0.38	4	YYYY
PROTEIN	G	20.00	3.40	40	PPPPPPPIPPPPPPPPPPPPPPPPPPPPP
CARBOHYDT	G	0.00	0.00	0	-
FAT	G	17.00	1.85	22	FFFFFFFIFFFFFFF
OLEIC A	G	6.70	2.33	27	OOOOOOOIOOOOOOOOOOOO
LINOL A	G	0.40	0.17	2	LL
SAT FAT A	G	7.00	2.09	25	SSSSSSSSISSSSSSSSS

166 ROAST BEEF, OVEN COOKED, MODERATELY FAT, LEAN AND FAT
ANALYSIS OF 85 GRAMS WHICH IS 3 OZ

NUTRIENT	UNIT	AMOUNT	INQ	% STD	0 10 20 30 40 50 60 70 80 90 100
ENERGY	KCAL	375.00	1.00	19	EEEEEEEEEEEE
VITAMIN A	IU	70.00	0.09	2	A
VITAMIN C	MG	0.00	0.00	0	-
THIAMIN	MG	0.05	0.27	5	TTT
RIBOFLAVN	MG	0.13	0.58	11	RRRRRRRR
NIACIN	MG	3.10	1.18	22	NNNNNNNNNNNNINNN
IRON	MG	2.20	0.73	14	IIIIIIIIII
CALCIUM	MG	8.00	0.05	1	K
PHOSPHRUS	MG	158.00	0.94	18	XXXXXXXXXXXI
POTASSIUM	MG	189.00	0.20	4	YYY
PROTEIN	G	17.00	1.81	34	PPPPPPPPPPPIPPPPPPPPP
CARBOHYDT	G	0.00	0.00	0	-
FAT	G	33.00	2.26	42	FFFFFFFFFFFIFFFFFFFFFFFFFFFFFF
OLEIC A	G	13.60	2.96	56	OOOOOOOOOOOIOOOOOOOOOOOOOOOOOOOOOOOOOO
LINOL A	G	0.80	0.21	4	LLL
SAT FAT A	G	14.00	2.62	49	SSSSSSSSSSSISSSSSSSSSSSSSSSSSSSSSSS

167 ROAST BEEF, OVEN COOKED, LEAN ONLY
ANALYSIS OF 51 GRAMS WHICH IS 1.8 OZ

NUTRIENT	UNIT	AMOUNT	INQ	% STD	0 10 20 30 40 50 60 70 80 90 100
ENERGY	KCAL	125.00	1.00	6	EEEE
VITAMIN A	IU	10.00	0.04	0	-
VITAMIN C	MG	0.00	0.00	0	
THIAMIN	MG	0.04	0.64	4	TTT
RIBOFLAVN	MG	0.11	1.47	9	RRRIRR
NIACIN	MG	2.60	2.97	19	NNNNINNNNNNNNN
IRON	MG	1.80	1.80	11	IIIIIIIII
CALCIUM	MG	6.00	0.11	1	K
PHOSPHRUS	MG	131.00	2.33	15	XXXXIXXXXXX
POTASSIUM	MG	161.00	0.52	3	YYY
PROTEIN	MG	14.00	4.48	28	PPPPIPPPPPPPPPPPPP
CARBOHYDT	G	0.00	0.00	0	
FAT	G	7.00	1.44	9	FFFFIFF
OLEIC A	G	2.50	1.63	10	OOOOIOOO
LINOL A	G	0.30	0.24	2	L
SAT FAT A	G	3.00	1.68	11	SSSSISSS

168 ROAST BEEF, OVEN COOKED, RELATIVELY LEAN, LEAN AND FAT
ANALYSIS OF 85 GRAMS WHICH IS 3 OZ

NUTRIENT	UNIT	AMOUNT	INQ	% STD	0 10 20 30 40 50 60 70 80 90 100
ENERGY	KCAL	165.00	1.00	8	EEEEEE
VITAMIN A	IU	10.00	0.03	0	-
VITAMIN C	MG	0.00	0.00	0	
THIAMIN	MG	0.06	0.73	6	TTTT
RIBOFLAVN	MG	0.19	1.92	16	RRRRRIRRRRRR
NIACIN	MG	4.50	3.90	32	NNNNNINNNNNNNNNNNNNNNN
IRON	MG	3.20	2.42	20	IIIIIIIIIIIIIII
CALCIUM	MG	11.00	0.15	1	K
PHOSPHRUS	MG	208.00	2.80	23	XXXXXIXXXXXXXXXX
POTASSIUM	MG	279.00	0.68	6	YYYY
PROTEIN	MG	25.00	6.06	50	PPPPPIPPPPPPPPPPPPPPPPPPPPPPPPPPPPPPPPPPPPPPP
CARBOHYDT	G	0.00	0.00	0	
FAT	G	7.00	1.09	9	FFFFFF
OLEIC A	G	2.70	1.34	11	OOOOOOIOO
LINOL A -	G	0.20	0.12	1	L
SAT FAT A	G	2.80	1.19	10	SSSSSIS

169 ROAST BEEF, OVEN COOKED, RELATIVELY LEAN, LEAN ONLY
ANALYSIS OF 78 GRAMS WHICH IS 2.8 OZ

NUTRIENT	UNIT	AMOUNT	INQ	% STD	0 10 20 30 40 50 60 70 80 90 100
ENERGY	KCAL	125.00	1.00	6	EEEEE
VITAMIN A	IU	0.00	0.00	0	-
VITAMIN C	MG	0.00	0.00	0	-
THIAMIN	MG	0.06	0.96	6	TTTT
RIBOFLAVN	MG	0.18	2.40	15	RRRR|RRRRRR
NIACIN	MG	4.30	4.91	31	NNNN|NNNNNNNNNNNNNNNNN
IRON	MG	3.00	3.00	19	IIII|IIIIIIIII
CALCIUM	MG	10.00	0.18	1	K
PHOSPHRUS	MG	199.00	3.54	22	XXXX|XXXXXXXXXX
POTASSIUM	MG	268.00	0.86	5	YYYY|
PROTEIN	G	24.00	7.68	48	PPPP|PPPPPPPPPPPPPPPPPPPP
CARBOHYDT	G	0.00	0.00	0	-
FAT	G	3.00	0.62	4	FFF |
OLEIC A	G	1.00	0.65	4	OOO |
LINOL A	G	0.10	0.08	1	-
SAT FAT A	G	0.67	0.67	4	SSS |

****

170 STEAK, SIRLOIN, BROILED, LEAN AND FAT, BONE REMOVED
ANALYSIS OF 85 GRAMS WHICH IS 3 OZ

NUTRIENT	UNIT	AMOUNT	INQ	% STD	0 10 20 30 40 50 60 70 80 90 100
ENERGY	KCAL	330.00	1.00	17	EEEEEEEEEE
VITAMIN A	IU	50.00	0.08	1	A
VITAMIN C	MG	0.00	0.00	0	-
THIAMIN	MG	0.05	0.30	5	TTT
RIBOFLAVN	MG	0.15	0.76	13	RRRRRRRR
NIACIN	MG	4.00	1.73	29	NNNNNNNNNN|NNNNNNNNN
IRON	MG	2.50	0.95	16	IIIIIIIIIII
CALCIUM	MG	9.00	0.06	1	K
PHOSPHRUS	MG	162.00	1.09	18	XXXXXXXXXX|X
POTASSIUM	MG	220.00	0.27	4	YYYY
PROTEIN	G	20.00	2.42	40	PPPPPPPPPP|PPPPPPPPPP
CARBOHYDT	G	0.00	0.00	0	-
FAT	G	27.00	2.10	35	FFFFFFFFFF|FFFFFFFFFFF
OLEIC A	G	11.10	2.75	45	OOOOOOOOOO|OOOOOOOOOOOOOOOOO
LINOL A	G	0.60	0.18	3	LL
SAT FAT A	G	11.30	2.40	40	SSSSSSSSSS|SSSSSSSSSSSSSSSSSS

****

171 STEAK, SIRLOIN, BROILED, LEAN ONLY, BONE REMOVED
ANALYSIS OF 56 GRAMS WHICH IS 2 OZ

```
                                0      10      20      30      40      50      60      70      80      90      100
                                                                                                        **************
NUTRIENT   UNIT   AMOUNT    INQ   % STD
ENERGY     KCAL   115.00   1.00     6   EEEEE
VITAMIN A  IU      10.00   0.04     0   -
VITAMIN C  MG       0.00   0.00     0   -
THIAMIN    MG       0.05   0.87     5   TTTT
RIBOFLAVN  MG       0.14   2.03    12   RRRRIRRRR
NIACIN     MG       3.60   4.47    26   NNNNINNNNNNNNNNNNNN
IRON       MG       2.20   2.39    14   IIIIIIIIIII
CALCIUM    MG       7.00   0.14     1   K
PHOSPHRUS  MG     146.00   2.82    16   XXXXIXXXXXXX
POTASSIUM  MG     202.00   0.70     4   YYY
PROTEIN    G       18.00   6.26    36   PPPPIPPPPPPPPPPPPPPPPPPPPP
CARBOHYDT  G        0.00   0.00     0   -
FAT        G        4.00   0.89     5   FFFFI
OLEIC A    G        1.60   1.14     7   OOOOO
LINOL A    G        0.20   0.17     1   L
SAT FAT A  G        1.80   1.10     6   SSSSS
*******************************************************
```

172 STEAK, ROUND, BRAISED, LEAN AND FAT, BONE REMOVED
ANALYSIS OF 85 GRAMS WHICH IS 3 OZ

```
                                0      10      20      30      40      50      60      70      80      90      100
                                                                                                        **************
NUTRIENT   UNIT   AMOUNT    INQ   % STD
ENERGY     KCAL   220.00   1.00    11   EEEEEEEE
VITAMIN A  IU      20.00   0.05     1   -
VITAMIN C  MG       0.00   0.00     0   -
THIAMIN    MG       0.07   0.64     7   TTTTT
RIBOFLAVN  MG       0.19   1.44    16   RRRRRRRIRRR
NIACIN     MG       4.80   3.12    34   NNNNNNNNINNNNNNNNNNNNNNNNN
IRON       MG       3.00   1.70    19   IIIIIIIIIIIIIII
CALCIUM    MG      10.00   0.10     1   K
PHOSPHRUS  MG     213.00   2.15    24   XXXXXXXIXXXXXXXX
POTASSIUM  MG     272.00   0.49     5   YYYY
PROTEIN    G       24.00   4.36    48   PPPPPPPIPPPPPPPPPPPPPPPPPPPPPPPPPPPPPPPP
CARBOHYDT  G        0.00   0.00     0   -
FAT        G       13.00   1.52    17   FFFFFFFIFFF
OLEIC A    G        5.20   1.93    21   OOOOOOOIOOOOOOO
LINOL A    G        0.40   0.18     2   LL
SAT FAT A  G        5.50   1.75    19   SSSSSSSSISSSSS
*******************************************************
```

173 STEAK, ROUND, BRAISED, LEAN ONLY, BONE REMOVED
ANALYSIS OF 68 GRAMS WHICH IS 2.4 OZ

```
                                          0    10   20   30   40   50   60   70   80   90   100
NUTRIENT   UNIT  AMOUNT   INQ   % STD
ENERGY     KCAL  130.00   1.00    7     EEEEE
VITAMIN A  IU     10.00   0.04    0     -
VITAMIN C  MG      0.00   0.00    0     -
THIAMIN    MG      0.05   0.77    5     TTTI
RIBOFLAVN  MG      0.16   2.05   13     RRRRIRRRRR
NIACIN     MG      4.10   4.51   29     NNNNINNNNNNNNNNNNNNN
IRON       MG      2.50   2.40   16     IIIIIIIIIIIII
CALCIUM    MG      9.00   0.15    1     K
PHOSPHRUS  MG    182.00   3.11   20     XXXXIXXXXXXXXX
POTASSIUM  MG    238.00   0.73    5     YYYI
PROTEIN    MG     21.00   6.46   42     PPPPIPPPPPPPPPPPPPPPPPPPPPPPPPP
CARBOHYDT  G       0.00   0.00    0     -
FAT        G       4.00   0.79    5     FFFI
OLEIC A    G       1.50   0.94    6     00000
LINOL A    G       0.20   0.15    1     L
SAT FAT A  G       1.70   0.92    6     SSSSS
***********************************************************
```

174 CORNED BEEF CANNED
ANALYSIS OF 85 GRAMS WHICH IS 3 OZ

```
                                          0    10   20   30   40   50   60   70   80   90   100
NUTRIENT   UNIT  AMOUNT   INQ   % STD
ENERGY     KCAL  185.00   1.00    9     EEEEEE
VITAMIN A  IU     30.00   0.08    1     A
VITAMIN C  MG      0.00   0.00    0     -
THIAMIN    MG      0.01   0.11    1     T
RIBOFLAVN  MG      0.20   1.80   17     RRRRRIRRRRR
NIACIN     MG      2.90   2.24   21     NNNNNINNNNNNNN
IRON       MG      3.70   2.50   23     IIIIIIIIIIIIIIIII
CALCIUM    MG     17.00   0.20    2     KK
PHOSPHRUS  MG     90.00   1.08   10     XXXXXXIX
POTASSIUM  MG     51.00   0.11    1     Y
PROTEIN    G      22.00   4.76   44     PPPPPIPPPPPPPPPPPPPPPPPPPPPPPPPPPPPP
CARBOHYDT  G       0.00   0.00    0     -
FAT        G      10.00   1.39   13     FFFFFIFFF
OLEIC A    G       4.50   1.99   18     00000I0000000
LINOL A    G       0.20   0.11    1     L
SAT FAT A  G       4.90   1.86   17     SSSSSISSSSSS
***********************************************************
```

175 CORNED BEEF HASH
ANALYSIS OF 220 GRAMS WHICH IS 1 CUP

NUTRIENT	UNIT	AMOUNT	INQ	% STD
ENERGY	KCAL	400.00	1.00	20
VITAMIN A	IU	0.00	0.00	0
VITAMIN C	MG	0.00	0.00	0
THIAMIN	MG	0.02	0.10	2
RIBOFLAVN	MG	0.20	0.83	17
NIACIN	MG	4.60	1.64	33
IRON	MG	4.40	1.38	28
CALCIUM	MG	29.00	0.16	3
PHOSPHRUS	MG	147.00	0.82	16
POTASSIUM	MG	440.00	0.44	9
PROTEIN	MG	19.00	1.90	38
CARBOHYDT	G	24.00	0.44	9
FAT	G	25.00	1.60	32
OLEIC A	G	10.50	2.22	44
LINOL A	G	0.50	0.13	3
SAT FAT A	G	11.90	2.09	42

176 CHIPPED BEEF, DRIED
ANALYSIS OF 71 GRAMS WHICH IS 2 1/2 OZ JAR

NUTRIENT	UNIT	AMOUNT	INQ	% STD
ENERGY	KCAL	145.00	1.00	7
VITAMIN A	IU	30.00	0.10	1
VITAMIN C	MG	0.00	0.00	0
THIAMIN	MG	0.05	0.69	5
RIBOFLAVN	MG	0.23	2.64	19
NIACIN	MG	2.70	2.66	19
IRON	MG	3.60	3.10	23
CALCIUM	MG	14.00	0.21	2
PHOSPHRUS	MG	287.00	4.40	32
POTASSIUM	MG	142.00	0.39	3
PROTEIN	MG	24.00	6.62	48
CARBOHYDT	G	0.00	0.00	0
FAT	G	4.00	0.71	5
OLEIC A	G	2.00	1.13	8
LINOL A	G	0.10	0.07	1
SAT FAT A	G	2.10	1.02	7

177 BEEF AND VEGETABLE STEW
ANALYSIS OF 245 GRAMS WHICH IS 1 CUP

NUTRIENT	UNIT	AMOUNT	INQ	% STD
ENERGY	KCAL	220.00	1.00	11
VITAMIN A	IU	2400.00	5.45	60
VITAMIN C	MG	17.00	2.58	28
THIAMIN	MG	0.15	1.36	15
RIBOFLAVN	MG	0.17	1.29	14
NIACIN	MG	4.70	3.05	34
IRON	MG	2.90	1.65	18
CALCIUM	MG	29.00	0.29	3
PHOSPHRUS	MG	184.00	1.86	20
POTASSIUM	MG	613.00	1.11	12
PROTEIN	G	16.00	2.91	32
CARBOHYDT	G	15.00	0.50	5
FAT	G	11.00	1.28	14
OLEIC A	G	4.50	1.67	18
LINOL A	G	0.20	0.09	1
SAT FAT A	G	4.90	1.56	17

178 BEEF POTPIE (HOME RECIPE)
ANALYSIS OF 210 GRAMS WHICH IS 1/3 OF 9-IN DIAM. PIE

NUTRIENT	UNIT	AMOUNT	INQ	% STD
ENERGY	KCAL	515.00	1.00	26
VITAMIN A	IU	1720.00	1.67	43
VITAMIN C	MG	6.00	0.39	10
THIAMIN	MG	0.30	1.17	30
RIBOFLAVN	MG	0.30	0.97	25
NIACIN	MG	5.50	1.53	39
IRON	MG	3.80	0.92	24
CALCIUM	MG	29.00	0.13	3
PHOSPHRUS	MG	149.00	0.64	17
POTASSIUM	MG	334.00	0.26	7
PROTEIN	G	21.00	1.63	42
CARBOHYDT	G	39.00	0.55	14
FAT	G	30.00	1.49	38
OLEIC A	G	12.80	2.03	52
LINOL A	G	6.70	1.30	33
SAT FAT A	G	7.90	1.08	28

179 CHILI CON CARNE WITH BEANS, CANNED
ANALYSIS OF 255 GRAMS WHICH IS 1 CUP

NUTRIENT	UNIT	AMOUNT	INQ	% STD
ENERGY	KCAL	340.00	1.00	17
VITAMIN A	IU	150.00	0.22	4
VITAMIN C	MG	0.00	0.08	0
THIAMIN	MG	0.08	0.47	8
RIBOFLAVN	MG	0.18	0.88	15
NIACIN	MG		1.39	24
IRON	MG	3.30	1.58	27
CALCIUM	MG	82.00	0.54	9
PHOSPHRUS	MG	321.00	2.10	36
POTASSIUM	MG	594.00	0.70	12
PROTEIN	G	19.00	2.24	38
CARBOHYDT	G	31.00	0.66	11
FAT	G	16.00	1.21	21
OLEIC A	G	6.80	1.63	28
LINOL A	G	0.30	0.09	2
SAT FAT A	G	7.50	1.55	26

180 CHOP SUEY WITH BEEF AND PORK (HOME RECIPE)
ANALYSIS OF 250 GRAMS WHICH IS 1 CUP

NUTRIENT	UNIT	AMOUNT	INQ	% STD
ENERGY	KCAL	300.00	1.00	15
VITAMIN A	IU	600.00	1.00	15
VITAMIN C	MG	33.00	3.67	55
THIAMIN	MG	0.28	1.87	28
RIBOFLAVN	MG	0.38	2.11	32
NIACIN	MG	5.00	2.38	36
IRON	MG	4.80	2.00	30
CALCIUM	MG	60.00	0.44	7
PHOSPHRUS	MG	248.00	1.84	28
POTASSIUM	MG	425.00	0.57	9
PROTEIN	G	26.00	3.47	52
CARBOHYDT	G	13.00	0.32	5
FAT	G	17.00	1.45	22
OLEIC A	G	6.20	1.69	25
LINOL A	G	0.70	0.23	4
SAT FAT A	G	8.50	1.99	30

181 HEART, BEEF, LEAN, BRAISED
ANALYSIS OF 85 GRAMS WHICH IS 3 OZ

NUTRIENT	UNIT	AMOUNT	INQ	% STD	0 10 20 30 40 50 60 70 80 90 100
ENERGY	KCAL	160.00	1.00	8	EEEEEE
VITAMIN A	IU	20.00	0.06	1	
VITAMIN C	MG	1.00	0.21	2	C
THIAMIN	MG	0.21	2.62	21	TTTT|TTTTTTTTTTT
RIBOFLAVN	MG	1.04	10.83	87	RRRR|RRRRRRRRRRRRRRRRRRRRRRRRRRRRRRRRRRRRRRRR
NIACIN	MG	6.50	5.80	46	NNNN|NNNNNNNNNNNNNNNNNNNNN
IRON	MG	5.00	3.91	31	IIII|IIIIIIIIIIIIIII
CALCIUM	MG	5.00	0.07	1	
PHOSPHRUS	MG	154.00	2.14	17	XXXXX|XXXXXXX
POTASSIUM	MG	197.00	0.49	4	YYY
PROTEIN	G	27.00	6.75	54	PPPP|PPPPPPPPPPPPPPPPPPPPPPP
CARBOHYDT	G		0.05	0	
FAT	G	5.00	0.80	6	FFFF|
OLEIC A	G	1.10	0.56	4	OOOO
LINOL A	G	0.60	0.38	3	LL
SAT FAT A	G	1.50	0.66	5	SSS|

182 LAMB CHOP, BROILED, LEAN AND FAT, BONE REMOVED
ANALYSIS OF 89 GRAMS WHICH IS 3.1 OZ

NUTRIENT	UNIT	AMOUNT	INQ	% STD	0 10 20 30 40 50 60 70 80 90 100
ENERGY	KCAL	360.00	1.00	18	EEEEEEEEEEE
VITAMIN A	IU	0.00	0.00	0	
VITAMIN C	MG	0.00	0.00	0	
THIAMIN	MG	0.11	0.61	11	TTTTTTT
RIBOFLAVN	MG	0.19	0.88	16	RRRRRRRRRRR
NIACIN	MG	4.10	1.63	29	NNNNNNNNNN|NNNNNNNNN
IRON	MG	1.00	0.35	6	IIIII
CALCIUM	MG	8.00	0.05	1	K
PHOSPHRUS	MG	139.00	0.86	15	XXXXXXXXXX
POTASSIUM	MG	200.00	0.22	4	YYY
PROTEIN	G	18.00	2.00	36	PPPPPPPPP|PPPPPPPPP
CARBOHYDT	G	0.00	0.00	0	
FAT	G	32.00	2.28	41	FFFFFFFFFF|FFFFFFFFFF
OLEIC A	G	12.10	2.74	49	OOOOOOOOOO|OOOOOOOOOOOOOOOOOOO
LINOL A	G	1.20	0.33	6	LLLLL
SAT FAT A	G	14.80	2.88	52	SSSSSSSSSS|SSSSSSSSSSSSS

183 LAMB CHOP, BROILED, LEAN ONLY, BONE REMOVED
ANALYSIS OF 57 GRAMS WHICH IS 2 OZ

NUTRIENT	UNIT	AMOUNT	INQ	% STD
ENERGY	KCAL	120.00	1.00	6
VITAMIN A	IU	0.00	0.00	0
VITAMIN C	MG	0.00	0.00	0
THIAMIN	MG	0.09	1.50	9
RIBOFLAVN	MG	0.15	2.08	13
NIACIN	MG	3.40	4.05	24
IRON	MG	1.10	1.15	7
CALCIUM	MG	6.00	0.11	1
PHOSPHRUS	MG	121.00	2.24	13
POTASSIUM	MG	174.00	0.58	3
PROTEIN	G	16.00	5.33	32
CARBOHYDT	G	0.00	0.00	0
FAT	G	6.00	1.28	8
OLEIC A	G	2.10	1.43	9
LINOL A	G	0.20	0.17	1
SAT FAT A	G	2.50	1.46	9

184 LEG OF LAMB, ROASTED, LEAN AND FAT
ANALYSIS OF 85 GRAMS WHICH IS 3 OZ

NUTRIENT	UNIT	AMOUNT	INQ	% STD
ENERGY	KCAL	235.00	1.00	12
VITAMIN A	IU	0.00	0.00	0
VITAMIN C	MG	0.00	0.00	0
THIAMIN	MG	0.13	1.11	13
RIBOFLAVN	MG	0.23	1.63	19
NIACIN	MG	4.70	2.86	34
IRON	MG	1.40	0.74	9
CALCIUM	MG	9.00	0.09	1
PHOSPHRUS	MG	177.00	1.67	20
POTASSIUM	MG	241.00	0.41	5
PROTEIN	G	22.00	3.74	44
CARBOHYDT	G	22.00	1.75	21
FAT	G	16.00	1.75	21
OLEIC A	G	6.60	2.08	24
LINOL A	G	0.60	0.26	3
SAT FAT A	G	7.30	2.18	26

185 LEG OF LAMB, ROASTED, LEAN ONLY
ANALYSIS OF 71 GRAMS WHICH IS 2.5 OZ

NUTRIENT	UNIT	AMOUNT	INQ	% STD	0 10 20 30 40 50 60 70 80 90 100
ENERGY	KCAL	130.00	1.00	7	EEEE
VITAMIN A	IU	0.00	0.00	0	-
VITAMIN C	MG	0.00	0.00	0	-
THIAMIN	MG	0.12	1.85	12	TTTTTTTT
RIBOFLAVN	MG	0.21	2.69	17	RRRRIRRRRRRRR
NIACIN	MG	4.40	4.84	31	NNNNINNNNNNNNNNNNNNNN
IRON	MG	1.40	1.35	9	IIIIII
CALCIUM	MG	9.00	0.15	1	K
PHOSPHRUS	MG	169.00	2.89	19	XXXXIXXXXXXXXX
POTASSIUM	MG	227.00	0.70	5	YYYYI
PROTEIN	G	20.00	6.15	40	PPPPIPPPPPPPPPPPPPPPPPPPPPPPPPP
CARBOHYDT	G	0.00	0.00	0	
FAT	G	5.00	0.99	6	FFFFF
OLEIC A	G	1.80	1.13	7	OOOOIO
LINOL A	G	0.20	0.15	1	L
SAT FAT A	G	2.10	1.13	7	SSSSIS

186 LAMB SHOULDER, ROASTED, LEAN AND FAT
ANALYSIS OF 85 GRAMS WHICH IS 3 OZ

NUTRIENT	UNIT	AMOUNT	INQ	% STD	0 10 20 30 40 50 60 70 80 90 100
ENERGY	KCAL	285.00	1.00	14	EEEEEEEEE
VITAMIN A	IU	0.00	0.00	0	-
VITAMIN C	MG	0.00	0.00	0	-
THIAMIN	MG	0.11	0.77	11	TTTTTTT
RIBOFLAVN	MG	0.20	1.17	17	RRRRRRRRRIRR
NIACIN	MG	4.00	2.01	29	NNNNNNNNNINNNNNNNNNN
IRON	MG	1.00	0.44	6	IIIII
CALCIUM	MG	9.00	0.07	1	K
PHOSPHRUS	MG	146.00	1.14	16	XXXXXXXXIXX
POTASSIUM	MG	206.00	0.29	4	YYY
PROTEIN	G	18.00	2.53	36	PPPPPPPPIPPPPPPPPPPPPPPP
CARBOHYDT	G	0.00	0.00	0	
FAT	G	23.00	2.07	29	FFFFFFFFIFFFFFFFFFFF
OLEIC A	G	8.80	2.52	36	OOOOOOOOIOOOOOOOOOOOOOOO
LINOL A	G	0.90	0.32	5	LLLL
SAT FAT A	G	10.80	2.66	38	SSSSSSSSISSSSSSSSSSSSSSSS

187 LAMB SHOULDER, ROASTED, LEAN ONLY
ANALYSIS OF 64 GRAMS WHICH IS 2.3 OZ

NUTRIENT	UNIT	AMOUNT	INQ	% STD
ENERGY	KCAL	130.00	1.00	7
VITAMIN A	IU	0.00	0.00	0
VITAMIN C	MG	0.00	0.00	0
THIAMIN	MG	0.00	1.54	10
RIBOFLAVN	MG	0.18	2.31	15
NIACIN	MG	3.70	4.07	26
IRON	MG	1.00	0.96	6
CALCIUM	MG	8.00	0.14	1
PHOSPHRUS	MG	140.00	2.39	16
POTASSIUM	MG	193.00	0.59	4
PROTEIN	G	17.00	5.23	34
CARBOHYDT	G	0.00	0.00	0
FAT	G	6.00	1.18	8
OLEIC A	G	2.30	1.44	9
LINOL A	G	0.20	0.15	1
SAT FAT A	G	1.94		13

188 LIVER, BEEF, FRIED
ANALYSIS OF 85 GRAMS WHICH IS 3 OZ

NUTRIENT	UNIT	AMOUNT	INQ	% STD
ENERGY	KCAL	195.00	1.00	10
VITAMIN A	IU	45390.00	116.38	1135
VITAMIN C	MG	23.00	3.93	38
THIAMIN	MG	0.22	2.26	22
RIBOFLAVN	MG	3.56	30.43	297
NIACIN	MG	14.00	10.26	100
IRON	MG	7.50	4.81	47
CALCIUM	MG	9.00	0.10	1
PHOSPHRUS	MG	405.00	4.62	45
POTASSIUM	MG	323.00	0.66	6
PROTEIN	G	22.00	4.51	44
CARBOHYDT	G	5.00	0.19	2
FAT	G	9.00	1.18	12
OLEIC A	G	3.50	1.47	14
LINOL A	G	0.90	0.46	5
SAT FAT A	G	2.50	0.90	9

189 HAM, LIGHT CURE, ROASTED, LEAN AND FAT
ANALYSIS OF 85 GRAMS WHICH IS 3 OZ

NUTRIENT	UNIT	AMOUNT	INQ	% STD	0 10 20 30 40 50 60 70 80 90 100
ENERGY	KCAL	245.00	1.00	12	EEEEEEEE
VITAMIN A	IU	0.00	0.00	0	
VITAMIN C	MG	0.00	0.00	0	-
THIAMIN	MG	0.40	3.27	40	TTTTTTTT|TTTTTTTTTTTTTTTTTT
RIBOFLAVN	MG	0.15	1.02	13	RRRRRRRRR
NIACIN	MG	3.10	1.81	22	NNNNNNNNN|NNNNNNNN
IRON	MG	2.20	1.12	14	IIIIIIIIIII
CALCIUM	MG	8.00	0.07	1	K
PHOSPHRUS	MG	146.00	1.32	16	XXXXXXXX|XXX
POTASSIUM	MG	199.00	0.32	4	YYY
PROTEIN	G	18.00	2.94	36	PPPPPPPP|PPPPPPPPPPPPPPPPPP
CARBOHYDT	G	0.00	0.00	0	-
FAT	G	19.00	1.99	24	FFFFFFF|FFFFFFFFF
OLEIC A	G	7.90	2.63	32	OOOOOOOOO|OOOOOOOOOOOOOOO
LINOL A	G	1.70	0.69	9	LLLLLL
SAT FAT A	G	6.80	1.95	24	SSSSSSSS|SSSSSSSS

190 LUNCHEON MEAT, BOILED HAM
ANALYSIS OF 28 GRAMS WHICH IS 1 OZ

NUTRIENT	UNIT	AMOUNT	INQ	% STD	0 10 20 30 40 50 60 70 80 90 100
ENERGY	KCAL	65.00	1.00	3	EEE
VITAMIN A	IU	0.00	0.00	0	
VITAMIN C	MG	0.00	0.00	0	-
THIAMIN	MG	0.12	3.69	12	TTTTTTTTT
RIBOFLAVN	MG	0.04	1.03	3	RRR
NIACIN	MG	0.70	1.54	5	NNN
IRON	MG	0.80	1.54	5	III
CALCIUM	MG	3.00	0.10	0	-
PHOSPHRUS	MG	47.00	1.61	5	XXX
POTASSIUM	MG	63.00	0.39	1	Y
PROTEIN	G	5.00	3.08	10	PP|PPPPP
CARBOHYDT	G	0.00	0.00	0	-
FAT	G	5.00	1.97	6	FF|FF
OLEIC A	G	2.00	2.51	8	OO|OOOO
LINOL A	G	0.40	0.62	2	LL
SAT FAT A	G	1.70	1.84	6	SS|SS

191 LUNCHEON MEAT, CANNED, SPICED OR UNSPICED
ANALYSIS OF 60 GRAMS WHICH IS 1 SLICE (3 BY 2 BY 1/2 IN)

NUTRIENT	UNIT	AMOUNT	INQ	% STD
ENERGY	KCAL	175.00	1.00	9
VITAMIN A	IU	0.00	0.00	0
VITAMIN C	MG	0.00	0.00	0
THIAMIN	MG	0.19	2.17	19
RIBOFLAVN	MG	0.13	1.24	11
NIACIN	MG	1.80	1.47	13
IRON	MG	1.30	0.93	8
CALCIUM	MG	5.00	0.06	1
PHOSPHRUS	MG	65.00	0.83	7
POTASSIUM	MG	133.00	0.30	3
PROTEIN	G	9.00	2.06	18
CARBOHYDT	G	1.00	0.04	0
FAT	G	15.00	2.20	19
OLEIC A	G	6.70	3.13	27
LINOL A	G	1.00	0.57	5
SAT FAT A	G	5.40	2.17	19

192 PORK CHOP, BROILED, LEAN AND FAT, BONE REMOVED
ANALYSIS OF 78 GRAMS WHICH IS 2.7 OZ

NUTRIENT	UNIT	AMOUNT	INQ	% STD
ENERGY	KCAL	305.00	1.00	15
VITAMIN A	IU	0.00	0.00	0
VITAMIN C	MG	0.00	0.00	0
THIAMIN	MG	0.75	4.92	75
RIBOFLAVN	MG	0.22	1.20	18
NIACIN	MG	4.50	2.11	32
IRON	MG	2.70	1.11	17
CALCIUM	MG	9.00	0.07	1
PHOSPHRUS	MG	209.00	1.52	23
POTASSIUM	MG	216.00	0.28	4
PROTEIN	G	19.00	2.49	38
CARBOHYDT	G	0.00	0.00	0
FAT	G	25.00	2.10	32
OLEIC A	G	10.40	2.78	42
LINOL A	G	2.20	0.72	11
SAT FAT A	G	8.90	2.05	31

193 PORK CHOP, BROILED, LEAN ONLY, BONE REMOVED
ANALYSIS OF 56 GRAMS WHICH IS 2 OZ

NUTRIENT	UNIT	AMOUNT	INQ	% STD	0 10 20 30 40 50 60 70 80 90 100
ENERGY	KCAL	150.00	1.00	8	EEEEE
VITAMIN A	IU	0.00	0.00	0	-
VITAMIN C	MG	0.00	0.00	0	-
THIAMIN	MG	0.63	8.40	63	TTTTT|TTTTTTTTTTTTTTTTTTTTTTTTTTT
RIBOFLAVN	MG	0.18	2.00	15	RRRRR|RRRRR
NIACIN	MG	3.80	3.62	27	NNNNN|NNNNNNNNNNNNNN
IRON	MG	2.00	1.83	14	IIIII|IIIII
CALCIUM	MG	7.00	0.10	1	K
PHOSPHRUS	MG	181.00	2.68	20	XXXXX|XXXXXXXXX
POTASSIUM	MG	192.00	0.51	4	YYY
PROTEIN	G	17.00	4.53	34	PPPP|PPPPPPPPPPPPPPPPP
CARBOHYDT	G	0.00	0.00	0	-
FAT	G	9.00	1.54	12	FFFFF|FFF
OLEIC A	G	3.60	1.96	15	OOOOO|OOOOOO
LINOL A	G	0.80	0.53	4	LLL
SAT FAT A	G	3.10	1.45	11	SSSSS|SSS

194 PORK ROAST, OVEN COOKED, LEAN AND FAT
ANALYSIS OF 85 GRAMS WHICH IS 3 OZ

NUTRIENT	UNIT	AMOUNT	INQ	% STD	0 10 20 30 40 50 60 70 80 90 100
ENERGY	KCAL	310.00	1.00	16	EEEEEEEEEE
VITAMIN A	IU	0.00	0.00	0	-
VITAMIN C	MG	0.00	0.00	0	-
THIAMIN	MG	0.78	5.03	78	TTTTTTTTTT|TTTTTTTTTTTTTTTTTTTTTTTTTTTTTTTTTTTTTTTTTTTTTTTTTTTTTTTTTTTTTTTTTTTT
RIBOFLAVN	MG	0.22	1.18	18	RRRRRRRRR|RRR
NIACIN	MG	4.80	2.21	34	NNNNNNNNNN|NNNNNNNNNNNNNNNNNN
IRON	MG	2.70	1.09	17	IIIIIIIIII|II
CALCIUM	MG	9.00	0.06	1	K
PHOSPHRUS	MG	218.00	1.56	24	XXXXXXXXXX|XXXXXXX
POTASSIUM	MG	233.00	0.30	5	YYYY
PROTEIN	G	21.00	2.71	42	PPPPPPPPPP|PPPPPPPPPPPPPPPPPPPPPP
CARBOHYDT	G	0.00	0.00	0	-
FAT	G	24.00	1.99	31	FFFFFFFFFF|FFFFFFFFFF
OLEIC A	G	10.20	2.69	42	OOOOOOOOOO|OOOOOOOOOOOOOOOOOOOO
LINOL A	G	2.20	0.71	11	LLLLLLLL
SAT FAT A	G	8.70	1.97	31	SSSSSSSSSS|SSSSSSSSSSSSS

195 PORK ROAST, OVEN COOKED, LEAN ONLY
ANALYSIS OF 68 GRAMS WHICH IS 2.4 OZ

NUTRIENT	UNIT	AMOUNT	INQ	% STD	0 10 20 30 40 50 60 70 80 90 100
ENERGY	KCAL	175.00	1.00	9	EEEEEE
VITAMIN A	IU	0.00	0.00	0	-
VITAMIN C	MG	0.00	0.00	0	-
THIAMIN	MG	0.73	8.34	73	TTTTTTTTTTTTTTTTTTTTTTTTTTTTTTTTTTTTTTTTTTTTTTTTTTTTTTTTTTTTTTTTTTTTTTTTT
RIBOFLAVN	MG	0.21	2.00	17	RRRRRR|RRRRRRR
NIACIN	MG	4.40	3.59	31	NNNNN|NNNNNNNNNNNNNNN
IRON	MG	2.60	1.86	16	IIIIII|IIIII
CALCIUM	MG	9.00	0.11	1	K
PHOSPHRUS	MG	211.00	2.68	23	XXXXXX|XXXXXXXXXXX
POTASSIUM	MG	224.00	0.51	4	YYYY
PROTEIN	G	20.00	4.57	40	PPPPP|PPPPPPPPPPPPPPPPPPPPP
CARBOHYDT	G	0.00	0.00	0	
FAT	G	10.00	1.47	13	FFFFFF|FFF
OLEIC A	G	4.10	1.91	17	OOOOOO|OOOOOO
LINOL A	G	0.80	0.46	4	LLL
SAT FAT A	G	3.50	1.40	12	SSSSSS|SSS

196 PORK SHOULDER, SIMMERED, LEAN AND FAT
ANALYSIS OF 85 GRAMS WHICH IS 3 OZ

NUTRIENT	UNIT	AMOUNT	INQ	% STD	0 10 20 30 40 50 60 70 80 90 100
ENERGY	KCAL	320.00	1.00	16	EEEEEEEEEE
VITAMIN A	IU	0.00	0.00	0	-
VITAMIN C	MG	0.00	0.00	0	-
THIAMIN	MG	0.46	2.88	46	TTTTTTTTTTTTTTTTTTTTTTTTTTTTTTTTTTTTTTTTTTTTTTT
RIBOFLAVN	MG	0.21	1.09	17	RRRRRR|RRRRRRR
NIACIN	MG	4.10	1.83	29	NNNNN|NNNNNNNNN
IRON	MG	2.60	1.02	16	IIIIII|IIIII
CALCIUM	MG	9.00	0.06	1	K
PHOSPHRUS	MG	118.00	0.82	13	XXXXXX|XXX
POTASSIUM	MG	158.00	0.20	3	YYY
PROTEIN	G	20.00	2.50	40	PPPPP|PPPPPPPPPPPPPPPP
CARBOHYDT	G	0.00	0.00	0	-
FAT	G	26.00	2.08	33	FFFFFF|FFFFFFFFFFFF
OLEIC A	G	10.90	2.78	44	OOOOOO|OOOOOOOOOOOOOOOOOOOO
LINOL A	G	2.30	0.72	12	LLLLLLLL
SAT FAT A	G	9.30	2.04	33	SSSSS|SSSSSSSSSSSS

197 PORK SHOULDER, SIMMERED, LEAN ONLY
ANALYSIS OF 63 GRAMS WHICH IS 2.2 OZ

NUTRIENT	UNIT	AMOUNT	INQ	% STD	0	10	20	30	40	50	60	70	80	90	100
ENERGY	KCAL	135.00	1.00	7	EEEEE										
VITAMIN A	IU	0.00	0.00	0	--										
VITAMIN C	MG	0.00	0.00	0	--										
THIAMIN	MG	0.42	6.22	42	TTTT	TTTTTTTTTTTTTTTTTT									
RIBOFLAVN	MG	0.19	2.35	16	RRRR	RRRRRRRR									
NIACIN	MG	3.70	3.92	26	NNNN	NNNNNNNNNNNNN									
IRON	MG	2.30	2.13	14	IIII	IIIIIII									
CALCIUM	MG	8.00	0.13	1	K										
PHOSPHRUS	MG	111.00	1.83	12	XXXX	XXXXX									
POTASSIUM	MG	146.00	0.43	3	YY										
PROTEIN	G	18.00	5.33	36	PPPP	PPPPPPPPPPPPPPPPPPPPPPPPPP									
CARBOHYDT	G	0.00	0.00	0	-										
FAT	G	6.00	1.14	8	FFFF	F									
OLEIC A	G	2.60	1.57	11	OOOO	OOO									
LINOL A	G	0.60	0.44	3	LL										
SAT FAT A	G	2.20	1.14	8	SSS	S									

198 BOLOGNA
ANALYSIS OF 28 GRAMS WHICH IS 1 SLICE

NUTRIENT	UNIT	AMOUNT	INQ	% STD	0	10	20	30	40	50	60	70	80	90	100
ENERGY	KCAL	85.00	1.00	4	EEE										
VITAMIN A	IU	0.00	0.00	0	--										
VITAMIN C	MG	0.00	0.00	0	--										
THIAMIN	MG	0.05	1.18	5	TTIT										
RIBOFLAVN	MG	0.06	1.18	5	RRIR										
NIACIN	MG	0.70	0.74	5	NNIN										
IRON	MG	0.50	0.74	3	III										
CALCIUM	MG	2.00	0.05	0	--										
PHOSPHRUS	MG	36.00	0.94	4	XXX										
POTASSIUM	MG	65.00	0.31	1	Y										
PROTEIN	G	3.00	1.41	6	PP|PP										
CARBOHYDT	G	0.00	0.00	0	-										
FAT	G	8.00	2.41	10	FF	FFFFF									
OLEIC A	G	3.40	3.27	14	OO	OOOOOOOO									
LINOL A	G	0.50	0.59	3	LL										
SAT FAT A	G	3.00	2.48	11	SS	SSSSS									

199 BRAUNSCHWEIGER
ANALYSIS OF 28 GRAMS WHICH IS 1 SLICE

NUTRIENT	UNIT	AMOUNT	INQ	% STD
ENERGY	KCAL	90.00	1.00	5
VITAMIN A	IU	1850.00	10.28	46
VITAMIN C	MG	0.00	0.00	0
THIAMIN	MG	0.05	1.11	5
RIBOFLAVN	MG	0.41	7.59	34
NIACIN	MG	2.30	3.65	16
IRON	MG	1.70	2.36	11
CALCIUM	MG	3.00	0.07	0
PHOSPHRUS	MG	69.00	1.70	8
POTASSIUM	MG	65.00	0.29	1
PROTEIN	G	4.00	1.78	8
CARBOHYDT	G	1.00	0.08	0
FAT	G	8.00	2.28	10
OLEIC A	G	3.40	3.08	14
LINOL A	G	0.80	0.89	4
SAT FAT A	G	2.60	2.03	9

200 BROWN AND SERVE SAUSAGES
ANALYSIS OF 17 GRAMS WHICH IS 1 LINK (10-11 PER 8-OZ PKG.)

NUTRIENT	UNIT	AMOUNT	INQ	% STD
ENERGY	KCAL	70.00	1.00	4
VITAMIN A	IU	0.00	0.00	0
VITAMIN C	MG	0.00	0.00	0
THIAMIN	MG	0.13	3.71	13
RIBOFLAVN	MG	0.06	1.43	5
NIACIN	MG	0.60	1.22	4
IRON	MG	0.40	0.71	3
CALCIUM	MG	1.00	0.03	0
PHOSPHRUS	MG	28.00	0.89	3
POTASSIUM	MG	46.00	0.26	1
PROTEIN	G	3.00	1.71	6
CARBOHYDT	G	0.00	0.00	0
FAT	G	6.00	2.20	8
OLEIC A	G	2.80	3.27	11
LINOL A	G	0.70	1.00	4
SAT FAT A	G	2.30	2.31	8

201 DEVILED HAM, CANNED
ANALYSIS OF 13 GRAMS WHICH IS 1 TBSP

NUTRIENT	UNIT	AMOUNT	INQ	% STD	0	10	20	30	40	50	60	70	80	90	100
ENERGY	KCAL	45.00	1.00	2	EE										
VITAMIN A	IU	0.00	0.00	0	I										
VITAMIN C	MG	0.00	0.00	0	I										
THIAMIN	MG	0.02	0.89	2	TT										
RIBOFLAVN	MG	0.01	0.37	1	RI										
NIACIN	MG	0.20	0.63	1	NI										
IRON	MG	0.30	0.83	2	II										
CALCIUM	MG	1.00	0.05	0	I										
PHOSPHRUS	MG	12.00	0.59	1	XI										
POTASSIUM	MG	29.00	0.26	1	I										
PROTEIN	G	2.00	1.78	4	PIP										
CARBOHYDT	G	0.00	0.00	0	I										
FAT	G	4.00	2.28	5	FIFF										
OLEIC A	G	1.80	3.27	7	O|OOOO										
LINOL A	G	0.40	0.89	2	LL										
SAT FAT A	G	1.50	2.34	5	S|SS										

202 FRANKFURTER
ANALYSIS OF 56 GRAMS WHICH IS 1 FRANKFURTER (8 PER 1-LB PKG.)

NUTRIENT	UNIT	AMOUNT	INQ	% STD	0	10	20	30	40	50	60	70	80	90	100
ENERGY	KCAL	170.00	1.00	9	EEEEEE										
VITAMIN A	IU	0.00	0.00	0	-										
VITAMIN C	MG	0.00	0.00	0	I										
THIAMIN	MG	0.08	0.94	8	TITTTTI										
RIBOFLAVN	MG	0.11	1.08	9	RRRRRR										
NIACIN	MG	1.40	1.18	10	NNNNNNIN										
IRON	MG	0.80	0.59	5	IIII										
CALCIUM	MG	3.00	0.04	0	I										
PHOSPHRUS	MG	57.00	0.75	6	XXXXX										
POTASSIUM	MG	123.00	0.29	2	YY										
PROTEIN	G	7.00	1.65	14	PPPPP|PPPP										
CARBOHYDT	G	1.00	0.04	0	I										
FAT	G	15.00	2.26	19	FFFFF|FFFFFFFF										
OLEIC A	G	6.50	3.12	27	OOOOO|OOOOOOOOOOOO										
LINOL A	G	1.20	0.71	6	LLLLL|										
SAT FAT A	G	5.60	2.31	20	SSSSS|SSSSSSSS										

```
100 ****************
 90
 80
 70
 60
 50
 40
 30
 20
 10
```

```
100 ****************
 90
 80
 70
 60
 50
 40
 30
 20
 10
```

203 POTTED MEAT, CANNED
ANALYSIS OF 13 GRAMS WHICH IS 1 TBSP

NUTRIENT	UNIT	AMOUNT	INQ	% STD	0
ENERGY	KCAL	30.00	1.00	2	E
VITAMIN A	IU	0.00	0.00	0	-
VITAMIN C	MG	0.00	0.00	0	-
THIAMIN	MG	0.00	0.00	0	I
RIBOFLAVN	MG	0.03	1.67	3	IR
NIACIN	MG	0.20	0.95	1	Z
IRON	MG	0.20	0.83	1	I
CALCIUM	MG	1.00	0.07	0	x
PHOSPHRUS	MG	13.00	0.96	1	I
POTASSIUM	MG	29.00	0.39	1	PP
PROTEIN	G	2.00	2.67	4	I
CARBOHYDT	G	0.00	0.00	0	-
FAT	G	2.00	1.71	3	IF
OLEIC A	G	1.40	3.81	6	IOOOO
LINOL A	G	0.10	0.33	1	-
SAT FAT A	G	1.40	3.27	5	ISSS

204 PORK LINK SAUSAGE
ANALYSIS OF 13 GRAMS WHICH IS 1 LINK (16 PER 1-LB PKG.)

NUTRIENT	UNIT	AMOUNT	INQ	% STD	0
ENERGY	KCAL	60.00	1.00	3	EE
VITAMIN A	IU	0.00	0.00	0	-I
VITAMIN C	MG	0.00	0.00	0	-I
THIAMIN	MG	0.10	3.33	10	TITTTTTT
RIBOFLAVN	MG	0.04	1.11	3	RIR
NIACIN	MG	0.50	1.19	4	NIN
IRON	MG	0.30	0.63	2	II
CALCIUM	MG	1.00	0.04	0	-I
PHOSPHRUS	MG	21.00	0.78	2	XX
POTASSIUM	MG	35.00	0.23	1	YI
PROTEIN	G	2.00	1.33	4	PIP
CARBOHYDT	G	0.00	0.00	0	-I
FAT	G	6.00	2.56	8	FIFFFF
OLEIC A	G	2.40	3.27	10	OIOOOOOO
LINOL A	G	0.50	0.83	3	LL
SAT FAT A	G	2.10	2.46	7	SISSSS

205 SALAMI, DRY TYPE
ANALYSIS OF 10 GRAMS WHICH IS 1 SLICE (12 PER 4-OZ PKG.)

NUTRIENT	UNIT	AMOUNT	INQ	% STD	0	10	20	30	40	50	60	70	80	90	100
ENERGY	KCAL	45.00	1.00	2	EE										
VITAMIN A	IU	0.00	0.00	0	-I										
VITAMIN C	MG	0.00	0.00	0	-I										
THIAMIN	MG	0.04	1.78	4	TIT										
RIBOFLAVN	MG	0.03	1.11	3	RR										
NIACIN	MG	0.50	1.59	4	NIN										
IRON	MG	0.40	1.11	3	II										
CALCIUM	MG	1.00	0.05	0	-I										
PHOSPHRUS	MG	28.00	1.38	3	XX										
POTASSIUM	MG	22.00	0.20	0	-I										
PROTEIN	G	2.00	1.78	4	PIP										
CARBOHYDT	G	0.00	0.00	0	-I										
FAT	G	4.00	2.28	5	FIFF										
OLEIC A	G	1.60	2.90	7	0I000										
LINOL A	G	0.10	0.22	1	-I										
SAT FAT A	G	1.60	2.50	6	SISS										

****

206 SALAMI, COOKED TYPE
ANALYSIS OF 28 GRAMS WHICH IS 1 SLICE (8 PER 8-OZ PKG.)

NUTRIENT	UNIT	AMOUNT	INQ	% STD	0	10	20	30	40	50	60	70	80	90	100
ENERGY	KCAL	90.00	1.00	5	EEEE										
VITAMIN A	IU	0.00	0.00	0	-I										
VITAMIN C	MG	0.00	0.00	0	-I										
THIAMIN	MG	0.07	1.56	7	TITITT										
RIBOFLAVN	MG	0.07	1.30	6	RRRIR										
NIACIN	MG	1.20	1.90	9	NNNINNN										
IRON	MG	0.70	0.97	4	IIII										
CALCIUM	MG	3.00	0.07	0	-I										
PHOSPHRUS	MG	57.00	1.41	6	XXXIX										
POTASSIUM	MG	63.00	0.28	1	Y-I										
PROTEIN	G	5.00	2.22	10	PPPIPPPP										
CARBOHYDT	G	0.00	0.00	0	-I										
FAT	G	7.00	1.99	9	FFFIFFF										
OLEIC A	G	3.00	2.72	12	000I000000										
LINOL A	G	0.20	0.22	1	L-I										
SAT FAT A	G	3.10	2.42	11	SSSISSSS										

****

207 VIENNA SAUSAGE
ANALYSIS OF 16 GRAMS WHICH IS 1 SAUSAGE (7 PER 4-OZ CAN)

```
                                        0   10   20   30   40   50   60   70   80   90  100
                                                                                         * * * * * * * * * * * * * * * * *
NUTRIENT    UNIT   AMOUNT   INQ   % STD
ENERGY      KCAL    40.00   1.00     2  EE
VITAMIN A   IU       0.00   0.00     0  - I
VITAMIN C   MG       0.00   0.00     0  - I
THIAMIN     MG       0.01   0.50     1  T I
RIBOFLAVN   MG       0.02   0.83     2  R I
NIACIN      MG       0.40   1.43     3  NN I
IRON        MG       0.30   0.94     2  II
CALCIUM     MG       1.00   0.06     0  - I
PHOSPHRUS   MG      24.00   1.33     3  XX I
POTASSIUM   MG      35.00   0.35     1  Y I
PROTEIN     G        2.00   2.00     4  P I P
CARBOHYDT   G        0.00   0.00     0  - I
FAT         G        3.00   1.92     4  F I F
OLEIC A     G        1.40   2.86     6  O I 000
LINOL A     G        0.20   0.50     1  L I
SAT FAT A   G        1.20   2.11     4  S I S
*************************************************************
```

208 VEAL CUTLET, BRAISED OR BROILED, BONE REMOVED
ANALYSIS OF 85 GRAMS WHICH IS 3 OZ

```
                                        0   10   20   30   40   50   60   70   80   90  100
                                                                                         * * * * * * * * * * * * * * * * *
NUTRIENT    UNIT   AMOUNT   INQ   % STD
ENERGY      KCAL   185.00   1.00     9  EEEEEE
VITAMIN A   IU       0.00   0.00     0  - I
VITAMIN C   MG       0.00   0.00     0  - I
THIAMIN     MG       0.06   0.65     6  TTTT I
RIBOFLAVN   MG       0.21   1.89    17  RRRRRR IRRRRRR
NIACIN      MG       4.60   3.55    33  NNNNNN INNNNNNNNNNNNNNNN
IRON        MG       2.70   1.82    17  IIIIII IIIIIII
CALCIUM     MG       9.00   0.11     1  K
PHOSPHRUS   MG     196.00   2.35    22  XXXXXX IXXXXXXXXXX
POTASSIUM   MG     258.00   0.56     5  YYYY I
PROTEIN     G       23.00   4.97    46  PPPPP IPPPPPPPPPPPPPPPPPPPPPPPPPPPP
CARBOHYDT   G        0.00   0.00     0  - I
FAT         G        9.00   1.25    12  FFFFFF IFF
OLEIC A     G        3.40   1.50    14  OOOOOO IOOOO
LINOL A     G        0.40   0.22     2  LL I
SAT FAT A   G        4.00   1.52    14  SSSSSS ISSSS
*************************************************************
```

209 VEAL RIB, ROASTED, BONE REMOVED
ANALYSIS OF 85 GRAMS WHICH IS 3 OZ

```
                                              0    10   20   30   40   50   60   70   80   90   100
                                                                                                *
                                                   *    *    *    *    *    *    *    *    *    *
NUTRIENT    UNIT    AMOUNT    INQ     % STD
ENERGY      KCAL    230.00    1.00      12    EEEEEEEE
VITAMIN A   IU        0.00    0.00       0    -
VITAMIN C   MG        0.00    0.00       0    -
THIAMIN     MG        0.11    0.96      11    TTTTTTTT
RIBOFLAVN   MG        0.26    1.88      22    RRRRRRRR|RRRRRRR
NIACIN      MG        6.60    4.10      47    NNNNNNNN|NNNNNNNNNNNNNNNNNNN
IRON        MG        2.90    1.58      18    IIIIIII|IIIIIII
CALCIUM     MG       10.00    0.10       1    K
PHOSPHRUS   MG      211.00    2.04      23    XXXXXXXX|XXXXXXXX
POTASSIUM   MG      259.00    0.45       5    YYYY
PROTEIN     G        23.00    4.00      46    PPPPPPPP|PPPPPPPPPPPPPPPPPPPPPPPPPPPP
CARBOHYDT   G         0.00    0.00       0    -
FAT         G        14.00    1.56      18    FFFFFFFF|FFFFF
OLEIC A     G         5.10    1.81      21    OOOOOOOO|OOOOOOO
LINOL A     G         0.60    0.26       3    LL
SAT FAT A   G         6.10    1.86      21    SSSSSSSS|SSSSSSS
************************************************
```

210 CHICKEN BREAST, FRIED, BONES REMOVED
ANALYSIS OF 79 GRAMS WHICH IS 2.8 OZ

```
                                              0    10   20   30   40   50   60   70   80   90   100
                                                                                                *
                                                   *    *    *    *    *    *    *    *    *    *
NUTRIENT    UNIT    AMOUNT    INQ     % STD
ENERGY      KCAL    160.00    1.00       8    EEEEE
VITAMIN A   IU       70.00    0.22       2    A
VITAMIN C   MG        0.00    0.00       0    -
THIAMIN     MG        0.04    0.50       4    TTT
RIBOFLAVN   MG        0.17    1.77      14    RRRRR|RRRRR
NIACIN      MG       11.60   10.36      83    NNNNN|NNNNNNNNNNNNNNNNNNNNNNNNNNNNNNNNNNNNNNNNNNNNNNNNNNNNNNNNNNNNNNNNNNNNNNNNNN
IRON        MG        1.30    1.02       8    IIIIII|
CALCIUM     MG        9.00    0.13       1    K
PHOSPHRUS   MG      218.00    3.03      24    XXXXX|XXXXXXXXXXXXXXXX
POTASSIUM   MG      343.00    0.86       7    YYYYY|
PROTEIN     G        26.00    6.50      52    PPPPP|PPPPPPPPPPPPPPPPPPPPPPPPPPPPPPPPPPPPPPPPPPPPP
CARBOHYDT   G         0.00    0.05       0    -
FAT         G         5.00    0.80       6    FFFFF|
OLEIC A     G         1.80    0.92       7    OOOOOO
LINOL A     G         1.10    0.69       6    LLLL|
SAT FAT A   G         1.40    0.61       5    SSSS|
************************************************
```

211 CHICKEN DRUMSTICK, FRIED, BONES REMOVED
ANALYSIS OF 38 GRAMS WHICH IS 1.3 OZ

NUTRIENT	UNIT	AMOUNT	INQ	% STD
ENERGY	KCAL	90.00	1.00	5
VITAMIN A	IU	50.00	0.28	1
VITAMIN C	MG	0.00	0.00	0
THIAMIN	MG	0.03	0.67	3
RIBOFLAVN	MG	0.15	2.78	13
NIACIN	MG	2.70	4.29	19
IRON	MG	0.90	1.25	6
CALCIUM	MG	6.00	0.15	1
PHOSPHRUS	MG	89.00	2.20	10
POTASSIUM	MG	122.00	0.54	2
PROTEIN	G	12.00	5.33	24
CARBOHYDT	G	0.00	0.00	0
FAT	G	4.00	1.14	5
OLEIC A	G	1.30	1.18	5
LINOL A	G	0.90	1.00	5
SAT FAT A	G	1.10	0.86	4

212 CHICKEN, HALF BROILER, BONES REMOVED
ANALYSIS OF 176 GRAMS WHICH IS 6.2 OZ

NUTRIENT	UNIT	AMOUNT	INQ	% STD
ENERGY	KCAL	240.00	1.00	12
VITAMIN A	IU	160.00	0.33	4
VITAMIN C	MG	0.00	0.00	0
THIAMIN	MG	0.09	0.75	9
RIBOFLAVN	MG	0.34	2.36	28
NIACIN	MG	15.50	9.23	111
IRON	MG	3.00	1.56	19
CALCIUM	MG	16.00	0.15	2
PHOSPHRUS	MG	355.00	3.29	39
POTASSIUM	MG	483.00	0.81	10
PROTEIN	G	42.00	7.00	84
CARBOHYDT	G	0.00	0.00	0
FAT	G	7.00	0.75	9
OLEIC A	G	2.50	0.85	10
LINOL A	G	1.30	0.54	7
SAT FAT A	G	2.20	0.64	8

```
213  CHICKEN, CANNED, BONELESS
ANALYSIS OF 85 GRAMS WHICH IS 3 OZ

                                                0      10        20        30        40        50        60        70        80        90        100
NUTRIENT   UNIT   AMOUNT   INQ    % STD
ENERGY     KCAL   170.00   1.00     9          EEEEEE                                                                                             *
VITAMIN A  IU     200.00   0.59     5          AAAA |                                                                                            *
VITAMIN C  MG       3.00   0.59     5          CCCC |                                                                                            *
THIAMIN    MG       0.03   0.35     3          TT   |                                                                                            *
RIBOFLAVN  MG       0.11   1.08     9          RRRRRR                                                                                            *
NIACIN     MG       3.70   3.11    26          NNNNNNN|NNNNNNNNNNNNNNN                                                                            *
IRON       MG       1.30   0.96     8          IIIIII |                                                                                           *
CALCIUM    MG      18.00   0.24     2          KK    |                                                                                            *
PHOSPHRUS  MG     210.00   2.75    23          XXXXXX|XXXXXXXXXXX                                                                                 *
POTASSIUM  MG     117.00   0.28     2          YY   |                                                                                            *
PROTEIN    MG      18.00   4.24    36          PPPPP|PPPPPPPPPPPPPPPPPPPPPPPPPPP                                                                  *
CARBOHYDT  G        0.00   0.00     0          -    |                                                                                            *
FAT        G       10.00   1.51    13          FFFFF|FFFF                                                                                        *
OLEIC A    G        3.80   1.82    16          OOOOO|OOOOO                                                                                        *
LINOL A    G        2.00   1.18    10          LLLLL|L                                                                                            *
SAT FAT A  G        3.20   1.32    11          SSSSSS|SS                                                                                          *
***************************************************************
```

```
14  CHICKEN A LA KING (HOME RECIPE)
NALYSIS OF 245 GRAMS WHICH IS 1 CUP

                                                0      10        20        30        40        50        60        70        80        90        100
NUTRIENT   UNIT   AMOUNT   INQ    % STD
ENERGY     KCAL   470.00   1.00    24          EEEEEEEEEEEEEEEE                                                                                   *
VITAMIN A  IU    1130.00   1.20    28          AAAAAAAAAAAAAAAAAA|AAAA                                                                            *
VITAMIN C  MG      12.00   0.85    20          CCCCCCCCCCCCCC                                                                                     *
THIAMIN    MG       0.10   0.43    10          TTTTTTT                                                                                            *
RIBOFLAVN  MG       0.42   1.49    35          RRRRRRRRRRRRRRRRRRR|RRRRRRRR                                                                       *
NIACIN     MG       5.40   1.64    39          NNNNNNNNNNNNNNNNNNN|NNNNNNNNNNNN                                                                   *
IRON       MG       2.50   0.66    16          IIIIIIIIIII                                                                                        *
CALCIUM    MG     127.00   0.60    14          KKKKKKKKKK                                                                                         *
PHOSPHRUS  MG     358.00   1.69    40          XXXXXXXXXXXXXXXXXXX|XXXXXXXXXXXXX                                                                  *
POTASSIUM  MG     404.00   0.34     8          YYYYYY                                                                                             *
PROTEIN    G       27.00   2.30    54          PPPPPPPPPPPPPPPPPPP|PPPPPPPPPPPPPPPPPPPPPPPPPP                                                     *
CARBOHYDT  G       12.00   0.19     4          HHH                                                                                                *
FAT        G       34.00   1.65    44          FFFFFFFFFFFFFFFFFFF|FFFFFFFFFFFFFFF                                                                *
OLEIC A    G       14.30   2.48    58          OOOOOOOOOOOOOOOOOOO|OOOOOOOOOOOOOOOOOOOOOOOOO                                                      *
LINOL A    G        3.00   0.70    17          LLLLLLLLLLLLL                                                                                      *
SAT FAT A  G       12.70   1.90    45          SSSSSSSSSSSSSSSSSSS|SSSSSSSSSSSSSSSS                                                               *
***************************************************************
```

215 CHICKEN AND NOODLES (HOME RECIPE)
ANALYSIS OF 240 GRAMS WHICH IS 1 CUP

NUTRIENT	UNIT	AMOUNT	INQ	% STD
ENERGY	KCAL	365.00	1.00	18
VITAMIN A	IU	430.00	0.59	11
VITAMIN C	MG	0.00	0.00	0
THIAMIN	MG	0.05	0.27	5
RIBOFLAVN	MG	0.17	0.78	14
NIACIN	MG	4.30	1.68	31
IRON	MG	2.20	0.75	14
CALCIUM	MG	26.00	0.16	3
PHOSPHRUS	MG	247.00	1.50	27
POTASSIUM	MG	149.00	0.16	3
PROTEIN	G	22.00	2.41	44
CARBOHYDT	G	26.00	0.52	9
FAT	G	18.00	1.26	23
OLEIC A	G	7.10	1.59	29
LINOL A	G	3.50	0.96	17
SAT FAT A	G	5.90	1.13	21

216 CHICKEN CHOW MEIN, CANNED
ANALYSIS OF 250 GRAMS WHICH IS 1 CUP

NUTRIENT	UNIT	AMOUNT	INQ	% STD
ENERGY	KCAL	95.00	1.00	5
VITAMIN A	IU	150.00	0.79	4
VITAMIN C	MG	13.00	4.56	22
THIAMIN	MG	0.05	1.05	5
RIBOFLAVN	MG	0.10	1.75	8
NIACIN	MG	1.00	1.50	7
IRON	MG	1.30	1.71	8
CALCIUM	MG	45.00	1.05	5
PHOSPHRUS	MG	85.00	1.99	9
POTASSIUM	MG	418.00	1.76	8
PROTEIN	G	7.00	2.95	14
CARBOHYDT	G	18.00	1.38	7
FAT	G	0.00	0.00	0
OLEIC A	G	14.60	12.55	60
LINOL A	G	3.40	3.58	17
SAT FAT A	G	13.00	9.60	46

217 CHICKEN CHOW MEIN (HOME RECIPE)
ANALYSIS OF 250 GRAMS WHICH IS 1 CUP

```
NUTRIENT    UNIT  AMOUNT  INQ   % STD  0        10        20        30        40        50        60        70        80        90       100
ENERGY      KCAL  255.00  1.00   13    EEEEEEEE                                                                                            *
VITAMIN A   IU    280.00  0.55    7    AAAAAA|                                                                                             *
VITAMIN C   MG     10.00  1.31   17    CCCCCCCCCC|CCC                                                                                      *
THIAMIN     MG      0.08  0.63    8    TTTTTT|                                                                                             *
RIBOFLAVN   MG      0.23  1.50   19    RRRRRRRRR|RRRR                                                                                      *
NIACIN      MG      4.30  2.41   31    NNNNNNNNN|NNNNNNNNNN                                                                                 *
IRON        MG      2.50  1.23   16    IIIIIIIII|III                                                                                       *
CALCIUM     MG     58.00  0.51    6    KKKKK                                                                                               *
PHOSPHRUS   MG    293.00  2.55   33    XXXXXXXXX|XXXXXXXXXXX                                                                               *
POTASSIUM   MG    473.00  0.74    9    YYYYYYYY|Y                                                                                          *
PROTEIN     G      31.00  4.86   62    PPPPPPPPP|PPPPPPPPPPPPPPPPPPPPPPPPPPPPPPPPPPPPPPPP                                                   *
CARBOHYDT   G      10.00  0.29    4    HHH                                                                                                 *
FAT         G      10.00  1.01   13    FFFFFFFFF|F                                                                                         *
OLEIC A     G       3.40  1.09   14    OOOOOOOOO|O                                                                                         *
LINOL A     G       3.10  1.22   16    LLLLLLLL|LL                                                                                         *
SAT FAT A   G       2.40  0.66    8    SSSSSSS|                                                                                            *
**********************************************************************************************************
```

218 CHICKEN POTPIE (HOME RECIPE)
ANALYSIS OF 232 GRAMS WHICH IS 1 PIECE OR 1/3 OF 9-IN DIAM. PIE

```
NUTRIENT    UNIT  AMOUNT   INQ   % STD  0        10        20        30        40        50        60        70        80        90       100
ENERGY      KCAL   545.00  1.00   27    EEEEEEEEEEEEEEEEEEEEEEEEEE                                                                          *
VITAMIN A   IU    3090.00  2.83   77    AAAAAAAAAAAAAAAA|AAAAAAAAAAAAAAAAAAAAAAAAAAAAAAAAAAAAAAAAAAAAAAAAAAAAAAAAAAAAAA                    *
VITAMIN C   MG       5.00  0.31    8    CCCCCC                                                                                             *
THIAMIN     MG       0.34  1.25   34    TTTTTTTTTTTTTTTTT|TTTTTTTTTTTTTTTTT                                                                 *
RIBOFLAVN   MG       0.31  0.95   26    RRRRRRRRRRRRR|RRRRRR                                                                                *
NIACIN      MG       5.50  1.44   39    NNNNNNNNNNNNNNNNN|NNNNNNNNNN|NNNNNNNN                                                               *
IRON        MG       3.00  0.69   19    IIIIIIIIIIIIIIIII|IIII                                                                              *
CALCIUM     MG      70.00  0.29    8    KKKKKK                                                                                             *
PHOSPHRUS   MG     232.00  0.95   26    XXXXXXXXXXXXX|XXXXXXXXXXXX|X                                                                        *
POTASSIUM   MG     343.00  0.25    7    YYYYY                                                                                              *
PROTEIN     G       23.00  1.69   46    PPPPPPPPPPPPPPPPP|PPPPPPPPPPPPPPPPPPPPPPPPPPPP|PPPPPPPPPP                                           *
CARBOHYDT   G       42.00  0.56   15    HHHHHHHHHH|HHHHH                                                                                    *
FAT         G       31.00  1.46   40    FFFFFFFFFFFFFFFFF|FFFFFFFFFFFFFFFFFFFF|FFFFFFFFF                                                    *
OLEIC A     G       10.90  1.63   44    OOOOOOOOOOOOOOOOO|OOOOOOOOOOOOOOOOOOOO|OOOOOOOOOOOOO                                                *
LINOL A     G        5.60  1.03   28    LLLLLLLLLLLLLLLLL|LLLLLLLLLLL                                                                       *
SAT FAT A   G       11.30  1.46   40    SSSSSSSSSSSSSSSSS|SSSSSSSSSSSSSSSSSSSS|SSSSSSSSS                                                    *
**********************************************************************************************************
```

219 TURKEY, DARK MEAT, FLESH ONLY, ROASTED
ANALYSIS OF 85 GRAMS WHICH IS 4 PIECES (2 1/2 BY 1 5/8 BY 1/4 IN.)

```
                                          0    10   20   30   40   50   60   70   80   90  100
```

NUTRIENT	UNIT	AMOUNT	INQ	% STD	
ENERGY	KCAL	175.00	1.00	9	EEEEEE
VITAMIN A	IU	50.00	0.14	1	A
VITAMIN C	MG	4.00	0.76	7	CCCCC
THIAMIN	MG	0.03	0.34	3	TT
RIBOFLAVN	MG	0.20	1.90	17	RRRRRIRRRRR
NIACIN	MG	3.60	2.94	26	NNNNNINNNNNNNNNNN
IRON	MG	2.00	1.43	13	IIIIIIIIIII
CALCIUM	MG	15.00	0.19	2	K
PHOSPHRUS	MG	29.00	0.37	3	XXX
POTASSIUM	MG	338.00	0.77	7	YYYY
PROTEIN	MG	26.00	5.94	52	PPPPPIPPPPPPPPPPPPPPPPPPPPPPPPPPPPPPPPPPPPPPPPP
CARBOHYDT	G	0.00		0	
FAT	G	7.00	1.03	9	FFFFFF
OLEIC A	G	1.50	0.70	6	OOOOO
LINOL A	G	1.50	0.86	8	LLLLLL
SAT FAT A	G	2.10	0.84	7	SSSSSI

220 TURKEY, LIGHT MEAT, FLESH ONLY, ROASTED
ANALYSIS OF 85 GRAMS WHICH IS 2 PIECES (4 BY 2 BY 1/4 IN.)

```
                                          0    10   20   30   40   50   60   70   80   90  100
```

NUTRIENT	UNIT	AMOUNT	INQ	% STD	
ENERGY	KCAL	150.00	1.00	8	EEEEE
VITAMIN A	IU	80.00	0.27	2	AA
VITAMIN C	MG	0.00	0.00	0	-
THIAMIN	MG	0.04	0.53	4	TTT
RIBOFLAVN	MG	0.12	1.33	10	RRRRRIRR
NIACIN	MG	9.40	8.95	67	NNNNNINNNNNNNNNNNNNNNNNNNNNNNNNNNNNNNNNNNNNNNNNNNNNNNNNNNNNNNNNNNNN
IRON	MG	1.00	0.83	6	IIIIII
CALCIUM	MG	9.00	0.13	1	K
PHOSPHRUS	MG	225.00	3.33	25	XXXXXIXXXXXXXXXX
POTASSIUM	MG	349.00	0.93	7	YYYYYY
PROTEIN	G	28.00	7.47	56	PPPPPIPPPPPPPPPPPPPPPPPPPPPPPPPPPPPPPPPPPPPPPPPPPPPP
CARBOHYDT	G	0.00	0.00	0	
FAT	G	3.00	0.51	4	FFF
OLEIC A	G	0.60	0.33	2	OO
LINOL A	G	0.70	0.47	4	LLL
SAT FAT A	G	0.90	0.42	3	SSS

221 TURKEY, LIGHT AND DARK MEAT CHOPPED
ANALYSIS OF 140 GRAMS WHICH IS 1 CUP

NUTRIENT	UNIT	AMOUNT	INQ	% STD
ENERGY	KCAL	265.00	1.00	13
VITAMIN A	IU	210.00	0.40	5
VITAMIN C	MG	0.00	0.00	0
THIAMIN	MG	0.07	0.53	7
RIBOFLAVN	MG	0.25	1.57	21
NIACIN	MG	10.80	5.82	77
IRON	MG	2.50	1.18	16
CALCIUM	MG	11.00	0.09	1
PHOSPHRUS	MG	351.00	2.94	39
POTASSIUM	MG	514.00	0.78	10
PROTEIN	G	44.00	6.64	88
CARBOHYDT	G	0.00	0.00	0
FAT	G	9.00	0.87	12
OLEIC A	G	1.70	0.52	7
LINOL A	G	1.80	0.68	9
SAT FAT A	G	2.50	0.66	9

222 TURKEY, LIGHT AND DARK
ANALYSIS OF 85 GRAMS WHICH IS 1.5 OZ EACH

NUTRIENT	UNIT	AMOUNT	INQ	% STD
ENERGY	KCAL	160.00	1.00	8
VITAMIN A	IU	130.00	0.41	3
VITAMIN C	MG	0.00	0.00	0
THIAMIN	MG	0.04	0.50	4
RIBOFLAVN	MG	0.15	1.56	13
NIACIN	MG	6.50	5.80	46
IRON	MG	1.50	1.17	9
CALCIUM	MG	7.00	0.10	1
PHOSPHRUS	MG	213.00	2.96	24
POTASSIUM	MG	312.00	0.78	6
PROTEIN	G	27.00	6.75	54
CARBOHYDT	G	0.00	0.00	0
FAT	G	5.00	0.80	6
OLEIC A	G	1.00	0.51	4
LINOL A	G	1.10	0.69	6
SAT FAT A	G	1.50	0.66	5

223 APPLE, RAW, UNPEELED, WITHOUT CORE
ANALYSIS OF 138 GRAMS WHICH IS 1--2 3/4-IN DIAM. APPLE

NUTRIENT	UNIT	AMOUNT	INQ	% STD
ENERGY	KCAL	80.00	1.00	4
VITAMIN A	IU	120.00	0.75	3
VITAMIN C	MG	6.00	2.50	10
THIAMIN	MG	0.04	1.00	4
RIBOFLAVN	MG	0.03	0.63	3
NIACIN	MG	0.10	0.18	1
IRON	MG	0.40	0.63	3
CALCIUM	MG	10.00	0.28	1
PHOSPHRUS	MG	14.00	0.39	2
POTASSIUM	MG	152.00	0.76	3
PROTEIN	G	0.00	0.00	0
CARBOHYDT	G	20.00	1.82	7
FAT	G	1.00	0.32	1
OLEIC A	G	0.00	0.00	0
LINOL A	G	0.00	0.00	0
SAT FAT A	G	0.00	0.00	0

224 APPLE, RAW, UNPEELED, WITHOUT CORE
ANALYSIS OF 212 GRAMS WHICH IS 1--3 1/4-IN DIAM. APPLE

NUTRIENT	UNIT	AMOUNT	INQ	% STD
ENERGY	KCAL	125.00	1.00	6
VITAMIN A	IU	190.00	0.76	5
VITAMIN C	MG	8.00	2.13	13
THIAMIN	MG	0.06	0.96	6
RIBOFLAVN	MG	0.04	0.53	3
NIACIN	MG	0.20	0.23	1
IRON	MG	0.60	0.60	4
CALCIUM	MG	15.00	0.27	2
PHOSPHRUS	MG	21.00	0.37	2
POTASSIUM	MG	233.00	0.75	5
PROTEIN	G	0.00	0.00	0
CARBOHYDT	G	31.00	1.80	11
FAT	G	1.00	0.21	1
OLEIC A	G	0.00	0.00	0
LINOL A	G	0.00	0.00	0
SAT FAT A	G	0.00	0.00	0

225 APPLEJUICE, BOTTLED OR CANNED
ANALYSIS OF 248 GRAMS WHICH IS 1 CUP

NUTRIENT	UNIT	AMOUNT	INQ	% STD	0 — 10 20 30 40 50 60 70 80 90 100
ENERGY	KCAL	120.00	1.00	6	EEEE
VITAMIN A	IU	0.00	0.00	0	-
VITAMIN C	MG	2.00	0.56	3	CCC
THIAMIN	MG	0.02	0.33	2	TT
RIBOFLAVN	MG	0.05	0.69	4	RRR
NIACIN	MG	0.20	0.24	1	N
IRON	MG	1.50	1.56	9	IIIIIIII
CALCIUM	MG	15.00	0.28	2	K
PHOSPHRUS	MG	22.00	0.41	2	XX
POTASSIUM	MG	250.00	0.83	5	YYYY
PROTEIN	G	0.00	0.00	0	-
CARBOHYDT	G	30.00	1.82	11	HHHH|HHHH
FAT	G	0.00	0.00	0	-
OLEIC A	G	0.00	0.00	0	-
LINOL A	G	0.00	0.00	0	-
SAT FAT A	G	0.00	0.00	0	-

226 APPLESAUCE, SWEETENED
ANALYSIS OF 255 GRAMS WHICH IS 1 CUP

NUTRIENT	UNIT	AMOUNT	INQ	% STD	0 — 10 20 30 40 50 60 70 80 90 100
ENERGY	KCAL	230.00	1.00	12	EEEEEEEE
VITAMIN A	IU	100.00	0.22	3	AA
VITAMIN C	MG	3.00	0.43	5	CCCC
THIAMIN	MG	0.05	0.43	5	TTTT
RIBOFLAVN	MG	0.03	0.22	3	RR
NIACIN	MG	0.10	0.06	1	N
IRON	MG	1.30	0.71	8	IIIIIII
CALCIUM	MG	10.00	0.10	1	K
PHOSPHRUS	MG	13.00	0.13	1	X
POTASSIUM	MG	166.00	0.29	3	YYY
PROTEIN	G	0.29	0.17	2	PP
CARBOHYDT	G	61.00	1.93	22	HHHHHHHH|HHHHHHHH
FAT	G	0.00	0.00	0	-
OLEIC A	G	0.00	0.00	0	-
LINOL A	G	0.00	0.00	0	-
SAT FAT A	G	0.00	0.00	0	-

227 APPLESAUCE, UNSWEETENED
ANALYSIS OF 244 GRAMS WHICH IS 1 CUP

Scale: 0 · 10 · 20 · 30 · 40 · 50 · 60 · 70 · 80 · 90 · 100

NUTRIENT	UNIT	AMOUNT	INQ	% STD	GRAPH
ENERGY	KCAL	100.00	1.00	5	EEEE
VITAMIN A	IU	100.00	0.50	3	AA
VITAMIN C	MG	2.00	0.67	3	CCC
THIAMIN	MG	0.05	1.00	5	TTT
RIBOFLAVN	MG	0.02	0.33	2	R
NIACIN	MG	0.10	0.14	1	N
IRON	MG	1.20	1.50	7	IIIIII
CALCIUM	MG	10.00	0.22	1	K
PHOSPHRUS	MG	12.00	0.27	1	X
POTASSIUM	MG	190.00	0.76	4	YYY
PROTEIN	G	0.00	0.00	0	-
CARBOHYDT	G	26.00	1.89	9	HHHIHHHH
FAT	G	0.00	0.00	0	-
OLEIC A	G	0.00	0.00	0	-
LINOL A	G	0.00	0.00	0	-
SAT FAT A	G	0.00	0.00	0	-

228 APRICOTS, RAW, WITHOUT PITS
ANALYSIS OF 107 GRAMS WHICH IS 3

Scale: 0 · 10 · 20 · 30 · 40 · 50 · 60 · 70 · 80 · 90 · 100

NUTRIENT	UNIT	AMOUNT	INQ	% STD	GRAPH
ENERGY	KCAL	55.00	1.00	3	EE
VITAMIN A	IU	2890.00	26.27	72	AIAAAAAAAAAAAAAAAAAAAAAAAAAAAAAAAAAAAAAAAAAAAAAAAAAAAAAAAAAAAAAAAAAAAAAA
VITAMIN C	MG	11.00	6.67	18	CICCCCCCCCCCC
THIAMIN	MG	0.03	0.67	3	TT
RIBOFLAVN	MG	0.04	1.09	3	RIR
NIACIN	MG	0.60	1.21	3	NIN
IRON	MG	0.50	1.56	4	III
CALCIUM	MG	18.00	1.14	3	KK
PHOSPHRUS	MG	25.00	0.73	2	XX
POTASSIUM	MG	301.00	1.01	3	YIYYY
PROTEIN	G	1.00	2.19	6	PP
CARBOHYDT	G	14.00	1.85	5	HIHH
FAT	G	0.00	0.00	0	-I
OLEIC A	G	0.00	0.00	0	-I
LINOL A	G	0.00	0.00	0	-I
SAT FAT A	G	0.00	0.00	0	-I

229 APRICOTS CANNED IN HEAVY SIRUP
ANALYSIS OF 258 GRAMS WHICH IS 1 CUP-HALVES AND SIRUP

```
NUTRIENT    UNIT  AMOUNT    INQ   % STD   0        10        20        30        40        50        60        70        80        90        100
ENERGY      KCAL  220.00   1.00     11   EEEEEEEE
VITAMIN A   IU   4490.00  10.20    112   AAAAAAAAIAAAAAAAAAAAAAAAAAAAAAAAAAAAAAAAAAAAAAAAAAAAAAAAAAAAAAAAAAAAAAAAAAAAAAAAAAAAAAAAAAAAAAAA * 112
VITAMIN C   MG    10.00   1.52     17   CCCCCCCICCCC
THIAMIN     MG     0.05   0.45      5   TTTT
RIBOFLAVN   MG     0.05   0.38      4   RRR
NIACIN      MG     1.00   0.65      7   NNNNNN
IRON        MG     0.80   0.45      5   IIII
CALCIUM     MG    28.00   0.28      3   KK
PHOSPHRUS   MG    39.00   0.39      4   XXX
POTASSIUM   MG   604.00   1.10     12   YYYYYYYIY
PROTEIN     G      2.00   0.36      4   PPP
CARBOHYDT   G     57.00   1.88     21   HHHHHHHIHHHHHHHH
FAT         G      0.00   0.00      0   -
OLEIC A     G      0.00   0.00      0   -
LINOL A     G      0.00   0.00      0   -
SAT FAT A   G      0.00   0.00      0   -
*******************************************
```

230 APRICOTS,DRIED, UNCOOKED
ANALYSIS OF 130 GRAMS WHICH IS 1 CUP-28 LARGE OR 37 MEDIUM HALVES

```
NUTRIENT    UNIT  AMOUNT     INQ   % STD   0        10        20        30        40        50        60        70        80        90        100
ENERGY      KCAL   340.00   1.00     17   EEEEEEEEEEE
VITAMIN A   IU   14170.00  20.84    354   AAAAAAAAAAAAIAAAAAAAAAAAICCCCCCC
VITAMIN C   MG     16.00   1.57     27   CCCCCCCCCCCCICCCCCCC
THIAMIN     MG      0.01   0.06      1   T
RIBOFLAVN   MG      0.21   1.03     17   RRRRRRRRRRRRR
NIACIN      MG      4.30   1.81     31   NNNNNNNNNNNNINNNNNNNNNNN
IRON        MG      7.20   2.65     45   IIIIIIIIIIIIIIIIIIIIIIIIIIIIIII
CALCIUM     MG     87.00   0.57     10   KKKKKKKK
PHOSPHRUS   MG    140.00   0.92     16   XXXXXXXXXXXX
POTASSIUM   MG   1273.00   1.50     25   YYYYYYYYYYYIYYYYY
PROTEIN     G      7.00   0.82     14   PPPPPPPPPP
CARBOHYDT   G     86.00   1.84     31   HHHHHHHHHHHHHIHHHHHHHHH
FAT         G      1.00   0.08      1   F
OLEIC A     G      0.00   0.00      0   -
LINOL A     G      0.00   0.00      0   -
SAT FAT A   G      0.00   0.00      0   -
*******************************************
```

231 APRICOTS, DRIED, COOKED, UNSWEETENED
ANALYSIS OF 250 GRAMS WHICH IS 1 CUP—FRUIT AND LIQUID

NUTRIENT	UNIT	AMOUNT	INQ	% STD
ENERGY	KCAL	215.00	1.00	11
VITAMIN A	IU	7500.00	17.44	188
VITAMIN C	MG	8.00	1.24	13
THIAMIN	MG	0.01	0.09	1
RIBOFLAVN	MG	0.13	1.01	11
NIACIN	MG	2.50	1.66	18
IRON	MG	4.50	2.62	28
CALCIUM	MG	55.00	0.57	6
PHOSPHRUS	MG	88.00	0.91	10
POTASSIUM	MG	795.00	1.48	16
PROTEIN	G	4.00	0.74	8
CARBOHYDT	G	54.00	1.83	20
FAT	G	1.00	0.12	1
OLEIC A	G	0.00	0.00	0
LINOL A	G	0.00	0.00	0
SAT FAT A	G	0.00	0.00	0

232 APRICOT NECTAR, CANNED
ANALYSIS OF 251 GRAMS WHICH IS 1 CUP

NUTRIENT	UNIT	AMOUNT	INQ	% STD
ENERGY	KCAL	145.00	1.00	7
VITAMIN A	IU	2380.00	8.21	59
VITAMIN C	MG	36.00	8.28	60
THIAMIN	MG	0.03	0.41	3
RIBOFLAVN	MG	0.03	0.34	3
NIACIN	MG	0.50	0.49	4
IRON	MG	0.50	0.43	3
CALCIUM	MG	23.00	0.35	3
PHOSPHRUS	MG	30.00	0.46	3
POTASSIUM	MG	379.00	1.05	8
PROTEIN	G	1.00	0.28	2
CARBOHYDT	G	37.00	1.86	13
FAT	G	0.00	0.00	0
OLEIC A	G	0.00	0.00	0
LINOL A	G	0.00	0.00	0
SAT FAT A	G	-	0.00	0.00	0

233 AVOCADOS, RAW, CALIFORNIA, WT. WITHOUT SKIN AND SEED
ANALYSIS OF 216 GRAMS WHICH IS 1--3 1/8-IN DIAM.

```
                                        0      10      20      30      40      50      60      70      80      90      100
NUTRIENT   UNIT   AMOUNT   INQ   % STD
ENERGY     KCAL   370.00   1.00   19   EEEEEEEEEEEEE
VITAMIN A  IU     630.00   0.85   16   AAAAAAAAAA |
VITAMIN C  MG     30.00    2.70   50   CCCCCCCCCCC|CCCCCCCCCCCCCCCCCCCCCCCCCC
THIAMIN    MG     0.24     1.30   24   TTTTTTTTTTTT|TTTTT
RIBOFLAVN  MG     0.43     1.94   36   RRRRRRRRRRRR|RRRRRRRRRRRRR
NIACIN     MG     3.50     1.35   25   NNNNNNNNNNNN|NNNNN
IRON       MG     1.30     0.44    8   IIIIIII
CALCIUM    MG     22.00    0.13    2   KK
PHOSPHRUS  MG     91.00    0.55   10   XXXXXXX
POTASSIUM  MG     1303.00  1.41   26   YYYYYYYYYYYY|YYYYY
PROTEIN    G      5.00     0.54   10   PPPPPPP
CARBOHYDT  G      13.00    0.26    5   HHH
FAT        G      37.00    2.56   47   FFFFFFFFFFFFF|FFFFFFFFFFFFFFFFFFFFFFFF
OLEIC A    G      22.00    4.85   90   OOOOOOOOOOOOO|OOOOOOOOOOOOOOOOOOOOOOOOOOOOOOOOOOOOOOOOOOOOOOOOOOOOOOOOOOOOOOOOOOOOOO
LINOL A    G      3.70     1.00   19   LLLLLLLLLLLLL
SAT FAT A  G      5.50     1.04   19   SSSSSSSSSSSSS
                                       **********
```

234 AVOCADOS, RAW, FLORIDA, WT. WITHOUT SKIN AND SEED
ANALYSIS OF 304 GRAMS WHICH IS 1--3 5/8-IN DIAM.

```
                                        0      10      20      30      40      50      60      70      80      90      100
NUTRIENT   UNIT   AMOUNT   INQ   % STD
ENERGY     KCAL   390.00   1.00   20   EEEEEEEEEEEEE
VITAMIN A  IU     880.00   1.13   22   AAAAAAAAAAAAA|AA
VITAMIN C  MG     43.00    3.68   72   CCCCCCCCCCC|CCCCCCCCCCCCCCCCCCCCCCCCCCCCCCCCCCCCCCCCCCCCCCCCC
THIAMIN    MG     0.33     1.69   33   TTTTTTTTTTTT|TTTTTTTTT
RIBOFLAVN  MG     0.61     2.61   51   RRRRRRRRRRRR|RRRRRRRRRRRRRRRRRRRRRRRRR
NIACIN     MG     4.90     1.79   35   NNNNNNNNNNNN|NNNNNNNNNNN
IRON       MG     1.80     0.58   11   IIIIIIIII
CALCIUM    MG     30.00    0.17    3   KKK
PHOSPHRUS  MG     128.00   0.73   14   XXXXXXXXXXX
POTASSIUM  MG     1836.00  1.88   37   YYYYYYYYYYYY|YYYYYYYYYYYYY
PROTEIN    G      4.00     0.41    8   PPPPPP
CARBOHYDT  G      27.00    0.50   10   HHHHHHHH
FAT        G      33.00    2.17   42   FFFFFFFFFFFFF|FFFFFFFFFFFFFFFFFFFFF
OLEIC A    G      15.70    3.29   64   OOOOOOOOOOOOO|OOOOOOOOOOOOOOOOOOOOOOOOOOOOOOOOOOOOOOOOOOOOOOO
LINOL A    G      5.30     1.36   27   LLLLLLLLLLLL|LLLL
SAT FAT A  G      6.70     1.21   24   SSSSSSSSSSSS|SSS
                                       **********
```

235 BANANA, RAW, WITHOUT PEEL
ANALYSIS OF 119 GRAMS WHICH IS 1--2.6 PER LB WITH PEEL

NUTRIENT	UNIT	AMOUNT	INQ	% STD	Chart (0 — 100)
ENERGY	KCAL	100.00	1.00	5	EEEE
VITAMIN A	IU	230.00	1.15	6	AAA|A
VITAMIN C	MG	12.00	4.00	20	CCC|CCCCCCCCCC
THIAMIN	MG	0.06	1.20	6	TTT|T
RIBOFLAVN	MG	0.07	1.17	6	RRR|R
NIACIN	MG	0.80	1.14	6	NNN|N
IRON	MG	0.80	1.00	5	III|I
CALCIUM	MG	10.00	0.22	1	K|
PHOSPHRUS	MG	31.00	0.69	3	XXX|
POTASSIUM	MG	440.00	1.76	9	YYY|YYY
PROTEIN	G	1.00	0.40	2	PP|
CARBOHYDT	G	26.00	1.89	9	HHH|HHHH
FAT	G	0.00	0.00	0	|
OLEIC A	G	0.00	0.00	0	|
LINOL A	G	0.00	0.00	0	|
SAT FAT A	G	0.00	0.00	0	|

236 BANANA FLAKES
ANALYSIS OF 6 GRAMS WHICH IS 1 TBSB

NUTRIENT	UNIT	AMOUNT	INQ	% STD	Chart (0 — 100)
ENERGY	KCAL	20.00	1.00	1	E
VITAMIN A	IU	50.00	1.25	1	A
VITAMIN C	MG	0.00	0.00	0	|
THIAMIN	MG	0.01	1.00	1	T
RIBOFLAVN	MG	0.01	0.83	1	R
NIACIN	MG	0.20	1.43	1	N
IRON	MG	0.20	1.25	1	I
CALCIUM	MG	2.00	0.22	0	X
PHOSPHRUS	MG	6.00	0.67	1	Y
POTASSIUM	MG	92.00	1.84	2	H
PROTEIN	G	0.00	0.00	0	|
CARBOHYDT	G	5.00	1.82	2	H
FAT	G	0.00	0.00	0	|
OLEIC A	G	0.00	0.00	0	|
LINOL A	G	0.00	0.00	0	|
SAT FAT A	G	0.00	0.00	0	|

237 BLACKBERRIES, RAW
ANALYSIS OF 144 GRAMS WHICH IS 1 CUP

NUTRIENT	UNIT	AMOUNT	INQ	% STD	0 · · 10 · · 20 · · 30 · · 40 · · 50 · · 60 · · 70 · · 80 · · 90 · · 100
ENERGY	KCAL	85.00	1.00	4	EEE
VITAMIN A	IU	290.00	1.71	7	AA│AAA
VITAMIN C	MG	30.00	11.76	50	CC│CCCCCCCCCCCCCCCCCCCCCCCCCCCC
THIAMIN	MG	0.04	0.94	4	TTT
RIBOFLAVN	MG	0.06	1.18	5	RR│R
NIACIN	MG	0.60	1.01	4	NNN
IRON	MG	1.30	1.91	8	II│IIII
CALCIUM	MG	46.00	1.20	5	KK│K
PHOSPHRUS	MG	27.00	0.71	3	XX│
POTASSIUM	MG	245.00	1.15	5	YY│Y
PROTEIN	G	2.00	0.94	4	PPP
CARBOHYDT	G	19.00	1.63	7	HH│HHH
FAT	G	1.00	0.30	1	F│
OLEIC A	G	0.00	0.00	0	─
LINOL A	G	0.00	0.00	0	─
SAT FAT A	G	0.00	0.00	0	─

238 BLUEBERRIES, RAW
ANALYSIS OF 145 GRAMS WHICH IS 1 CUP

NUTRIENT	UNIT	AMOUNT	INQ	% STD	0 · · 10 · · 20 · · 30 · · 40 · · 50 · · 60 · · 70 · · 80 · · 90 · · 100
ENERGY	KCAL	90.00	1.00	5	EEEE
VITAMIN A	IU	150.00	0.83	4	AAA│
VITAMIN C	MG	20.00	7.41	33	CCC│CCCCCCCCCCCCCCCCCC
THIAMIN	MG	0.04	0.89	4	TTT│
RIBO LAVN	MG	0.09	1.67	8	RRR│RR
NIACIN	MG	0.70	1.11	5	NNNN
IRON	MG	1.50	2.08	9	III│IIII
CALCIUM	MG	22.00	0.54	2	KK│
PHOSPHRUS	MG	19.00	0.47	2	XX│
POTASSIUM	MG	117.00	0.52	2	YY│
PROTEIN	G	1.00	0.44	2	PP│
CARBOHYDT	G	22.00	1.78	8	HHH│HH
FAT	G	1.00	0.28	1	F│
OLEIC A	G	0.00	0.00	0	─
LINOL A	G	0.00	0.00	0	─
SAT FAT A	G	0.00	0.00	0	─

239 CHERRIES, SOUR, RED, PITTED, CANNED, WATER PACK
ANALYSIS OF 244 GRAMS WHICH IS 1 CUP

NUTRIENT	UNIT	AMOUNT	INQ	% STD	0 10 20 30 40 50 60 70 80 90 100
ENERGY	KCAL	105.00	1.00	5	EEEE
VITAMIN A	IU	1660.00	7.90	42	AAA AAAAAAAAAAAAAAAAAAAA
VITAMIN C	MG	12.00	3.81	20	CCC CCCCCCCCCC
THIAMIN	MG	0.07	1.33	7	TTT TT
RIBOFLAVN	MG	0.05	0.79	4	RRR I
NIACIN	MG	0.50	0.68	4	NNN I
IRON	MG	0.70	0.83	4	III I
CALCIUM	MG	37.00	0.78	4	KKK I
PHOSPHRUS	MG	32.00	0.68	4	XXX I
POTASSIUM	MG	317.00	1.21	6	YYY I
PROTEIN	G	2.00	0.76	4	PPP I
CARBOHYDT	G	26.00	1.80	9	HHH HHHH
FAT	G	0.00	0.00	0	—
OLEIC A	G	0.00	0.00	0	I
LINOL A	G	0.00	0.00	0	I
SAT FAT A	G	0.00	0.00	0	—

240 CHERRIES, SWEET, RAW, WITHOUT PITS AND STEMS
ANALYSIS OF 68 GRAMS WHICH IS 10 CHERRIES

NUTRIENT	UNIT	AMOUNT	INQ	% STD	0 10 20 30 40 50 60 70 80 90 100
ENERGY	KCAL	45.00	1.00	2	EE
VITAMIN A	IU	70.00	0.78	2	AI
VITAMIN C	MG	7.00	5.19	12	CICCCCCCC
THIAMIN	MG	0.03	0.78	2	TT
RIBOFLAVN	MG	0.04	1.33	3	RIR
NIACIN	MG	0.30	0.95	2	NN
IRON	MG	0.30	0.83	2	II
CALCIUM	MG	15.00	0.74	1	KI
PHOSPHRUS	MG	13.00	0.64	1	XI
POTASSIUM	MG	129.00	1.15	3	YY
PROTEIN	G	1.00	0.89	2	PP
CARBOHYDT	G	12.00	1.94	4	HIH
FAT	G	0.00	0.00	0	—I
OLEIC A	G	0.00	0.00	0	—I
LINOL A	G	0.00	0.00	0	—I
SAT FAT A	G	0.00	0.00	0	—I

241 CRANBERRY JUICE COCKTAIL, BOTTLED, SWEETENED
ANALYSIS OF 253 GRAMS WHICH IS 1 CUP

NUTRIENT	UNIT	AMOUNT	INQ	% STD
ENERGY	KCAL	165.00	1.00	8
VITAMIN A	IU	0.00	0.00	0
VITAMIN C	MG	81.00	16.36	135
THIAMIN	MG	0.03	0.36	3
RIBOFLAVN	MG	0.03	0.30	3
NIACIN	MG	0.10	0.09	1
IRON	MG	0.80	0.61	5
CALCIUM	MG	13.00	0.18	1
PHOSPHRUS	MG	8.00	0.11	1
POTASSIUM	MG	25.00	0.06	1
PROTEIN	G	0.00	0.00	0
CARBOHYDT	G	42.00	1.85	15
FAT	G	0.00	0.00	0
OLEIC A	G	0.00	0.00	0
LINOL A	G	0.00	0.00	0
SAT FAT A	G	0.00	0.00	0

242 CRANBERRY SAUCE, SWEETENED, CANNED, STRAINED
ANALYSIS OF 277 GRAMS WHICH IS 1 CUP

NUTRIENT	UNIT	AMOUNT	INQ	% STD
ENERGY	KCAL	405.00	1.00	20
VITAMIN A	IU	60.00	0.07	2
VITAMIN C	MG	6.00	0.49	10
THIAMIN	MG	0.03	0.15	3
RIBOFLAVN	MG	0.03	0.12	3
NIACIN	MG	0.10	0.04	1
IRON	MG	0.60	0.19	4
CALCIUM	MG	17.00	0.09	2
PHOSPHRUS	MG	11.00	0.06	1
POTASSIUM	MG	83.00	0.08	2
PROTEIN	G	0.00	0.00	0
CARBOHYDT	G	104.00	1.87	38
FAT	G	1.00	0.06	1
OLEIC A	G	0.00	0.00	0
LINOL A	G	0.00	0.00	0
SAT FAT A	G	0.00	0.00	0

243 DATES, WHOLE, WITHOUT PITS
ANALYSIS OF 80 GRAMS WHICH IS 10 DATES

NUTRIENT	UNIT	AMOUNT	INQ	% STD	
ENERGY	KCAL	220.00	1.00	11	EEEEEEEE
VITAMIN A	IU	40.00	0.09	1	A
VITAMIN C	MG	0.00	0.00	0	-
THIAMIN	MG	0.07	0.64	7	TTTTT
RIBOFLAVN	MG	0.08	0.61	7	RRRRR
NIACIN	MG	1.80	1.17	13	NNNNNNNN N
IRON	MG	2.40	1.36	15	IIIIIIIIIII
CALCIUM	MG	47.00	0.47	5	KKKK
PHOSPHRUS	MG	50.00	0.51	6	XXXX
POTASSIUM	MG	518.00	0.94	10	YYYYYYY
PROTEIN	G	2.00	0.36	4	PPP
CARBOHYDT	G	58.00	1.92	21	HHHHHHH HHHHHHHH
FAT	G	0.00	0.00	0	-
OLEIC A	G	0.00	0.00	0	-
LINOL A	G	0.00	0.00	0	-
SAT FAT A	G	0.00	0.00	0	-

244 DATES, CHOPPED
ANALYSIS OF 178 GRAMS WHICH IS 1 CUP

NUTRIENT	UNIT	AMOUNT	INQ	% STD	
ENERGY	KCAL	490.00	1.00	25	EEEEEEEEEEEEEEEEEE
VITAMIN A	IU	90.00	0.09	2	AA
VITAMIN C	MG	0.00	0.00	0	-
THIAMIN	MG	0.16	0.65	16	TTTTTTTTTTT
RIBOFLAVN	MG	0.18	0.61	15	RRRRRRRRRR
NIACIN	MG	3.90	1.14	28	NNNNNNNNNNNNNNNNNNN NN
IRON	MG	5.30	1.35	33	IIIIIIIIIIIIIIIIIIIIIII
CALCIUM	MG	105.00	0.48	12	KKKKKKKK
PHOSPHRUS	MG	112.00	0.51	12	XXXXXXXXX
POTASSIUM	MG	1153.00	0.94	23	YYYYYYYYYYYYYYYYY
PROTEIN	G	4.00	0.33	8	PPPPP
CARBOHYDT	G	130.00	1.93	47	HHHHHHHHHHHHHHHHHH HHHHHHHHHHHHHHHHHH
FAT	G	1.00	0.05	1	F
OLEIC A	G	0.00	0.00	0	-
LINOL A	G	0.00	0.00	0	-
SAT FAT A	G	0.00	0.00	0	-

245 FRUIT COCKTAIL CANNED IN HEAVY SYRUP
ANALYSIS OF 255 GRAMS WHICH IS 1 CUP

```
                                    0   10   20   30   40   50   60   70   80   90  100
                                                                                     ***************
NUTRIENT   UNIT   AMOUNT   INQ  % STD
ENERGY     KCAL   195.00   1.00   10   EEEEEEE
VITAMIN A  IU     360.00   0.92    9   AAAAAAA|
VITAMIN C  MG       5.00   0.85    8   CCCCCCC|
THIAMIN    MG       0.05   0.51    5   TTT|
RIBOFLAVN  MG       0.03   0.26    3   RR|
NIACIN     MG       1.00   0.73    7   NNNNNN|
IRON       MG       1.00   0.64    6   IIIII|
CALCIUM    MG      23.00   0.26    3   KK|
PHOSPHRUS  MG      31.00   0.35    3   XXX|
POTASSIUM  MG     411.00   0.84    8   YYYYYY|
PROTEIN    G        1.00   0.21    2   PP|
CARBOHYDT  G       50.00   1.86   18   HHHHHH|HHHHHHH
FAT        G        0.00   0.00    0   -|
OLEIC A    G        0.00   0.00    0   -|
LINOL A    G        0.00   0.00    0   -|
SAT FAT A  G        0.00   0.00    0   -|
************************************************************
```

246 GRAPEFRUIT, RAW, PINK OR RED, WT WITHOUT PEEL AND MEMBRANES
ANALYSIS OF 123 GRAMS WHICH IS 1/2 MEDIUM (3 3/4-IN DIAM.) GRAPEFRUIT

```
                                    0   10   20   30   40   50   60   70   80   90  100
                                                                                     ***************
NUTRIENT   UNIT   AMOUNT   INQ  % STD
ENERGY     KCAL    50.00   1.00    3   EE
VITAMIN A  IU     540.00   5.40   14   AIAAAAAAAA
VITAMIN C  MG      44.00  29.33   73   CICCCCCCCCCCCCCCCCCCCCCCCCCCCCCCCCCCCCCCCCCCCCCCCCCCCCCCCCCCCCCC
THIAMIN    MG       0.05   2.00    5   TITT
RIBOFLAVN  MG       0.02   0.67    2   RI
NIACIN     MG       0.20   0.57    1   NI
IRON       MG       0.50   1.25    3   III
CALCIUM    MG      20.00   0.89    2   KK
PHOSPHRUS  MG      20.00   0.89    2   XX
POTASSIUM  MG     166.00   1.33    3   YIY
PROTEIN    G        1.00   0.80    2   PP
CARBOHYDT  G       13.00   1.89    5   HIHH
FAT        G        0.00   0.00    0   -I
OLEIC A    G        0.00   0.00    0   -I
LINOL A    G        0.00   0.00    0   -I
SAT FAT A  G        0.00   0.00    0   -I
*******************************************************************
```

247 GRAPEFRUIT, RAW, WHITE, WT WITHOUT PEEL AND MEMBRANES
ANALYSIS OF 118 GRAMS WHICH IS 1/2 MEDIUM (3 3/4-IN DIAM.) GRAPEFRUIT

NUTRIENT	UNIT	AMOUNT	INQ	% STD	0 10 20 30 40 50 60 70 80 90 100
ENERGY	KCAL	45.00	1.00	2	EE
VITAMIN A	IU	10.00	0.11	0	—
VITAMIN C	MG	44.00	32.59	73	C|CCCCCCCCCCCCCCCCCCCCCCCCCCCCCCCCCCCCC
THIAMIN	MG	0.05	2.22	5	T|TT
RIBOFLAVN	MG	0.02	0.74	1	R|
NIACIN	MG	0.20	0.63	1	N|
IRON	MG	0.50	1.39	3	I|I
CALCIUM	MG	19.00	0.94	2	K|K
PHOSPHRUS	MG	19.00	0.94	2	X|X
POTASSIUM	MG	159.00	1.41	3	Y|IY
PROTEIN	G	1.00	0.89	2	P|P
CARBOHYDT	G	12.00	1.94	4	H|IH
FAT	G	0.00	0.00	0	—|
OLEIC A	G	0.00	0.00	0	—|
LINOL A	G	0.00	0.00	0	—|
SAT FAT A	G	0.00	0.00	0	—|

248 GRAPEFRUIT, CANNED, SECTIONS WITH SIRUP
ANALYSIS OF 254 GRAMS WHICH IS 1 CUP

NUTRIENT	UNIT	AMOUNT	INQ	% STD	0 10 20 30 40 50 60 70 80 90 100
ENERGY	KCAL	180.00	1.00	9	EEEEEE
VITAMIN A	IU	30.00	0.08	1	A
VITAMIN C	MG	76.00	14.07	127	CCCCC|CCCCCCCCCCCCCCCCCCCCCCCCCCCCCCCCCCCCCCCCCCCCCCCCCCCCCCCCCCCCCCC * 127
THIAMIN	MG	0.08	0.89	8	TTTTT|
RIBOFLAVN	MG	0.05	0.46	4	RRR|
NIACIN	MG	0.50	0.40	4	NNN|
IRON	MG	0.80	0.56	5	IIII|
CALCIUM	MG	33.00	0.41	4	KKK|
PHOSPHRUS	MG	36.00	0.44	4	XXX|
POTASSIUM	MG	343.00	0.76	7	YYYY|
PROTEIN	G	2.00	0.44	4	PPP|
CARBOHYDT	G	45.00	1.82	16	HHHHHH|IHHHHHH
FAT	G	0.00	0.00	0	—|
OLEIC A	G	0.00	0.00	0	—|
LINOL A	G	0.00	0.00	0	—|
SAT FAT A	G	0.00	0.00	0	—|

249 GRAPEFRUIT JUICE, RAW
ANALYSIS OF 246 GRAMS WHICH IS 1 CUP

NUTRIENT	UNIT	AMOUNT	INQ	% STD	
ENERGY	KCAL	95.00	1.00	5	EEEE
VITAMIN A	IU	0.00	0.00	0	-
VITAMIN C	MG	93.00	32.63	155	CCCCCCCCCCCCCCCCCCCCCCCCCCCCCCCCCCCCCCCCCCCCCCCCCCCCCCCCCCCCCCCCCCCCCCCCCCCCCCCCCCCCCCCC * 155
THIAMIN	MG	0.10	2.11	10	TTT|TTT
RIBOFLAVN	MG	0.05	0.88	4	RRR|
NIACIN	MG	0.50	0.75	4	NNN|
IRON	MG	0.50	0.66	3	III|
CALCIUM	MG	22.00	0.51	2	KK|
PHOSPHRUS	MG	37.00	0.87	4	XXX|
POTASSIUM	MG	399.00	1.68	8	YYY|YY
PROTEIN	G	1.00	0.42	2	PP|
CARBOHYDT	G	23.00	1.76	0	HHH|HHH
FAT	G	0.00	0.00	0	-|
OLEIC A	G	0.00	0.00	0	-|
LINOL A	G	0.00	0.00	0	-|
SAT FAT A	G	0.00	0.00	0	-

0 10 20 30 40 50 60 70 80 90 100

250 GRAPEFRUIT JUICE, CANNED, UNSWEETENED
ANALYSIS OF 247 GRAMS WHICH IS 1 CUP

NUTRIENT	UNIT	AMOUNT	INQ	% STD	
ENERGY	KCAL	100.00	1.00	5	EEEE
VITAMIN A	IU	20.00	0.10	1	EEEE
VITAMIN C	MG	84.00	28.00	140	CCCCCCCCCCCCCCCCCCCCCCCCCCCCCCCCCCCCCCCCCCCCCCCCCCCCCCCCCCCCCCCCCCCCCCCCCCCCCCCCCCCCC * 140
THIAMIN	MG	0.07	1.40	7	TTT|TT
RIBOFLAVN	MG	0.05	0.83	4	RRR|
NIACIN	MG	0.50	0.71	4	NNN|
IRON	MG	1.00	1.25	6	III|I
CALCIUM	MG	20.00	0.44	2	KK|
PHOSPHRUS	MG	35.00	0.78	4	XXX|
POTASSIUM	MG	400.00	1.60	8	YYY|YY
PROTEIN	G	1.00	0.40	2	PP|
CARBOHYDT	G	24.00	1.75	9	HHH|HHH
FAT	G	0.00	0.00	0	-|
OLEIC A	G	0.00	0.00	0	-|
LINOL A	G	0.00	0.00	0	-|
SAT FAT A	G	0.00	0.00	0	-

0 10 20 30 40 50 60 70 80 90 100

251 GRAPEFRUIT JUICE, CANNED, SWEETENED
ANALYSIS OF 250 GRAMS WHICH IS 1 CUP

NUTRIENT	UNIT	AMOUNT	INQ	% STD
ENERGY	KCAL	135.00	1.00	7
VITAMIN A	IU	30.00	0.11	1
VITAMIN C	MG	78.00	19.26	130
THIAMIN	MG	0.08	1.19	8
RIBOFLAVN	MG	0.05	0.62	4
NIACIN	MG	0.50	0.53	4
IRON	MG	1.00	0.93	6
CALCIUM	MG	20.00	0.33	2
PHOSPHRUS	MG	35.00	0.58	4
POTASSIUM	MG	405.00	1.20	8
PROTEIN	G	1.00	0.30	2
CARBOHYDT	G	32.00	1.72	12
FAT	G	0.00	0.00	0
OLEIC A	G	0.00	0.00	0
LINOL A	G	0.00	0.00	0
SAT FAT A	G	0.00	0.00	0

252 GRAPEFRUIT JUICE, FROZEN, CONCENTRATED, UNSWEETENED, UNDILUTED
ANALYSIS OF 207 GRAMS WHICH IS 1--6-FL OZ CAN

NUTRIENT	UNIT	AMOUNT	INQ	% STD
ENERGY	KCAL	300.00	1.00	15
VITAMIN A	IU	60.00	0.10	2
VITAMIN C	MG	286.00	31.78	477
THIAMIN	MG	0.29	1.93	29
RIBOFLAVN	MG	0.12	0.67	10
NIACIN	MG	1.40	0.67	10
IRON	MG	0.80	0.33	5
CALCIUM	MG	70.00	0.52	8
PHOSPHRUS	MG	124.00	0.92	14
POTASSIUM	MG	1250.00	1.67	25
PROTEIN	G	4.00	0.53	8
CARBOHYDT	G	72.00	1.75	26
FAT	G	1.00	0.09	1
OLEIC A	G	0.00	0.00	0
LINOL A	G	0.00	0.00	0
SAT FAT A	G	0.00	0.00	0

253 GRAPEFRUIT JUICE, FROZEN, CONCENTRATE, UNSWEETENED, DILUTED
ANALYSIS OF 247 GRAMS WHICH IS 1 CUP

NUTRIENT	UNIT	AMOUNT	INQ	% STD	0	10	20	30	40	50	60	70	80	90	100	
ENERGY	KCAL	100.00	1.00	5	EEEE											
VITAMIN A	IU	20.00	0.10	1	-											
VITAMIN C	MG	96.00	32.00	160	CCC|CCCCCCCCCCCCCCCCCCCCCCCCCCCCCCCCCCCCCCCCCCCCCCCCCCCCCCCCCCCCCCCCCCCCCCCCCCCCCCCC										* 160
THIAMIN	MG	0.10	2.00	10	TTT|TTTT											
RIBOFLAVN	MG	0.04	0.67	3	RRR|											
NIACIN	MG	0.50	0.71	4	NNN|											
IRON	MG	0.20	0.25	1	I |											
CALCIUM	MG	25.00	0.56	3	KK |											
PHOSPHRUS	MG	42.00	0.93	5	XXXX											
POTASSIUM	MG	420.00	1.68	8	YYY|YYY											
PROTEIN	G	1.00	0.40	2	PP |											
CARBOHYDT	G	24.00	1.75	9	HHH|HHH											
FAT	G	0.00	0.00	0	- |											
OLEIC A	G	0.00	0.00	0	- |											
LINOL A	G	0.00	0.00	0	- |											
SAT FAT A	G	0.00	0.00	0	-											

254 GRAPEFRUIT JUICE, DEHYDRATED CRYSTALS, PREPARED WITH WATER
ANALYSIS OF 247 GRAMS WHICH IS 1 CUP

NUTRIENT	UNIT	AMOUNT	INQ	% STD	0	10	20	30	40	50	60	70	80	90	100	
ENERGY	KCAL	100.00	1.00	5	EEEE											
VITAMIN A	IU	20.00	0.10	1	-											
VITAMIN C	MG	91.00	30.33	152	CCC|CCCCCCCCCCCCCCCCCCCCCCCCCCCCCCCCCCCCCCCCCCCCCCCCCCCCCCCCCCCCCCCCCCCCCCCCCCCC										* 152
THIAMIN	MG	0.10	2.00	10	TTT|TTTT											
RIBOFLAVN	MG	0.05	0.83	4	RRR|											
NIACIN	MG	0.50	0.71	4	NNN|											
IRON	MG	0.20	0.25	1	I |											
CALCIUM	MG	22.00	0.49	2	KK |											
PHOSPHRUS	MG	40.00	0.89	4	XXXX											
POTASSIUM	MG	412.00	1.65	8	YYY|YYY											
PROTEIN	G	1.00	0.40	2	PP |											
CARBOHYDT	G	24.00	1.75	9	HHH|HHH											
FAT	G	0.00	0.00	0	- |											
OLEIC A	G	0.00	0.00	0	- |											
LINOL A	G	0.00	0.00	0	- |											
SAT FAT A	G	0.00	0.00	0	-											

255 GRAPES, THOMPSON SEEDLESS
ANALYSIS OF 50 GRAMS WHICH IS 10 GRAPES

NUTRIENT	UNIT	AMOUNT	INQ	% STD	0
ENERGY	KCAL	35.00	1.00	2	E
VITAMIN A	IU	50.00	0.71	1	A
VITAMIN C	MG	2.00	1.90	3	CC
THIAMIN	MG	0.03	1.71	3	IT
RIBOFLAVN	MG	0.02	0.95	2	R
NIACIN	MG	0.20	0.82	1	N
IRON	MG	0.20	0.71	1	I
CALCIUM	MG	6.00	0.38	1	X
PHOSPHRUS	MG	10.00	0.63	1	Y
POTASSIUM	MG	87.00	0.99	2	-
PROTEIN	G	0.00	0.00	0	I
CARBOHYDT	G	9.00	1.87	3	HH
FAT	G	0.00	0.00	0	-
OLEIC A	G	0.00	0.00	0	-
LINOL A	G	0.00	0.00	0	-
SAT FAT A	G	0.00	0.00	0	-

256 GRAPES, TOKAY AND EMPEROR, WITH SEEDS
ANALYSIS OF 60 GRAMS WHICH IS 10 GRAPES

NUTRIENT	UNIT	AMOUNT	INQ	% STD	0
ENERGY	KCAL	40.00	1.00	2	EE
VITAMIN A	IU	60.00	0.75	2	AI
VITAMIN C	MG	2.00	1.67	3	CIC
THIAMIN	MG	0.03	1.50	3	TT
RIBOFLAVN	MG	0.02	0.83	2	RI
NIACIN	MG	0.20	0.71	1	NI
IRON	MG	0.20	0.63	1	II
CALCIUM	MG	7.00	0.39	1	KI
PHOSPHRUS	MG	11.00	0.61	1	XI
POTASSIUM	MG	99.00	0.99	2	YY
PROTEIN	G	0.00	0.00	0	-I
CARBOHYDT	G	10.00	1.82	4	HIH
FAT	G	0.00	0.00	0	-I
OLEIC A	G	0.00	0.00	0	-I
LINOL A	G	0.00	0.00	0	-I
SAT FAT A	G	0.00	0.00	0	-I

257 GRAPEJUICE, CANNED OR BOTTLED
ANALYSIS OF 253 GRAMS WHICH IS 1 CUP

NUTRIENT	UNIT	AMOUNT	INQ	% STD	PROFILE (0–100)
ENERGY	KCAL	165.00	1.00	8	EEEEEE
VITAMIN A	IU	0.00	0.00	0	-
VITAMIN C	MG	0.10	1.21	10	TTTTTTTT
THIAMIN	MG	0.05	0.51	4	RRR
RIBOFLAVN	MG	0.05	0.43	4	NNN
NIACIN	MG	0.50	0.61	5	IIII
IRON	MG	0.80	0.38	3	KK
CALCIUM	MG	28.00	0.40	3	XXX
PHOSPHRUS	MG	30.00	0.71	6	YYYY
POTASSIUM	MG	293.00	0.24	2	PP
PROTEIN	G	1.00	1.85	15	HHHHHH HHHHH
CARBOHYDT	G	42.00	0.00	0	-
FAT	G	0.00	0.00	0	-
OLEIC A	G	0.00	0.00	0	-
LINOL A	G	0.00	0.00	0	-
SAT FAT A	G	0.00	0.00	0	-

258 GRAPEJUICE, FROZEN CONCENTRATE, SWEETENED, UNDILUTED
ANALYSIS OF 216 GRAMS WHICH IS 1--6FL OZ CAN

NUTRIENT	UNIT	AMOUNT	INQ	% STD	PROFILE (0–100)
ENERGY	KCAL	395.00	1.00	20	EEEEEEEEEEEEE
VITAMIN A	IU	40.00	0.05	1	A
VITAMIN C	MG	32.00	2.70	53	CCCCCCCCCCCCCCCCCCCCCCCCCCCC
THIAMIN	MG	0.13	0.66	13	TTTTTTTTTTT
RIBOFLAVN	MG	0.22	0.93	18	RRRRRRRRRR
NIACIN	MG	1.50	0.54	11	NNNNNNNNN
IRON	MG	0.90	0.28	6	IIIII
CALCIUM	MG	22.00	0.12	2	KK
PHOSPHRUS	MG	32.00	0.18	4	XXX
POTASSIUM	MG	255.00	0.26	5	YYYY
PROTEIN	G	1.00	0.10	2	PP
CARBOHYDT	G	100.00	1.84	36	HHHHHHHHHHHHHHHHH HHHHHHHHHHHHH
FAT	G	0.00	0.00	0	-
OLEIC A	G	0.00	0.00	0	-
LINOL A	G	0.00	0.00	0	-
SAT FAT A	G	0.00	0.00	0	-

259 GRAPEJUICE, FROZEN CONCENTRATE, SWEETENED, DILUTED
ANALYSIS OF 250 GRAMS WHICH IS 1 CUP

NUTRIENT	UNIT	AMOUNT	INQ	% STD
ENERGY	KCAL	135.00	1.00	7
VITAMIN A	IU	10.00	0.04	0
VITAMIN C	MG	10.00	2.47	17
THIAMIN	MG	0.05	0.74	5
RIBOFLAVN	MG	0.08	0.99	7
NIACIN	MG	0.50	0.53	4
IRON	MG	0.30	0.28	2
CALCIUM	MG	8.00	0.13	1
PHOSPHRUS	MG	10.00	0.16	1
POTASSIUM	MG	85.00	0.25	2
PROTEIN	G	1.00	0.30	2
CARBOHYDT	G	33.00	1.78	12
FAT	G	0.00	0.00	0
OLEIC A	G	0.00	0.00	0
LINOL A	G	0.00	0.00	0
SAT FAT A	G	0.00	0.00	0

260 GRAPE DRINK CANNED
ANALYSIS OF 250 GRAMS WHICH IS 1 CUP

NUTRIENT	UNIT	AMOUNT	INQ	% STD
ENERGY	KCAL	135.00	1.00	7
VITAMIN A	IU	0.00	0.00	0
VITAMIN C	MG	0.00	0.00	0
THIAMIN	MG	0.03	0.44	3
RIBOFLAVN	MG	0.03	0.37	3
NIACIN	MG	0.30	0.32	2
IRON	MG	0.30	0.28	2
CALCIUM	MG	8.00	0.13	1
PHOSPHRUS	MG	10.00	0.16	1
POTASSIUM	MG	88.00	0.26	2
PROTEIN	G	0.00	0.00	0
CARBOHYDT	G	35.00	1.89	13
FAT	G	0.00	0.00	0
OLEIC A	G	0.00	0.00	0
LINOL A	G	0.00	0.00	0
SAT FAT A	G	0.00	0.00	0

261 LEMON, RAW, WT WITHOUT PEEL AND SEEDS
ANALYSIS OF 74 GRAMS WHICH IS 1 LEMON (ABOUT 4 PER LB WITH PEEL AND SEEDS)

NUTRIENT	UNIT	AMOUNT	INQ	% STD
ENERGY	KCAL	20.00	1.00	1
VITAMIN A	IU	10.00	0.25	0
VITAMIN C	MG	39.00	65.00	65
THIAMIN	MG	0.03	3.00	3
RIBOFLAVN	MG	0.01	0.83	1
NIACIN	MG	0.10	0.71	1
IRON	MG	0.40	2.50	3
CALCIUM	MG	19.00	2.11	2
PHOSPHRUS	MG	12.00	1.33	1
POTASSIUM	MG	102.00	2.04	2
PROTEIN	G	1.00	2.00	2
CARBOHYDT	G	6.00	2.18	2
FAT	G	0.00	0.00	0
OLEIC A	G	0.00	0.00	0
LINOL A	G	0.00	0.00	0
SAT FAT A	G	0.00	0.00	0

262 LEMON JUICE, RAW
ANALYSIS OF 244 GRAMS WHICH IS 1 CUP

NUTRIENT	UNIT	AMOUNT	INQ	% STD
ENERGY	KCAL	60.00	1.00	3
VITAMIN A	IU	50.00	0.42	1
VITAMIN C	MG	112.00	62.22	187
THIAMIN	MG	0.07	2.33	7
RIBOFLAVN	MG	0.02	0.56	2
NIACIN	MG	0.20	0.48	1
IRON	MG	0.50	1.04	3
CALCIUM	MG	17.00	0.63	2
PHOSPHRUS	MG	24.00	0.89	3
POTASSIUM	MG	344.00	2.29	7
PROTEIN	G	1.00	0.67	2
CARBOHYDT	G	20.00	2.42	7
FAT	G	0.00	0.00	0
OLEIC A	G	0.00	0.00	0
LINOL A	G	0.00	0.00	0
SAT FAT A	G	0.00	0.00	0

263 LEMON JUICE, CANNED OR BOTTLED, UNSWEETENED
ANALYSIS OF 244 GRAMS WHICH IS 1 CUP

NUTRIENT	UNIT	AMOUNT	INQ	% STD	0	10	20	30	40	50	60	70	80	90	100
ENERGY	KCAL	55.00	1.00	3	EE										*
VITAMIN A	IU	50.00	0.45	1	AI										
VITAMIN C	MG	102.00	61.82	170	CICCCCCCCCCCCCCCCCCCCCCCCCCCCCCCCCCCCCCCCCCCCCCCCCCCCCCCCCCCCCCCCCCCCC *170
THIAMIN	MG	0.07	2.55	7	TITTTT
RIBOFLAVN	MG	0.02	0.61	2	RI
NIACIN	MG	0.05	0.52	1	NI
IRON	MG	0.50	1.14	3	III
CALCIUM	MG	17.00	0.69	2	KK
PHOSPHRUS	MG	24.00	0.97	3	XX
POTASSIUM	MG	344.00	2.50	7	YIYYYY
PROTEIN	G	1.00	0.73	2	PP
CARBOHYDT	G	19.00	2.51	7	HIHHHH
FAT	G	0.00	0.00	0	-I
OLEIC A	G	0.00	0.00	0	-I
LINOL A	G	0.00	0.00	0	-I
SAT FAT A	G	0.00	0.00	0	-I

****

264 LEMON JUICE, FROZEN, SINGLE STRENGTH, UNSWEETENED
ANALYSIS OF 183 GRAMS WHICH IS 1--6-FL OZ CAN

NUTRIENT	UNIT	AMOUNT	INQ	% STD	0	10	20	30	40	50	60	70	80	90	100
ENERGY	KCAL	40.00	1.00	2	EE										*
VITAMIN A	IU	40.00	0.50	1	AI										
VITAMIN C	MG	81.00	67.50	135	CICCCCCCCCCCCCCCCCCCCCCCCCCCCCCCCCCCCCCCCCCCCCCCCCCCCCCCCCCCCCCCCCCCC *135
THIAMIN	MG	0.05	2.50	5	TITT
RIBOFLAVN	MG	0.02	0.83	2	RI
NIACIN	MG	0.20	0.71	1	NI
IRON	MG	0.50	1.56	3	III
CALCIUM	MG	13.00	0.72	1	KI
PHOSPHRUS	MG	16.00	0.89	2	XI
POTASSIUM	MG	258.00	2.58	5	YIYY
PROTEIN	G	1.00	1.00	2	PP
CARBOHYDT	G	13.00	2.36	5	HIHH
FAT	G	0.00	0.00	0	-I
OLEIC A	G	0.00	0.00	0	-I
LINOL A	G	0.00	0.00	0	-I
SAT FAT A	G	0.00	0.00	0	-I

****

265 LEMONADE CONCENTRATE, FROZEN, UNDILUTED
ANALYSIS OF 219 GRAMS WHICH IS 1--6-FL OZ CAN

NUTRIENT	UNIT	AMOUNT	INQ	% STD
ENERGY	KCAL	425.00	1.00	21
VITAMIN A	IU	40.00	0.05	1
VITAMIN C	MG	66.00	5.18	110
THIAMIN	MG	0.05	0.24	5
RIBOFLAVN	MG	0.06	0.24	5
NIACIN	MG	0.70	0.24	5
IRON	MG	0.40	0.12	3
CALCIUM	MG	9.00	0.05	1
PHOSPHRUS	MG	13.00	0.07	1
POTASSIUM	MG	153.00	0.14	3
PROTEIN	G	0.00	0.00	0
CARBOHYDT	G	112.00	1.92	41
FAT	G	0.00	0.00	0
OLEIC A	G	0.00	0.00	0
LINOL A	G	0.00	0.00	0
SAT FAT A	G	0.00	0.00	0

266 LEMONADE CONCENTRATE, FROZEN, DILUTED
ANALYSIS OF 248 GRAMS WHICH IS 1 CUP

NUTRIENT	UNIT	AMOUNT	INQ	% STD
ENERGY	KCAL	105.00	1.00	5
VITAMIN A	IU	10.00	0.05	0
VITAMIN C	MG	17.00	5.40	28
THIAMIN	MG	0.01	0.19	1
RIBOFLAVN	MG	0.02	0.32	2
NIACIN	MG	0.20	0.27	1
IRON	MG	0.10	0.12	1
CALCIUM	MG	2.00	0.04	0
PHOSPHRUS	MG	3.00	0.06	0
POTASSIUM	MG	40.00	0.15	1
PROTEIN	G	0.00	0.00	0
CARBOHYDT	G	28.00	1.94	10
FAT	G	0.00	0.00	0
OLEIC A	G	0.00	0.00	0
LINOL A	G	0.00	0.00	0
SAT FAT A	G	0.00	0.00	0

267 LIMEADE CONCENTRATE, FROZEN, UNDILUTED
ANALYSIS OF 218 GRAMS WHICH IS 1--6-FL OZ CAN

```
                                    0      10      20      30      40      50      60      70      80      90      100
                                                                                                                    * ** ** ** ** ** ** ** ** * *
NUTRIENT    UNIT    AMOUNT   INQ    % STD
ENERGY      KCAL    410.00   1.00   21    EEEEEEEEEEEEEE
VITAMIN A   IU        0.00   0.00   43    -
VITAMIN C   MG       26.00   2.11    2    CCCCCCCCCCCCCC|CCCCCCCCCCCCCCCCCCCCC
THIAMIN     MG        0.02   0.10    2    TT
RIBOFLAVN   MG        0.02   0.08    2    R
NIACIN      MG        0.20   0.07    1    N
IRON        MG        0.20   0.06    1    I
CALCIUM     MG       11.00   0.06    1    K
PHOSPHRUS   MG       13.00   0.07    1    X
POTASSIUM   MG      129.00   0.13    3    YY
PROTEIN     G         0.00   0.00    0
CARBOHYDT   G       108.00   1.92   39    HHHHHHHHHHHHHHHH|HHHHHHHHHHHHHHH
FAT         G         0.00   0.00    0    I
OLEIC A     G         0.00   0.00    0    I
LINOL A     G         0.00   0.00    0    I
SAT FAT A   G         0.00   0.00    0    I
*******************************************************
```

268 LIMEADE CONCENTRATE, FROZEN, DILUTED
ANALYSIS OF 247 GRAMS WHICH IS 1 CUP

```
                                    0      10      20      30      40      50      60      70      80      90      100
                                                                                                                    * ** ** ** ** ** ** ** ** * *
NUTRIENT    UNIT    AMOUNT   INQ    % STD
ENERGY      KCAL    100.00   1.00    5    EEEE
VITAMIN A   IU        0.00   0.00    0    -
VITAMIN C   MG        6.00   2.00   10    CCC|CCCC
THIAMIN     MG        0.00   0.00    0    -
RIBOFLAVN   MG        0.00   0.00    0    -
NIACIN      MG        0.00   0.00    0    -
IRON        MG        0.00   0.00    0    -
CALCIUM     MG        3.00   0.07    0    Y
PHOSPHRUS   MG        3.00   0.07    0    Y
POTASSIUM   MG       32.00   0.13    1    Y
PROTEIN     G         0.00   0.00    0    -
CARBOHYDT   G        27.00   1.96   10    HHH|HHHH
FAT         G         0.00   0.00    0    I
OLEIC A     G         0.00   0.00    0    I
LINOL A     G         0.00   0.00    0    I
SAT FAT A   G         0.00   0.00    0    I
*******************************************************
```

269 LIMEJUICE, RAW
ANALYSIS OF 246 GRAMS WHICH IS 1 CUP

NUTRIENT	UNIT	AMOUNT	INQ	% STD	0	10	20	30	40	50	60	70	80	90	100	
ENERGY	KCAL	65.00	1.00	3	EEE										*	
VITAMIN A	IU	20.00	0.15	1	- I										*	
VITAMIN C	MG	79.00	40.51	132	CCCCCCCCCCCCCCCCCCCCCCCCCCCCCCCCCCCCCCCCCCCCCCCCCCCCCCCCCCCCCCC * 132											
THIAMIN	MG	0.05	1.54	5	TT|T										*	
RIBOFLAVN	MG	0.02	0.51	2	R I										*	
NIACIN	MG	0.20	0.44	1	N I										*	
IRON	MG	0.50	0.96	3	III										*	
CALCIUM	MG	22.00	0.75	2	KK|										*	
PHOSPHRUS	MG	27.00	0.92	3	XX|										*	
POTASSIUM	MG	256.00	1.58	5	YY|Y										*	
PROTEIN	G	1.00	0.62	2	PP|										*	
CARBOHYDT	G	22.00	2.46	8	HH|HHH										*	
FAT	G	0.00	0.00	0	- I										*	
OLEIC A	G	0.00	0.00	0	- I										*	
LINOL A	G	0.00	0.00	0	- I										*	
SAT FAT A	G	0.00	0.00	0	- I										*	

270 LIMEJUICE, CANNED, UNSWEETENED
ANALYSIS OF 246 GRAMS WHICH IS 1 CUP

NUTRIENT	UNIT	AMOUNT	INQ	% STD	0	10	20	30	40	50	60	70	80	90	100	
ENERGY	KCAL	65.00	1.00	3	EEE										*	
VITAMIN A	IU	20.00	0.15	1	- I										*	
VITAMIN C	MG	52.00	26.67	87	CCCCCCCCCCCCCCCCCCCCCCCCCCCCCCCCCCCCCCCCCCC										*	
THIAMIN	MG	0.05	1.54	5	TT|T										*	
RIBOFLAVN	MG	0.02	0.51	2	R I										*	
NIACIN	MG	0.20	0.44	1	N I										*	
IRON	MG	0.50	0.96	3	III										*	
CALCIUM	MG	22.00	0.75	2	KK|										*	
PHOSPHRUS	MG	27.00	0.92	3	XX|										*	
POTASSIUM	MG	256.00	1.58	5	YY|Y										*	
PROTEIN	G	1.00	0.62	2	PP|										*	
CARBOHYDT	G	22.00	2.46	8	HH|HHH										*	
FAT	G	0.00	0.00	0	- I										*	
OLEIC A	G	0.00	0.00	0	- I										*	
LINOL A	G	0.00	0.00	0	- I										*	
SAT FAT A	G	0.00	0.00	0	- I										*	

271 CANTALOUP, WT WITHOUT RIND AND SEEDS
ANALYSIS OF 272 GRAMS WHICH IS 1/2 OF A 5-IN DIAM. MELON

NUTRIENT	UNIT	AMOUNT	INQ	% STD
ENERGY	KCAL	80.00	1.00	4
VITAMIN A	IU	9240.00	57.75	231
VITAMIN C	MG	90.00	37.50	150
THIAMIN	MG	0.11	2.75	11
RIBOFLAVN	MG	0.08	1.67	7
NIACIN	MG	1.60	2.86	11
IRON	MG	1.10	1.72	7
CALCIUM	MG	38.00	1.06	4
PHOSPHRUS	MG	44.00	1.22	5
POTASSIUM	MG	682.00	3.41	14
PROTEIN	G	2.00	1.00	4
CARBOHYDT	G	20.00	1.82	7
FAT	G	0.00	0.00	0
OLEIC A	G	0.00	0.00	0
LINOL A	G	0.00	0.00	0
SAT FAT A	G	0.00	0.00	0

272 HONEYDEW MELON, WT WITHOUT RIND AND SEEDS
ANALYSIS OF 149 GRAMS WHICH IS 1/10 OF A 6 1/2-IN DIAM. MELON

NUTRIENT	UNIT	AMOUNT	INQ	% STD
ENERGY	KCAL	50.00	1.00	3
VITAMIN A	IU	60.00	0.60	2
VITAMIN C	MG	34.00	22.67	57
THIAMIN	MG	0.06	2.40	6
RIBOFLAVN	MG	0.04	1.33	3
NIACIN	MG	0.90	2.57	6
IRON	MG	0.60	1.50	6
CALCIUM	MG	21.00	0.93	4
PHOSPHRUS	MG	24.00	1.07	2
POTASSIUM	MG	374.00	2.99	7
PROTEIN	G	1.00	0.80	2
CARBOHYDT	G	11.00	1.60	4
FAT	G	0.00	0.00	0
OLEIC A	G	0.00	0.00	0
LINOL A	G	0.00	0.00	0
SAT FAT A	G	0.00	0.00	0

273 ORANGE, RAW, WT WITHOUT PEEL AND SEEDS
ANALYSIS OF 131 GRAMS WHICH IS 1--2 5/8-IN DIAM.

NUTRIENT	UNIT	AMOUNT	INQ	% STD
ENERGY	KCAL	65.00	1.00	3
VITAMIN A	IU	260.00	2.00	7
VITAMIN C	MG	66.00	33.85	110
THIAMIN	MG	0.13	4.00	13
RIBOFLAVN	MG	0.05	1.28	4
NIACIN	MG	0.50	1.10	4
IRON	MG	0.50	0.96	3
CALCIUM	MG	54.00	1.85	6
PHOSPHRUS	MG	26.00	0.89	3
POTASSIUM	MG	263.00	1.62	5
PROTEIN	G	1.00	0.62	2
CARBOHYDT	G	16.00	1.79	6
FAT	G	0.00	0.00	0
OLEIC A	G	0.00	0.00	0
LINOL A	G	0.00	0.00	0
SAT FAT A	G	0.00	0.00	0

274 ORANGE SECTIONS WITHOUT MEMBRANES, RAW
ANALYSIS OF 180 GRAMS WHICH IS 1 CUP

NUTRIENT	UNIT	AMOUNT	INQ	% STD
ENERGY	KCAL	90.00	1.00	5
VITAMIN A	IU	360.00	2.00	9
VITAMIN C	MG	90.00	33.33	150
THIAMIN	MG	0.18	4.00	18
RIBOFLAVN	MG	0.07	1.30	6
NIACIN	MG	0.70	1.11	5
IRON	MG	0.70	0.97	4
CALCIUM	MG	74.00	1.83	8
PHOSPHRUS	MG	36.00	0.89	4
POTASSIUM	MG	360.00	1.60	7
PROTEIN	G	2.00	0.89	4
CARBOHYDT	G	22.00	1.78	8
FAT	G	0.00	0.00	0
OLEIC A	G	0.00	0.00	0
LINOL A	G	0.00	0.00	0
SAT FAT A	G	0.00	0.00	0

275 ORANGE JUICE, FRESH
ANALYSIS OF 248 GRAMS WHICH IS 1 CUP

NUTRIENT	UNIT	AMOUNT	INQ	% STD
ENERGY	KCAL	110.00	1.00	6
VITAMIN A	IU	500.00	2.27	13
VITAMIN C	MG	124.00	37.58	207
THIAMIN	MG	0.22	4.00	22
RIBOFLAVN	MG	0.07	1.06	6
NIACIN	MG	1.00	1.30	7
IRON	MG	0.50	0.57	3
CALCIUM	MG	27.00	0.55	3
PHOSPHRUS	MG	42.00	0.85	5
POTASSIUM	MG	496.00	1.80	10
PROTEIN	G	2.00	0.73	4
CARBOHYDT	G	26.00	1.72	9
FAT	G	0.00	0.00	0
OLEIC A	G	0.00	0.00	0
LINOL A	G	0.00	0.00	0
SAT FAT A	G	0.00	0.00	0

276 ORANGE JUICE, CANNED, UNSWEETENED
ANALYSIS OF 249 GRAMS WHICH IS 1 CUP

NUTRIENT	UNIT	AMOUNT	INQ	% STD
ENERGY	KCAL	120.00	1.00	6
VITAMIN A	IU	500.00	2.08	13
VITAMIN C	MG	100.00	27.78	167
THIAMIN	MG	0.17	2.83	17
RIBOFLAVN	MG	0.05	0.69	4
NIACIN	MG	0.70	0.83	5
IRON	MG	1.00	1.04	6
CALCIUM	MG	25.00	0.46	3
PHOSPHRUS	MG	45.00	0.83	5
POTASSIUM	MG	496.00	1.65	10
PROTEIN	G	2.00	0.67	4
CARBOHYDT	G	28.00	1.70	10
FAT	G	0.00	0.00	0
OLEIC A	G	0.00	0.00	0
LINOL A	G	0.00	0.00	0
SAT FAT A	G	0.00	0.00	0

277 ORANGE JUICE, FROZEN CONCENTRATE, UNDILUTED
ANALYSIS OF 213 GRAMS WHICH IS 1--6-FL OZ CAN

NUTRIENT	UNIT	AMOUNT	INQ	% STD
ENERGY	KCAL	360.00	1.00	18
VITAMIN A	IU	1620.00	2.25	41
VITAMIN C	MG	360.00	33.33	600
THIAMIN	MG	0.68	3.78	68
RIBOFLAVN	MG	0.11	0.51	9
NIACIN	MG	2.80	1.11	20
IRON	MG	0.90	0.31	6
CALCIUM	MG	75.00	0.46	8
PHOSPHRUS	MG	126.00	0.78	14
POTASSIUM	MG	1500.00	1.67	30
PROTEIN	G	5.00	0.56	10
CARBOHYDT	G	87.00	1.76	32
FAT	G	0.00	0.00	0
OLEIC A	G	0.00	0.00	0
LINOL A	G	0.00	0.00	0
SAT FAT A	G	0.00	0.00	0

278 ORANGE JUICE, FROZEN CONCENTRATE, DILUTED
ANALYSIS OF 249 GRAMS WHICH IS 1 CUP

NUTRIENT	UNIT	AMOUNT	INQ	% STD
ENERGY	KCAL	120.00	1.00	6
VITAMIN A	IU	540.00	2.25	14
VITAMIN C	MG	120.00	33.33	200
THIAMIN	MG	0.23	3.83	23
RIBOFLAVN	MG	0.03	0.42	3
NIACIN	MG	0.90	1.07	6
IRON	MG	0.20	0.21	1
CALCIUM	MG	25.00	0.46	3
PHOSPHRUS	MG	42.00	0.78	5
POTASSIUM	MG	505.00	1.68	10
PROTEIN	G	2.00	0.67	4
CARBOHYDT	G	29.00	1.76	11
FAT	G	0.00	0.00	0
OLEIC A	G	0.00	0.00	0
LINOL A	G	0.00	0.00	0
SAT FAT A	G	0.00	0.00	0

279 ORANGE JUICE, DEHYDRATED CRYSTALS, PREPARED WITH WATER
ANALYSIS OF 248 GRAMS WHICH IS 1 CUP

NUTRIENT	UNIT	AMOUNT	INQ	% STD
ENERGY	KCAL	115.00	1.00	6
VITAMIN A	IU	500.00	2.17	13
VITAMIN C	MG	109.00	31.59	182
THIAMIN	MG	0.20	3.48	20
RIBOFLAVN	MG	0.07	1.01	6
NIACIN	MG	1.00	1.24	7
IRON	MG	0.50	0.54	3
CALCIUM	MG	25.00	0.48	3
PHOSPHRUS	MG	40.00	0.77	4
POTASSIUM	MG	518.00	1.80	10
PROTEIN	G	1.00	0.35	2
CARBOHYDT	G	27.00	1.71	10
FAT	G	0.00	0.00	0
OLEIC A	G	0.00	0.00	0
LINOL A	G	0.00	0.00	0
SAT FAT A	G	0.00	0.00	0

280 ORANGE AND GRAPEFRUIT JUICE, FROZEN CONCENTRATE, UNDILUTED
ANALYSIS OF 210 GRAMS WHICH IS 1--6 FL OZ CAN

NUTRIENT	UNIT	AMOUNT	INQ	% STD
ENERGY	KCAL	330.00	1.00	17
VITAMIN A	IU	800.00	1.21	20
VITAMIN C	MG	302.00	30.51	503
THIAMIN	MG	0.48	2.91	48
RIBOFLAVN	MG	0.06	0.30	5
NIACIN	MG	2.30	1.00	16
IRON	MG	0.80	0.30	5
CALCIUM	MG	61.00	0.41	7
PHOSPHRUS	MG	99.00	0.67	11
POTASSIUM	MG	1308.00	1.59	26
PROTEIN	G	4.00	0.48	8
CARBOHYDT	G	78.00	1.72	28
FAT	G	1.00	0.08	1
OLEIC A	G	0.00	0.00	0
LINOL A	G	0.00	0.00	0
SAT FAT A	G	0.00	0.00	0

281 ORANGE AND GRAPEFRUIT JUICE, FROZEN CONCENTRATE, DILUTED
ANALYSIS OF 248 GRAMS WHICH IS 1 CUP

NUTRIENT	UNIT	AMOUNT	INQ	% STD
ENERGY	KCAL	110.00	1.00	6
VITAMIN A	IU	270.00	1.23	7
VITAMIN C	MG	102.00	30.91	170
THIAMIN	MG	0.15	2.73	15
RIBOFLAVN	MG	0.02	0.30	2
NIACIN	MG	0.70	0.91	5
IRON	MG	0.20	0.23	1
CALCIUM	MG	20.00	0.40	2
PHOSPHRUS	MG	32.00	0.65	4
POTASSIUM	MG	439.00	1.60	9
PROTEIN	G	1.00	0.36	2
CARBOHYDT	G	26.00	1.72	9
FAT	G	0.00	0.00	0
OLEIC A	G	0.00	0.00	0
LINOL A	G	0.00	0.00	0
SAT FAT A	G	0.00	0.00	0

(Bar chart scale: 0 10 20 30 40 50 60 70 80 90 100; VITAMIN C extends to * 170)

282 PAPAYAS, RAW, 1/2 INCH CUBES
ANALYSIS OF 140 GRAMS WHICH IS 1 CUP

NUTRIENT	UNIT	AMOUNT	INQ	% STD
ENERGY	KCAL	55.00	1.00	3
VITAMIN A	IU	2450.00	22.27	61
VITAMIN C	MG	78.00	47.27	130
THIAMIN	MG	0.06	2.18	6
RIBOFLAVN	MG	0.06	1.82	5
NIACIN	MG	0.40	1.04	3
IRON	MG	0.40	0.91	3
CALCIUM	MG	28.00	1.13	3
PHOSPHRUS	MG	22.00	0.89	2
POTASSIUM	MG	328.00	2.39	7
PROTEIN	G	1.00	0.73	2
CARBOHYDT	G	14.00	1.85	5
FAT	G	0.00	0.00	0
OLEIC A	G	0.00	0.00	0
LINOL A	G	0.00	0.00	0
SAT FAT A	G	0.00	0.00	0

(Bar chart scale: 0 10 20 30 40 50 60 70 80 90 100; VITAMIN C extends to * 130)

283 PEACHES, RAW, WT FOR PEELED AND PITTED
ANALYSIS OF 100 GRAMS WHICH IS 1--2 1/2-IN DIAM. PEACH

NUTRIENT	UNIT	AMOUNT	INQ	% STD	0 ... 100
ENERGY	KCAL	40.00	1.00	2	EE
VITAMIN A	IU	1330.00	16.63	33	A|AAAAAAAAAAAAAAAAAAAAA
VITAMIN C	MG	7.00	5.83	12	C|CCCCCC
THIAMIN	MG	0.05	1.00	2	T|T
RIBOFLAVN	MG	0.05	2.08	4	R|R
NIACIN	MG	1.00	3.57	7	N|NNNN
IRON	MG	0.50	1.56	3	I|II
CALCIUM	MG	9.00	0.50	1	K|
PHOSPHRUS	MG	19.00	1.06	2	X|X
POTASSIUM	MG	202.00	2.02	4	Y|Y
PROTEIN	G	1.00	1.00	2	P|P
CARBOHYDT	G	10.00	1.82	4	H|H
FAT	G	0.00	0.00	0	-|
OLEIC A	G	0.00	0.00	0	-|
LINOL A	G	0.00	0.00	0	-|
SAT FAT A	G	0.00	0.00	0	-|

284 PEACHES, RAW, SLICED
ANALYSIS OF 170 GRAMS WHICH IS 1 CUP

NUTRIENT	UNIT	AMOUNT	INQ	% STD	0 ... 100
ENERGY	KCAL	65.00	1.00	3	EEE
VITAMIN A	IU	2260.00	17.38	57	AA|AAAAAAAAAAAAAAAAAAAAAAAAAAAAAAAAAAAAAAAAAAAAAAAA
VITAMIN C	MG	12.00	6.15	20	CC|CCCCCCCCCCCCCC
THIAMIN	MG	0.03	0.92	3	TT|T
RIBOFLAVN	MG	0.09	2.31	8	RR|RRK
NIACIN	MG	1.70	3.74	12	NN|NNNNNNN
IRON	MG	0.90	1.73	6	II|II
CALCIUM	MG	15.00	0.51	2	K|I
PHOSPHRUS	MG	32.00	1.09	4	XXX
POTASSIUM	MG	343.00	2.11	7	YY|YY
PROTEIN	G	1.00	0.62	2	PP|
CARBOHYDT	G	16.00	1.79	6	HH|HH
FAT	G	0.00	0.00	0	-|I
OLEIC A	G	0.00	0.00	0	-|I
LINOL A	G	0.00	0.00	0	-|I
SAT FAT A	G	0.00	0.00	0	-|I

285 PEACHES, CANNED, SYRUP PACK
ANALYSIS OF 256 GRAMS WHICH IS 1 CUP (SOLIDS AND LIQUID)

NUTRIENT	UNIT	AMOUNT	INQ	% STD
ENERGY	KCAL	200.00	1.00	10
VITAMIN A	IU	1100.00	2.75	28
VITAMIN C	MG	8.00	1.33	13
THIAMIN	MG	0.03	0.30	3
RIBOFLAVN	MG	0.05	0.42	4
NIACIN	MG	1.50	1.07	11
IRON	MG	0.80	0.50	5
CALCIUM	MG	10.00	0.11	1
PHOSPHRUS	MG	31.00	0.34	3
POTASSIUM	MG	333.00	0.67	7
PROTEIN	G	1.00	0.20	2
CARBOHYDT	G	51.00	1.85	19
FAT	G	0.00	0.00	0
OLEIC A	G	0.00	0.00	0
LINOL A	G	0.00	0.00	0
SAT FAT A	G	0.00	0.00	0

286 PEACHES, CANNED, WATER PACK
ANALYSIS OF 244 GRAMS WHICH IS 1 CUP (SOLIDS AND LIQUID)

NUTRIENT	UNIT	AMOUNT	INQ	% STD
ENERGY	KCAL	75.00	1.00	4
VITAMIN A	IU	1100.00	7.33	28
VITAMIN C	MG	7.00	3.11	12
THIAMIN	MG	0.02	0.53	2
RIBOFLAVN	MG	0.07	1.56	6
NIACIN	MG	1.50	2.86	11
IRON	MG	0.70	1.17	4
CALCIUM	MG	10.00	0.30	1
PHOSPHRUS	MG	32.00	0.95	4
POTASSIUM	MG	334.00	1.78	7
PROTEIN	G	1.00	0.53	2
CARBOHYDT	G	20.00	1.94	7
FAT	G	0.00	0.00	0
OLEIC A	G	0.00	0.00	0
LINOL A	G	0.00	0.00	0
SAT FAT A	G	0.00	0.00	0

287 PEACHES, DRIED, UNCOOKED
ANALYSIS OF 160 GRAMS WHICH IS 1 CUP

NUTRIENT	UNIT	AMOUNT	INQ	% STD
ENERGY	KCAL	420.00	1.00	21
VITAMIN A	IU	6240.00	7.43	156
VITAMIN C	MG	29.00	2.30	48
THIAMIN	MG	0.02	0.10	2
RIBOFLAVN	MG	0.30	1.19	25
NIACIN	MG	8.50	2.89	61
IRON	MG	9.60	2.86	60
CALCIUM	MG	77.00	0.41	9
PHOSPHRUS	MG	187.00	0.99	21
POTASSIUM	MG	1520.00	1.45	30
PROTEIN	G	5.00	0.48	10
CARBOHYDT	G	109.00	1.89	40
FAT	G	1.00	0.06	1
OLEIC A	G	0.00	0.00	0
LINOL A	G	0.00	0.00	0
SAT FAT A	G	0.00	0.00	0

288 PEACHES, DRIED, COOKED, UNSWEETENED
ANALYSIS OF 250 GRAMS WHICH IS 1 CUP (HALVES AND JUICE)

NUTRIENT	UNIT	AMOUNT	INQ	% STD
ENERGY	KCAL	205.00	1.00	10
VITAMIN A	IU	3050.00	7.44	76
VITAMIN C	MG	5.00	0.81	8
THIAMIN	MG	0.01	0.10	1
RIBOFLAVN	MG	0.15	1.22	13
NIACIN	MG	3.80	2.65	27
IRON	MG	4.80	2.93	30
CALCIUM	MG	38.00	0.41	4
PHOSPHRUS	MG	93.00	1.01	10
POTASSIUM	MG	743.00	1.45	15
PROTEIN	G	3.00	0.59	6
CARBOHYDT	G	54.00	1.92	20
FAT	G	1.00	0.13	1
OLEIC A	G	0.00	0.00	0
LINOL A	G	0.00	0.00	0
SAT FAT A	G	0.00	0.00	0

289 PEACHES, FROZEN, SLICED, SWEETENED
ANALYSIS OF 284 GRAMS WHICH IS 1--10-OZ CONTAINER

NUTRIENT	UNIT	AMOUNT	INQ	% STD
ENERGY	KCAL	250.00	1.00	13
VITAMIN A	IU	1850.00	3.70	46
VITAMIN C	MG	116.00	15.47	193
THIAMIN	MG	0.11	0.24	3
RIBOFLAVN	MG	0.11	0.73	9
NIACIN	MG	2.00	1.14	14
IRON	MG	1.40	0.70	9
CALCIUM	MG	11.00	0.10	1
PHOSPHRUS	MG	37.00	0.33	4
POTASSIUM	MG	352.00	0.56	7
PROTEIN	G	1.00	0.16	2
CARBOHYDT	G	64.00	1.86	23
FAT	G	0.00	0.00	0
OLEIC A	G	0.00	0.00	0
LINOL A	G	0.00	0.00	0
SAT FAT A	G	0.00	0.00	0

(Bar chart scale: 0 10 20 30 40 50 60 70 80 90 100; VITAMIN C bar extends off scale marked *193)

290 PEACHES, FROZEN, SLICED, SWEETENED
ANALYSIS OF 250 GRAMS WHICH IS 1 CUP

NUTRIENT	UNIT	AMOUNT	INQ	% STD
ENERGY	KCAL	220.00	1.00	11
VITAMIN A	IU	1630.00	3.70	41
VITAMIN C	MG	103.00	15.61	172
THIAMIN	MG	0.03	0.27	3
RIBOFLAVN	MG	0.10	0.76	8
NIACIN	MG	1.80	1.17	13
IRON	MG	1.30	0.74	8
CALCIUM	MG	10.00	0.10	1
PHOSPHRUS	MG	33.00	0.33	4
POTASSIUM	MG	310.00	0.56	6
PROTEIN	G	1.00	0.18	2
CARBOHYDT	G	57.00	1.88	21
FAT	G	0.00	0.00	0
OLEIC A	G	0.00	0.00	0
LINOL A	G	0.00	0.00	0
SAT FAT A	G	0.00	0.00	0

(Bar chart scale: 0 10 20 30 40 50 60 70 80 90 100; VITAMIN C bar extends off scale marked *172)

291 PEARS, BARTLETT, RAW, CORED WITH SKIN
ANALYSIS OF 164 GRAMS WHICH IS 1--2 1/2-IN DIAM. PEAR

NUTRIENT	UNIT	AMOUNT	INQ	% STD	0 10 20 30 40 50 60 70 80 90 100
ENERGY	KCAL	100.00	1.00	5	EEEE
VITAMIN A	IU	30.00	0.15	1	A
VITAMIN C	MG	7.00	2.33	12	CCC|CCCCC
THIAMIN	MG	0.03	0.60	3	TT
RIBOFLAVN	MG	0.07	1.17	6	RRR|R
NIACIN	MG	0.20	0.29	1	N
IRON	MG	0.50	0.63	3	III
CALCIUM	MG	13.00	0.29	1	K
PHOSPHRUS	MG	18.00	0.40	2	XX
POTASSIUM	MG	213.00	0.85	4	YYY
PROTEIN	G	1.00	0.40	2	PP
CARBOHYDT	G	25.00	1.82	9	HHH|HHH
FAT	G	1.00	0.26	1	F
OLEIC A	G	0.00	0.00	0	-
LINOL A	G	0.00	0.00	0	-
SAT FAT A	G	0.00	0.00	0	-

292 PEARS, BOSC, RAW, CORED WITH SKIN
ANALYSIS OF 141 GRAMS WHICH IS 1--2 1/2-IN DIAM. PEAR

NUTRIENT	UNIT	AMOUNT	INQ	% STD	0 10 20 30 40 50 60 70 80 90 100
ENERGY	KCAL	85.00	1.00	4	EEE
VITAMIN A	IU	30.00	0.18	1	A
VITAMIN C	MG	6.00	2.35	10	CC|CCCCC
THIAMIN	MG	0.03	0.71	3	TT
RIBOFLAVN	MG	0.06	1.18	5	RRR|R
NIACIN	MG	0.10	0.17	1	N
IRON	MG	0.40	0.59	3	II
CALCIUM	MG	11.00	0.29	1	K
PHOSPHRUS	MG	16.00	0.42	2	X
POTASSIUM	MG	83.00	0.39	2	Y
PROTEIN	G	1.00	0.47	2	PP
CARBOHYDT	G	22.00	1.88	8	HH|HHH
FAT	G	1.00	0.30	1	F
OLEIC A	G	0.00	0.00	0	-
LINOL A	G	0.00	0.00	0	-
SAT FAT A	G	0.00	0.00	0	-

293 PEARS, D'ANJOU, RAW, CORED WITH SKIN
ANALYSIS OF 200 GRAMS WHICH IS 1--3-IN DIAM. PEAR

NUTRIENT	UNIT	AMOUNT	INQ	% STD	0 10 20 30 40 50 60 70 80 90 100
ENERGY	KCAL	120.00	1.00	6	EEEEE
VITAMIN A	IU	40.00	0.17	1	A
VITAMIN C	MG	8.00	2.22	13	CCCCICCCCCC
THIAMIN	MG	0.04	0.67	4	TTT
RIBOFLAVN	MG	0.08	1.11	7	RRRR
NIACIN	MG	0.20	0.24	1	N
IRON	MG	0.60	0.63	4	III
CALCIUM	MG	16.00	0.30	2	K
PHOSPHRUS	MG	22.00	0.41	2	XX
POTASSIUM	MG	260.00	0.87	5	YYYI
PROTEIN	G	1.00	0.33	2	PP
CARBOHYDT	G	31.00	1.88	11	HHHHIHHHH
FAT	G	1.00	0.21	1	F
OLEIC A	G	0.00	0.00	0	-
LINOL A	G	0.00	0.00	0	-
SAT FAT A	G	0.00	0.00	0	-

294 PEARS, CANNED, HEAVY SYRUP PACK (SOLIDS AND LIQUID)
ANALYSIS OF 255 GRAMS WHICH IS 1 CUP (SOLIDS AND LIQUID)

NUTRIENT	UNIT	AMOUNT	INQ	% STD	0 10 20 30 40 50 60 70 80 90 100
ENERGY	KCAL	195.00	1.00	10	EEEEEEE
VITAMIN A	IU	10.00	0.03	0	-
VITAMIN C	MG	3.00	0.51	5	CCCC
THIAMIN	MG	0.03	0.31	3	TT
RIBOFLAVN	MG	0.05	0.43	4	RRR
NIACIN	MG	0.30	0.22	2	NN
IRON	MG	0.50	0.32	3	III
CALCIUM	MG	13.00	0.15	1	K
PHOSPHRUS	MG	18.00	0.21	2	XX
POTASSIUM	MG	214.00	0.44	4	YYY
PROTEIN	G	1.00	0.21	2	PP
CARBOHYDT	G	50.00	1.86	18	HHHHHHHIHHHHHHH
FAT	G	1.00	0.13	1	F
OLEIC A	G	0.00	0.00	0	-
LINOL A	G	0.00	0.00	0	-
SAT FAT A	G	0.00	0.00	0	-

295 PINEAPPLE, RAW, DICED
ANALYSIS OF 155 GRAMS WHICH IS 1 CUP

NUTRIENT	UNIT	AMOUNT	INQ	% STD	0	10	20	30	40	50	60	70	80	90	100
ENERGY	KCAL	80.00	1.00	4	EEE										
VITAMIN A	IU	110.00	0.69	3	AAI										
VITAMIN C	MG	26.00	10.83	43	CCICCCCCCCCCCCCCCCCCCCCCCCCCCCCCC										
THIAMIN	MG	0.14	3.50	14	TTITTTTTTT										
RIBOFLAVN	MG	0.05	1.04	4	RRR										
NIACIN	MG	0.30	0.54	2	NNI										
IRON	MG	0.80	1.25	5	IIII										
CALCIUM	MG	26.00	0.72	3	KKI										
PHOSPHRUS	MG	12.00	0.33	1	X I										
POTASSIUM	MG	226.00	1.13	5	YYIY										
PROTEIN	G	1.00	0.50	2	PPI										
CARBOHYDT	G	21.00	1.91	8	MHIHHH										
FAT	G	0.00	0.00	0	- I										
OLEIC A	G	0.00	0.00	0	- I										
LINOL A	G	0.00	0.00	0	- I										
SAT FAT A	G	0.00	0.00	0	- I										

296 PINEAPPLE, CANNED, CRUSHED, CHUNKS, TIDBITS, HEAVY SYRUP PACK
ANALYSIS OF 255 GRAMS WHICH IS 1 CUP (SOLIDS AND LIQUID)

NUTRIENT	UNIT	AMOUNT	INQ	% STD	0	10	20	30	40	50	60	70	80	90	100
ENERGY	KCAL	190.00	1.00	10	EEEEEEE										
VITAMIN A	IU	130.00	0.34	3	AAA										
VITAMIN C	MG	18.00	3.16	30	CCCCCCCICCCCCCCCCCCCCCCC										
THIAMIN	MG	0.20	2.11	20	TTTTTTTITTTTTTT										
RIBOFLAVN	MG	0.05	0.44	4	RRR										
NIACIN	MG	0.50	0.38	4	NNN										
IKON	MG	0.80	0.53	5	IIII										
CALCIUM	MG	28.00	0.33	3	KK										
PHOSPHRUS	MG	13.00	0.15	1	X I										
POTASSIUM	MG	245.00	0.52	5	YYYY										
PROTEIN	G	1.00	0.21	2	PP I										
CARBOHYDT	G	49.00	1.88	18	HHHHHHHIHHHHHH										
FAT	G	0.00	0.00	0	- I										
OLEIC A	G	0.00	0.00	0	- I										
LINOL A	G	0.00	0.00	0	- I										
SAT FAT A	G	0.00	0.00	0	- I										

297 PINEAPPLE, CANNED, LARGE SLICE, HEAVY SYRUP PACK
ANALYSIS OF 105 GRAMS WHICH IS 1SLICE, 2 1/4 TBSP LIQUID

NUTRIENT	UNIT	AMOUNT	INQ	% STD
ENERGY	KCAL	80.00	1.00	4
VITAMIN A	IU	50.00	0.31	1
VITAMIN C	MG	7.00	2.92	12
THIAMIN	MG	0.08	2.00	8
RIBOFLAVN	MG	0.02	0.42	2
NIACIN	MG	0.20	0.36	1
IRON	MG	0.30	0.47	2
CALCIUM	MG	12.00	0.33	1
PHOSPHRUS	MG	5.00	0.14	1
POTASSIUM	MG	101.00	0.50	2
PROTEIN	G	0.00	0.00	0
CARBOHYDT	G	20.00	1.82	7
FAT	G	0.00	0.00	0
OLEIC A	G	0.00	0.00	0
LINOL A	G	0.00	0.00	0
SAT FAT A	G	0.00	0.00	0

98 PINEAPPLE, CANNED, MEDIUM SLICE, HEAVY SYRUP PACK
NALYSIS OF 58 GRAMS WHICH IS 1 SLICE, 1 1/4 TBSP LIQUID

NUTRIENT	UNIT	AMOUNT	INQ	% STD
ENERGY	KCAL	45.00	1.00	2
VITAMIN A	IU	30.00	0.33	1
VITAMIN C	MG	4.00	2.96	7
THIAMIN	MG	0.05	2.22	5
RIBOFLAVN	MG	0.01	0.37	1
NIACIN	MG	0.10	0.32	1
IRON	MG	0.20	0.56	1
CALCIUM	MG	6.00	0.30	1
PHOSPHRUS	MG	3.00	0.15	1
POTASSIUM	MG	56.00	0.50	1
PROTEIN	G	0.00	0.00	0
CARBOHYDT	G	11.00	1.78	4
FAT	G	0.00	0.00	0
OLEIC A	G	0.00	0.00	0
LINOL A	G	0.00	0.00	0
SAT FAT A	G	0.00	0.00	0

299 PINEAPPLE JUICE, UNSWEETENED, CANNED
ANALYSIS OF 250 GRAMS WHICH IS 1 CUP

```
                                   0    10   20   30   40   50   60   70   80   90   100
NUTRIENT   UNIT   AMOUNT   INQ   % STD
ENERGY     KCAL   140.00   1.00    7   EEEEE                                            *
VITAMIN A  IU     130.00   0.46    3   AAA
VITAMIN C  MG      80.00  19.05  133   CCCCC|CCCCCCCCCCCCCCCCCCCCCCCCCCCCCCCCCCCCCCCCCCCC * 133
THIAMIN    MG       0.13   1.86   13   TTTTT|TTTT
RIBOFLAVN  MG       0.05   0.60    4   RRR  |
NIACIN     MG       0.50   0.51    4   NNN  |
IRON       MG       0.80   0.71    5   IIII |
CALCIUM    MG      38.00   0.60    4   KKK  |
PHOSPHRUS  MG      23.00   0.37    3   XX   |
POTASSIUM  MG     373.00   1.07    7   YYYYY|
PROTEIN    G        1.00   0.29    2   PP   |
CARBOHYDT  G       34.00   1.77   12   HHHHH|HHHH
FAT        G        0.00   0.00    0        |
OLEIC A    G        0.00   0.00    0        |
LINOL A    G        0.00   0.00    0        |
SAT FAT A  G        0.00   0.00    0        |
```

300 PLUMS, JAPANESE AND HYBRID, RAW, WITHOUT PITS
ANALYSIS OF 66 GRAMS WHICH IS 1--2 1/8-IN DIAM. PLUM

```
                                   0    10   20   30   40   50   60   70   80   90   100
NUTRIENT   UNIT   AMOUNT   INQ   % STD
ENERGY     KCAL    30.00   1.00    2   E
VITAMIN A  IU     160.00   2.67    4   IAA
VITAMIN C  MG       4.00   4.44    7   ICCCC
THIAMIN    MG       0.02   1.33    2   IT
RIBOFLAVN  MG       0.02   1.11    2   R
NIACIN     MG       0.30   1.43    2   IN
IRON       MG       0.30   1.25    2   II
CALCIUM    MG       8.00   0.59    1   IK
PHOSPHRUS  MG      12.00   0.89    1   X
POTASSIUM  MG     112.00   1.49    2   IY
PROTEIN    G        0.00   0.00    0   I
CARBOHYDT  G        8.00   1.94    3   IH
FAT        G        0.00   0.00    0   I
OLEIC A    G        0.00   0.00    0   I
LINOL A    G        0.00   0.00    0   I
SAT FAT A  G        0.00   0.00    0   I
```

301 PLUMS, PRUNE-TYPE, RAW, WITHOUT PITS
ANALYSIS OF 28 GRAMS WHICH IS 1--1 1/2-IN DIAM. PLUM

```
                                    0    10    20    30    40    50    60    70    80    90   100
                                    *     *     *     *     *     *     *     *     *     *     *
NUTRIENT   UNIT  AMOUNT    INQ  % STD
ENERGY     KCAL   20.00   1.00    1   E
VITAMIN A  IU     80.00   2.00    2   IA
VITAMIN C  MG      1.00   1.67    2   C
THIAMIN    MG      0.01   1.00    1   T
RIBOFLAVN  MG      0.01   0.83    1   R
NIACIN     MG      0.10   0.71    1   N
IRON       MG      0.10   0.63    1   I
CALCIUM    MG      3.00   0.33    0   -
PHOSPHRUS  MG      5.00   0.56    1   Y
POTASSIUM  MG     48.00   0.96    0   Y
PROTEIN    G       0.00   0.00    0   -
CARBOHYDT  G       6.00   2.18    2   IH
FAT        G       0.00   0.00    0   -
OLEIC A    G       0.00   0.00    0   -
LINOL A    G       0.00   0.00    0   -
SAT FAT A  G       0.00   0.00    0   -
***********************************
```

302 PLUMS, CANNED, HEAVY SYRUP PACK (WITH PITS AND LIQUID)
ANALYSIS OF 272 GRAMS WHICH IS 1 CUP (WITH PITS AND LIQUID)

```
                                    0    10    20    30    40    50    60    70    80    90   100
                                    *     *     *     *     *     *     *     *     *     *     *
NUTRIENT   UNIT  AMOUNT    INQ  % STD
ENERGY     KCAL   215.00   1.00   11   EEEEEEEE
VITAMIN A  IU    3130.00   7.28   78   AAAAAAAAIAAAAAAAAAAAAAAAAAAAAAAAAAAAAAAAAAAAAAAAAAAAAAAAAAAAAAAAAAAAAAAAAAA
VITAMIN C  MG      5.00    0.78    8   CCCCCCC
THIAMIN    MG      0.05    0.47    5   TTTT
RIBOFLAVN  MG      0.05    0.39    4   RRR
NIACIN     MG      1.00    0.66    7   NNNNNN
IRON       MG      2.30    1.34   14   IIIIIIIIIIIII
CALCIUM    MG     23.00    0.24    3   KK
PHOSPHRUS  MG     26.00    0.27    3   XX
POTASSIUM  MG    367.00    0.68    7   YYYYY
PROTEIN    G       1.00    0.19    2   PP
CARBOHYDT  G      56.00    1.89   20   HHHHHHHHIHHHHHHH
FAT        G       0.00    0.00    0   -
OLEIC A    G       0.00    0.00    0   -
LINOL A    G       0.00    0.00    0   -
SAT FAT A  G       0.00    0.00    0   -
***********************************
```

303 PLUMS, CANNED, HEAVY SYRUP PACK
ANALYSIS OF 140 GRAMS WHICH IS 3 PLUMS (WITH PITS) AND 2 3/4 TBSP LIQUID

NUTRIENT	UNIT	AMOUNT	INQ	% STD	0 10 20 30 40
ENERGY	KCAL	110.00	1.00	6	EEEE
VITAMIN A	IU	1610.00	7.32	40	AAA|AAAAAAAAAAAAAAAAAAAAAAAAAAAA
VITAMIN C	MG	3.00	0.91	5	CCCC
THIAMIN	MG	0.03	0.55	3	TT|
RIBOFLAVN	MG	0.03	0.45	3	RR|
NIACIN	MG	0.50	0.65	4	NNN|
IRON	MG	1.20	1.36	7	III|II
CALCIUM	MG	12.00	0.24	1	K|
PHOSPHRUS	MG	13.00	0.26	1	X|
POTASSIUM	MG	189.00	0.69	4	YYY|
PROTEIN	G	1.00	0.36	2	PP|
CARBOHYDT	G	29.00	1.92	11	HHH|HHHH
FAT	G	0.00	0.00	0	|
OLEIC A	G	0.00	0.00	0	|
LINOL A	G	0.00	0.00	0	|
SAT FAT A	G	0.00	0.00	0	|

304 PRUNES, DRIED, "SOFTENIZED," WITH PITS, UNCOOKED
ANALYSIS OF 49 GRAMS WHICH IS 4 EXTRA LARGE OR 5 LARGE PRUNES

NUTRIENT	UNIT	AMOUNT	INQ	% STD	0 10 20 30 40
ENERGY	KCAL	110.00	1.00	6	EEEE
VITAMIN A	IU	690.00	3.14	17	AAA|AAAAAAAAA
VITAMIN C	MG	1.00	0.30	2	C|
THIAMIN	MG	0.04	0.73	4	TTT|
RIBOFLAVN	MG	0.07	1.06	6	RRR|R
NIACIN	MG	0.70	0.91	5	NNNN|
IRON	MG	1.70	1.93	11	III|IIIII
CALCIUM	MG	22.00	0.44	2	KK|
PHOSPHRUS	MG	34.00	0.69	4	XXX|
POTASSIUM	MG	298.00	1.08	6	YYY|Y
PROTEIN	G	1.00	0.36	2	PP|
CARBOHYDT	G	29.00	1.92	11	HHH|HHHH
FAT	G	0.00	0.00	0	|
OLEIC A	G	0.00	0.00	0	|
LINOL A	G	0.00	0.00	0	|
SAT FAT A	G	0.00	0.00	0	|

305 PRUNES, DRIED, "SOFTENIZED," WITH PITS, COOKED, UNSWEETENED
ANALYSIS OF 250 GRAMS WHICH IS 1 CUP (FRUIT AND LIQUID)

```
NUTRIENT   UNIT  AMOUNT    INQ  % STD  0        10        20        30        40        50        60        70        80        90       100
                                                                                                                                          *
ENERGY     KCAL   255.00  1.00    13  EEEEEEEE                                                                                            *
VITAMIN A  IU    1590.00  3.12    40  AAAAAAAA|AAAAAAAAAAAAAAAAAAAAAAA                                                                    *
VITAMIN C  MG       2.00  0.26     3  CCC                                                                                                 *
THIAMIN    MG       0.07  0.55     7  TTTTT|                                                                                              *
RIBOFLAVN  MG       0.15  0.98    13  RRRRRRRRR                                                                                           *
NIACIN     MG       1.50  0.84    11  NNNNNNNNN|                                                                                          *
IRON       MG       3.80  1.86    24  IIIIIIIII|IIIIIIIII                                                                                 *
CALCIUM    MG      51.00  0.44     6  KKKKK                                                                                               *
PHOSPHRUS  MG      79.00  0.69     9  XXXXXXX|                                                                                            *
POTASSIUM  MG     695.00  1.09    14  YYYYYYYYY|Y                                                                                         *
PROTEIN    G        2.00  0.31     4  PPP                                                                                                 *
CARBOHYDT  G       67.00  1.91    24  HHHHHHHHH|HHHHHHHH                                                                                  *
FAT        G        1.00  0.10     1  F                                                                                                   *
OLEIC A    G        0.00  0.00     0  -                                                                                                   *
LINOL A    G        0.00  0.00     0  -                                                                                                   *
SAT FAT A  G        0.00  0.00     0  -                                                                                                   *
*************************************************************************************************************************************
```

306 PRUNE JUICE, CANNED OR BOTTLED
ANALYSIS OF 256 GRAMS WHICH IS 1 CUP

```
NUTRIENT   UNIT  AMOUNT    INQ  % STD  0        10        20        30        40        50        60        70        80        90       100
                                                                                                                                          *
ENERGY     KCAL   195.00  1.00    10  EEEEEE                                                                                              *
VITAMIN A  IU    1540.00  3.95    39  AAAAAAA|AAAAAAAAAAAAAAAAAAAAAAA                                                                     *
VITAMIN C  MG       5.00  0.85     8  CCCCCCC|                                                                                            *
THIAMIN    MG       0.03  0.31     3  TT                                                                                                  *
RIBOFLAVN  MG       0.03  0.26     3  RR                                                                                                  *
NIACIN     MG       1.00  0.73     7  NNNNN                                                                                               *
IRON       MG       1.80  1.15    11  IIIIIII|I                                                                                           *
CALCIUM    MG      36.00  0.41     4  KKK                                                                                                 *
PHOSPHRUS  MG      51.00  0.58     6  XXXXX                                                                                               *
POTASSIUM  MG     602.00  1.23    12  YYYYYYY|YY                                                                                          *
PROTEIN    G        1.00  0.21     2  PP                                                                                                  *
CARBOHYDT  G       49.00  1.83    18  HHHHHHH|HHHHH                                                                                       *
FAT        G        0.00  0.00     0  -                                                                                                   *
OLEIC A    G        0.00  0.00     0  -                                                                                                   *
LINOL A    G        0.00  0.00     0  -                                                                                                   *
SAT FAT A  G        0.00  0.00     0  -                                                                                                   *
*************************************************************************************************************************************
```

307 RAISINS, SEEDLESS
ANALYSIS OF 145 GRAMS WHICH IS 1 CUP

NUTRIENT	UNIT	AMOUNT	INQ	% STD
ENERGY	KCAL	420.00	1.00	21
VITAMIN A	IU	30.00	0.04	1
VITAMIN C	MG	1.00	0.08	2
THIAMIN	MG	0.16	0.76	16
RIBOFLAVN	MG	0.12	0.48	10
NIACIN	MG	0.70	0.24	5
IRON	MG	5.10	1.52	32
CALCIUM	MG	90.00	0.48	10
PHOSPHRUS	MG	146.00	0.77	16
POTASSIUM	MG	1106.00	1.05	22
PROTEIN	G	4.00	0.38	8
CARBOHYDT	G	112.00	1.94	41
FAT	G	0.00	0.00	0
OLEIC A	G	0.00	0.00	0
LINOL A	G	0.00	0.00	0
SAT FAT A	G	0.00	0.00	0

308 RAISINS, SEEDLESS
ANALYSIS OF 14 GRAMS WHICH IS 1/2 OZ PACKET OR 1 1/2 TBSP

NUTRIENT	UNIT	AMOUNT	INQ	% STD
ENERGY	KCAL	40.00	1.00	2
VITAMIN A	IU	0.00	0.00	0
VITAMIN C	MG	0.00	0.00	0
THIAMIN	MG	0.02	1.00	2
RIBOFLAVN	MG	0.01	0.42	1
NIACIN	MG	0.10	0.36	1
IRON	MG	0.50	1.56	3
CALCIUM	MG	9.00	0.50	1
PHOSPHRUS	MG	14.00	0.78	2
POTASSIUM	MG	107.00	1.07	2
PROTEIN	G	0.00	0.00	0
CARBOHYDT	G	11.00	2.00	4
FAT	G	0.00	0.00	0
OLEIC A	G	0.00	0.00	0
LINOL A	G	0.00	0.00	0
SAT FAT A	G	0.00	0.00	0

309 RASPBERRIES, RED, RAW, WHOLE
ANALYSIS OF 123 GRAMS WHICH IS 1 CUP

NUTRIENT	UNIT	AMOUNT	ING	% STD
ENERGY	KCAL	70.00	1.00	4
VITAMIN A	IU	160.00	1.14	4
VITAMIN C	MG	31.00	14.76	52
THIAMIN	MG	0.04	1.14	4
RIBOFLAVN	MG	0.11	2.62	9
NIACIN	MG	1.10	2.24	8
IRON	MG	1.10	1.96	7
CALCIUM	MG	27.00	0.86	3
PHOSPHRUS	MG	27.00	0.86	3
POTASSIUM	MG	207.00	1.18	4
PROTEIN	G	1.00	0.57	2
CARBOHYDT	G	17.00	1.77	6
FAT	G	1.00	0.37	1
OLEIC A	G	0.00	0.00	0
LINOL A	G	0.00	0.00	0
SAT FAT A	G	0.00	0.00	0

310 RASPBERRIES, RED, FROZEN, SWEETENED
ANALYSIS OF 284 GRAMS WHICH IS 1--10-OZ CONTAINER

NUTRIENT	UNIT	AMOUNT	ING	% STD
ENERGY	KCAL	280.00	1.00	14
VITAMIN A	IU	200.00	0.36	5
VITAMIN C	MG	60.00	7.14	100
THIAMIN	MG	0.06	0.43	6
RIBOFLAVN	MG	0.17	1.01	14
NIACIN	MG	1.70	0.87	12
IRON	MG	1.70	0.76	11
CALCIUM	MG	37.00	0.29	4
PHOSPHRUS	MG	48.00	0.38	5
POTASSIUM	MG	284.00	0.41	6
PROTEIN	G	2.00	0.29	4
CARBOHYDT	G	70.00	1.82	25
FAT	G	1.00	0.09	1
OLEIC A	G	0.00	0.00	0
LINOL A	G	0.00	0.00	0
SAT FAT A	G	0.00	0.00	0

```
                    100 * * * * * * * * * * * * * * *                    100 * * * * * * * * * * * * * * *

                     90                                                   90

                     80                                                   80

                     70                                                   70

                     60                                                   60

                     50                                                   50

                     40                                                   40

                     30                                                   30

                     20                                                   20

                     10                                                   10
```

311 RHUBARB, COOKED, ADDED SUGAR
ANALYSIS OF 270 GRAMS WHICH IS 1 CUP

NUTRIENT	UNIT	AMOUNT	INQ	% STD	0
ENERGY	KCAL	380.00	1.00	19	EEEEEEEEEEEE
VITAMIN A	IU	220.00	0.29	6	AAAA
VITAMIN C	MG	16.00	1.40	27	CCCCCCCCCCCCCC ICCCCCC
THIAMIN	MG	0.05	0.26	5	TTTT
RIBOFLAVN	MG	0.14	0.61	12	RRRRRRRR
NIACIN	MG	0.80	0.30	6	NNNNN
IRON	MG	1.60	0.53	10	IIIIIIII
CALCIUM	MG	211.00	1.23	23	KKKKKKKKKKKKKKK IKKKK
PHOSPHRUS	MG	41.00	0.24	5	XXXX
POTASSIUM	MG	546.00	0.58	11	YYYYYYY
PROTEIN	G	1.00	0.11	2	PP
CARBUHYDT	G	97.00	1.86	35	HHHHHHHHHHHHHHHH IHHHHHHHHHHHHHH
FAT	G	0.00	0.00	0	-
OLEIC A	G	0.00	0.00	0	-
LINOL A	G	0.00	0.00	0	-
SAT FAT A	G	0.00	0.00	0	-

312 RHUBARB, FROZEN, COOKED, SWEETENED
ANALYSIS OF 270 GRAMS WHICH IS 1 CUP

NUTRIENT	UNIT	AMOUNT	INQ	% STD	0
ENERGY	KCAL	385.00	1.00	19	EEEEEEEEEEEE
VITAMIN A	IU	190.00	0.25	5	AAAA
VITAMIN C	MG	16.00	1.39	27	CCCCCCCCCCCCCC ICCCCC
THIAMIN	MG	0.05	0.26	5	TTTT
RIBOFLAVN	MG	0.11	0.48	9	RRRRRR
NIACIN	MG	0.50	0.19	4	NNN
IRON	MG	1.90	0.62	12	IIIIIIIII
CALCIUM	MG	211.00	1.22	23	KKKKKKKKKKKKKKK IKKKK
PHOSPHRUS	MG	32.00	0.18	4	XXX
POTASSIUM	MG	475.00	0.49	10	YYYYYYY
PROTEIN	G	1.00	0.10	2	PP
CARBUHYDT	G	98.00	1.85	36	HHHHHHHHHHHHHHHH IHHHHHHHHHHHHHHHH
FAT	G	1.00	0.07	1	F
OLEIC A	G	0.00	0.00	0	-
LINOL A	G	0.00	0.00	0	-
SAT FAT A	G	0.00	0.00	0	-

313 STRAWBERRIES, RAW, WHOLE, CAPPED
ANALYSIS OF 149 GRAMS WHICH IS 1 CUP

```
NUTRIENT    UNIT  AMOUNT   INQ    % STD    0          10        20        30        40        50        60        70        80        90       100
ENERGY      KCAL   55.00   1.00      3     EE                                                                                                        *
VITAMIN A   IU     90.00   0.82      2     AA                                                                                                        *
VITAMIN C   MG     88.00  53.33    147     CICCCCCCCCCCCCCCCCCCCCCCCCCCCCCCCCCCCCCCCCCCCCCCCCCCCCCCCCCCCCCCCCCCC *147
THIAMIN     MG      0.04   1.45      4     TIT                                                                                                       *
RIBOFLAVN   MG      0.10   3.03      8     RIRRRRR                                                                                                   *
NIACIN      MG      0.90   2.34      6     NINNN                                                                                                     *
IRON        MG      1.50   3.41      9     IIIIIIII                                                                                                  *
CALCIUM     MG     31.00   1.25      3     KIK                                                                                                       *
PHOSPHRUS   MG     31.00   1.25      3     XIX                                                                                                       *
POTASSIUM   MG    244.00   1.77      5     YIYY                                                                                                      *
PROTEIN     G       1.00   0.73      2     PP                                                                                                        *
CARBOHYDT   G      13.00   1.72      5     HIHH                                                                                                      *
FAT         G       1.00   0.47      1     FI                                                                                                        *
OLEIC A     G       0.00   0.00      0     -I                                                                                                        *
LINOL A     G       0.00   0.00      0     -I                                                                                                        *
SAT FAT A   G       0.00   0.00      0     -I                                                                                                        *
```

314 STRAWBERRIES, FROZEN, SWEETENED, SLICED
ANALYSIS OF 284 GRAMS WHICH IS 1--10-OZ CONTAINER

```
NUTRIENT    UNIT  AMOUNT   INQ    % STD    0          10        20        30        40        50        60        70        80        90       100
ENERGY      KCAL  310.00   1.00     16     EEEEEEEEEE                                                                                                *
VITAMIN A   IU     90.00   0.15      2     AA                                                                                                        *
VITAMIN C   MG    151.00  16.24    252     CCCCCCCCCCICCCCCCCCCCCCCCCCCCCCCCCCCCCCCCCCCCCCCCCCCCCCCCCCCCCCCCCCCCCCCCCCCC *252
THIAMIN     MG      0.06   0.39      6     TTTT                                                                                                      *
RIBOFLAVN   MG      0.17   0.91     14     RRRRRRRRRR                                                                                                *
NIACIN      MG      1.40   0.65     10     NNNNNNNN                                                                                                  *
IRON        MG      2.00   0.81     13     IIIIIIIII                                                                                                 *
CALCIUM     MG     40.00   0.29      4     KKKK                                                                                                      *
PHOSPHRUS   MG     48.00   0.34      5     XXXX                                                                                                      *
POTASSIUM   MG    318.00   0.41      6     YYYY                                                                                                      *
PROTEIN     G       1.00   0.13      2     PP                                                                                                        *
CARBOHYDT   G      79.00   1.85     29     HHHHHHHHHHHHHHHHHHHH                                                                                       *
FAT         G       1.00   0.08      1     F                                                                                                         *
OLEIC A     G       0.00   0.00      0     -                                                                                                         *
LINOL A     G       0.00   0.00      0     -                                                                                                         *
SAT FAT A   G       0.00   0.00      0     -                                                                                                         *
```

315 STRAWBERRIES, FROZEN, SWEETENED, WHOLE
ANALYSIS OF 454 GRAMS WHICH IS 1-LB CONTAINER

NUTRIENT	UNIT	AMOUNT	INQ	% STD	0 10 20 30 40 50 60 70 80 90 100
ENERGY	KCAL	415.00	1.00	21	EEEEEEEEEEEEE
VITAMIN A	IU	140.00	0.17	4	AAA
VITAMIN C	MG	249.00	20.00	415	CCCCCCCCCCCCCCCC|CCCCCCCCCCCCCCCCCCCCCCCCCCCCCCCCCCCCCCCCCCCC * 415
THIAMIN	MG	0.09	0.43	9	TTTTTT
RIBOFLAVN	MG	0.27	1.08	23	RRRRRRRRRRRRRRR|R
NIACIN	MG	2.30	0.79	16	NNNNNNNNNNNN
IRON	MG	2.70	0.81	17	IIIIIIIIIIIIIII
CALCIUM	MG	59.00	0.32	7	KKKKK
PHOSPHRUS	MG	73.00	0.39	8	XXXXXX
POTASSIUM	MG	472.00	0.45	9	YYYYYYY
PROTEIN	G	2.00	0.19	4	PPP
CARBOHYDT	G	107.00	1.88	39	HHHHHHHHHHHHHHHH|HHHHHHHHHHHHH
FAT	G	1.00	0.06	1	F
OLEIC A	G	0.00	0.00	0	-
LINOL A	G	0.00	0.00	0	-
SAT FAT A	G	0.00	0.00	0	-

316 TANGERINE, RAW, WT WITHOUT PEEL
ANALYSIS OF 86 GRAMS WHICH IS 1 (2 3/8 IN DIAM.) TANGERINE

NUTRIENT	UNIT	AMOUNT	INQ	% STD	0 10 20 30 40 50 60 70 80 90 100
ENERGY	KCAL	40.00	1.00	2	EE
VITAMIN A	IU	360.00	4.50	9	AIAAAAA
VITAMIN C	MG	27.00	22.50	45	CICCCCCCCCCCCCCCCCCCCCCCCCCCCCCCC
THIAMIN	MG	0.05	2.50	5	TITT
RIBOFLAVN	MG	0.02	0.83	2	RI
NIACIN	MG	0.10	0.36	1	NI
IRON	MG	0.30	0.94	2	II
CALCIUM	MG	34.00	1.89	4	KIK
PHOSPHRUS	MG	15.00	0.83	2	XI
POTASSIUM	MG	108.00	1.08	2	YY
PROTEIN	G	1.00	1.00	2	PP
CARBOHYDT	G	10.00	1.82	4	HIH
FAT	G	0.00	0.00	0	-I
OLEIC A	G	0.00	0.00	0	-I
LINOL A	G	0.00	0.00	0	-I
SAT FAT A	G	0.00	0.00	0	-I

317 TANGERINE JUICE, CANNED, SWEETENED
ANALYSIS OF 249 GRAMS WHICH IS 1 CUP

NUTRIENT	UNIT	AMOUNT	INQ	% STD
ENERGY	KCAL	125.00	1.00	6
VITAMIN A	IU	1040.00	4.16	26
VITAMIN C	MG	54.00	14.40	90
THIAMIN	MG	0.15	0.67	4
RIBOFLAVN	MG	0.05	0.23	1
NIACIN	MG	0.20	0.20	1
IRON	MG	0.50	0.50	3
CALCIUM	MG	44.00	0.78	5
PHOSPHRUS	MG	35.00	0.62	4
POTASSIUM	MG	440.00	1.41	9
PROTEIN	G	1.00	0.32	2
CARBOHYDT	G	30.00	1.75	11
FAT	G	0.00	0.00	0
OLEIC A	G	0.00	0.00	0
LINOL A	G	0.00	0.00	0
SAT FAT A	G	0.00	0.00	0

318 WATERMELON, WT WITHOUT RIND AND SEEDS
ANALYSIS OF 426 GRAMS WHICH IS 1/16 OF 33 LB MELON

NUTRIENT	UNIT	AMOUNT	INQ	% STD
ENERGY	KCAL	110.00	1.00	6
VITAMIN A	IU	2510.00	11.41	63
VITAMIN C	MG	30.00	9.09	50
THIAMIN	MG	0.13	2.36	13
RIBOFLAVN	MG	0.13	1.97	11
NIACIN	MG	0.90	1.17	6
IRON	MG	2.10	2.39	13
CALCIUM	MG	30.00	0.61	3
PHOSPHRUS	MG	43.00	0.87	5
POTASSIUM	MG	426.00	1.55	9
PROTEIN	G	2.00	0.73	4
CARBOHYDT	G	27.00	1.79	10
FAT	G	1.00	0.23	1
OLEIC A	G	0.00	0.00	0
LINOL A	G	0.00	0.00	0
SAT FAT A	G	0.00	0.00	0

319 BAGEL, MADE WITH EGG
ANALYSIS OF 55 GRAMS WHICH IS 1--3-IN DIAM.

NUTRIENT	UNIT	AMOUNT	INQ	% STD
ENERGY	KCAL	165.00	1.00	8
VITAMIN A	IU	30.00	0.09	1
VITAMIN C	MG	0.00	0.00	0
THIAMIN	MG	0.14	1.70	14
RIBOFLAVN	MG	0.10	1.01	8
NIACIN	MG	1.20	1.04	9
IRON	MG	1.20	0.91	7
CALCIUM	MG	9.00	0.12	1
PHOSPHRUS	MG	43.00	0.58	5
POTASSIUM	MG	41.00	0.10	1
PROTEIN	G	6.00	1.45	12
CARBOHYDT	G	28.00	1.23	10
FAT	G	2.00	0.31	3
OLEIC A	G	0.90	0.45	4
LINOL A	G	0.80	0.48	4
SAT FAT A	G	0.50	0.21	2

320 BAGEL, MADE WITH WATER
ANALYSIS OF 55 GRAMS WHICH IS 1--3-IN DIAM.

NUTRIENT	UNIT	AMOUNT	INQ	% STD
ENERGY	KCAL	165.00	1.00	8
VITAMIN A	IU	0.00	0.00	0
VITAMIN C	MG	0.00	0.00	0
THIAMIN	MG	0.15	1.82	15
RIBOFLAVN	MG	0.11	1.11	9
NIACIN	MG	1.40	1.21	10
IRON	MG	1.20	0.91	7
CALCIUM	MG	8.00	0.11	1
PHOSPHRUS	MG	41.00	0.55	5
POTASSIUM	MG	42.00	0.10	1
PROTEIN	G	6.00	1.45	12
CARBOHYDT	G	30.00	1.32	11
FAT	G	1.00	0.16	1
OLEIC A	G	0.40	0.20	2
LINOL A	G	0.60	0.36	3
SAT FAT A	G	0.20	0.09	1

321 BARLEY, PEARLED, UNCOOKED
ANALYSIS OF 200 GRAMS WHICH IS 1 CUP

NUTRIENT	UNIT	AMOUNT	INQ	% STD
ENERGY	KCAL	700.00	1.00	35
VITAMIN A	IU	0.00	0.00	0
VITAMIN C	MG	0.00	0.00	0
THIAMIN	MG	0.24	0.69	24
RIBOFLAVN	MG	0.10	0.24	8
NIACIN	MG	6.20	1.27	44
IRON	MG	4.00	0.71	25
CALCIUM	MG	32.00	0.10	4
PHOSPHRUS	MG	378.00	1.20	42
POTASSIUM	MG	320.00	0.18	6
PROTEIN	G	16.00	0.91	32
CARBOHYDT	G	158.00	1.64	57
FAT	G	2.00	0.07	3
OLEIC A	G	0.20	0.02	1
LINOL A	G	0.80	0.11	4
SAT FAT A	G	0.30	0.03	1

322 BISCUITS, BAKING POWDER, HOME RECIPE
ANALYSIS OF 28 GRAMS WHICH IS 2-IN DIAM. BISCUIT

NUTRIENT	UNIT	AMOUNT	INQ	% STD
ENERGY	KCAL	105.00	1.00	5
VITAMIN A	IU	0.00	0.00	0
VITAMIN C	MG	0.00	0.00	0
THIAMIN	MG	0.08	1.52	8
RIBOFLAVN	MG	0.08	1.27	7
NIACIN	MG	0.70	0.95	5
IRON	MG	0.40	0.48	3
CALCIUM	MG	34.00	0.72	4
PHOSPHRUS	MG	49.00	1.04	5
POTASSIUM	MG	33.00	0.13	1
PROTEIN	G	2.00	0.76	4
CARBOHYDT	G	13.00	0.90	5
FAT	G	5.00	1.22	6
OLEIC A	G	2.00	1.55	8
LINOL A	G	1.20	1.14	6
SAT FAT A	G	1.20	0.80	4

323 BISCUITS, BAKING POWDER, MADE FROM MIX
ANALYSIS OF 28 GRAMS WHICH IS 2-IN DIAM. BISCUIT

```
                                          0        10        20        30        40        50        60        70        80        90       100
                                                                                                                                        *****************
```

NUTRIENT	UNIT	AMOUNT	INQ	% STD	
ENERGY	KCAL	90.00	1.00	5	
VITAMIN A	IU	0.00	0.00	0	EEEE
VITAMIN C	MG	0.00	0.00	0	-	
THIAMIN	MG	0.09	2.00	9	TTT|TTT
RIBOFLAVN	MG	0.08	1.48	7	RRRIR
NIACIN	MG	0.80	1.27	6	NNNIN
IRON	MG	0.60	0.83	4	III|
CALCIUM	MG	19.00	0.47	2	KK	
PHOSPHRUS	MG	65.00	1.60	7	XXXIXX
POTASSIUM	MG	32.00	0.14	1	Y	
PROTEIN	G	2.00	0.89	4	PPPI
CARBOHYDT	G	15.00	1.21	5	HHHH
FAT	G	3.00	0.85	4	FFFI
OLEIC A	G	1.10	1.00	4	OOOO
LINOL A	G	0.70	0.78	4	LLLI
SAT FAT A	G	0.60	0.47	2	SS	

```
*************************************************
```

324 BREADCRUMBS (ENRICHED), DRY, GRATED
ANALYSIS OF 100 GRAMS WHICH IS 1CUP

```
                                          0        10        20        30        40        50        60        70        80        90       100
                                                                                                                                        *****************
```

NUTRIENT	UNIT	AMOUNT	INQ	% STD	
ENERGY	KCAL	390.00	1.00	20	EEEEEEEEEEEEEE
VITAMIN A	IU	0.00	0.00	0	-	
VITAMIN C	MG	0.00	0.00	0	-	
THIAMIN	MG	0.35	1.79	35	TTTTTTTTTTTTTTT|TTTTTTTTTTTTT
RIBOFLAVN	MG	0.35	1.50	29	RRRRRRRRRRRRRR|RRRRRRRRR
NIACIN	MG	4.80	1.76	34	NNNNNNNNNNNNNNN|NNNNNNNNNNN
IRON	MG	3.60	1.15	23	IIIIIIIIIIIIIIII|II
CALCIUM	MG	122.00	0.70	14	KKKKKKKKKKK
PHOSPHRUS	MG	141.00	0.80	16	XXXXXXXXXXXX
POTASSIUM	MG	152.00	0.16	3	YY	
PROTEIN	G	13.00	1.33	26	PPPPPPPPPPPPPP|PPPP
CARBOHYDT	G	73.00	1.36	27	HHHHHHHHHHHHHH|HHHH
FAT	G	5.00	0.33	6	FFFFF
OLEIC A	G	1.60	0.33	7	OOOOO
LINOL A	G	1.40	0.36	7	LLLLLL
SAT FAT A	G	1.00	0.18	4	SSS	

```
*************************************************
```

325 BOSTON BROWN BREAD, CANNED
ANALYSIS OF 45 GRAMS WHICH IS 1--3 1/4 BY 1/2 IN. SLICE

NUTRIENT	UNIT	AMOUNT	INQ	% STD
ENERGY	KCAL	95.00	1.00	5
VITAMIN A	IU	0.00	0.00	0
VITAMIN C	MG	0.00	0.00	0
THIAMIN	MG	0.06	1.26	6
RIBOFLAVN	MG	0.04	0.70	3
NIACIN	MG	0.70	1.05	5
IRON	MG	0.90	1.18	6
CALCIUM	MG	41.00	0.96	5
PHOSPHRUS	MG	72.00	1.68	8
POTASSIUM	MG	131.00	0.55	3
PROTEIN	G	2.00	0.84	4
CARBOHYDT	G	21.00	1.61	8
FAT	G	1.00	0.27	1
OLEIC A	G	0.20	0.17	1
LINOL A	G	0.20	0.21	1
SAT FAT A	G	0.10	0.07	0

326 CRACKED-WHEAT BREAD
ANALYSIS OF 454 GRAMS WHICH IS 1 LB LOAF

NUTRIENT	UNIT	AMOUNT	INQ	% STD
ENERGY	KCAL	1195.00	1.00	60
VITAMIN A	IU	0.00	0.00	0
VITAMIN C	MG	0.00	0.00	0
THIAMIN	MG	1.52	2.54	152
RIBOFLAVN	MG	1.13	1.58	94
NIACIN	MG	14.40	1.72	103
IRON	MG	9.50	0.99	59
CALCIUM	MG	399.00	0.74	44
PHOSPHRUS	MG	581.00	1.08	65
POTASSIUM	MG	608.00	0.20	12
PROTEIN	G	39.00	1.31	78
CARBOHYDT	G	236.00	1.44	86
FAT	G	10.00	0.21	13
OLEIC A	G	3.00	0.20	12
LINOL A	G	3.90	0.33	20
SAT FAT A	G	2.20	0.13	8

327 CRACKED-WHEAT BREAD
ANALYSIS OF 25 GRAMS WHICH IS 1 SLICE (18 PER 1LB LOAF)

NUTRIENT	UNIT	AMOUNT	INQ	% STD
ENERGY	KCAL	65.00	1.00	3
VITAMIN A	IU	0.00	0.00	0
VITAMIN C	MG	0.00	0.00	0
THIAMIN	MG	0.08	2.46	8
RIBOFLAVN	MG	0.06	1.54	5
NIACIN	MG	0.80	1.76	6
IRON	MG	0.50	0.96	3
CALCIUM	MG	22.00	0.75	2
PHOSPHRUS	MG	32.00	1.09	4
POTASSIUM	MG	34.00	0.21	1
PROTEIN	G	2.00	1.23	4
CARBOHYDT	G	13.00	1.45	5
FAT	G	1.00	0.39	1
OLEIC A	G	0.20	0.25	1
LINOL A	G	0.20	0.31	1
SAT FAT A	G	0.10	0.11	0

328 FRENCH OR VIENNA BREAD
ANALYSIS OF 454 GRAMS WHICH IS 1 LB LOAF

NUTRIENT	UNIT	AMOUNT	INQ	% STD
ENERGY	KCAL	1315.00	1.00	66
VITAMIN A	IU	0.00	0.00	0
VITAMIN C	MG	0.00	0.00	0
THIAMIN	MG	1.80	2.74	180
RIBOFLAVN	MG	1.10	1.39	92
NIACIN	MG	15.00	1.63	107
IRON	MG	10.00	0.95	63
CALCIUM	MG	195.00	0.33	22
PHOSPHRUS	MG	386.00	0.65	43
POTASSIUM	MG	408.00	0.12	8
PROTEIN	G	41.00	1.25	82
CARBOHYDT	G	251.00	1.39	91
FAT	G	14.00	0.27	18
OLEIC A	G	4.70	0.29	19
LINOL A	G	4.60	0.35	23
SAT FAT A	G	3.20	0.17	11

329 FRENCH BREAD
ANALYSIS OF 35 GRAMS WHICH IS 5 BY 2 1/2 BY 1 IN SLICE

NUTRIENT	UNIT	AMOUNT	INQ	% STD	0	10	20	30	40	50	60	70	80	90	100
ENERGY	KCAL	100.00	1.00	5	EEEE										*
VITAMIN A	IU	0.00	0.00	0	-										*
VITAMIN C	MG	0.00	0.00	0	-										*
THIAMIN	MG	0.14	2.80	14	TTT|TTTTTT										*
RIBOFLAVN	MG	0.08	1.33	7	RRR|R										*
NIACIN	MG	1.20	1.71	9	NNN|NNN										*
IRON	MG	0.80	1.00	5	IIII										*
CALCIUM	MG	15.00	0.33	2	K										*
PHOSPHRUS	MG	30.00	0.67	3	XXX|										*
POTASSIUM	MG	32.00	0.13	1	Y|										*
PROTEIN	G	3.00	1.20	6	PPP|P										*
CARBOHYDT	G	19.00	1.38	7	HHH|HH										*
FAT	G	1.00	0.26	1	F										*
OLEIC A	G	0.40	0.33	2	O										*
LINOL A	G	0.40	0.40	2	LL										*
SAT FAT A	G	0.20	0.14	1	S										*

330 VIENNA BREAD
ANALYSIS OF 25 GRAMS WHICH IS 4 3/4 BY 4 BY 1/2 IN SLICE

NUTRIENT	UNIT	AMOUNT	INQ	% STD	0	10	20	30	40	50	60	70	80	90	100
ENERGY	KCAL	75.00	1.00	4	EEE										*
VITAMIN A	IU	0.00	0.00	0	-										*
VITAMIN C	MG	0.00	0.00	0	-										*
THIAMIN	MG	0.10	2.67	10	TT|TTTTT										*
RIBOFLAVN	MG	0.06	1.33	6	RR|R										*
NIACIN	MG	0.80	1.52	6	NN|NN										*
IRON	MG	0.60	1.00	4	III										*
CALCIUM	MG	11.00	0.33	1	K										*
PHOSPHRUS	MG	21.00	0.62	2	XX|										*
POTASSIUM	MG	23.00	0.12	0	-|										*
PROTEIN	G	2.00	1.07	4	PPP										*
CARBOHYDT	G	14.00	1.36	5	HH|H										*
FAT	G	1.00	0.34	1	F										*
OLEIC A	G	0.30	0.33	1	O										*
LINOL A	G	0.40	0.40	2	L|										*
SAT FAT A	G	0.20	0.19	1	S										*

331 ITALIAN BREAD
ANALYSIS OF 454 GRAMS WHICH IS 1 LB LOAF

NUTRIENT	UNIT	AMOUNT	INQ	% STD
ENERGY	KCAL	1250.00	1.00	63
VITAMIN A	IU	0.00	0.00	0
VITAMIN C	MG	0.00	0.00	0
THIAMIN	MG	1.80	2.88	180
RIBOFLAVN	MG	1.10	1.47	92
NIACIN	MG	15.00	1.71	107
IRON	MG	10.00	1.00	63
CALCIUM	MG	77.00	0.14	9
PHOSPHRUS	MG	349.00	0.62	39
POTASSIUM	MG	336.00	0.11	7
PROTEIN	G	41.00	1.31	82
CARBOHYDT	G	256.00	1.49	93
FAT	G	4.00	0.08	5
OLEIC A	G	0.30	0.02	1
LINOL A	G	1.50	0.12	8
SAT FAT A	G	0.60	0.03	2

Scale: 0 10 20 30 40 50 60 70 80 90 100
(THIAMIN ∗180, NIACIN ∗107)

332 ITALIAN BREAD
ANALYSIS OF 30 GRAMS WHICH IS 4 1/2 BY 3 1/4 BY 3/4 IN SLICE

NUTRIENT	UNIT	AMOUNT	INQ	% STD
ENERGY	KCAL	85.00	1.00	4
VITAMIN A	IU	0.00	0.00	0
VITAMIN C	MG	0.00	0.00	0
THIAMIN	MG	0.12	2.82	12
RIBOFLAVN	MG	0.07	1.37	6
NIACIN	MG	1.00	1.68	7
IRON	MG	0.70	1.03	4
CALCIUM	MG	5.00	0.13	1
PHOSPHRUS	MG	23.00	0.60	3
POTASSIUM	MG	22.00	0.10	0
PROTEIN	G	3.00	1.41	6
CARBOHYDT	G	17.00	1.45	6
FAT	G	0.00	0.00	0
OLEIC A	G	0.00	0.00	0
LINOL A	G	0.10	0.12	1
SAT FAT A	G	0.00	0.00	0

Scale: 0 10 20 30 40 50 60 70 80 90 100

333 RAISIN BREAD
ANALYSIS OF 454 GRAMS WHICH IS 1 LB LOAF

NUTRIENT	UNIT	AMOUNT	INQ	% STD
ENERGY	KCAL	1190.00	1.00	59
VITAMIN A	IU	0.00	0.00	0
VITAMIN C	MG	0.00	0.00	0
THIAMIN	MG	1.70	2.86	170
RIBOFLAVN	MG	1.07	1.50	89
NIACIN	MG	10.70	1.28	76
IRON	MG	10.00	1.05	63
CALCIUM	MG	322.00	0.60	36
PHOSPHRUS	MG	395.00	0.74	44
POTASSIUM	MG	1057.00	0.36	21
PROTEIN	G	30.00	1.01	60
CARBOHYDT	G	243.00	1.49	88
FAT	G	13.00	0.28	17
OLEIC A	G	4.70	0.32	19
LINOL A	G	3.90	0.33	20
SAT FAT A	G	3.00	0.18	11

334 RAISIN BREAD
ANALYSIS OF 25 GRAMS WHICH IS 1 SLICE (18 PER 1LB LOAF)

NUTRIENT	UNIT	AMOUNT	INQ	% STD
ENERGY	KCAL	65.00	1.00	3
VITAMIN A	IU	0.00	0.00	0
VITAMIN C	MG	0.00	0.00	0
THIAMIN	MG	0.09	2.77	9
RIBOFLAVN	MG	0.06	1.54	5
NIACIN	MG	0.60	1.32	4
IRON	MG	0.60	1.15	4
CALCIUM	MG	18.00	0.62	2
PHOSPHRUS	MG	22.00	0.75	2
POTASSIUM	MG	58.00	0.36	1
PROTEIN	G	2.00	1.23	4
CARBOHYDT	G	13.00	1.45	5
FAT	G	1.00	0.39	1
OLEIC A	G	0.30	0.38	1
LINOL A	G	0.20	0.31	1
SAT FAT A	G	0.20	0.22	1

335 RYE BREAD, AMERICAN, LIGHT
ANALYSIS OF 454 GRAMS WHICH IS 1 LB LOAF

NUTRIENT	UNIT	AMOUNT	INQ	% STD	0 10 20 30 40 50 60 70 80 90 100
ENERGY	KCAL	1100.00	1.00	55	EEEEEEEEEEEEEEEEEEEEEEEEEEEEEEEEEEEEEEEEEEEEEEEEEEEEEEEE *
VITAMIN A	IU	0.00	0.00	0	- *
VITAMIN C	MG	0.00	0.00	0	- *
THIAMIN	MG	1.35	2.45	135	TTTTTTTTTTTTTTTTTTTTTTTTTTTTTTTTTTTTTTTTTTTTTTTTTTTTTTTTTTTTTTTTTTTTTTTTTTTTTTTTTTTTTTTTTTTTTTTTTTTTTTTTTTTTTTTTTTTTTTTTTTTTTTTTTTTT *135
RIBOFLAVN	MG	0.98	1.48	82	RRRRRRRRRRRRRRRRRRRRRRRRRRRRRRRRRRRRRRRRRRRRRRRRRRRRRRRRRRRRRRRRRRRRRRRRRRRRRRRRRRR *
NIACIN	MG	12.90	1.68	92	NNNNNNNNNNNNNNNNNNNNNNNNNNNNNNNNNNNNNNNNNNNNNNNNNNNNNNNNNNNNNNNNNNNNNNNNNNNNNNNNNNNNNNNNNNNN *
IRON	MG	9.10	1.03	57	IIIIIIIIIIIIIIIIIIIIIIIIIIIIIIIIIIIIIIIIIIIIIIIIIIIIIIIII *
CALCIUM	MG	340.00	0.69	38	KKKKKKKKKKKKKKKKKKKKKKKKKKKKKKKKKKKKKK *
PHOSPHRUS	MG	667.00	1.35	74	XXXXXXXXXXXXXXXXXXXXXXXXXXXXXXXXXXXXXXXXXXXXXXXXXXXXXXXXXXXXXXXXXXXXXXXXXXXX *
POTASSIUM	MG	658.00	0.24	13	YYYYYYYYYYYYY *
PROTEIN	G	41.00	1.49	82	PPPPPPPPPPPPPPPPPPPPPPPPPPPPPPPPPPPPPPPPPPPPPPPPPPPPPPPPPPPPPPPPPPPPPPPPPPPPPPPPPPPP *
CARBOHYDT	G	236.00	1.56	86	HHHHHHHHHHHHHHHHHHHHHHHHHHHHHHHHHHHHHHHHHHHHHHHHHHHHHHHHHHHHHHHHHHHHHHHHHHHHHHHHHHHHHHHH *
FAT	G	5.00	0.12	6	FFFF *
OLEIC A	G	0.50	0.04	2	OO *
LINOL A	G	2.20	0.20	11	LLLLLLLLL *
SAT FAT A	G	0.70	0.04	2	SS *

****

336 RYE BREAD, AMERICAN, LIGHT
ANALYSIS OF 25 GRAMS WHICH IS 5 BY 4 BY 3/8 IN SLICE

NUTRIENT	UNIT	AMOUNT	INQ	% STD	0 10 20 30 40 50 60 70 80 90 100
ENERGY	KCAL	60.00	1.00	3	EE *
VITAMIN A	IU	0.00	0.00	0	- I *
VITAMIN C	MG	0.00	0.00	0	- I *
THIAMIN	MG	0.07	2.33	7	TITTTT *
RIBOFLAVN	MG	0.05	1.39	4	RIR *
NIACIN	MG	0.70	1.67	5	NNN *
IRON	MG	0.50	1.04	3	III *
CALCIUM	MG	19.00	0.70	2	KK *
PHOSPHRUS	MG	37.00	1.37	4	XIX *
POTASSIUM	MG	36.00	0.24	1	YI *
PROTEIN	G	2.00	1.33	4	PIP *
CARBOHYDT	G	13.00	1.58	5	HIHH *
FAT	G	0.00	0.00	0	- I *
OLEIC A	G	0.00	0.00	0	- I *
LINOL A	G	0.10	0.17	1	- I *
SAT FAT A	G	0.00	0.00	0	- I *

****

337 RYE BREAD, PUMPERNICKEL
ANALYSIS OF 454 GRAMS WHICH IS 1 LB LOAF

NUTRIENT	UNIT	AMOUNT	INQ	% STD
ENERGY	KCAL	1115.00	1.00	56
VITAMIN A	IU	0.00	0.00	0
VITAMIN C	MG	0.00	0.00	0
THIAMIN	MG	1.30	2.33	130
RIBOFLAVN	MG	0.93	1.39	78
NIACIN	MG	8.50	1.09	61
IRON	MG	11.80	1.32	74
CALCIUM	MG	381.00	0.76	42
PHOSPHRUS	MG	1039.00	2.07	115
POTASSIUM	MG	2059.00	0.74	41
PROTEIN	G	41.00	1.47	82
CARBOHYDT	G	241.00	1.57	88
FAT	G	5.00	0.11	6
OLEIC A	G	0.50	0.04	2
LINOL A	G	2.40	0.22	12
SAT FAT A	G	0.70	0.04	2

338 RYE BREAD, PUMPERNICKEL
ANALYSIS OF 32 GRAMS WHICH IS 5 BY 4 BY 3/8 IN SLICE

NUTRIENT	UNIT	AMOUNT	INQ	% STD
ENERGY	KCAL	80.00	1.00	4
VITAMIN A	IU	0.00	0.00	0
VITAMIN C	MG	0.00	0.00	0
THIAMIN	MG	0.09	2.25	9
RIBOFLAVN	MG	0.07	1.46	6
NIACIN	MG	0.60	1.07	4
IRON	MG	0.80	1.25	5
CALCIUM	MG	27.00	0.75	3
PHOSPHRUS	MG	73.00	2.03	8
POTASSIUM	MG	145.00	0.73	3
PROTEIN	G	3.00	1.50	6
CARBOHYDT	G	17.00	1.55	6
FAT	G	0.00	0.00	0
OLEIC A	G	0.00	0.00	0
LINOL A	G	0.20	0.25	1
SAT FAT A	G	0.10	0.09	0

339 WHITE BREAD, SOFT-CRUMB TYPE
ANALYSIS OF 454 GRAMS WHICH IS 1 LB LOAF

NUTRIENT	UNIT	AMOUNT	INQ	% STD
ENERGY	KCAL	1225.00	1.00	61
VITAMIN A	IU	0.00	0.00	0
VITAMIN C	MG	0.00	0.00	0
THIAMIN	MG	1.80	2.94	180
RIBOFLAVN	MG	1.10	1.50	92
NIACIN	MG	15.00	1.75	107
IRON	MG	11.30	1.15	71
CALCIUM	MG	381.00	0.69	42
PHOSPHRUS	MG	440.00	0.80	49
POTASSIUM	MG	476.00	0.16	10
PROTEIN	G	39.00	1.27	78
CARBOHYDT	G	229.00	1.36	83
FAT	G	15.00	0.31	19
OLEIC A	G	5.30	0.35	22
LINOL A	G	4.60	0.38	23
SAT FAT A	G	3.40	0.19	12

340 WHITE BREAD, SOFT-CRUMB TYPE
ANALYSIS OF 25 GRAMS WHICH IS 1 SLICE (18 PER 1LB LOAF)

NUTRIENT	UNIT	AMOUNT	INQ	% STD
ENERGY	KCAL	70.00	1.00	4
VITAMIN A	IU	0.00	0.00	0
VITAMIN C	MG	0.00	0.00	0
THIAMIN	MG	0.10	2.86	10
RIBOFLAVN	MG	0.06	1.43	5
NIACIN	MG	0.80	1.63	6
IRON	MG	0.60	1.07	4
CALCIUM	MG	21.00	0.67	2
PHOSPHRUS	MG	24.00	0.76	3
POTASSIUM	MG	26.00	0.15	1
PROTEIN	G	2.00	1.14	4
CARBOHYDT	G	13.00	1.35	5
FAT	G	1.00	0.37	1
OLEIC A	G	0.30	0.35	1
LINOL A	G	0.30	0.43	2
SAT FAT A	G	0.20	0.20	1

```
341 WHITE BREAD, SOFT-CRUMB TYPE, TOASTED
ANALYSIS OF 22 GRAMS WHICH IS 1 SLICE (18 PER 1LB LOAF)

NUTRIENT   UNIT  AMOUNT   INQ  % STD  0        10   20   30   40   50   60   70   80   90   100
ENERGY     KCAL   70.00  1.00    4    EEE                                                   *
VITAMIN A  IU      0.00  0.00    0    - I                                                   *
VITAMIN C  MG      0.00  0.00    0    - I                                                   *
THIAMIN    MG      0.08  2.29    8    TTITTT                                                *
RIBOFLAVN  MG      0.06  1.43    5    RRIR                                                  *
NIACIN     MG      0.80  1.63    6    NNINN                                                 *
IRON       MG      0.60  1.07    4    III                                                   *
CALCIUM    MG     21.00  0.67    2    KKI                                                   *
PHOSPHRUS  MG     24.00  0.76    3    XXI                                                   *
POTASSIUM  MG     26.00  0.15    1    - I                                                   *
PROTEIN    G       2.00  1.14    4    PPP                                                   *
CARBOHYDT  G      13.00  1.35    5    HHIH                                                  *
FAT        G       1.00  0.37    1    F                                                     *
OLEIC A    G       0.30  0.35    1    O I                                                   *
LINOL A    G       0.30  0.43    2    L I                                                   *
SAT FAT A  G       0.20  0.20    1    S I                                                   *
********************************************
```

```
342 WHITE BREAD, SOFT-CRUMB TYPE
ANALYSIS OF 20 GRAMS WHICH IS 1 SLICE (22 PER 1LB LOAF)

NUTRIENT   UNIT  AMOUNT   INQ  % STD  0        10   20   30   40   50   60   70   80   90   100
ENERGY     KCAL   55.00  1.00    3    EE                                                    *
VITAMIN A  IU      0.00  0.00    0    - I                                                   *
VITAMIN C  MG      0.00  0.00    0    - I                                                   *
THIAMIN    MG      0.08  2.91    8    TITTTT                                                *
RIBOFLAVN  MG      0.05  1.52    4    RIR                                                   *
NIACIN     MG      0.70  1.82    5    NINN                                                  *
IRON       MG      0.50  1.14    3    III                                                   *
CALCIUM    MG     17.00  0.69    2    KK                                                    *
PHOSPHRUS  MG     19.00  0.77    2    XX                                                    *
POTASSIUM  MG     21.00  0.15    0    - I                                                   *
PROTEIN    G       2.00  1.45    4    PIP                                                   *
CARBOHYDT  G      10.00  1.32    4    HIH                                                   *
FAT        G       1.00  0.47    1    FI                                                    *
OLEIC A    G       0.20  0.30    1    OI                                                    *
LINOL A    G       0.20  0.36    1    LI                                                    *
SAT FAT A  G       0.20  0.26    1    SI                                                    *
********************************************
```

343 WHITE BREAD, SOFT-CRUMB TYPE, TOASTED
ANALYSIS OF 17 GRAMS WHICH IS 1 SLICE (22 PER 1LB LOAF)

NUTRIENT	UNIT	AMOUNT	INQ	% STD
ENERGY	KCAL	55.00	1.00	3
VITAMIN A	IU	0.00	0.00	0
VITAMIN C	MG	0.00	0.00	0
THIAMIN	MG	0.06	2.18	6
RIBOFLAVN	MG	0.05	1.52	4
NIACIN	MG	0.70	1.82	5
IRON	MG	0.50	1.14	3
CALCIUM	MG	17.00	0.69	2
PHOSPHRUS	MG	19.00	0.77	2
POTASSIUM	MG	21.00	0.15	0
PROTEIN	G	2.00	1.45	4
CARBOHYDT	G	10.00	1.32	4
FAT	G	1.00	0.47	1
OLEIC A	G	0.20	0.30	1
LINOL A	G	0.20	0.36	1
SAT FAT A	G	0.20	0.26	1

344 WHITE BREAD, SOFT-CRUMB TYPE
ANALYSIS OF 680 GRAMS WHICH IS 1 1/2 LB LOAF

NUTRIENT	UNIT	AMOUNT	INQ	% STD
ENERGY	KCAL	1835.00	1.00	92
VITAMIN A	IU	0.00	0.00	0
VITAMIN C	MG	0.00	0.00	0
THIAMIN	MG	2.70	2.94	270
RIBOFLAVN	MG	1.65	1.50	138
NIACIN	MG	22.50	1.75	161
IRON	MG	17.00	1.16	106
CALCIUM	MG	571.00	0.69	63
PHOSPHRUS	MG	660.00	0.80	73
POTASSIUM	MG	714.00	0.16	14
PROTEIN	G	59.00	1.29	118
CARBOHYDT	G	343.00	1.36	125
FAT	G	22.00	0.31	28
OLEIC A	G	7.90	0.35	32
LINOL A	G	6.90	0.38	34
SAT FAT A	G	5.20	0.20	18

345 WHITE BREAD, SOFT-CRUMB TYPE
ANALYSIS OF 28 GRAMS WHICH IS 1 SLICE (24 PER 1 1/2 LB LOAF)

NUTRIENT	UNIT	AMOUNT	INQ	% STD	0 10 20 ... 100
ENERGY	KCAL	75.00	1.00	4	EEE
VITAMIN A	IU	0.00	0.00	0	-
VITAMIN C	MG	0.00	0.00	0	-
THIAMIN	MG	0.11	2.93	11	TT|TTTTT
RIBOFLAVN	MG	0.07	1.56	6	RR|RR
NIACIN	MG	0.90	1.71	6	NN|NN
IRON	MG	0.70	1.17	4	II|I
CALCIUM	MG	24.00	0.71	3	KK|
PHOSPHRUS	MG	27.00	0.80	3	XX|
POTASSIUM	MG	29.00	0.15	1	-|
PROTEIN	G	2.00	1.07	4	PPP
CARBOHYDT	G	14.00	1.36	5	HH|H
FAT	G	1.00	0.33	1	F|
OLEIC A	G	0.30	0.33	1	O|
LINOL A	G	0.30	0.40	2	L|
SAT FAT A	G	0.20	0.19	1	S|

346 WHITE BREAD, SOFT-CRUMB TYPE, TOASTED
ANALYSIS OF 24 GRAMS WHICH IS 1 SLICE (24 PER 1 1/2 LB LOAF)

NUTRIENT	UNIT	AMOUNT	INQ	% STD	0 10 20 ... 100
ENERGY	KCAL	75.00	1.00	4	EEE
VITAMIN A	IU	0.00	0.00	0	-
VITAMIN C	MG	0.00	0.00	0	-
THIAMIN	MG	0.09	2.40	9	TT|TTT
RIBOFLAVN	MG	0.07	1.56	6	RR|RR
NIACIN	MG	0.90	1.71	6	NN|NN
IRON	MG	0.70	1.17	4	II|I
CALCIUM	MG	24.00	0.71	3	KK|
PHOSPHRUS	MG	27.00	0.80	3	XX|
POTASSIUM	MG	29.00	0.15	1	-|
PROTEIN	G	2.00	1.07	4	PPP
CARBOHYDT	G	14.00	1.36	5	HH|H
FAT	G	1.00	0.34	1	F|
OLEIC A	G	0.30	0.33	1	O|
LINOL A	G	0.30	0.40	2	L|
SAT FAT A	G	0.20	0.19	1	S|

347 WHITE BREAD, SOFT-CRUMB TYPE
ANALYSIS OF 24 GRAMS WHICH IS 1 SLICE (28 PER 1 1/2 LB LOAF)

NUTRIENT	UNIT	AMOUNT	INQ	% STD	0	10	20	30	40	50	60	70	80	90	100
ENERGY	KCAL	65.00	1.00	3	EEE										
VITAMIN A	IU	0.00	0.00	0	-|										
VITAMIN C	MG	0.00	0.00	0	-|										
THIAMIN	MG	0.10	3.08	10	TT|TT|TT										
RIBOFLAVN	MG	0.06	1.54	5	RR|R										
NIACIN	MG	0.80	1.76	6	NN|NN										
IRON	MG	0.60	1.15	4	III										
CALCIUM	MG	20.00	0.68	2	KK|										
PHOSPHRUS	MG	23.00	0.79	3	XX|										
POTASSIUM	MG	25.00	0.15	1	-|										
PROTEIN	G	2.00	1.23	4	PPP										
CARBOHYDT	G	12.00	1.34	4	HHH										
FAT	G	1.00	0.39	1	F|										
OLEIC A	G	0.30	0.38	1	O|										
LINOL A	G	0.20	0.31	1	L|										
SAT FAT A	G	0.20	0.22	1	S|										

348 WHITE BREAD, SOFT-CRUMB TYPE, TOASTED
ANALYSIS OF 21 GRAMS WHICH IS 1 SLICE (28 PER 1 1/2 LB LOAF)

NUTRIENT	UNIT	AMOUNT	INQ	% STD	0	10	20	30	40	50	60	70	80	90	100
ENERGY	KCAL	65.00	1.00	3	EEE										
VITAMIN A	IU	0.00	0.00	0	-|										
VITAMIN C	MG	0.00	0.00	0	-|										
THIAMIN	MG	0.08	2.46	8	TT|TT										
RIBOFLAVN	MG	0.06	1.54	5	RR|R										
NIACIN	MG	0.80	1.76	6	NN|NN										
IRON	MG	0.60	1.15	4	III										
CALCIUM	MG	20.00	0.68	2	KK|										
PHOSPHRUS	MG	23.00	0.79	3	XX|										
POTASSIUM	MG	25.00	0.15	1	-|										
PROTEIN	G	2.00	1.23	4	PPP										
CARBOHYDT	G	12.00	1.34	4	HHH										
FAT	G	1.00	0.39	1	F|										
OLEIC A	G	0.30	0.38	1	O|										
LINOL A	G	0.20	0.31	1	L|										
SAT FAT A	G	0.20	0.22	1	S|										

349 WHITE BREAD, SOFT-CRUMB TYPE, CUBES
ANALYSIS OF 30 GRAMS WHICH IS 1 CUP

```
                                                       0        10        20        30        40        50        60        70        80        90       100
```

NUTRIENT	UNIT	AMOUNT	INQ	% STD	
ENERGY	KCAL	80.00	1.00	4	EEE
VITAMIN A	IU	0.00	0.00	0	-
VITAMIN C	MG	0.00	0.00	0	-
THIAMIN	MG	0.12	3.00	12	TTITTTTTT
RIBOFLAVN	MG	0.07	1.46	6	RRIRR
NIACIN	MG	1.00	1.79	7	NNINNN
IRON	MG	0.80	1.25	5	IIIII
CALCIUM	MG	25.00	0.69	3	KKI
PHOSPHRUS	MG	29.00	0.81	3	XXX
POTASSIUM	MG	32.00	0.16	1	Y
PROTEIN	G	3.00	1.50	6	PPIPP
CARBOHYDT	G	15.00	1.36	5	HHIH
FAT	G	1.00	0.32	1	F
OLEIC A	G	0.30	0.31	1	O
LINOL A	G	0.30	0.37	2	L
SAT FAT A	G	0.20	0.18	1	S

350 WHITE BREAD, SOFT-CRUMB TYPE, CRUMBS
ANALYSIS OF 45 GRAMS WHICH IS 1 CUP

```
                                                       0        10        20        30        40        50        60        70        80        90       100
```

NUTRIENT	UNIT	AMOUNT	INQ	% STD	
ENERGY	KCAL	120.00	1.00	6	EEEEE
VITAMIN A	IU	0.00	0.00	0	-
VITAMIN C	MG	0.00	0.00	0	-
THIAMIN	MG	0.18	3.00	18	TTTITTTTTTTT
RIBOFLAVN	MG	0.11	1.53	9	RRRRIRR
NIACIN	MG	1.50	1.79	11	NNNNINNNN
IRON	MG	1.10	1.15	7	IIIIII
CALCIUM	MG	38.00	0.70	4	KKK
PHOSPHRUS	MG	44.00	0.81	5	XXXXI
POTASSIUM	MG	47.00	0.16	1	Y
PROTEIN	G	4.00	1.33	8	PPPPIP
CARBOHYDT	G	23.00	1.39	8	HHHHIHH
FAT	G	1.00	0.21	1	F
OLEIC A	G	0.50	0.34	2	OO
LINOL A	G	0.50	0.42	3	LL
SAT FAT A	G	0.30	0.18	1	S

351 WHITE BREAD, FIRM-CRUMB TYPE
ANALYSIS OF 454 GRAMS WHICH IS 1 LB LOAF

NUTRIENT	UNIT	AMOUNT	INQ	% STD
ENERGY	KCAL	1245.00	1.00	62
VITAMIN A	IU	0.00	0.00	0
VITAMIN C	MG	0.00	0.00	0
THIAMIN	MG	1.80	2.89	180
RIBOFLAVN	MG	1.10	1.47	92
NIACIN	MG	15.00	1.72	107
IRON	MG	11.30	1.13	71
CALCIUM	MG	435.00	0.78	48
PHOSPHRUS	MG	463.00	0.83	51
POTASSIUM	MG	549.00	0.18	11
PROTEIN	G	41.00	1.32	82
CARBOHYDT	G	228.00	1.33	83
FAT	G	17.00	0.35	22
OLEIC A	G	5.90	0.39	24
LINOL A	G	5.20	0.42	26
SAT FAT A	G	3.90	0.22	14

352 WHITE BREAD, FIRM-CRUMB TYPE
ANALYSIS OF 23 GRAMS WHICH IS 1 SLICE (20 PER 1LB LOAF)

NUTRIENT	UNIT	AMOUNT	INQ	% STD
ENERGY	KCAL	65.00	1.00	3
VITAMIN A	IU	0.00	0.00	0
VITAMIN C	MG	0.00	0.00	0
THIAMIN	MG	0.09	2.77	9
RIBOFLAVN	MG	0.06	1.54	5
NIACIN	MG	0.80	1.76	6
IRON	MG	0.60	1.15	4
CALCIUM	MG	22.00	0.75	2
PHOSPHRUS	MG	23.00	0.79	3
POTASSIUM	MG	28.00	0.17	1
PROTEIN	G	2.00	1.23	4
CARBOHYDT	G	12.00	1.34	4
FAT	G	1.00	0.39	1
OLEIC A	G	0.30	0.38	1
LINOL A	G	0.30	0.46	2
SAT FAT A	G	0.20	0.22	1

353 WHITE BREAD, FIRM-CRUMB TYPE, TOASTED
ANALYSIS OF 20 GRAMS WHICH IS 1 SLICE (20 PER 1LB LOAF)

NUTRIENT	UNIT	AMOUNT	INQ	% STD
ENERGY	KCAL	65.00	1.00	3
VITAMIN A	IU	0.00	0.00	0
VITAMIN C	MG	0.00	0.00	0
THIAMIN	MG	0.07	2.15	7
RIBOFLAVN	MG	0.06	1.54	5
NIACIN	MG	0.80	1.76	6
IRON	MG	0.60	1.15	4
CALCIUM	MG	22.00	0.75	2
PHOSPHRUS	MG	23.00	0.79	3
POTASSIUM	MG	28.00	0.17	1
PROTEIN	G	2.00	1.23	4
CARBOHYDT	G	12.00	1.34	4
FAT	G	1.00	0.39	1
OLEIC A	G	0.30	0.38	1
LINOL A	G	0.30	0.46	2
SAT FAT A	G	0.20	0.22	1

```
        0    10   20   30   40   50   60   70   80   90   100
ENERGY    EEE
VITAMIN A - I
VITAMIN C - I
THIAMIN   TI|TTT
RIBOFLAVN RR|R
NIACIN    NN|NN
IRON      II|I
CALCIUM   KK|
PHOSPHRUS XX|
POTASSIUM - |
PROTEIN   PPP
CARBOHYDT HHH
FAT       F |
OLEIC A   O |
LINOL A   L |
SAT FAT A S |
**************
```

354 WHITE BREAD, FIRM-CRUMB TYPE
ANALYSIS OF 907 GRAMS WHICH IS 2 LB LOAF

NUTRIENT	UNIT	AMOUNT	INQ	% STD
ENERGY	KCAL	2495.00	1.00	125
VITAMIN A	IU	0.00	0.00	0
VITAMIN C	MG	0.00	0.00	0
THIAMIN	MG	3.60	2.89	360
RIBOFLAVN	MG	2.20	1.47	183
NIACIN	MG	30.00	1.72	214
IRON	MG	22.70	1.14	142
CALCIUM	MG	871.00	0.78	97
PHOSPHRUS	MG	925.00	0.82	103
POTASSIUM	MG	1097.00	0.18	22
PROTEIN	G	82.00	1.31	164
CARBOHYDT	G	455.00	1.33	165
FAT	G	34.00	0.35	44
OLEIC A	G	11.80	0.39	48
LINOL A	G	10.40	0.42	52
SAT FAT A	G	7.70	0.22	27

```
        0    10   20   30   40   50   60   70   80   90   100
ENERGY    EEEEEEEEEEEEEEEEEEEEEEEEEEEEEEEEEEEEEEEEEEEEEEEEEEEEEEEEEE * 125
VITAMIN A *
VITAMIN C *
THIAMIN   TTTTTTTTTTTTTTTTTTTTTTTTTTTTTTTTTTTTTTTTTTTTTTT * 360
RIBOFLAVN RRRRRRRRRRRRRRRRRRRRRRRRRRRRRRRRRRRRRRRRRRRRRRR * 183
NIACIN    NNNNNNNNNNNNNNNNNNNNNNNNNNNNNNNNNNNNNNNNNNNNNNN * 214
IRON      IIIIIIIIIIIIIIIIIIIIIIIIIIIIIIIIIIIIIIIIIIIIIII * 142
CALCIUM   KKKKKKKKKKKKKKKKKKKKKKKKKKKKKKKKKKKKKKKKKKK * 97
PHOSPHRUS XXXXXXXXXXXXXXXXXXXXXXXXXXXXXXXXXXXXXXXXXXXXXXX * 103
POTASSIUM YYYYYYYYYYYY * 22
PROTEIN   PPPPPPPPPPPPPPPPPPPPPPPPPPPPPPPPPPPPPPPPPPPPPPPPPPPPP * 164
CARBOHYDT HHHHHHHHHHHHHHHHHHHHHHHHHHHHHHHHHHHHHHHHHHHHHHHHHHHH * 165
FAT       FFFFFFFFFFFFFFFFFFFFFFFFFFFFFFF *
OLEIC A   OOOOOOOOOOOOOOOOOOOOOOOOOOOOOOOOO *
LINOL A   LLLLLLLLLLLLLLLLLLLLLLLLLLLLLLLLLLL *
SAT FAT A SSSSSSSSSSSSSSSSSS *
**************
```

355 WHITE BREAD, FIRM-CRUMB TYPE
ANALYSIS OF 27 GRAMS WHICH IS 1 SLICE (34 PER 2 LB LOAF)

NUTRIENT	UNIT	AMOUNT	INQ	% STD
ENERGY	KCAL	75.00	1.00	4
VITAMIN A	IU	0.00	0.00	0
VITAMIN C	MG	0.00	0.00	0
THIAMIN	MG	0.11	2.93	11
RIBOFLAVN	MG	0.06	1.33	5
NIACIN	MG	0.90	1.71	6
IRON	MG	0.70	1.17	4
CALCIUM	MG	26.00	0.77	3
PHOSPHRUS	MG	28.00	0.83	3
POTASSIUM	MG	33.00	0.18	1
PROTEIN	G	2.00	1.07	4
CARBOHYDT	G	14.00	1.36	5
FAT	G	1.00	0.34	1
OLEIC A	G	0.30	0.33	1
LINOL A	G	0.30	0.40	2
SAT FAT A	G	0.20	0.19	1

356 WHITE BREAD, FIRM-CRUMB TYPE, TOASTED
ANALYSIS OF 23 GRAMS WHICH IS 1 SLICE (34 PER 2 LB LOAF)

NUTRIENT	UNIT	AMOUNT	INQ	% STD
ENERGY	KCAL	75.00	1.00	4
VITAMIN A	IU	0.00	0.00	0
VITAMIN C	MG	0.00	0.00	0
THIAMIN	MG	0.09	2.40	9
RIBOFLAVN	MG	0.06	1.33	5
NIACIN	MG	0.90	1.71	6
IRON	MG	0.70	1.17	4
CALCIUM	MG	26.00	0.77	3
PHOSPHRUS	MG	28.00	0.83	3
POTASSIUM	MG	33.00	0.18	1
PROTEIN	G	2.00	1.07	4
CARBOHYDT	G	14.00	1.36	5
FAT	G	1.00	0.34	1
OLEIC A	G	0.30	0.33	1
LINOL A	G	0.30	0.40	2
SAT FAT A	G	0.20	0.19	1

357 WHOLE-WHEAT BREAD, SOFT-CRUMB TYPE
ANALYSIS OF 454 GRAMS WHICH IS 1 LB LOAF

NUTRIENT	UNIT	AMOUNT	INQ	% STD
ENERGY	KCAL	1095.00	1.00	55
VITAMIN A	IU	0.00	0.00	0
VITAMIN C	MG	0.00	0.00	0
THIAMIN	MG	1.37	2.50	137
RIBOFLAVN	MG	0.45	0.68	38
NIACIN	MG	12.70	1.66	91
IRON	MG	13.60	1.55	85
CALCIUM	MG	381.00	0.77	42
PHOSPHRUS	MG	1152.00	2.34	128
POTASSIUM	MG	1161.00	0.42	23
PROTEIN	G	41.00	1.50	82
CARBOHYDT	G	224.00	1.49	81
FAT	G	12.00	0.28	15
OLEIC A	G	2.90	0.22	12
LINOL A	G	4.20	0.38	21
SAT FAT A	G	2.20	0.14	8

358 WHOLE-WHEAT BREAD, SOFT-CRUMB TYPE
ANALYSIS OF 28 GRAMS WHICH IS 1 SLICE (16 PER 1 LB LOAF)

NUTRIENT	UNIT	AMOUNT	INQ	% STD
ENERGY	KCAL	65.00	1.00	3
VITAMIN A	IU	0.00	0.00	0
VITAMIN C	MG	0.00	0.00	0
THIAMIN	MG	0.09	2.77	9
RIBOFLAVN	MG	0.03	0.77	3
NIACIN	MG	0.80	1.76	6
IRON	MG	0.80	1.54	5
CALCIUM	MG	24.00	0.82	3
PHOSPHRUS	MG	71.00	2.43	8
POTASSIUM	MG	72.00	0.44	1
PROTEIN	G	3.00	1.85	6
CARBOHYDT	G	14.00	1.57	5
FAT	G	1.00	0.39	1
OLEIC A	G	0.20	0.25	1
LINOL A	G	0.20	0.31	1
SAT FAT A	G	0.10	0.11	0

359 WHOLE-WHEAT BREAD, SOFT-CRUMB TYPE, TOASTED
ANALYSIS OF 24 GRAMS WHICH IS 1 SLICE (16 PER 1 LB LOAF)

NUTRIENT	UNIT	AMOUNT	INQ	% STD
ENERGY	KCAL	65.00	1.00	3
VITAMIN A	IU	0.00	0.00	0
VITAMIN C	MG	0.00	0.00	0
THIAMIN	MG	0.07	2.15	7
RIBOFLAVN	MG	0.03	0.77	3
NIACIN	MG	0.80	1.76	6
IRON	MG	0.80	1.54	5
CALCIUM	MG	24.00	0.82	3
PHOSPHRUS	MG	71.00	2.43	8
POTASSIUM	MG	72.00	0.44	1
PROTEIN	G	3.00	1.85	6
CARBOHYDT	G	14.00	1.57	5
FAT	G	1.00	0.39	1
OLEIC A	G	0.20	0.25	1
LINOL A	G	0.20	0.31	1
SAT FAT A	G	0.10	0.11	0

360 WHOLE-WHEAT BREAD, FIRM-CRUMB TYPE
ANALYSIS OF 454 GRAMS WHICH IS 1 LB LOAF

NUTRIENT	UNIT	AMOUNT	INQ	% STD
ENERGY	KCAL	1100.00	1.00	55
VITAMIN A	IU	0.00	0.00	0
VITAMIN C	MG	0.00	0.00	0
THIAMIN	MG	1.17	2.13	117
RIBOFLAVN	MG	0.54	0.82	45
NIACIN	MG	12.70	1.65	91
IRON	MG	13.60	1.55	85
CALCIUM	MG	449.00	0.91	50
PHOSPHRUS	MG	1034.00	2.09	115
POTASSIUM	MG	1238.00	0.45	25
PROTEIN	G	48.00	1.75	96
CARBOHYDT	G	216.00	1.43	79
FAT	G	14.00	0.33	18
OLEIC A	G	3.30	0.24	13
LINOL A	G	4.90	0.45	24
SAT FAT A	G	2.50	0.16	9

361 WHOLE-WHEAT BREAD, FIRM-CRUMB TYPE
ANALYSIS OF 25 GRAMS WHICH IS 1 SLICE (18 PER 1 LB LOAF)

NUTRIENT	UNIT	AMOUNT	INQ	% STD
ENERGY	KCAL	60.00	1.00	3
VITAMIN A	IU	0.00	0.00	0
VITAMIN C	MG	0.00	0.00	0
THIAMIN	MG	0.06	2.00	6
RIBOFLAVN	MG	0.03	0.83	3
NIACIN	MG	0.70	1.67	5
IRON	MG	0.80	1.67	5
CALCIUM	MG	25.00	0.93	3
PHOSPHRUS	MG	57.00	2.11	6
POTASSIUM	MG	68.00	0.45	1
PROTEIN	G	3.00	2.00	6
CARBOHYDT	G	12.00	1.45	4
FAT	G	1.00	0.43	1
OLEIC A	G	0.20	0.27	1
LINOL A	G	0.30	0.50	2
SAT FAT A	G	0.10	0.12	0

362 WHOLE-WHEAT BREAD, FIRM-CRUMB TYPE, TOASTED
ANALYSIS OF 21 GRAMS WHICH IS 1 SLICE (18 PER 1 LB LOAF)

NUTRIENT	UNIT	AMOUNT	INQ	% STD
ENERGY	KCAL	60.00	1.00	3
VITAMIN A	IU	0.00	0.00	0
VITAMIN C	MG	0.00	0.00	0
THIAMIN	MG	0.05	1.67	5
RIBOFLAVN	MG	0.03	0.83	3
NIACIN	MG	0.70	1.67	5
IRON	MG	0.80	1.67	5
CALCIUM	MG	25.00	0.93	3
PHOSPHRUS	MG	57.00	2.11	6
POTASSIUM	MG	68.00	0.45	1
PROTEIN	G	3.00	2.00	6
CARBOHYDT	G	12.00	1.45	4
FAT	G	1.00	0.43	1
OLEIC A	G	0.20	0.27	1
LINOL A	G	0.30	0.50	2
SAT FAT A	G	0.10	0.12	0

363 CORN GRITS, COOKED, ENRICHED
ANALYSIS OF 245 GRAMS WHICH IS 1 CUP

NUTRIENT	UNIT	AMOUNT	INQ	% STD	0
ENERGY	KCAL	125.00	1.00	6	EEEEE
VITAMIN A	IU	0.00	0.00	0	-
VITAMIN C	MG	0.00	0.00	0	-
THIAMIN	MG	0.10	1.60	10	TTTTITTT
RIBOFLAVN	MG	0.07	0.93	6	RRRRR
NIACIN	MG	1.00	1.14	7	NNNNIN
IRON	MG	0.70	0.70	4	IIIII
CALCIUM	MG	2.00	0.04	0	-
PHOSPHRUS	MG	25.00	0.44	3	XX
POTASSIUM	MG	27.00	0.09	1	-
PROTEIN	G	3.00	0.96	6	PPPPP
CARBOHYDT	G	27.00	1.57	10	HHHHIHHH
FAT	G	0.00	0.00	0	-
OLEIC A	G	0.00	0.00	0	-
LINOL A	G	0.10	0.08	1	-
SAT FAT A	G	0.00	0.00	0	-

364 CORN GRITS, COOKED, UNENRICHED
ANALYSIS OF 245 GRAMS WHICH IS 1 CUP

NUTRIENT	UNIT	AMOUNT	INQ	% STD	0
ENERGY	KCAL	125.00	1.00	6	EEEEE
VITAMIN A	IU	0.00	0.00	0	-
VITAMIN C	MG	0.00	0.00	0	-
THIAMIN	MG	0.05	0.80	5	TTTTI
RIBOFLAVN	MG	0.02	0.27	2	R
NIACIN	MG	0.50	0.57	4	NNN
IRON	MG	0.20	0.20	1	I
CALCIUM	MG	2.00	0.04	0	-
PHOSPHRUS	MG	25.00	0.44	3	XX
POTASSIUM	MG	27.00	0.09	1	-
PROTEIN	G	3.00	0.96	6	PPPPP
CARBOHYDT	G	27.00	1.57	10	HHHHIHHH
FAT	G	0.00	0.00	0	-
OLEIC A	G	0.00	0.00	0	-
LINOL A	G	0.10	0.08	1	-
SAT FAT A	G	0.00	0.00	0	-

365 FARINA, QUICK-COOKING, ENRICHED, COOKED
ANALYSIS OF 245 GRAMS WHICH IS 1 CUP

NUTRIENT	UNIT	AMOUNT	INQ	% STD	0 10 20 ... 100
ENERGY	KCAL	105.00	1.00	5	EEEE
VITAMIN A	IU	0.00	0.00	0	-
VITAMIN C	MG	0.00	0.00	0	-
THIAMIN	MG	0.12	2.29	12	TTTITTTTTT
RIBOFLAVN	MG	0.07	1.11	6	RRRIR
NIACIN	MG	1.00	1.36	7	NNNINN
IRON	MG	0.00	0.00	0	-
CALCIUM	MG	147.00	3.11	16	KKKIKKKKKKKK
PHOSPHRUS	MG	113.00	2.39	13	XXXIXXXXXX
POTASSIUM	MG	25.00	0.10	1	-
PROTEIN	G	3.00	1.14	6	PPPIP
CARBOHYDT	G	22.00	1.52	8	HHHIHH
FAT	G	0.00	0.00	0	-
OLEIC A	G	0.00	0.00	0	-
LINOL A	G	0.10	0.10	1	-
SAT FAT A	G	0.00	0.00	0	-

366 OATMEAL OR ROLLED OATS, COOKED
ANALYSIS OF 240 GRAMS WHICH IS 1 CUP

NUTRIENT	UNIT	AMOUNT	INQ	% STD	0 10 20 ... 100
ENERGY	KCAL	130.00	1.00	7	EEEE
VITAMIN A	IU	0.00	0.00	0	-
VITAMIN C	MG	0.00	0.00	0	-
THIAMIN	MG	0.19	2.92	19	TTTITTTTTTTTT
RIBOFLAVN	MG	0.05	0.64	4	RRR
NIACIN	MG	0.20	0.22	1	N
IRON	MG	1.40	1.35	9	IIIIIII
CALCIUM	MG	22.00	0.38	2	KK
PHOSPHRUS	MG	137.00	2.34	15	XXXXIXXXXXXX
POTASSIUM	MG	146.00	0.45	3	YY
PROTEIN	G	5.00	1.54	10	PPPPIPPP
CARBOHYDT	G	23.00	1.29	8	HHHHIHH
FAT	G	2.00	0.39	3	FF
OLEIC A	G	0.80	0.50	3	OOO
LINOL A	G	0.90	0.69	5	LLLLI
SAT FAT A	G	0.40	0.22	1	S

367 WHEAT, ROLLED, COOKED
ANALYSIS OF 240 GRAMS WHICH IS 1 CUP

NUTRIENT	UNIT	AMOUNT	INQ	% STD
ENERGY	KCAL	180.00	1.00	9
VITAMIN A	IU	0.00	0.00	0
VITAMIN C	MG	0.00	0.00	0
THIAMIN	MG	0.17	1.89	17
RIBOFLAVN	MG	0.07	0.65	6
NIACIN	MG	2.20	1.75	16
IRON	MG	1.70	1.18	11
CALCIUM	MG	19.00	0.23	2
PHOSPHRUS	MG	182.00	2.25	20
POTASSIUM	MG	202.00	0.45	4
PROTEIN	G	5.00	1.11	10
CARBOHYDT	G	41.00	1.66	15
FAT	G	1.00	0.14	1
OLEIC A	G	0.00	0.00	0
LINOL A	G	0.00	0.00	0
SAT FAT A	G	0.00	0.00	0

368 WHEAT, WHOLE-MEAL, COOKED
ANALYSIS OF 245 GRAMS WHICH IS 1 CUP

NUTRIENT	UNIT	AMOUNT	INQ	% STD
ENERGY	KCAL	110.00	1.00	6
VITAMIN A	IU	0.00	0.00	0
VITAMIN C	MG	0.00	0.00	0
THIAMIN	MG	0.15	2.73	15
RIBOFLAVN	MG	0.05	0.76	4
NIACIN	MG	1.50	1.95	11
IRON	MG	1.20	1.36	7
CALCIUM	MG	17.00	0.34	2
PHOSPHRUS	MG	127.00	2.57	14
POTASSIUM	MG	118.00	0.43	2
PROTEIN	G	4.00	1.45	8
CARBOHYDT	G	23.00	1.52	8
FAT	G	1.00	0.23	1
OLEIC A	G	0.00	0.00	0
LINOL A	G	0.00	0.00	0
SAT FAT A	G	0.00	0.00	0

369 BRAN FLAKES (40% BRAN), ADDED SUGAR, SALT, IRON AND VITAMINS
ANALYSIS OF 35 GRAMS WHICH IS 1 CUP

```
                                      0    10   20   30   40   50   60   70   80   90  100
                                                                                        *  *  *  *  *  *  *  *  *  *  *  *  *
NUTRIENT   UNIT  AMOUNT    INQ   %STD
ENERGY     KCAL   105.00   1.00    5  EEEE
VITAMIN A  IU    1650.00   7.86   41  AAAIAAAAAAAAAAAAAAAAAAAA
VITAMIN C  MG      12.00   3.81   20  CCCICCCCCCCCC
THIAMIN    MG       0.41   7.81   41  TTTITTTTTTTTTTTTTTTT
RIBOFLAVN  MG       0.49   7.78   41  RRRIRRRRRRRRRRRRRRRR
NIACIN     MG       4.10   5.58   29  NNNINNNNNNNNNNNN
IRON       MG       5.60   6.67   35  IIIIIIIIIIIIIIIII
CALCIUM    MG      19.00   0.40    2  KK
PHOSPHRUS  MG     125.00   2.65   14  XXXIXXXXXX
POTASSIUM  MG     137.00   0.52    3  YY
PROTEIN    G        4.00   1.52    8  PPPIPP
CARBOHYDT  G       28.00   1.94   10  HHHIHHHH
FAT        G        1.00   0.24    1  F
OLEIC A    G        0.00   0.00    0  -
LINOL A    G        0.00   0.00    0  -
SAT FAT A  G        0.00   0.00    0  -
************************************************************
```

370 BRAN FLAKES WITH RAISINS, ADDED SUGAR, SALT, IRON AND VITAMINS
ANALYSIS OF 50 GRAMS WHICH IS 1 CUP

```
                                      0    10   20   30   40   50   60   70   80   90  100
                                                                                        *  *  *  *  *  *  *  *  *  *  *  *  *
NUTRIENT   UNIT  AMOUNT    INQ   %STD
ENERGY     KCAL   145.00   1.00    7  EEEEE
VITAMIN A  IU    2350.00   8.10   59  AAAAIAAAAAAAAAAAAAAAAAAAAAAAAAAAAAAAAAAAAAAAAAAAAA
VITAMIN C  MG      18.00   4.14   30  CCCCICCCCCCCCCCCCC
THIAMIN    MG       0.58   8.00   58  TTTTITTTTTTTTTTTTTTTTTTTTTTTTT
RIBOFLAVN  MG       0.71   8.16   59  RRRRIRRRRRRRRRRRRRRRRRRRRRRRRRRRR
NIACIN     MG       5.80   5.71   41  NNNNINNNNNNNNNNNNNN
IRON       MG       6.90   5.95   43  IIIIIIIIIIIIIIIIIIIII
CALCIUM    MG      28.00   0.43    3  KK
PHOSPHRUS  MG     146.00   2.24   16  XXXXIXXXXXX
POTASSIUM  MG     154.00   0.42    3  YY
PROTEIN    G        4.00   1.10    8  PPPPP
CARBOHYDT  G       40.00   2.01   15  HHHHIHHHHH
FAT        G        1.00   0.18    1  F
OLEIC A    G        0.00   0.00    0  -
LINOL A    G        0.00   0.00    0  -
SAT FAT A  G        0.00   0.00    0  -
************************************************************
```

371 CORN FLAKES, PLAIN, ADDED SUGAR, SALT, IRON, VITAMINS
ANALYSIS OF 25 GRAMS WHICH IS 1 CUP

NUTRIENT	UNIT	AMOUNT	INQ	% STD	0 10 20 30 40 50 60 70 80 90 100
ENERGY	KCAL	95.00	1.00	5	EEEE
VITAMIN A	IU	1180.00	6.21	30	AAAIAAAAAAAAAAAAAAAAAA
VITAMIN C	MG	9.00	3.16	15	CCCICCCCCC
THIAMIN	MG	0.29	6.11	29	TTTITTTTTTTTTTTTTTTTT
RIBOFLAVN	MG	0.35	6.14	29	RRRIRRRRRRRRRRRRRRRRRR
NIACIN	MG	2.90	4.36	21	NNNINNNNNNNNNN
IRON	MG	0.60	0.79	4	III
CALCIUM	MG	0.00	0.00	0	-
PHOSPHRUS	MG	0.00	0.21	1	X
POTASSIUM	MG	9.00	0.13	1	-
PROTEIN	G	2.00	0.84	4	PPP
CARBOHYDT	G	21.00	1.61	8	HHHIHH
FAT	G	0.00	0.00	0	-
OLEIC A	G	0.00	0.00	0	-
LINOL A	G	0.00	0.00	0	-
SAT FAT A	G	0.00	0.00	0	-

372 CORN FLAKES, SUGAR-COATED, ADDED SALT, IRON, VITAMINS
ANALYSIS OF 40 GRAMS WHICH IS 1 CUP

NUTRIENT	UNIT	AMOUNT	INQ	% STD	0 10 20 30 40 50 60 70 80 90 100
ENERGY	KCAL	155.00	1.00	8	EEEEE
VITAMIN A	IU	1880.00	6.06	47	AAAAIAAAAAAAAAAAAAAAAAAAAAAAAAAAAAAAAAAAAAA
VITAMIN C	MG	14.00	3.01	23	CCCCICCCCCCCCCCC
THIAMIN	MG	0.46	5.94	46	TTTITTTTTTTTTTTTTTTTTTTTTTTTTTTTTTTTTTTTTTT
RIBOFLAVN	MG	0.56	6.02	47	RRRRIRRRRRRRRRRRRRRRRRRRRRRRRRRRRRRRRRR
NIACIN	MG	4.60	4.24	33	NNNNINNNNNNNNNNNNNNNNN
IRON	MG	1.00	0.81	6	IIIII
CALCIUM	MG	1.00	0.01	0	-
PHOSPHRUS	MG	10.00	0.14	1	X
POTASSIUM	MG	27.00	0.07	1	-
PROTEIN	G	2.00	0.52	4	PPP
CARBOHYDT	G	37.00	1.74	13	HHHHIHHHHH
FAT	G	0.00	0.00	0	-
OLEIC A	G	0.00	0.00	0	-
LINOL A	G	0.00	0.00	0	-
SAT FAT A	G	0.00	0.00	0	-

373 PUFFED CORN, PLAIN, ADDED SUGAR, SALT, IRON, VITAMINS
ANALYSIS OF 20 GRAMS WHICH IS 1 CUP

NUTRIENT	UNIT	AMOUNT	INQ	% STD	0 10 20 30 40 50 60 70 80 90 100
ENERGY	KCAL	80.00	1.00	4	EEE
VITAMIN A	IU	940.00	5.88	24	AA|AAAAAAAAAAAAAA
VITAMIN C	MG	7.00	2.92	12	CC|CCCCC
THIAMIN	MG	0.23	5.75	23	TT|TTTTTTTTTTTTT
RIBOFLAVN	MG	0.28	5.83	23	RR|RRRRRRRRRRRRRR
NIACIN	MG	2.30	4.11	16	NN|NNNNNNNNN
IRON	MG	2.30	3.59	14	II|IIIIIIIII
CALCIUM	MG	4.00	0.11	0	-|
PHOSPHRUS	MG	18.00	0.50	2	XX|
POTASSIUM	MG	13.00	0.07	0	-|
PROTEIN	G	2.00	1.45	4	PPP
CARBOHYDT	G	16.00	0.32	6	HH|HH
FAT	G	1.00	0.20	1	F|
OLEIC A	G	0.20	0.50	1	-|
LINOL A	G	0.40	0.00	2	LL|
SAT FAT A	G	0.00	0.00	0	-|

374 SHREDDED CORN, ADDED SUGAR, SALT, IRON, THIAMIN, NIACIN
ANALYSIS OF 25 GRAMS WHICH IS 1 CUP

NUTRIENT	UNIT	AMOUNT	INQ	% STD	0 10 20 30 40 50 60 70 80 90 100
ENERGY	KCAL	95.00	1.00	5	EEEE
VITAMIN A	IU	0.00	0.00	0	-|
VITAMIN C	MG	0.00	0.00	0	-|
THIAMIN	MG	0.11	2.32	11	TT|TTTTT
RIBOFLAVN	MG	0.05	0.88	4	RRR|
NIACIN	MG	0.50	0.79	4	NNN|
IRON	MG	0.60	0.79	4	III|
CALCIUM	MG	1.00	0.02	0	-|
PHOSPHRUS	MG	10.00	0.23	1	X|
POTASSIUM	MG	17.00	0.07	0	-|
PROTEIN	G	2.00	0.84	4	PPP|
CARBOHYDT	G	22.00	1.68	8	HHH|HH
FAT	G	0.00	0.00	0	-|
OLEIC A	G	0.00	0.00	0	-|
LINOL A	G	0.00	0.00	0	-|
SAT FAT A	G	0.00	0.00	0	-|

375 PUFFED OATS, ADDED SUGAR, SALT, MINERALS, VITAMINS
ANALYSIS OF 25 GRAMS WHICH IS 1 CUP

NUTRIENT	UNIT	AMOUNT	INQ	% STD
ENERGY	KCAL	100.00	1.00	5
VITAMIN A	IU	1180.00	5.90	30
VITAMIN C	MG	9.00	3.00	15
THIAMIN	MG	0.29	5.80	29
RIBOFLAVN	MG	0.35	5.83	29
NIACIN	MG	2.90	4.14	21
IRON	MG	2.90	3.63	18
CALCIUM	MG	44.00	0.98	5
PHOSPHRUS	MG	102.00	2.27	11
POTASSIUM	MG	0.00	0.00	0
PROTEIN	G	3.00	1.20	6
CARBOHYDT	G	19.00	1.38	7
FAT	G	1.00	0.26	1
OLEIC A	G	0.20	0.16	1
LINOL A	G	0.50	0.50	3
SAT FAT A	G	0.20	0.14	1

376 PUFFED RICE, PLAIN, ADDED IRON, THIAMIN, NIACIN
ANALYSIS OF 15 GRAMS WHICH IS 1 CUP

NUTRIENT	UNIT	AMOUNT	INQ	% STD
ENERGY	KCAL	60.00	1.00	3
VITAMIN A	IU	0.00	0.00	0
VITAMIN C	MG	0.00	0.00	0
THIAMIN	MG	0.07	2.33	7
RIBOFLAVN	MG	0.01	0.28	1
NIACIN	MG	0.70	1.67	5
IRON	MG	0.30	0.63	2
CALCIUM	MG	3.00	0.11	0
PHOSPHRUS	MG	14.00	0.52	2
POTASSIUM	MG	15.00	0.10	0
PROTEIN	G	1.00	0.67	2
CARBOHYDT	G	13.00	1.58	5
FAT	G	0.00	0.00	0
OLEIC A	G	0.00	0.00	0
LINOL A	G	0.00	0.00	0
SAT FAT A	G	0.00	0.00	0

```
377 PUFFED RICE, PRESWEETENED, ADDED SALT, IRON, VITAMINS
ANALYSIS OF 28 GRAMS WHICH IS 1 CUP

                                      0    10    20    30    40    50    60    70    80    90    100
NUTRIENT  UNIT  AMOUNT    INQ   % STD
ENERGY    KCAL  115.00    1.00    6   EEEEE                                                    *
VITAMIN A IU   1250.00    5.43   31   AAAAIAAAAAAAAAAAAAAAAAA                                  *
VITAMIN C MG     15.00    4.35   25   CCCCICCCCCCCCCC                                          *
THIAMIN   MG      0.38    6.61   38   TTTTITTTTTTTTTTTTTTTTTTTTTTTT                            *
RIBOFLAVN MG      0.43    6.23   36   RRRRIRRRRRRRRRRRRRRRRRRR                                 *
NIACIN    MG      5.00    6.21   36   NNNNINNNNNNNNNNNNNNNNNN                                  *
IRON      MG      1.10    1.20    7   IIIIII                                                   *
CALCIUM   MG      3.00    0.06    0   -                                                        *
PHOSPHRUS MG     14.00    0.27    2   X                                                        *
POTASSIUM MG     43.00    0.15    0   Y                                                        *
PROTEIN   G       1.00    0.35    2   PP                                                       *
CARBOHYDT G      26.00    1.64    9   HHHHIHHH                                                 *
FAT       G       0.00    0.00    0   -                                                        *
OLEIC A   G       0.00    0.00    0   -                                                        *
LINOL A   G       0.00    0.00    0   -                                                        *
SAT FAT A G       0.00    0.00    0   -                                                        *
******************************************************************************************
```

```
378 WHEAT FLAKES, ADDED SUGAR, SALT, IRON, VITAMINS
ANALYSIS OF 30 GRAMS WHICH IS 1 CUP

                                      0    10    20    30    40    50    60    70    80    90    100
NUTRIENT  UNIT  AMOUNT    INQ   % STD
ENERGY    KCAL  105.00    1.00    5   EEE                                                      *
VITAMIN A IU   1410.00    6.71   35   AAAIAAAAAAAAAAAAAAAAA                                    *
VITAMIN C MG     11.00    3.49   18   CCCICCCCCCCCCC                                           *
THIAMIN   MG      0.35    6.67   35   TTTITTTTTTTTTTTTTTTT                                     *
RIBOFLAVN MG      0.42    6.67   35   RRRIRRRRRRRRRRRRRRRRR                                    *
NIACIN    MG      3.50    4.76   25   NNNINNNNNNNNNNNN                                         *
IRON      MG      0.00    0.25    0   K-                                                       *
CALCIUM   MG     12.00    0.25    1   XXXIXXX                                                  *
PHOSPHRUS MG     83.00    1.76    9   Y-                                                       *
POTASSIUM MG     81.00    0.31    2   PPPIP                                                    *
PROTEIN   G       3.00    1.14    6   HHHIHHH                                                  *
CARBOHYDT G      24.00    1.66    9   -                                                        *
FAT       G       0.00    0.00    0   -                                                        *
OLEIC A   G       0.00    0.00    0   -                                                        *
LINOL A   G       0.00    0.00    0   -                                                        *
SAT FAT A G       0.00    0.00    0   -                                                        *
******************************************************************************************
```

379 PUFFED WHEAT, PLAIN, ADDED IRON, THIAMIN, NIACIN
ANALYSIS OF 15 GRAMS WHICH IS 1 CUP

```
                                              10   20   30   40   50   60   70   80   90  100
NUTRIENT   UNIT  AMOUNT   INQ   % STD  0                                                    ********************
ENERGY     KCAL   55.00  1.00    3     EE
VITAMIN A  IU      0.00  0.00    0     -I
VITAMIN C  MG      0.00  0.00    0     -I
THIAMIN    MG      0.08  2.91    8     TITTTT
RIBOFLAVN  MG      0.03  0.91    3     RR
NIACIN     MG      1.20  3.12    9     NINNNNN
IRON       MG      0.60  1.36    4     III
CALCIUM    MG      4.00  0.16    0     -I
PHOSPHRUS  MG     48.00  1.94    5     XIXX
POTASSIUM  MG     51.00  0.37    1     YI
PROTEIN    G       2.00  1.45    4     PIP
CARBOHYDT  G      12.00  1.59    4     HIH
FAT        G       0.00  0.00    0     -I
OLEIC A    G       0.00  0.00    0     -I
LINOL A    G       0.00  0.00    0     -I
SAT FAT A  G       0.00  0.00    0     -I
************************************************
```

380 PUFFED WHEAT, PRESWEETENED, ADDED SALT, IRON, VITAMINS
ANALYSIS OF 38 GRAMS WHICH IS 1 CUP

```
                                              10   20   30   40   50   60   70   80   90  100
NUTRIENT   UNIT  AMOUNT   INQ   % STD  0                                                    ********************
ENERGY     KCAL  140.00  1.00    7     EEEEEE
VITAMIN A  IU   1680.00  6.00   42     AAAAAIAAAAAAAAAAAAAAAAAAAAAAAAAAAAAAAAAAA
VITAMIN C  MG     20.00  4.76   33     CCCCICCCCCCCCCCCCCCCCCCCCCCCCCCCC
THIAMIN    MG            7.14   50     TTTTITTTTTTTTTTTTTTTTTTTTTTTTTTTTTTTTTTTTTTTTTTT
RIBOFLAVN  MG      0.57  6.79   48     RRRRIRRRRRRRRRRRRRRRRRRRRRRRRRRRRRRRRRRRRRRRR
NIACIN     MG      6.70  6.84   48     NNNNINNNNNNNNNNNNNNNNNNNNNNNNNNNNNNNNNNNNNNNN
IRON       MG      1.60  1.43   10     IIIIIIII
CALCIUM    MG      7.00  0.11    1     K
PHOSPHRUS  MG     52.00  0.83    6     XXXXXI
POTASSIUM  MG     63.00  0.18    1     Y
PROTEIN    G       3.00  0.86    6     PPPPPI
CARBOHYDT  G      33.00  1.71   12     HHHHHIHHHH
FAT        G       0.00  0.00    0     -I
OLEIC A    G       0.00  0.00    0     -I
LINOL A    G       0.00  0.00    0     -I
SAT FAT A  G       0.00  0.00    0     -I
************************************************
```

381 SHREDDED WHEAT, PLAIN
ANALYSIS OF 25 GRAMS WHICH IS 1 LARGE BISCUIT OR 1/2 CUP SMALL BISCUITS

NUTRIENT	UNIT	AMOUNT	INQ	% STD	0 10 20 30 40 50 60 70 80 90 100
ENERGY	KCAL	90.00	1.00	5	EEEE
VITAMIN A	IU	0.00	0.00	0	-
VITAMIN C	MG	0.00	0.00	0	-
THIAMIN	MG	0.06	1.33	6	TTTIT
RIBOFLAVN	MG	0.03	0.56	3	RR
NIACIN	MG	1.10	1.75	8	NNNINN
IRON	MG	0.90	1.25	6	IIIII
CALCIUM	MG	11.00	0.27	1	K
PHOSPHRUS	MG	97.00	2.40	11	XXXIXXXXX
POTASSIUM	MG	87.00	0.39	2	Y
PROTEIN	G	2.00	0.89	4	PPPI
CARBOHYDT	G	20.00	1.62	7	HHHIHH
FAT	G	1.00	0.28	1	F
OLEIC A	G	0.20	0.18	1	O
LINOL A	G	0.20	0.22	1	L
SAT FAT A	G	0.00	0.00	0	-

382 WHEAT GERM, WITHOUT SALT AND SUGAR, TOASTED
ANALYSIS OF 6 GRAMS WHICH IS 1 TBSP

NUTRIENT	UNIT	AMOUNT	INQ	% STD	0 10 20 30 40 50 60 70 80 90 100
ENERGY	KCAL	25.00	1.00	1	E
VITAMIN A	IU	10.00	0.20	0	-
VITAMIN C	MG	1.00	1.33	2	C
THIAMIN	MG	0.11	8.80	11	ITTTTTT
RIBOFLAVN	MG	0.05	3.33	4	IRR
NIACIN	MG	0.30	1.71	2	N
IRON	MG	0.50	2.50	3	III
CALCIUM	MG	3.00	0.27	0	-
PHOSPHRUS	MG	70.00	6.22	8	IXXXXX
POTASSIUM	MG	57.00	0.91	1	Y
PROTEIN	G	2.00	3.20	4	IPP
CARBOHYDT	G	3.00	0.87	1	H
FAT	G	1.00	1.03	1	F
OLEIC A	G	0.20	0.65	1	O
LINOL A	G	0.10	1.20	2	L
SAT FAT A	G	0.10	0.28	0	-

383 BUCKWHEAT FLOUR,LIGHT,SIFTED
ANALYSIS OF 98 GRAMS WHICH IS 1 CUP

NUTRIENT	UNIT	AMOUNT	INQ	% STD
ENERGY	KCAL	340.00	1.00	17
VITAMIN A	IU	0.00	0.00	0
VITAMIN C	MG	0.00	0.00	0
THIAMIN	MG	0.08	0.47	8
RIBOFLAVN	MG	0.04	0.20	3
NIACIN	MG	0.40	0.17	3
IRON	MG	1.30	0.37	6
CALCIUM	MG	11.00	0.07	1
PHOSPHRUS	MG	86.00	0.56	10
POTASSIUM	MG	314.00	0.37	6
PROTEIN	G	6.00	0.71	12
CARBOHYDT	G	78.00	1.67	28
FAT	G	1.00	0.08	1
OLEIC A	G	0.40	0.10	2
LINOL A	G	0.12	0.12	2
SAT FAT A	G	0.20	0.04	1

384 BULGUR,CANNED,SEASONED
ANALYSIS OF 135 GRAMS WHICH IS 1 CUP

NUTRIENT	UNIT	AMOUNT	INQ	% STD
ENERGY	KCAL	245.00	1.00	12
VITAMIN A	IU	0.00	0.00	0
VITAMIN C	MG	0.00	0.00	0
THIAMIN	MG	0.08	0.65	8
RIBOFLAVN	MG	0.05	0.34	4
NIACIN	MG	4.10	2.39	29
IRON	MG	1.90	0.97	12
CALCIUM	MG	27.00	0.24	3
PHOSPHRUS	MG	263.00	2.39	29
POTASSIUM	MG	151.00	0.25	3
PROTEIN	G	8.00	1.31	16
CARBOHYDT	G	44.00	1.31	16
FAT	G	4.00	0.42	5
OLEIC A	G	1.40	0.47	6
LINOL A	G	1.40	0.57	7
SAT FAT A	G	1.40	0.40	5

385 ANGELFOOD CAKE
ANALYSIS OF 635 GRAMS WHICH IS 1 WHOLE CAKE,9 3/4-IN DIAM. TUBE CAKE

NUTRIENT	UNIT	AMOUNT	INQ	% STD		0	10	20	30	40	50	60	70	80	90	100
ENERGY	KCAL	1645.00	1.00	82		EEEEEEEEEEEEEEEEEEEEEEEEEEEEEEEEEEEEEEEEEEEEEEEEEEEEEEEEEEEEEEEEEEEEEEEEEEEEEEEEEE										
VITAMIN A	IU	0.00	0.00	0		-										
VITAMIN C	MG	0.00	0.00	0		-										
THIAMIN	MG	0.37	0.45	37		TTTTTTTTTTTTTTTTTTTTTTTTTTTTTTTTTTTTT										
RIBOFLAVN	MG	0.95	0.96	79		RRRRRRRRRRRRRRRRRRRRRRRRRRRRRRRRRRRRRRRRRRRRRRRRRRRRRRRRRRRRRRRRRRRRRRRRRRRRRRRR										
NIACIN	MG	3.60	0.31	26		NNNNNNNNNNNNNNNNNNNNNNNNNN										
IRON	MG	2.50	0.19	16		IIIIIIIIIIIIIIII										
CALCIUM	MG	603.00	0.81	67		KKKKKKKKKKKKKKKKKKKKKKKKKKKKKKKKKKKKKKKKKKKKKKKKKKKKKKKKKKKKKKKKKKKKK										
PHOSPHRUS	MG	756.00	1.02	84		XXXXXXXXXXXXXXXXXXXXXXXXXXXXXXXXXXXXXXXXXXXXXXXXXXXXXXXXXXXXXXXXXXXXXXXXXXXXXXXXXXXXXX	X									
POTASSIUM	MG	381.00	0.09	8		YYYYYYYY										
PROTEIN	G	36.00	0.88	72		PPPPPPPPPPPPPPPPPPPPPPPPPPPPPPPPPPPPPPPPPPPPPPPPPPPPPPPPPPPPPPPPPPPPPPPPPP										
CARBOHYDT	G	377.00	1.67	137		HHHHHHHHHHHHHHHHHHHHHHHHHHHHHHHHHHHHHHHHHHHHHHHHHHHHHHHHHHHHHHHHHHHHHHHHHHHHHHHHHHHHH	HHHHHHHHHHHHHHHHHHHHHHH							*137
FAT	G	1.00	0.02	1		F										
OLEIC A	G	0.00	0.00	0		-										
LINOL A	G	0.00	0.00	0		-										
SAT FAT A	G	0.00	0.00	0		-										

386 ANGELFOOD CAKE
ANALYSIS OF 53 GRAMS WHICH IS 1 PIECE,1/12 CAKE

NUTRIENT	UNIT	AMOUNT	INQ	% STD		0	10	20	30	40	50	60	70	80	90	100
ENERGY	KCAL	135.00	1.00	7		EEEEE										
VITAMIN A	IU	0.00	0.00	0		-										
VITAMIN C	MG	0.00	0.00	0		-										
THIAMIN	MG	0.03	0.44	3		TT										
RIBOFLAVN	MG	0.08	0.99	7		RRRR										
NIACIN	MG	0.30	0.32	2		NN										
IRON	MG	0.20	0.19	1		I										
CALCIUM	MG	50.00	0.82	6		KKKK										
PHOSPHRUS	MG	63.00	1.04	7		XXXX|X										
POTASSIUM	MG	32.00	0.09	1		Y										
PROTEIN	G	3.00	0.89	6		PPPP										
CARBOHYDT	G	32.00	1.72	12		HHHH|HHHH										
FAT	G	0.00	0.00	0		-										
OLEIC A	G	0.00	0.00	0		-										
LINOL A	G	0.00	0.00	0		-										
SAT FAT A	G	0.00	0.00	0		-										

387 COFFEECAKE
ANALYSIS OF 430 GRAMS WHICH IS 1 WHOLE CAKE (7 3/4 BY 5 5/8 BY 1 1/4 IN)

NUTRIENT	UNIT	AMOUNT	INQ	%STD
ENERGY	KCAL	1385.00	1.00	69
VITAMIN A	IU	690.00	0.25	17
VITAMIN C	MG	1.00	0.02	2
THIAMIN	MG	0.82	1.18	82
RIBOFLAVN	MG	0.91	1.10	76
NIACIN	MG	7.70	0.79	55
IRON	MG	6.90	0.62	43
CALCIUM	MG	262.00	0.42	29
PHOSPHRUS	MG	748.00	1.20	83
POTASSIUM	MG	469.00	0.14	9
PROTEIN	G	27.00	0.78	54
CARBOHYDT	G	225.00	1.18	82
FAT	G	41.00	0.76	53
OLEIC A	G	16.30	0.96	67
LINOL A	G	8.80	0.64	44
SAT FAT A	G	11.70	0.59	41

388 COFFEECAKE
ANALYSIS OF 72 GRAMS WHICH IS 1 PIECE, 1/6 CAKE

NUTRIENT	UNIT	AMOUNT	INQ	%STD
ENERGY	KCAL	230.00	1.00	12
VITAMIN A	IU	120.00	0.26	3
VITAMIN C	MG	0.00	0.00	0
THIAMIN	MG	0.14	1.22	14
RIBOFLAVN	MG	0.15	1.09	13
NIACIN	MG	1.30	0.81	9
IRON	MG	1.20	0.65	7
CALCIUM	MG	44.00	0.43	5
PHOSPHRUS	MG	125.00	1.21	14
POTASSIUM	MG	78.00	0.14	2
PROTEIN	G	5.00	0.87	10
CARBOHYDT	G	38.00	1.20	14
FAT	G	7.00	0.78	11
OLEIC A	G	2.70	0.96	9
LINOL A	G	1.50	0.65	8
SAT FAT A	G	2.00	0.61	7

389 CUPCAKES WITHOUT ICING
ANALYSIS OF 25 GRAMS WHICH IS 1 CAKE 2 1/2 IN DIAM.

NUTRIENT	UNIT	AMOUNT	INQ	% STD	0	10	20	30	40	50	60	70	80	90	100
ENERGY	KCAL	90.00	1.00	5	EEEE										*********
VITAMIN A	IU	40.00	0.22	1	A										
VITAMIN C	MG	0.00	0.00	0	-										
THIAMIN	MG	0.05	1.11	5	TTTT										
RIBOFLAVN	MG	0.05	0.93	4	RRR										
NIACIN	MG	0.40	0.63	3	NN										
IRON	MG	0.30	0.42	2	II										
CALCIUM	MG	40.00	0.99	4	KKKK										
PHOSPHRUS	MG	59.00	1.46	7	XXXIX										
POTASSIUM	MG	21.00	0.09	0	-										
PROTEIN	G	1.00	0.44	2	PP										
CARBOHYDT	G	14.00	1.13	5	HHHH										
FAT	G	3.00	0.85	4	FFF										
OLEIC A	G	1.20	1.09	5	OOOO										
LINOL A	G	0.70	0.78	4	LLL										
SAT FAT A	G	0.80	0.62	3	SS										

390 CUPCAKES WITH CHOCOLATE ICING
ANALYSIS OF 36 GRAMS WHICH IS 1 CAKE 2 1/2 IN DIAM.

NUTRIENT	UNIT	AMOUNT	INQ	% STD	0	10	20	30	40	50	60	70	80	90	100
ENERGY	KCAL	130.00	1.00	7	EEEEE										*********
VITAMIN A	IU	60.00	0.23	2	A										
VITAMIN C	MG	0.00	0.00	0	-										
THIAMIN	MG	0.05	0.77	5	TTTT										
RIBOFLAVN	MG	0.06	0.77	5	RRRR										
NIACIN	MG	0.40	0.44	3	NN										
IRON	MG	0.40	0.38	3	II										
CALCIUM	MG	47.00	0.80	5	KKKK										
PHOSPHRUS	MG	71.00	1.21	8	XXXIX										
POTASSIUM	MG	42.00	0.13	1	Y										
PROTEIN	G	2.00	0.62	4	PPP										
CARBOHYDT	G	21.00	1.17	8	HHHHIH										
FAT	G	5.00	0.99	6	FFFFF										
OLEIC A	G	1.60	1.00	7	OOOOO										
LINOL A	G	0.60	0.46	3	LL										
SAT FAT A	G	2.00	1.08	7	SSSSIS										

391 DEVILSFOOD CAKE WITH CHOCOLATE ICING
ANALYSIS OF 1107 GRAMS WHICH IS WHOLE 2 LAYER CAKE (8 OR 9 IN DIAM)

NUTRIENT	UNIT	AMOUNT	INQ	% STD
ENERGY	KCAL	3755.00	1.00	188
VITAMIN A	IU	1660.00	0.22	42
VITAMIN C	MG	1.00	0.01	2
THIAMIN	MG	1.06	0.56	106
RIBOFLAVN	MG	1.65	0.73	138
NIACIN	MG	10.10	0.38	72
IRON	MG	16.60	0.55	104
CALCIUM	MG	653.00	0.39	73
PHOSPHRUS	MG	1162.00	0.69	129
POTASSIUM	MG	1439.00	0.15	29
PROTEIN	G	49.00	0.52	98
CARBOHYDT	G	645.00	1.25	235
FAT	G	136.00	0.93	174
OLEIC A	G	44.90	0.98	183
LINOL A	G	17.00	0.45	85
SAT FAT A	G	50.00	0.93	175

392 DEVILSFOOD CAKE WITH CHOCOLATE ICING
ANALYSIS OF 69 GRAMS WHICH IS 1 PIECE 1/6 OF CAKE

NUTRIENT	UNIT	AMOUNT	INQ	% STD
ENERGY	KCAL	235.00	1.00	12
VITAMIN A	IU	100.00	0.21	3
VITAMIN C	MG	0.00	0.00	0
THIAMIN	MG	0.07	0.60	7
RIBOFLAVN	MG	0.60	0.71	8
NIACIN	MG	0.60	0.36	4
IRON	MG	1.00	0.53	6
CALCIUM	MG	41.00	0.39	5
PHOSPHRUS	MG	72.00	0.68	8
POTASSIUM	MG	90.00	0.15	2
PROTEIN	G	3.00	0.51	6
CARBOHYDT	G	40.00	1.24	15
FAT	G	8.00	0.87	10
OLEIC A	G	2.80	0.97	11
LINOL A	G	1.10	0.47	6
SAT FAT A	G	3.10	0.93	11

393 DEVILSFOOD CUPCAKE WITH CHOCOLATE ICING
ANALYSIS OF 35 GRAMS WHICH IS 1 CUPCAKE,2 1/2-IN DIAM

```
NUTRIENT   UNIT   AMOUNT   INQ    % STD  0        10        20        30        40        50        60        70        80        90        100
ENERGY     KCAL   120.00   1.00     6    EEEE  -                                                                                      *
VITAMIN A  IU      50.00   0.21     1    A     -                                                                                      *
VITAMIN C  MG       0.00   0.00     0    -     -                                                                                      *
THIAMIN    MG       0.03   0.50     3    TT    -                                                                                      *
RIBOFLAVN  MG       0.05   0.69     4    RRR   -                                                                                      *
NIACIN     MG       0.30   0.36     2    NN    -                                                                                      *
IRON       MG       0.50   0.52     3    III   -                                                                                      *
CALCIUM    MG      21.00   0.39     2    KK    -                                                                                      *
PHOSPHRUS  MG      37.00   0.69     4    XXX   -                                                                                      *
POTASSIUM  MG      46.00   0.15     1    Y     -                                                                                      *
PROTEIN    G        2.00   0.67     4    PPP   -                                                                                      *
CARBOHYDT  G       20.00   1.21     7    HHHHH -                                                                                      *
FAT        G        4.00   0.85     5    FFFF  -                                                                                      *
OLEIC A    G        1.40   0.95     6    OOOOO -                                                                                      *
LINOL A    G        0.50   0.42     3    LL    -                                                                                      *
SAT FAT A  G        1.60   0.94     6    SSSS  -                                                                                      *
*******************************************
```

394 GINGERBREAD
ANALYSIS OF 570 GRAMS WHICH IS 1 WHOLE CAKE (8-IN SQUARE)

```
NUTRIENT   UNIT   AMOUNT    INQ    % STD  0        10        20        30        40        50        60        70        80        90        100
ENERGY     KCAL  1575.00   1.00    79    EEEEEEEEEEEEEEEEEEEEEEEEEEEEEEEEEEEEEEEEEEEEEEEEEEEEEEEEEEEEEEEEEEEE                         *
VITAMIN A  IU       0.00   0.00     0    -                                                                                           *
VITAMIN C  MG       0.00   0.00     0    -                                                                                           *
THIAMIN    MG       0.84   1.07    84    TTTTTTTTTTTTTTTTTTTTTTTTTTTTTTTTTTTTTTTTTTTTTTTTTTTTTTTTTTTTTTTTTTTTTTTT                     *
RIBOFLAVN  MG       1.00   1.06    83    RRRRRRRRRRRRRRRRRRRRRRRRRRRRRRRRRRRRRRRRRRRRRRRRRRRRRRRRRRRRRRRRRRRRRRRRR  RRRR            *
NIACIN     MG       7.40   0.67    53    NNNNNNNNNNNNNNNNNNNNNNNNNNNNNNNNNNNNNNNNNNNNNNNNN                                           *
IRON       MG       8.60   0.68    54    IIIIIIIIIIIIIIIIIIIIIIIIIIIIIIIIIIIIIIIIIIIIIIIIIIIII                                       *
CALCIUM    MG     513.00   0.72    57    KKKKKKKKKKKKKKKKKKKKKKKKKKKKKKKKKKKKKKKKKKKKKKKKKKKKKKK                                     *
PHOSPHRUS  MG     570.00   0.80    63    XXXXXXXXXXXXXXXXXXXXXXXXXXXXXXXXXXXXXXXXXXXXXXXXXXXXXXXXXXXXX                               *
POTASSIUM  MG    1562.00   0.40    31    YYYYYYYYYYYYYYYYYYYYYYYYYYYYYY                                                              *
PROTEIN    G      18.00   0.46    36    PPPPPPPPPPPPPPPPPPPPPPPPPPPPPPPPPP                                                          *
CARBOHYDT  G     291.00   1.34   106    HHHHHHHHHHHHHHHHHHHHHHHHHHHHHHHHHHHHHHHHHHHHHHHHHHHHHHHHHHHHHHHHHHHHHHHHHHHHHHHHHHHHHHHHHHHHHHHHHHHHHHH *106
FAT        G      39.00   0.63    50    FFFFFFFFFFFFFFFFFFFFFFFFFFFFFFFFFFFFFFFFFFFFFFFFFF                                          *
OLEIC A    G      16.60   0.86    68    OOOOOOOOOOOOOOOOOOOOOOOOOOOOOOOOOOOOOOOOOOOOOOOOOOOOOOOOOOOOOOOOOOOO                         *
LINOL A    G      10.00   0.63    50    LLLLLLLLLLLLLLLLLLLLLLLLLLLLLLLLLLLLLLLLLLLLLLLLLL                                          *
SAT FAT A  G       9.70   0.43    34    SSSSSSSSSSSSSSSSSSSSSSSSSSSSSSSSSS                                                          *
*******************************************
```

395 GINGERBREAD
ANALYSIS OF 63 GRAMS WHICH IS 1 PIECE, 1/9 OF CAKE

NUTRIENT	UNIT	AMOUNT	INQ	% STD	
ENERGY	KCAL	175.00	1.00	9	EEEEEE
VITAMIN A	IU	0.00	0.00	0	-
VITAMIN C	MG	0.00	0.00	0	-
THIAMIN	MG	0.09	1.03	9	TTTTTT
RIBOFLAVN	MG	0.11	1.05	9	RRRRRR
NIACIN	MG	0.80	0.65	6	NNNN
IRON	MG	0.90	0.64	6	IIIII
CALCIUM	MG	57.00	0.72	6	KKKKK
PHOSPHRUS	MG	63.00	0.80	7	XXXXXX
POTASSIUM	MG	173.00	0.40	3	YYY
PROTEIN	G	2.00	0.46	4	PPP
CARBOHYDT	G	32.00	1.33	12	HHHHHH HH
FAT	G	4.00	0.59	5	FFFF
OLEIC A	G	1.80	0.84	7	OOOOOO
LINOL A	G	1.10	0.63	6	LLLL
SAT FAT A	G	1.10	0.44	4	SSS

396 WHITE CAKE, 2 LAYER WITH CHOCOLATE ICING
ANALYSIS OF 1140 GRAMS WHICH IS 1 WHOLE CAKE (8 OR 9 IN DIAM)

NUTRIENT	UNIT	AMOUNT	INQ	% STD	
ENERGY	KCAL	4000.00	1.00	200	EEEEE...EEEE * 200
VITAMIN A	IU	680.00	0.09	17	AAAAAAAAA
VITAMIN C	MG	2.00	0.02	3	CCC
THIAMIN	MG	1.50	0.75	150	TTTTT...TTT *150
RIBOFLAVN	MG	1.77	0.74	148	RRRRR...RRR *148
NIACIN	MG	12.50	0.45	89	NNNNN...NNN
IRON	MG	11.40	0.36	71	IIIII...III
CALCIUM	MG	1129.00	0.63	125	KKKKK...KKK *125
PHOSPHRUS	MG	2041.00	1.13	227	XXXXX...XXX *227
POTASSIUM	MG	1322.00	0.13	26	YYYYY...YYY
PROTEIN	G	44.00	0.44	88	PPPPP...PPP
CARBOHYDT	G	716.00	1.30	260	HHHHH...HHH *260
FAT	G	122.00	0.78	156	FFFFF...FFF *156
OLEIC A	G	46.40	0.95	189	OOOOO...OOO *189
LINOL A	G	20.00	0.50	100	LLLLL...LLL
SAT FAT A	G	48.20	0.85	169	SSSSS...SSS *169

Scale: 0   10   20   30   40   50   60   70   80   90   100

397 WHITE CAKE WITH CHOCOLATE ICING
ANALYSIS OF 71 GRAMS WHICH IS 1 PIECE, 1/16 OF CAKE

NUTRIENT	UNIT	AMOUNT	INQ	% STD
ENERGY	KCAL	250.00	1.00	13
VITAMIN A	IU	40.00	0.08	1
VITAMIN C	MG	0.00	0.00	0
THIAMIN	MG	0.00	0.72	9
RIBOFLAVN	MG	0.11	0.73	9
NIACIN	MG	0.80	0.46	6
IRON	MG	0.70	0.35	4
CALCIUM	MG	70.00	0.62	8
PHOSPHRUS	MG	127.00	1.13	14
POTASSIUM	MG	82.00	0.13	2
PROTEIN	G	3.00	0.48	6
CARBOHYDT	G	45.00	1.31	16
FAT	G	8.00	0.82	10
OLEIC A	G	2.90	0.95	12
LINOL A	G	1.20	0.48	6
SAT FAT A	G	3.00	0.84	11

```
                    0        10    20    30    40    50    60    70    80    90   100
ENERGY              EEEEEEEEE
VITAMIN A           A
VITAMIN C           -
THIAMIN             TTTTTT
RIBOFLAVN           RRRRRR
NIACIN              NNNN
IRON                IIII
CALCIUM             KKKKK
PHOSPHRUS           XXXXXXXXX|X
POTASSIUM           Y
PROTEIN             PPPP
CARBOHYDT           HHHHHHHHH|HHH
FAT                 FFFFFFF
OLEIC A             OOOOOOOO|
LINOL A             LLLLL
SAT FAT A           SSSSSSS|
********************
```

398 YELLOW CAKE, 2 LAYER WITH CHOCOLATE ICING
ANALYSIS OF 1108 GRAMS WHICH IS 1 WHOLE CAKE (8 OR 9 IN DIAM)

NUTRIENT	UNIT	AMOUNT	INQ	% STD
ENERGY	KCAL	3735.00	1.00	187
VITAMIN A	IU	1550.00	0.21	39
VITAMIN C	MG	2.00	0.02	3
THIAMIN	MG	1.24	0.66	124
RIBOFLAVN	MG	1.67	0.75	139
NIACIN	MG	10.60	0.41	76
IRON	MG	12.20	0.41	76
CALCIUM	MG	1008.00	0.60	112
PHOSPHRUS	MG	2017.00	1.20	224
POTASSIUM	MG	1208.00	0.13	24
PROTEIN	G	45.00	0.48	90
CARBOHYDT	G	638.00	1.24	232
FAT	G	125.00	0.86	160
OLEIC A	G	47.80	1.04	195
LINOL A	G	20.30	0.54	102
SAT FAT A	G	47.80	0.90	168

```
          0        10    20    30    40    50    60    70    80    90   100
ENERGY    EEEEEEEEEEEEEEEEEEEEEEEEEEEEEEEEEEEEEEEEEEEEEEEEEEEEEEEEEEEEEE * 187
VITAMIN A AAAAAAAAAAAAAAAAAAAAAAAAA
VITAMIN C CCC
THIAMIN   TTTTTTTTTTTTTTTTTTTTTTTTTTTTTTTTTTTTTTTTTTTTTTTTTTTTTTTTT * 124
RIBOFLAVN RRRRRRRRRRRRRRRRRRRRRRRRRRRRRRRRRRRRRRRRRRRRRRRRRRRRRRRRRRRR * 139
NIACIN    NNNNNNNNNNNNNNNNNNNNNNNNNNNNNNNNNNNNNN
IRON      IIIIIIIIIIIIIIIIIIIIIIIIIIIIIIIIIIIIII
CALCIUM   KKKKKKKKKKKKKKKKKKKKKKKKKKKKKKKKKKKKKKKKKKKKKKKKKKKKKKKKK * 112
PHOSPHRUS XXXXXXXXXXXXXXXXXXXXXXXXXXXXXXXXXXXXXXXXXXXXXXXXXXXXXXXXXXXX * 224
POTASSIUM YYYYYYYYYYYY
PROTEIN   PPPPPPPPPPPPPPPPPPPPPPPPPPPPPPPPPPPPPPPPPPPPPP *
CARBOHYDT HHHHHHHHHHHHHHHHHHHHHHHHHHHHHHHHHHHHHHHHHHHHHHHHHHHHHHHHHHHH * 232
FAT       FFFFFFFFFFFFFFFFFFFFFFFFFFFFFFFFFFFFFFFFFFFFFFFFFFFFFFFFF * 160
OLEIC A   OOOOOOOOOOOOOOOOOOOOOOOOOOOOOOOOOOOOOOOOOOOOOOOOOOOOOOOOOOOO * 195
LINOL A   LLLLLLLLLLLLLLLLLLLLLLLLLLLLLLLLLLLLLLLLLLLLLLLLLLLL * 102
SAT FAT A SSSSSSSSSSSSSSSSSSSSSSSSSSSSSSSSSSSSSSSSSSSSSSSSSSSSSSSSSSS * 168
*******************
```

399 YELLOW CAKE WITH CHOCOLATE ICING
ANALYSIS OF 69 GRAMS WHICH IS 1 PIECE 1/16 OF CAKE

NUTRIENT	UNIT	AMOUNT	INQ	% STD
ENERGY	KCAL	235.00	1.00	12
VITAMIN A	IU	100.00	0.21	3
VITAMIN C	MG	0.00	0.00	0
THIAMIN	MG	0.08	0.68	8
RIBOFLAVN	MG	0.10	0.71	8
NIACIN	MG	0.70	0.43	5
IRON	MG	0.80	0.43	5
CALCIUM	MG	63.00	0.60	7
PHOSPHRUS	MG	126.00	1.19	14
POTASSIUM	MG	75.00	0.13	2
PROTEIN	G	3.00	0.51	6
CARBOHYDT	G	40.00	1.24	15
FAT	G	8.00	0.87	10
OLEIC A	G	3.00	1.04	12
LINOL A	G	1.30	0.55	7
SAT FAT A	G	0.90	0.90	11

400 BOSTON CREAM PIE WITH CUSTARD FILLING
ANALYSIS OF 825 GRAMS WHICH IS 1 WHOLE CAKE (8 IN DIAM)

NUTRIENT	UNIT	AMOUNT	INQ	% STD
ENERGY	KCAL	2490.00	1.00	125
VITAMIN A	IU	1730.00	0.35	43
VITAMIN C	MG	2.00	0.03	3
THIAMIN	MG	1.04	0.84	104
RIBOFLAVN	MG	1.27	0.85	106
NIACIN	MG	9.60	0.55	69
IRON	MG	8.20	0.41	51
CALCIUM	MG	553.00	0.49	61
PHOSPHRUS	MG	833.00	0.74	93
POTASSIUM	MG	734.00	0.12	15
PROTEIN	G	41.00	0.66	82
CARBOHYDT	G	412.00	1.20	150
FAT	G	78.00	0.80	100
OLEIC A	G	30.10	0.99	123
LINOL A	G	15.20	0.61	76
SAT FAT A	G	23.00	0.65	81

401 BOSTON CREAM PIE WITH CUSTARD FILLING
ANALYSIS OF 69 GRAMS WHICH IS 1 PIECE 1/12 CAKE

NUTRIENT	UNIT	AMOUNT	INQ	% STD
ENERGY	KCAL	210.00	1.00	11
VITAMIN A	IU	140.00	0.33	4
VITAMIN C	MG	0.00	0.00	0
THIAMIN	MG	0.09	0.86	9
RIBOFLAVN	MG	0.11	0.87	9
NIACIN	MG	0.80	0.54	6
IRON	MG	0.70	0.42	4
CALCIUM	MG	46.00	0.49	5
PHOSPHRUS	MG	70.00	0.74	8
POTASSIUM	MG	61.00	0.12	1
PROTEIN	G	3.00	0.57	6
CARBOHYDT	G	34.00	1.18	12
FAT	G	6.00	0.73	8
OLEIC A	G	2.50	0.97	10
LINOL A	G	1.30	0.62	7
SAT FAT A	G	1.90	0.63	7

402 FRUIT CAKE, DARK
ANALYSIS OF 454 GRAMS WHICH IS 1 LOAF 1 LB.

NUTRIENT	UNIT	AMOUNT	INQ	% STD
ENERGY	KCAL	1720.00	1.00	86
VITAMIN A	IU	540.00	0.16	14
VITAMIN C	MG	2.00	0.04	3
THIAMIN	MG	0.72	0.84	72
RIBOFLAVN	MG	0.73	0.71	61
NIACIN	MG	4.90	0.41	35
IRON	MG	11.80	0.86	74
CALCIUM	MG	327.00	0.42	36
PHOSPHRUS	MG	513.00	0.66	57
POTASSIUM	MG	2250.00	0.52	45
PROTEIN	G	22.00	0.51	44
CARBOHYDT	G	271.00	1.15	99
FAT	G	69.00	1.03	88
OLEIC A	G	33.50	1.59	137
LINOL A	G	14.80	0.86	74
SAT FAT A	G	14.40	0.59	51

403 FRUIT CAKE, DARK
ANALYSIS OF 15 GRAMS WHICH IS 1 SLICE 1/30 OF LOAF

NUTRIENT	UNIT	AMOUNT	INQ	% STD
ENERGY	KCAL	55.00	1.00	3
VITAMIN A	IU	20.00	0.18	1
VITAMIN C	MG	0.00	0.00	0
THIAMIN	MG	0.02	0.73	2
RIBOFLAVN	MG	0.02	0.61	2
NIACIN	MG	0.20	0.52	1
IRON	MG	0.40	0.91	3
CALCIUM	MG	11.00	0.44	1
PHOSPHRUS	MG	17.00	0.69	2
POTASSIUM	MG	74.00	0.54	1
PROTEIN	G	1.00	0.73	2
CARBOHYDT	G	9.00	1.19	3
FAT	G	2.00	0.93	3
OLEIC A	G	1.10	1.63	4
LINOL A	G	0.50	0.91	3
SAT FAT A	G	0.50	0.64	2

404 SHEET CAKE, WITHOUT ICING
ANALYSIS OF 777 GRAMS WHICH IS 1 WHOLE CAKE 9-IN. SQUARE

NUTRIENT	UNIT	AMOUNT	INQ	% STD
ENERGY	KCAL	2830.00	1.00	141
VITAMIN A	IU	1320.00	0.23	33
VITAMIN C	MG	2.00	0.02	3
THIAMIN	MG	1.21	0.86	121
RIBOFLAVN	MG	1.40	0.82	117
NIACIN	MG	10.20	0.51	73
IRON	MG	8.50	0.38	53
CALCIUM	MG	497.00	0.39	55
PHOSPHRUS	MG	793.00	0.62	88
POTASSIUM	MG	614.00	0.09	12
PROTEIN	G	35.00	0.49	70
CARBOHYDT	G	434.00	1.12	158
FAT	G	106.00	0.98	138
OLEIC A	G	44.40	1.28	181
LINOL A	G	23.90	0.84	120
SAT FAT A	G	29.50	0.73	104

405 SHEET CAKE, WITHOUT ICING
ANALYSIS OF 86 GRAMS WHICH IS 1 PIECE,1/9 OF CAKE

NUTRIENT	UNIT	AMOUNT	INQ	% STD
ENERGY	KCAL	315.00	1.00	16
VITAMIN A	IU	150.00	0.24	0
VITAMIN C	MG	0.00	0.00	0
THIAMIN	MG	0.13	0.83	13
RIBOFLAVN	MG	0.15	0.79	13
NIACIN	MG	1.10	0.50	8
IRON	MG	0.90	0.36	6
CALCIUM	MG	55.00	0.39	6
PHOSPHRUS	MG	88.00	0.62	10
POTASSIUM	MG	68.00	0.09	1
PROTEIN	G	4.00	0.51	8
CARBOHYDT	G	48.00	1.11	17
FAT	G	12.00	0.98	15
OLEIC A	G	4.90	1.27	20
LINOL A	G	2.60	0.83	13
SAT FAT A	G	3.30	0.74	12

```
          0    10   20   30   40   50   60   70   80   90  100
ENERGY    EEEEEEEEEE
VITAMIN A AAA
VITAMIN C -
THIAMIN   TTTTTTTT
RIBOFLAVN RRRRRRRR
NIACIN    NNNNN
IRON      IIIII
CALCIUM   KKKKK
PHOSPHRUS XXXXXXX
POTASSIUM Y
PROTEIN   PPPPP
CARBOHYDT HHHHHHHHHHH H
FAT       FFFFFFFFFF
OLEIC A   OOOOOOOOOOOOO OOO
LINOL A   LLLLLLLLL
SAT FAT A SSSSSSSS
```

406 SHEET CAKE WITH UNCOOKED WHITE ICING
ANALYSIS OF 1096 GRAMS WHICH IS 1 WHOLE CAKE 9-IN SQUARE

NUTRIENT	UNIT	AMOUNT	INQ	% STD
ENERGY	KCAL	4020.00	1.00	201
VITAMIN A	IU	2190.00	0.27	55
VITAMIN C	MG	2.00	0.02	3
THIAMIN	MG	1.22	0.61	122
RIBOFLAVN	MG	1.47	0.61	123
NIACIN	MG	10.20	0.36	73
IRON	MG	8.20	0.25	51
CALCIUM	MG	548.00	0.30	61
PHOSPHRUS	MG	822.00	0.45	91
POTASSIUM	MG	669.00	0.07	13
PROTEIN	G	37.00	0.37	74
CARBOHYDT	G	694.00	1.26	252
FAT	G	129.00	0.82	165
OLEIC A	G	49.50	1.01	202
LINOL A	G	24.40	0.61	122
SAT FAT A	G	42.20	0.74	148

```
          0    10   20   30   40   50   60   70   80   90  100
ENERGY    EEEEEEEEEEEEEEEEEEEEEEEEEEEEEEEEEEEEEEEEEEEEEEEEEEEEEE *201
VITAMIN A AAAAAAAAAAAAAAAAAAAAAAAAAAAAAAA
VITAMIN C CCC
THIAMIN   TTTTTTTTTTTTTTTTTTTTTTTTTTTTTTTTTTTTTTTTTTTTTTTTTTTTTTTTTTTTT *122
RIBOFLAVN RRRRRRRRRRRRRRRRRRRRRRRRRRRRRRRRRRRRRRRRRRRRRRRRRRRRRRRRRRRRRR *123
NIACIN    NNNNNNNNNNNNNNNNNNNNNNNNNNNNNNNNNNNNNNN
IRON      IIIIIIIIIIIIIIIIIIIIIIIIIII
CALCIUM   KKKKKKKKKKKKKKKKKKKKKKKKKKKKKKKK
PHOSPHRUS XXXXXXXXXXXXXXXXXXXXXXXXXXXXXXXXXXXXXXXXXXXXXXXXX
POTASSIUM YYYYYYYYYYYY
PROTEIN   PPPPPPPPPPPPPPPPPPPPPPPPPPPPPPPPPPPPPP
CARBOHYDT HHHHHHHHHHHHHHHHHHHHHHHHHHHHHHHHHHHHHHHHHHHHHHHHHHHHHHHHHHHHHHH *252
FAT       FFFFFFFFFFFFFFFFFFFFFFFFFFFFFFFFFFFFFFFFFFFFFFFFFFFFFFFFFFFFFFF *165
OLEIC A   OOOOOOOOOOOOOOOOOOOOOOOOOOOOOOOOOOOOOOOOOOOOOOOOOOOOOOOOOOOOOOO *202
LINOL A   LLLLLLLLLLLLLLLLLLLLLLLLLLLLLLLLLLLLLLLLLLLLLLLLLLLLLLLLLLLLLLL *122
SAT FAT A SSSSSSSSSSSSSSSSSSSSSSSSSSSSSSSSSSSSSSSSSSSSSSSSSSSSSSSSSSSSSSS *148
```

407 SHEETCAKE WITH UNCOOKED WHITE ICING
ANALYSIS OF 121 GRAMS WHICH IS 1 PIECE,1/9 OF CAKE

NUTRIENT	UNIT	AMOUNT	INQ	% STD
ENERGY	KCAL	445.00	1.00	22
VITAMIN A	IU	240.00	0.27	6
VITAMIN C	MG	0.00	0.00	0
THIAMIN	MG	0.14	0.63	14
RIBOFLAVN	MG	0.16	0.60	13
NIACIN	MG	1.10	0.35	8
IRON	MG	0.80	0.22	5
CALCIUM	MG	61.00	0.30	7
PHOSPHRUS	MG	91.00	0.45	10
POTASSIUM	MG	74.00	0.07	1
PROTEIN	G	4.00	0.36	8
CARBOHYDT	G	77.00	1.26	28
FAT	G	14.00	0.81	18
OLEIC A	G	5.50	1.01	22
LINOL A	G	2.70	0.61	14
SAT FAT A	G	4.70	0.74	16

408 POUNDCAKE
ANALYSIS OF 565 GRAMS WHICH IS 1 LOAF,8 1/2 BY 3 1/2 BY 3 1/4 IN.

NUTRIENT	UNIT	AMOUNT	INQ	% STD
ENERGY	KCAL	2725.00	1.00	136
VITAMIN A	IU	1410.00	0.26	35
VITAMIN C	MG	0.00	0.00	0
THIAMIN	MG	0.90	0.66	90
RIBOFLAVN	MG	0.99	0.61	83
NIACIN	MG	7.30	0.38	52
IRON	MG	7.90	0.36	49
CALCIUM	MG	107.00	0.09	12
PHOSPHRUS	MG	418.00	0.34	46
POTASSIUM	MG	345.00	0.05	7
PROTEIN	G	31.00	0.46	62
CARBOHYDT	G	273.00	0.73	99
FAT	G	170.00	1.60	218
OLEIC A	G	73.10	2.19	298
LINOL A	G	39.60	1.45	198
SAT FAT A	G	42.90	1.10	151

409 POUNDCAKE
ANALYSIS OF 33 GRAMS WHICH IS 1 SLICE, 1/17 OF LOAF

NUTRIENT	UNIT	AMOUNT	INQ	% STD	0	10
ENERGY	KCAL	160.00	1.00	8	EEEEE	
VITAMIN A	IU	80.00	0.25	2	AA	
VITAMIN C	MG	0.00	0.00	0	-	
THIAMIN	MG	0.05	0.63	5	TTTT	
RIBOFLAVN	MG	0.06	0.63	5	RRRR	
NIACIN	MG	0.40	0.36	3	NN	
IRON	MG	0.50	0.39	3	III	
CALCIUM	MG	6.00	0.08	1	K	
PHOSPHRUS	MG	24.00	0.33	3	XX	
POTASSIUM	MG	20.00	0.05	0	-	
PROTEIN	G	2.00	0.50	4	PPP	
CARBOHYDT	G	16.00	0.73	6	HHHHH	
FAT	G	10.00	1.60	13	FFFFIFFFF	
OLEIC A	G	4.30	2.19	18	OOOOOIOOOOOOOO	
LINOL A	G	2.30	1.44	12	LLLLILLL	
SAT FAT A	G	2.50	1.10	9	SSSSIS	

(scale: 0 10 20 30 40 50 60 70 80 90 100)

410 SPONGECAKE
ANALYSIS OF 790 GRAMS WHICH IS 1 WHOLE CAKE (9 3/4-IN DIAM. TUBE)

NUTRIENT	UNIT	AMOUNT	INQ	% STD	0
ENERGY	KCAL	2345.00	1.00	117	EEEEEEEEEEEEEEEEEEEEEEEEEEEEEEEEEEEEEEEEEEEEEEEEEEEEEEEEEE * 117
VITAMIN A	IU	3560.00	0.76	89	AAAAAAAAAAAAAAAAAAAAAAAAAAAAAAAAAAAAAAAAAAAA
VITAMIN C	MG	0.00	0.00	0	-
THIAMIN	MG	1.10	0.94	110	TTTTTTTTTTTTTTTTTTTTTTTTTTTTTTTTTTTTTTTTTTTTTTTTTTTTTT * 110
RIBOFLAVN	MG	1.64	1.17	137	RRRRRRRRRRRRRRRRRRRRRRRRRRRRRRRRRRRRRRRRRRRRRRRRRRRRRRRRRRRRRRRRRRRRRR * 137
NIACIN	MG	7.40	0.45	53	NNNNNNNNNNNNNNNNNNNNNNNNNN
IRON	MG	13.40	0.71	84	IIIIIIIIIIIIIIIIIIIIIIIIIIIIIIIIIIIIIIIIII
CALCIUM	MG	237.00	0.22	26	KKKKKKKKKKKKK
PHOSPHRUS	MG	885.00	0.84	98	XXXXXXXXXXXXXXXXXXXXXXXXXXXXXXXXXXXXXXXXXXXXXXXXX
POTASSIUM	MG	687.00	0.12	14	YYYYYYY
PROTEIN	G	60.00	1.02	120	PPPPPPPPPPPPPPPPPPPPPPPPPPPPPPPPPPPPPPPPPPPPPPPPPPPPPPPPPPPPP * 120
CARBOHYDT	G	427.00	1.32	155	HHHHHHHHHHHHHHHHHHHHHHHHHHHHHHHHHHHHHHHHHHHHHHHHHHHHHHHHHHHHHHHHHHHHHHHHHHHHHHH * 155
FAT	G	45.00	0.49	58	FFFFFFFFFFFFFFFFFFFFFFFFFFFFF
OLEIC A	G	15.80	0.55	64	OOOOOOOOOOOOOOOOOOOOOOOOOOOOOOOO
LINOL A	G	5.70	0.24	29	LLLLLLLLLLLLLL
SAT FAT A	G	13.10	0.39	46	SSSSSSSSSSSSSSSSSSSSSSS

(scale: 0 10 20 30 40 50 60 70 80 90 100)

```
                                        100 * * * * * * * * * * * * * * * * * *                    100 * * * * * * * * * * * * * * * * *

                                         90                                                         90

                                         80                                                         80

                                         70                                                         70

                                         60                                                         60

                                         50                                                         50

                                         40                                                         40

                                         30                                                         30

                                         20                                                         20

411  SPONGECAKE
ANALYSIS OF 66 GRAMS WHICH IS 1 PIECE, 1/12 OF CAKE

NUTRIENT    UNIT   AMOUNT    INQ    % STD   0                 10
ENERGY      KCAL   195.00    1.00    10     EEEEEEE
VITAMIN A   IU     300.00    0.77     8     AAAAA    |
VITAMIN C   MG       0.00    0.00     0     -        |
THIAMIN     MG       0.09    0.92     9     TTTTTT   |
RIBOFLAVN   MG       0.14    1.20    12     RRRRRRR R
NIACIN      MG       0.60    0.44     4     NNN      |
IRON        MG       1.10    0.71     7     IIIIII   |
CALCIUM     MG      20.00    0.23     2     KK       |
PHOSPHRUS   MG      74.00    0.84     8     XXXXXXX  |
POTASSIUM   MG      57.00    0.12     1     Y        |
PROTEIN     G        5.00    1.03    10     PPPPPPP  |
CARBOHYDT   G       36.00    1.34    13     HHHHHHH HH
FAT         G        4.00    0.53     5     FFFF     |
OLEIC A     G        1.30    0.54     5     OOOO     |
LINOL A     G        0.50    0.26     3     LL       |
SAT FAT A   G        1.10    0.40     4     SSS      |
************************************************************

412  BROWNIES WITH NUTS,HOME PREPARED
ANALYSIS OF 20 GRAMS WHICH IS 1 BROWNIE,1 3/4 BY 1 3/4 BY 7/8 IN.

NUTRIENT    UNIT   AMOUNT    INQ    % STD   0                 10          20          30
ENERGY      KCAL    95.00    1.00     5     EEEE
VITAMIN A   IU      40.00    0.21     1     A   |
VITAMIN C   MG       0.00    0.00     0     -   |
THIAMIN     MG       0.04    0.84     4     TTT |
RIBOFLAVN   MG       0.03    0.53     3     RR  |
NIACIN      MG       0.20    0.30     1     N   |
IRON        MG       0.40    0.53     3     II  |
CALCIUM     MG       8.00    0.19     1     K   |
PHOSPHRUS   MG      30.00    0.70     3     XXX |
POTASSIUM   MG      38.00    0.16     1     Y   |
PROTEIN     G        1.00    0.42     2     PP  |
CARBOHYDT   G       10.00    0.77     4     HHH |
FAT         G        6.00    1.62     8     FFFIFF
OLEIC A     G        3.00    2.58    12     OOO1OOOOOO
LINOL A     G        1.20    1.26     6     LLLIL
SAT FAT A   G        1.50    1.11     5     SSSS
************************************************************
```

413 BROWNIES WITH NUTS,COMMERCIAL RECIPE
ANALYSIS OF 20 GRAMS WHICH IS 1 BROWNIE,1 3/4 BY 1 3/4 BY 7/8 IN

NUTRIENT	UNIT	AMOUNT	INQ	% STD	0 10 20 30 40 50 60 70 80 90 100
ENERGY	KCAL	85.00	1.00	4	EEE
VITAMIN A	IU	20.00	0.12	1	-
VITAMIN C	MG	0.00	0.00	0	-
THIAMIN	MG	0.03	0.71	3	TT
RIBOFLAVN	MG	0.02	0.39	2	R
NIACIN	MG	0.20	0.34	1	N
IRON	MG	0.40	0.59	3	II
CALCIUM	MG	9.00	0.24	1	K
PHOSPHRUS	MG	27.00	0.71	3	XX
POTASSIUM	MG	34.00	0.16	1	Y
PROTEIN	G	1.00	0.47	2	PP
CARBOHYDT	G	13.00	1.11	5	HHH
FAT	G	4.00	1.21	5	FFIF
OLEIC A	G	1.40	1.34	6	OOIOO
LINOL A	G	1.30	1.53	7	LLILL
SAT FAT A	G	0.90	0.74	3	SSS

414 BROWNIES FROZEN,WITH CHOCOLATE ICING
ANALYSIS OF 25 GRAMS WHICH IS 1 BROWNIE,1 1/2 BY 1 3/4 BY 7/8 IN

NUTRIENT	UNIT	AMOUNT	INQ	% STD	0 10 20 30 40 50 60 70 80 90 100
ENERGY	KCAL	105.00	1.00	5	EEEE
VITAMIN A	IU	50.00	0.24	1	A
VITAMIN C	MG	0.00	0.00	0	-
THIAMIN	MG	0.03	0.57	3	TT
RIBOFLAVN	MG	0.03	0.48	3	RR
NIACIN	MG	0.20	0.27	1	N
IRON	MG	0.40	0.48	3	II
CALCIUM	MG	10.00	0.21	1	K
PHOSPHRUS	MG	31.00	0.66	3	XXX
POTASSIUM	MG	44.00	0.17	1	Y
PROTEIN	G	1.00	0.38	2	PP
CARBOHYDT	G	15.00	1.04	5	HHHH
FAT	G	5.00	1.22	6	FFFIF
OLEIC A	G	2.20	1.71	9	OOOIOOO
LINOL A	G	0.70	0.67	4	LLLI
SAT FAT A	G	2.00	1.34	7	SSSISS

415 CHOCOLATE CHIP COOKIES,COMMERCIAL RECIPE
ANALYSIS OF 42 GRAMS WHICH IS 4 COOKIES,2 1/4-IN DIAM,3/8-IN THICK

```
                                    0    10   20   30   40   50   60   70   80   90   100
                                                                                     *************
NUTRIENT   UNIT  AMOUNT   INQ  % STD
ENERGY     KCAL  200.00  1.00   10  EEEEEEE
VITAMIN A  IU     50.00  0.13    1  A
VITAMIN C  MG      0.00  0.00    0  -
THIAMIN    MG      0.17  1.00   10  TTTTTTT
RIBOFLAVN  MG      0.42  1.42   14  RRRRRRRIRRR
NIACIN     MG      0.90  0.64    6  NNNNN
IRON       MG      1.00  0.63    6  IIIII
CALCIUM    MG     16.00  0.18    2  K
PHOSPHRUS  MG     48.00  0.53    5  XXXX
POTASSIUM  MG     56.00  0.11    1  Y
PROTEIN    G       2.00  0.40    4  PPP
CARBOHYDT  G      29.00  1.05   11  HHHHHHH
FAT        G       9.00  1.15   12  FFFFFFFIF
OLEIC A    G       2.90  1.18   12  OOOOOOOIO
LINOL A    G       2.20  1.10   11  LLLLLLLIL
SAT FAT A  G       2.80  0.98   10  SSSSSSS
************************************************
```

416 CHOCOLATE CHIP COOKIES,HOME RECIPE
ANALYSIS OF 40 GRAMS WHICH IS 4 COOKIES,2 1/3-IN DIAM

```
                                    0    10   20   30   40   50   60   70   80   90   100
                                                                                     *************
NUTRIENT   UNIT  AMOUNT   INQ  % STD
ENERGY     KCAL  205.00  1.00   10  EEEEEEE
VITAMIN A  IU     40.00  0.10    1  A
VITAMIN C  MG      0.00  0.00    0  -
THIAMIN    MG      0.06  0.59    6  TTTT
RIBOFLAVN  MG      0.06  0.49    5  RRRR
NIACIN     MG      0.50  0.35    4  NNN
IRON       MG      0.80  0.49    5  IIII
CALCIUM    MG     14.00  0.15    2  K
PHOSPHRUS  MG     40.00  0.43    4  XXXX
POTASSIUM  MG     47.00  0.09    1  Y
PROTEIN    G       2.00  0.39    4  PPP
CARBOHYDT  G      24.00  0.85    9  HHHHHHH
FAT        G      12.00  1.50   15  FFFFFFFIFFFF
OLEIC A    G       4.50  1.79   18  OOOOOOOIOOOOOOO
LINOL A    G       2.90  1.41   15  LLLLLLLILLLL
SAT FAT A  G       3.50  1.20   12  SSSSSSSISS
************************************************
```

417 FIGBARS
ANALYSIS OF 56 GRAMS WHICH IS 4 COOKIES,1 5/8 BY 1 5/8 BY 3/8 IN.

NUTRIENT	UNIT	AMOUNT	INQ	% STD	0 ... 100
ENERGY	KCAL	200.00	1.00	10	EEEEEEE
VITAMIN A	IU	60.00	0.15	2	A
VITAMIN C	MG	0.00	0.00	0	-
THIAMIN	MG	0.04	0.40	4	TTT
RIBOFLAVN	MG	0.14	1.17	12	RRRRRRR|R
NIACIN	MG	0.90	0.64	6	NNNNN
IRON	MG	1.00	0.63	6	IIIII
CALCIUM	MG	44.00	0.49	5	KKKK
PHOSPHRUS	MG	34.00	0.38	4	XXX
POTASSIUM	MG	111.00	0.22	2	YY
PROTEIN	G	2.00	0.40	4	PPP
CARBOHYDT	G	42.00	1.53	15	HHHHHHH|HHHH
FAT	G	3.00	0.38	4	FFF
OLEIC A	G	1.20	0.49	5	OOOO
LINOL A	G	0.70	0.35	4	LLL
SAT FAT A	G	0.80	0.28	3	SS

418 GINGERSNAPS
ANALYSIS OF 28 GRAMS WHICH IS 4 COOKIES, 1/4-IN THICK

NUTRIENT	UNIT	AMOUNT	INQ	% STD	0 ... 100
ENERGY	KCAL	90.00	1.00	5	EEE
VITAMIN A	IU	20.00	0.11	1	-
VITAMIN C	MG	0.00	0.00	0	-
THIAMIN	MG	0.08	1.78	8	TTTITT
RIBOFLAVN	MG	0.06	1.11	5	RRRR
NIACIN	MG	0.70	1.11	5	NNNN
IRON	MG	0.70	0.97	4	IIII
CALCIUM	MG	20.00	0.49	2	KK
PHOSPHRUS	MG	13.00	0.32	1	X
POTASSIUM	MG	129.00	0.57	3	YY
PROTEIN	G	2.00	0.89	4	PPP
CARBOHYDT	G	22.00	1.78	8	HHH|HH
FAT	G	2.00	0.57	3	FF
OLEIC A	G	1.00	0.91	4	OOO
LINOL A	G	0.60	0.67	3	LL
SAT FAT A	G	0.70	0.55	2	SS

419 MACAROONS
ANALYSIS OF 38 GRAMS WHICH IS 2 COOKIES, 2 3/4-IN DIAM., 1/4-IN. THICK

NUTRIENT	UNIT	AMOUNT	INQ	% STD	0 10 20 30 40 50 60 70 80 90 100
ENERGY	KCAL	180.00	1.00	9	EEEEEE
VITAMIN A	IU	0.00	0.00	0	-
VITAMIN C	MG	0.00	0.00	0	-
THIAMIN	MG	0.02	0.22	2	TT
RIBOFLAVN	MG	0.06	0.56	5	RRRR
NIACIN	MG	0.20	0.16	1	N
IRON	MG	0.30	0.21	2	II
CALCIUM	MG	10.00	0.12	1	K
PHOSPHRUS	MG	32.00	0.40	4	XXX
POTASSIUM	MG	176.00	0.39	4	YYY
PROTEIN	G	2.00	0.44	4	PPP
CARBOHYDT	G	25.00	1.01	9	HHHHHHH
FAT	G	9.00	1.28	12	FFFFFFF
OLEIC A	G	1.90	0.86	8	OOOOOO
LINOL A	G	0.40	0.22	2	LL
SAT FAT A	G	6.00	2.34	21	SSSSSSISSSSSSSSSSS

420 OATMEAL COOKIES WITH RASINS
ANALYSIS OF 52 GRAMS WHICH IS 4 COOKIES, 2 5/8-IN DIAM, 1/4-IN THICK

NUTRIENT	UNIT	AMOUNT	INQ	% STD	0 10 20 30 40 50 60 70 80 90 100
ENERGY	KCAL	235.00	1.00	12	EEEEEEEE
VITAMIN A	IU	30.00	0.06	1	A
VITAMIN C	MG	0.00	0.00	0	-
THIAMIN	MG	0.15	1.28	15	TTTTTTTTTTTT
RIBOFLAVN	MG	0.10	0.71	8	RRRRRR
NIACIN	MG	1.00	0.61	7	NNNNN
IRON	MG	1.40	0.74	9	IIIIIII
CALCIUM	MG	11.00	0.10	1	K
PHOSPHRUS	MG	53.00	0.50	6	XXXXX
POTASSIUM	MG	192.00	0.33	4	YYY
PROTEIN	G	3.00	0.51	6	PPPP
CARBOHYDT	G	38.00	1.18	14	HHHHHHHHHH
FAT	G	8.00	0.87	10	FFFFFFFF
OLEIC A	G	3.30	1.15	13	OOOOOOOOOO
LINOL A	G	2.00	0.85	10	LLLLLLLL
SAT FAT A	G	2.00	0.60	7	SSSSS

421 PLAIN COOKIES, COMMERCIAL RECIPE
ANALYSIS OF 48 GRAMS WHICH IS 4 COOKIES, 2 1/2-IN DIAM., 1/4-IN THICK

NUTRIENT	UNIT	AMOUNT	INQ	% STD
ENERGY	KCAL	240.00	1.00	12
VITAMIN A	IU	36.00	0.06	1
VITAMIN C	MG	0.00	0.00	0
THIAMIN	MG	0.10	0.83	10
RIBOFLAVN	MG	0.08	0.56	7
NIACIN	MG	0.90	0.54	6
IRON	MG	0.60	0.31	4
CALCIUM	MG	17.00	0.16	2
PHOSPHRUS	MG	35.00	0.32	4
POTASSIUM	MG	23.00	0.04	0
PROTEIN	G	2.00	0.33	4
CARBOHYDT	G	31.00	0.94	11
FAT	G	12.00	1.28	15
OLEIC A	G	5.20	1.77	21
LINOL A	G	2.90	1.21	15
SAT FAT A	G	3.00	0.88	11

422 SANDWICH TYPE COOKIES (CHOCOLATE OR VANILLA)
ANALYSIS OF 40 GRAMS WHICH IS 4 COOKIES 1 3/4-IN DIAM., 3/8-IN THICK

NUTRIENT	UNIT	AMOUNT	INQ	% STD
ENERGY	KCAL	200.00	1.00	10
VITAMIN A	IU	0.00	0.00	0
VITAMIN C	MG	0.00	0.00	0
THIAMIN	MG	0.06	0.60	6
RIBOFLAVN	MG	0.10	0.83	8
NIACIN	MG	0.70	0.50	5
IRON	MG	0.70	0.44	4
CALCIUM	MG	10.00	0.11	1
PHOSPHRUS	MG	96.00	1.07	11
POTASSIUM	MG	15.00	0.03	0
PROTEIN	G	2.00	0.40	4
CARBOHYDT	G	28.00	1.02	10
FAT	G	9.00	1.15	12
OLEIC A	G	3.90	1.59	16
LINOL A	G	2.20	1.10	11
SAT FAT A	G	2.20	0.77	8

423 VANILLA WAFERS
ANALYSIS OF 40 GRAMS WHICH IS 10 COOKIES,1 3/4-IN DIAM.,1/4-IN THICK

NUTRIENT	UNIT	AMOUNT	INQ	% STD
ENERGY	KCAL	185.00	1.00	9
VITAMIN A	IU	50.00	0.14	1
VITAMIN C	MG	0.00	0.00	0
THIAMIN	MG	0.10	1.08	10
RIBOFLAVN	MG	0.09	0.81	8
NIACIN	MG	0.80	0.62	6
IRON	MG	0.60	0.41	4
CALCIUM	MG	16.00	0.19	2
PHOSPHRUS	MG	25.00	0.30	3
POTASSIUM	MG	29.00	0.06	1
PROTEIN	G	2.00	0.43	4
CARBOHYDT	G	30.00	1.18	11
FAT	G	6.00	0.83	8
OLEIC A	G	4.00	1.77	16
LINOL A	G	0.40	0.22	2
SAT FAT A	G	1.60	0.61	6

424 CORNMEAL,WHOLE-GROUND,UNBOLTED,DRY FORM
ANALYSIS OF 122 GRAMS WHICH IS 1 CUP

NUTRIENT	UNIT	AMOUNT	INQ	% STD
ENERGY	KCAL	435.00	1.00	22
VITAMIN A	IU	620.00	0.71	16
VITAMIN C	MG	0.00	0.00	0
THIAMIN	MG	0.46	2.11	46
RIBOFLAVN	MG	0.13	0.50	11
NIACIN	MG	2.40	0.79	17
IRON	MG	2.90	0.83	18
CALCIUM	MG	24.00	0.12	3
PHOSPHRUS	MG	312.00	1.59	35
POTASSIUM	MG	346.00	0.32	7
PROTEIN	G	11.00	1.01	22
CARBOHYDT	G	90.00	1.50	33
FAT	G	5.00	0.29	6
OLEIC A	G	1.00	0.19	4
LINOL A	G	2.50	0.57	13
SAT FAT A	G	0.50	0.08	2

425 CORNMEAL,BOLTED,DRY FORM
ANALYSIS OF 122 GRAMS WHICH IS 1 CUP

```
                                0         10        20        30        40        50        60        70        80        90       100
NUTRIENT   UNIT   AMOUNT   ING  % STD     *         *         *         *         *         *         *         *         *         *
ENERGY     KCAL   440.00   1.00   22      EEEEEEEEEEEEEEEEE
VITAMIN A  IU     590.00   0.67   15      AAAAAAAAAAA
VITAMIN C  MG       0.00   0.00    0      -
THIAMIN    MG       0.37   1.68   37      TTTTTTTTTTTTTTTTTT|TTTTTTTTTT
RIBOFLAVN  MG       0.10   0.38    8      RRRRRRR
NIACIN     MG       2.30   0.75   16      NNNNNNNNNNNN
IRON       MG       2.20   0.63   14      IIIIIIIIIII
CALCIUM    MG      21.00   0.11    2      KK
PHOSPHRUS  MG     272.00   1.37   30      XXXXXXXXXXXXXXXXXXXXXX|XXXXX
POTASSIUM  MG     303.00   0.28    6      YYYYY
PRUTEIN    G       11.00   1.00   22      PPPPPPPPPPPPPPPPP
CARBOHYDT  G       91.00   1.50   33      HHHHHHHHHHHHHHHHHHHHHHHHH|HHHHHHHH
FAT        G        4.00   0.23    5      FFFF
OLEIC A    G        0.90   0.17    4      OOO
LINOL A    G        2.10   0.48   11      LLLLLLLL
SAT FAT A  G        0.50   0.08    2      S
**********************************************************
```

426 CORNMEAL,DEGERMED,ENRICHED DRY FORM
ANALYSIS OF 138 GRAMS WHICH IS 1 CUP

```
                                0         10        20        30        40        50        60        70        80        90       100
NUTRIENT   UNIT   AMOUNT   ING  % STD     *         *         *         *         *         *         *         *         *         *
ENERGY     KCAL   500.00   1.00   25      EEEEEEEEEEEEEEEEEEE
VITAMIN A  IU     610.00   0.61   15      AAAAAAAAAAA
VITAMIN C  MG       0.00   0.00    0      -
THIAMIN    MG       0.61   2.44   61      TTTTTTTTTTTTTTTTTT|TTTTTTTTTTTTTTTTTT|TTTTTTTTTTTTTTT
RIBOFLAVN  MG       0.36   1.20   30      RRRRRRRRRRRRRRRRRRRRRR|RRRR
NIACIN     MG       4.80   1.37   34      NNNNNNNNNNNNNNNNNNNNNNNNN|NNNNNNN
IRON       MG       4.00   1.00   25      IIIIIIIIIIIIIIIIIIIII
CALCIUM    MG       8.00   0.04    1      K
PHOSPHRUS  MG     137.00   0.61   15      XXXXXXXXXXX
POTASSIUM  MG     166.00   0.13    3      YYY
PROTEIN    G       11.00   0.88   22      PPPPPPPPPPPPPPPPP
CARBOHYDT  G      108.00   1.57   39      HHHHHHHHHHHHHHHHHHHHHHHHHHHHH|HHHHHHHHHH
FAT        G        2.00   0.10    3      FF
OLEIC A    G        0.40   0.07    2      O
LINOL A    G        0.90   0.18    5      LLLL
SAT FAT A  G        0.20   0.03    1      S
**********************************************************
```

427 CORNMEAL,DEGERMED,ENRICHED,COOKED
ANALYSIS OF 240 GRAMS WHICH IS 1 CUP

NUTRIENT	UNIT	AMOUNT	INQ	% STD
ENERGY	KCAL	120.00	1.00	6
VITAMIN A	IU	140.00	0.58	4
VITAMIN C	MG	0.00	0.00	0
THIAMIN	MG	0.14	2.33	14
RIBOFLAVN	MG	0.10	1.39	8
NIACIN	MG	1.20	1.43	9
IRON	MG	1.00	1.04	6
CALCIUM	MG	2.00	0.04	0
PHOSPHRUS	MG	34.00	0.63	4
POTASSIUM	MG	38.00	0.13	1
PROTEIN	G	3.00	1.00	6
CARBOHYDT	G	26.00	1.58	9
FAT	G	0.00	0.00	0
OLEIC A	G	0.10	0.07	0
LINOL A	G	0.20	0.17	1
SAT FAT A	G	0.00	0.00	0

428 CORNMEAL,DEGERMED, UNENRICHED, DRY FORM
ANALYSIS OF 138 GRAMS WHICH IS 1 CUP

NUTRIENT	UNIT	AMOUNT	INQ	% STD
ENERGY	KCAL	500.00	1.00	25
VITAMIN A	IU	610.00	0.61	15
VITAMIN C	MG	0.00	0.00	0
THIAMIN	MG	0.19	0.76	19
RIBOFLAVN	MG	0.07	0.23	6
NIACIN	MG	1.40	0.40	10
IRON	MG	1.50	0.38	9
CALCIUM	MG	8.00	0.04	1
PHOSPHRUS	MG	137.00	0.61	15
POTASSIUM	MG	166.00	0.13	3
PROTEIN	G	11.00	0.88	22
CARBOHYDT	G	108.00	1.57	39
FAT	G	2.00	0.10	3
OLEIC A	G	0.40	0.07	2
LINOL A	G	0.90	0.18	5
SAT FAT A	G	0.20	0.03	1

429 CORNMEAL,DEGERMED, UNENRICHED, COOKED
ANALYSIS OF 240 GRAMS WHICH IS 1 CUP

NUTRIENT	UNIT	AMOUNT	INQ	% STD	0	10	20	30	40	50	60	70	80	90	100
ENERGY	KCAL	120.00	1.00	6	EEEEE										*
VITAMIN A	IU	140.00	0.58	4	AAA										*
VITAMIN C	MG	0.00	0.00	0	-										*
THIAMIN	MG	0.02	0.83	5	TTTT										*
RIBOFLAVN	MG	0.02	0.28	2	R										*
NIACIN	MG	0.20	0.24	1	N										*
IRON	MG	0.50	0.52	3	III										*
CALCIUM	MG	2.00	0.04	0	-										*
PHOSPHRUS	MG	34.00	0.63	4	XXX										*
POTASSIUM	MG	38.00	0.13	1	Y										*
PROTEIN	G	3.00	1.00	6	PPPPP										*
CARBOHYDT	G	26.00	1.58	9	HHHH HHH										*
FAT	G	0.00	0.00	0	-										*
OLEIC A	G	0.10	0.07	0	-										*
LINOL A	G	0.20	0.17	1	L										*
SAT FAT A	G	0.00	0.00	0	-										*

430 GRAHAM CRACKERS PLAIN
ANALYSIS OF 14 GRAMS WHICH IS 2 CRACKERS

NUTRIENT	UNIT	AMOUNT	INQ	% STD	0	10	20	30	40	50	60	70	80	90	100
ENERGY	KCAL	55.00	1.00	3	EE										*
VITAMIN A	IU	0.00	0.00	0	-										*
VITAMIN C	MG	0.00	0.00	0	-										*
THIAMIN	MG	0.02	0.73	2	TT										*
RIBOFLAVN	MG	0.08	2.42	7	RIRRR										*
NIACIN	MG	0.50	1.30	4	NIN										*
IRON	MG	0.50	1.14	3	III										*
CALCIUM	MG	6.00	0.24	1	KI										*
PHOSPHRUS	MG	21.00	0.85	2	XX										*
POTASSIUM	MG	55.00	0.40	1	YI										*
PROTEIN	G	1.00	0.73	2	PP										*
CARBOHYDT	G	10.00	1.32	4	HIH										*
FAT	G	1.00	0.47	1	FI										*
OLEIC A	G	0.50	0.74	2	OO										*
LINOL A	G	0.30	0.55	2	LI										*
SAT FAT A	G	0.30	0.38	1	SI										*

431 RYE WAFERS, WHOLE GRAIN,
ANALYSIS OF 13 GRAMS WHICH IS 2 WAFERS, 1 7/8 BY 3 1/2-IN.

NUTRIENT	UNIT	AMOUNT	INQ	% STD	Graph
ENERGY	KCAL	45.00	1.00	2	EE
VITAMIN A	IU	0.00	0.00	0	-I
VITAMIN C	MG	0.00	0.00	0	-I
THIAMIN	MG	0.04	1.78	4	TIT
RIBOFLAVN	MG	0.03	1.11	3	RR
NIACIN	MG	0.20	0.63	1	NI
IRON	MG	0.50	1.39	3	III
CALCIUM	MG	7.00	0.35	1	KI
PHOSPHRUS	MG	50.00	2.47	6	XIXX
POTASSIUM	MG	78.00	0.69	2	YI
PROTEIN	G	2.00	1.78	4	PIP
CARBOHYDT	G	10.00	1.62	4	HIH
FAT	G	0.00	0.00	0	-I
OLEIC A	G	0.00	0.00	0	-I
LINOL A	G	0.00	0.00	0	-I
SAT FAT A	G	0.00	0.00	0	-I

432 SALTINES
ANALYSIS OF 11 GRAMS WHICH IS 4 CRACKERS OR 1 PACKET

NUTRIENT	UNIT	AMOUNT	INQ	% STD	Graph
ENERGY	KCAL	50.00	1.00	3	EE
VITAMIN A	IU	0.00	0.00	0	-I
VITAMIN C	MG	0.00	0.00	0	-I
THIAMIN	MG	0.05	2.00	5	TITT
RIBOFLAVN	MG	0.05	1.67	4	RIR
NIACIN	MG	0.40	1.14	3	NN
IRON	MG	0.50	1.25	3	III
CALCIUM	MG	2.00	0.09	0	-I
PHOSPHRUS	MG	10.00	0.44	1	XI
POTASSIUM	MG	13.00	0.10	0	-I
PROTEIN	G	1.00	0.80	2	PP
CARBOHYDT	G	8.00	1.16	3	HH
FAT	G	1.00	0.51	1	FI
OLEIC A	G	0.50	0.82	2	OO
LINOL A	G	0.40	0.80	2	LL
SAT FAT A	G	0.30	0.42	1	SI

433 DANISH PASTRY WITHOUT FRUIT OR NUTS
ANALYSIS OF 340 GRAMS WHICH IS 1 RING, 12 OZ.

```
NUTRIENT   UNIT   AMOUNT    INQ   % STD   0        10        20        30        40        50        60        70        80        90       100
ENERGY     KCAL   1435.00   1.00    72    EEEEEEEEEEEEEEEEEEEEEEEEEEEEEEEEEEEEEEEEEEEEEEEEEEEEEEEEEEEEEEEEEEEEEEEEEEE                                         *
VITAMIN A  IU     1050.00   0.37    26    AAAAAAAAAAAAAAAAAAAAAAAAAA                                                                                 *
VITAMIN C  MG        0.00   0.00     0    -                                                                                                          *
THIAMIN    MG        0.97   1.35    97    TTTTTTTTTTTTTTTTTTTTTTTTTTTTTTTTTTTTTTTTTTTTTTTTTTTTTTTTTTTTTTTTTTTTTTTTTTTTTTTTTTTTTTTTTTTTTTTTTT           *
RIBOFLAVN  MG        1.01   1.17    84    RRRRRRRRRRRRRRRRRRRRRRRRRRRRRRRRRRRRRRRRRRRRRRRRRRRRRRRRRRRRRRRRRRRRRRRRRRRRRRRRRRRR                           *
NIACIN     MG        8.60   0.86    61    NNNNNNNNNNNNNNNNNNNNNNNNNNNNNNNNNNNNNNNNNNNNNNNNNNNNNNNNNNNNNN                                               *
IRON       MG        6.10   0.53    38    IIIIIIIIIIIIIIIIIIIIIIIIIIIIIIIIIIIIII                                                                      *
CALCIUM    MG      170.00   0.26    19    KKKKKKKKKKKKKKKKKKK                                                                                         *
PHOSPHRUS  MG      371.00   0.57    41    XXXXXXXXXXXXXXXXXXXXXXXXXXXXXXXXXXXXXXXXX                                                                   *
POTASSIUM  MG      381.00   0.11     8    YYYYYY                                                                                                      *
PROTEIN    G       25.00    0.70    50    PPPPPPPPPPPPPPPPPPPPPPPPPPPPPPPPPPPPPPPPPPPPPPPPPPP                                                          *
CARBOHYDT  G      155.00    0.79    56    HHHHHHHHHHHHHHHHHHHHHHHHHHHHHHHHHHHHHHHHHHHHHHHHHHHHHHHHHH                                                    *
FAT        G       80.00    1.43   103    FFFFFFFFFFFFFFFFFFFFFFFFFFFFFFFFFFFFFFFFFFFFFFFFFFFFFFFFFFFFFFFFFFFFFFFFFFFFFFFFFFFFFFFFFFFFFFFFFFFFFFF   *103
OLEIC A    G       31.70    1.80   129    OOOOOOOOOOOOOOOOOOOOOOOOOOOOOOOOOOOOOOOOOOOOOOOOOOOOOOOOOOOOOOOOOOOOOOOOOOOOOOOOOOOOOOOOOOOOOOOOOOOOOOOOOOOOOOOOOOOOOOOOOOOOOOOOOOO   *129
LINOL A    G       16.50    1.15    83    LLLLLLLLLLLLLLLLLLLLLLLLLLLLLLLLLLLLLLLLLLLLLLLLLLLLLLLLLLLLLLLLLLLLLLLLLLLLLLLLLLLLL                         *
SAT FAT A  G       24.30    1.19    85    SSSSSSSSSSSSSSSSSSSSSSSSSSSSSSSSSSSSSSSSSSSSSSSSSSSSSSSSSSSSSSSSSSSSSSSSSSSSSSSSSSSSSSS                       *
********************************************************************************************
```

434 DANISH PASTRY WITHOUT FRUIT OR NUTS
ANALYSIS OF 65 GRAMS WHICH IS 1 ROUND PIECE 4 1/4-IN DIAM BY 1-IN. THICK

```
NUTRIENT   UNIT   AMOUNT   INQ   % STD   0        10        20        30        40        50        60        70        80        90       100
ENERGY     KCAL   275.00   1.00    14    EEEEEEEEEE                                                                                                  *
VITAMIN A  IU     200.00   0.36     5    AAAA                                                                                                        *
VITAMIN C  MG       0.00   0.00     0    -                                                                                                           *
THIAMIN    MG       0.18   1.31    18    TTTTTTTTTTTTTTTTTT                                                                                          *
RIBOFLAVN  MG       0.19   1.15    16    RRRRRRRRRRRRRRRR                                                                                            *
NIACIN     MG       1.70   0.88    12    NNNNNNNNNNNN                                                                                                *
IRON       MG       1.20   0.55     7    IIIIIII                                                                                                     *
CALCIUM    MG      33.00   0.27     4    KKK                                                                                                         *
PHOSPHRUS  MG      71.00   0.57     8    XXXXXXX                                                                                                     *
POTASSIUM  MG      73.00   0.11     1    Y                                                                                                           *
PROTEIN    G        5.00   0.73    10    PPPPPPPP                                                                                                    *
CARBOHYDT  G       30.00   0.79    11    HHHHHHHHHHH                                                                                                 *
FAT        G       15.00   1.40    19    FFFFFFFFFFFFFFFFFFF                                                                                         *
OLEIC A    G        6.10   1.81    25    OOOOOOOOOOOIOOOOOOOOOOOOO                                                                                    *
LINOL A    G        3.20   1.16    16    LLLLLLLLLLLLLLLL                                                                                            *
SAT FAT A  G        4.70   1.20    16    SSSSSSSSSSISS                                                                                               *
********************************************************************************************
```

435 DANISH PASTRY WITHOUT FRUIT OR NUTS
ANALYSIS OF 28 GRAMS WHICH IS 1 OZ

NUTRIENT	UNIT	AMOUNT	INQ	% STD	
ENERGY	KCAL	120.00	1.00	6	EEEEE
VITAMIN A	IU	90.00	0.38	2	AA
VITAMIN C	MG	0.00	0.00	0	-
THIAMIN	MG	0.08	1.33	8	TTTTT
RIBOFLAVN	MG	0.08	1.11	7	RRRRR
NIACIN	MG	0.70	0.83	5	NNNN
IRON	MG	0.50	0.52	3	III
CALCIUM	MG	14.00	0.26	2	K
PHOSPHRUS	MG	31.00	0.57	3	XXX
POTASSIUM	MG	32.00	0.11	1	Y
PROTEIN	G	2.00	0.67	4	PPP
CARBOHYDT	G	13.00	0.79	5	HHHH
FAT	G	7.00	1.50	9	FFFFIFF
OLEIC A	G	2.70	1.84	11	000010000
LINOL A	G	1.40	1.17	7	LLLIL
SAT FAT A	G	2.00	1.17	7	SSSSIS

436 DOUGHNUTS, CAKE TYPE
ANALYSIS OF 25 GRAMS WHICH IS 1 DOUGHNUT, PLAIN,2 1/2-IN DIAM, 1 IN HIGH

NUTRIENT	UNIT	AMOUNT	INQ	% STD	
ENERGY	KCAL	100.00	1.00	5	EEEE
VITAMIN A	IU	20.00	0.10	1	-
VITAMIN C	MG	0.00	0.00	0	-
THIAMIN	MG	0.05	1.00	5	TTTT
RIBOFLAVN	MG	0.05	0.83	4	RRRI
NIACIN	MG	0.40	0.57	3	NN
IRON	MG	0.40	0.50	3	II
CALCIUM	MG	10.00	0.22	1	K
PHOSPHRUS	MG	48.00	1.07	5	XXXX
POTASSIUM	MG	23.00	0.09	0	-
PROTEIN	G	1.00	0.40	2	PP
CARBOHYDT	G	13.00	0.95	5	HHHH
FAT	G	5.00	1.28	6	FFFIF
OLEIC A	G	2.00	1.63	8	000I000
LINOL A	G	1.10	1.10	6	LLLL
SAT FAT A	G	1.20	0.84	4	SSSI

437 DOUGHNUTS, YEAST-LEAVENED,GLAZED,
ANALYSIS OF 50 GRAMS WHICH IS 1 DOUGHNUT, 3 3/4-IN DIAM., 1 1/4-IN HIGH

Scale: 0 10 20 30 40 50 60 70 80 90 100

NUTRIENT	UNIT	AMOUNT	INQ	% STD	PROFILE
ENERGY	KCAL	205.00	1.00	10	EEEEEEE
VITAMIN A	IU	25.00	0.06	1	A
VITAMIN C	MG	0.00	0.00	0	-
THIAMIN	MG	0.10	0.98	10	TTTTTTT
RIBOFLAVN	MG	0.10	0.81	8	RRRRRR
NIACIN	MG	0.80	0.56	6	NNNNN
IRON	MG	0.60	0.37	4	III
CALCIUM	MG	16.00	0.17	2	K
PHOSPHRUS	MG	33.00	0.36	4	XXX
POTASSIUM	MG	34.00	0.07	1	Y
PROTEIN	G	3.00	0.59	6	PPPPP
CARBOHYDT	G	22.00	0.78	8	HHHHHH
FAT	G	11.00	1.38	14	FFFFFFFFF
OLEIC A	G	5.80	2.31	24	OOOOOOOOOOOOOOOO
LINOL A	G	3.30	1.61	17	LLLLLLLLLLL
SAT FAT A	G	3.30	1.13	12	SSSSSSS

438 MACARONI,ENRICHED, COOKED FIRM STAGE (HOT)
ANALYSIS OF 130 GRAMS WHICH IS 1 CUP

Scale: 0 10 20 30 40 50 60 70 80 90 100

NUTRIENT	UNIT	AMOUNT	INQ	% STD	PROFILE
ENERGY	KCAL	190.00	1.00	10	EEEEEEE
VITAMIN A	IU	0.00	0.00	0	-
VITAMIN C	MG	0.00	0.00	0	-
THIAMIN	MG	0.23	2.42	23	TTTTTTTTTTTTTTT
RIBOFLAVN	MG	0.13	1.14	11	RRRRRRR
NIACIN	MG	1.80	1.35	13	NNNNNNNNN
IRON	MG	1.40	0.92	9	IIIIIII
CALCIUM	MG	14.00	0.16	2	K
PHOSPHRUS	MG	85.00	0.99	9	XXXXXXX
POTASSIUM	MG	103.00	0.22	2	YY
PROTEIN	G	7.00	1.47	14	PPPPPPPPP
CARBOHYDT	G	39.00	1.49	14	HHHHHHHHH
FAT	G	1.00	0.13	1	F
OLEIC A	G	0.00	0.00	0	-
LINOL A	G	0.00	0.00	0	-
SAT FAT A	G	0.00	0.00	0	-

439 MACARONI,ENRICHED TENDER STAGE,COLD
ANALYSIS OF 105 GRAMS WHICH IS 1 CUP

NUTRIENT	UNIT	AMOUNT	INQ	% STD	0 10 20 ... 100
ENERGY	KCAL	115.00	1.00	6	EEEEE
VITAMIN A	IU	0.00	0.00	0	-
VITAMIN C	MG	0.00	0.00	0	-
THIAMIN	MG	0.15	2.61	15	TTTTITTTTTT
RIBOFLAVN	MG	0.08	1.16	7	RRRR
NIACIN	MG	1.20	1.49	9	NNNNINN
IRON	MG	0.90	0.98	6	IIIII
CALCIUM	MG	8.00	0.15	1	K
PHOSPHRUS	MG	53.00	1.02	6	XXXXX
POTASSIUM	MG	64.00	0.22	1	Y
PROTEIN	G	4.00	1.39	8	PPPPIP
CARBOHYDT	G	24.00	1.52	9	HHHHIHH
FAT	G	0.00	0.00	0	I
OLEIC A	G	0.00	0.00	0	I
LINOL A	G	0.00	0.00	0	I
SAT FAT A	G	0.00	0.00	0	I

440 MACARONI,ENRICHED,TENDER STAGE, HOT
ANALYSIS OF 140 GRAMS WHICH IS 1 CUP

NUTRIENT	UNIT	AMOUNT	INQ	% STD	0 10 20 ... 100
ENERGY	KCAL	155.00	1.00	8	EEEEE
VITAMIN A	IU	0.00	0.00	0	-
VITAMIN C	MG	0.00	0.00	0	-
THIAMIN	MG	0.20	2.58	20	TTTTTITTTTTTTT
RIBOFLAVN	MG	0.11	1.18	9	RRRRIR
NIACIN	MG	1.50	1.38	11	NNNNNINNN
IRON	MG	1.30	1.05	8	IIIIIII
CALCIUM	MG	11.00	0.16	1	K
PHOSPHRUS	MG	70.00	1.00	8	XXXXXX
POTASSIUM	MG	85.00	0.22	2	Y
PROTEIN	G	5.00	1.29	10	PPPPPIPP
CARBOHYDT	G	32.00	1.50	12	HHHHHIHHH
FAT	G	1.00	0.17	1	F
OLEIC A	G	0.00	0.00	0	I
LINOL A	G	0.00	0.00	0	I
SAT FAT A	G	0.00	0.00	0	I

441 MACARONI (ENRICHED) AND CHEESE, CANNED
ANALYSIS OF 240 GRAMS WHICH IS 1 CUP

NUTRIENT	UNIT	AMOUNT	INQ	% STD	0 · · · 10 · · · 20 · · · 30 · · · 40 · · · 50 · · · 60 · · · 70 · · · 80 · · · 90 · · · 100
ENERGY	KCAL	230.00	1.00	12	EEEEEEEE
VITAMIN A	IU	260.00	0.57	7	AAAA
VITAMIN C	MG	0.00	0.00	0	
THIAMIN	MG	0.12	1.04	12	TTTTTTTT
RIBOFLAVN	MG	0.24	1.74	20	RRRRRRRR RRRRRRR
NIACIN	MG	1.00	0.62	7	NNNNNN
IRON	MG	1.00	0.54	6	IIIII
CALCIUM	MG	199.00	1.92	22	KKKKKKKK KKKKKKKK
PHOSPHRUS	MG	182.00	1.76	20	XXXXXXXX XXXXXXX
POTASSIUM	MG	139.00	0.24	3	YY
PROTEIN	G	9.00	1.57	18	PPPPPPPP PPPPP
CARBOHYDT	G	26.00	0.82	9	HHHHHHH
FAT	G	10.00	1.11	13	FFFFFFFF F
OLEIC A	G	3.10	1.10	13	OOOOOOOO O
LINOL A	G	1.40	0.61	7	LLLLLL
SAT FAT A	G	4.20	1.28	15	SSSSSSSS SSS

442 MACARONI (ENRICHED) AND CHEESE, HOME RECIPE
ANALYSIS OF 200 GRAMS WHICH IS 1 CUP

NUTRIENT	UNIT	AMOUNT	INQ	% STD	0 · · · 10 · · · 20 · · · 30 · · · 40 · · · 50 · · · 60 · · · 70 · · · 80 · · · 90 · · · 100
ENERGY	KCAL	430.00	1.00	22	EEEEEEEE EEEEEEEE EEEE
VITAMIN A	IU	860.00	1.00	22	AAAAAAAA AAAAAAAA AAAA
VITAMIN C	MG	0.00	0.00	0	
THIAMIN	MG	0.20	0.93	20	TTTTTTTT TTTTTTTT
RIBOFLAVN	MG	0.40	1.55	33	RRRRRRRR RRRRRRRR RRRRRRRR R
NIACIN	MG	1.80	0.60	13	NNNNNNNN NNNN
IRON	MG	1.80	0.52	11	IIIIIIII II
CALCIUM	MG	362.00	1.87	40	KKKKKKKK KKKKKKKK KKKKKKKK KKKKKKKK
PHOSPHRUS	MG	322.00	1.66	36	XXXXXXXX XXXXXXXX XXXXXXXX XXXX
POTASSIUM	MG	240.00	0.22	5	YYYY
PROTEIN	G	17.00	1.58	34	PPPPPPPP PPPPPPPP PPPPPPPP PP
CARBOHYDT	G	40.00	0.68	15	HHHHHHHH HHH
FAT	G	22.00	1.31	28	FFFFFFFF FFFFFFFF FFFFFF
OLEIC A	G	8.80	1.67	36	OOOOOOOO OOOOOOOO OOOOOOOO OOOO
LINOL A	G	2.90	0.67	15	LLLLLLLL LLL
SAT FAT A	G	8.90	1.45	31	SSSSSSSS SSSSSSSS SSSSSSSS S

```
                                                                              100 ****************
                                       90        80        70        60        50        40        30        20        10
```

443 BLUEBERRY MUFFINS, HOME RECIPE
ANALYSIS OF 40 GRAMS WHICH IS 1 MUFFIN, 2 3/8-IN DIAM, 1 1/2-IM HIGH

NUTRIENT	UNIT	AMOUNT	INQ	% STD	
ENERGY	KCAL	110.00	1.00	6	EEEE
VITAMIN A	IU	90.00	0.41	2	AA	
VITAMIN C	MG	0.00	0.00	0	-	
THIAMIN	MG	0.09	1.64	9	TTT|TTT
RIBOFLAVN	MG	0.10	1.52	8	RRR|RRR
NIACIN	MG	0.70	0.91	5	NNNN
IRON	MG	0.60	0.68	4	III|
CALCIUM	MG	34.00	0.69	4	KKK|
PHOSPHRUS	MG	53.00	1.07	6	XXX|X
POTASSIUM	MG	46.00	0.17	1	Y	
PROTEIN	G	3.00	1.09	6	PPP|P
CARBOHYDT	G	17.00	1.12	6	HHH|H
FAT	G	4.00	0.93	5	FFFF
OLEIC A	G	1.40	1.04	6	OOO|O
LINOL A	G	0.70	0.64	4	LLL|
SAT FAT A	G	1.10	0.70	4	SSS|

```
                                                                              100 ****************
                                       90        80        70        60        50        40        30        20        10
```

444 BRAN MUFFINS, HOME RECIPE
ANALYSIS OF 40 GRAMS WHICH IS 1 MUFFIN 2 3/8-IN DIAM., 1 1/2-IN HIGH

NUTRIENT	UNIT	AMOUNT	INQ	% STD	
ENERGY	KCAL	105.00	1.00	5	EEEE
VITAMIN A	IU	90.00	0.43	2	AA	
VITAMIN C	MG	0.00	0.00	0	-	
THIAMIN	MG	0.07	1.33	7	TTT|TTT
RIBOFLAVN	MG	0.10	1.59	8	RRR|RRR
NIACIN	MG	1.70	2.31	12	NNN|NNNNNN
IRON	MG	1.50	1.79	9	III|IIIII
CALCIUM	MG	57.00	1.21	6	KKK|IK
PHOSPHRUS	MG	162.00	3.43	18	XXX|XXXXXXXXXX
POTASSIUM	MG	172.00	0.66	3	YYY|
PROTEIN	G	3.00	1.14	6	PPP|P
CARBOHYDT	G	17.00	1.18	6	HHH|H
FAT	G	4.00	0.98	5	FFFF
OLEIC A	G	1.40	1.09	6	OOO|O
LINOL A	G	0.80	0.76	4	LLL|
SAT FAT A	G	1.20	0.80	4	SSS|

445 CORN MUFFINS, HOME RECIPE
ANALYSIS OF 40 GRAMS WHICH IS 1 MUFFIN 2 3/8-IN DIAM., 1 1/2-IN HIGH

NUTRIENT	UNIT	AMOUNT	INQ	% STD	0 10 20 30 40 50 60 70 80 90 100
ENERGY	KCAL	125.00	1.00	6	EEEEE
VITAMIN A	IU	120.00	0.48	3	AA
VITAMIN C	MG	0.00	0.00	0	-
THIAMIN	MG	0.10	1.60	10	TTTTITT
RIBOFLAVN	MG	0.10	1.33	8	RRRRIRR
NIACIN	MG	0.70	0.80	5	NNNNI
IRON	MG	0.70	0.70	4	IIIII
CALCIUM	MG	42.00	0.75	5	KKKKI
PHOSPHRUS	MG	68.00	1.21	8	XXXXIX
POTASSIUM	MG	54.00	0.17	1	Y
PROTEIN	G	3.00	0.96	6	PPPPP
CARBOHYDT	G	19.00	1.11	7	HHHHIH
FAT	G	4.00	0.82	5	FFFFI
OLEIC A	G	1.60	1.04	7	OOOOO
LINOL A	G	0.90	0.72	5	LLLLI
SAT FAT A	G	1.20	0.67	4	SSS

446 PLAIN MUFFIN, HOME RECIPE
ANALYSIS OF 40 GRAMS WHICH IS 1 MUFFIN, 3-IN DIAM, 1 1/2-IN HIGH

NUTRIENT	UNIT	AMOUNT	INQ	% STD	0 10 20 30 40 50 60 70 80 90 100
ENERGY	KCAL	120.00	1.00	6	EEEEE
VITAMIN A	IU	40.00	0.17	1	A
VITAMIN C	MG	0.00	0.00	0	-
THIAMIN	MG	0.09	1.50	9	TTTTITT
RIBOFLAVN	MG	0.12	1.67	10	RRRRIRRR
NIACIN	MG	0.90	1.07	6	NNNNN
IRON	MG	0.60	0.63	4	III
CALCIUM	MG	42.00	0.78	5	KKKKI
PHOSPHRUS	MG	60.00	1.11	7	XXXXX
POTASSIUM	MG	50.00	0.17	1	Y
PROTEIN	G	3.00	1.00	6	PPPPP
CARBOHYDT	G	17.00	1.03	6	HHHHH
FAT	G	4.00	0.85	5	FFFFI
OLEIC A	G	1.70	1.16	7	OOOOIO
LINOL A	G	1.00	0.83	5	LLLLI
SAT FAT A	G	1.00	0.58	4	SSS

447 CORN MUFFIN MIX, EGG, MILK
ANALYSIS OF 40 GRAMS WHICH IS 1 MUFFIN, 2 3/8-IN DIAM., 11/2 IN HIGH

NUTRIENT	UNIT	AMOUNT	INQ	% STD	0 10 20 30 ... 100
ENERGY	KCAL	130.00	1.00	7	EEEEE
VITAMIN A	IU	100.00	0.38	3	AA
VITAMIN C	MG	0.00	0.00	0	-
THIAMIN	MG	0.08	1.23	8	TTTTIT
RIBOFLAVN	MG	0.09	1.15	8	RRRIR
NIACIN	MG	0.70	0.77	5	NNNN
IRON	MG	0.60	0.58	4	III
CALCIUM	MG	96.00	1.64	11	KKKKIKKKK
PHOSPHRUS	MG	152.00	2.60	17	XXXXIXXXXXXXX
POTASSIUM	MG	44.00	0.14	1	Y
PROTEIN	G	3.00	0.92	6	PPPPP
CARBOHYDT	G	20.00	1.12	7	HHHHH
FAT	G	4.00	0.79	5	FFFF
OLEIC A	G	1.70	1.07	7	OOOOIO
LINOL A	G	0.90	0.69	5	LLLL
SAT FAT A	G	1.20	0.65	4	SSS

448 EGG NOODLES, ENRICHED, COOKED
ANALYSIS OF 160 GRAMS WHICH IS 1 CUP

NUTRIENT	UNIT	AMOUNT	INQ	% STD	0 10 20 30 ... 100
ENERGY	KCAL	200.00	1.00	10	EEEEEE
VITAMIN A	IU	110.00	0.28	3	AA
VITAMIN C	MG	0.00	0.00	0	-
THIAMIN	MG	0.22	2.20	22	TTTTTTITTTTTTTT
RIBOFLAVN	MG	0.13	1.08	11	RRRRRRIR
NIACIN	MG	1.90	1.36	14	NNNNNNIINNN
IRON	MG	1.40	0.88	9	IIIIIII
CALCIUM	MG	16.00	0.18	2	K
PHOSPHRUS	MG	94.00	1.04	10	XXXXXXX
POTASSIUM	MG	70.00	0.14	1	Y
PROTEIN	G	7.00	1.40	14	PPPPPPIPPP
CARBOHYDT	G	37.00	1.35	13	HHHHHHIHHH
FAT	G	2.00	0.26	3	FF
OLEIC A	G	0.00	0.00	0	-
LINOL A	G	0.00	0.00	0	-
SAT FAT A	G	0.00	0.00	0	-

449 NOODLES, CHOW MEIN, CANNED
ANALYSIS OF 45 GRAMS WHICH IS 1 CUP

NUTRIENT	UNIT	AMOUNT	INQ	% STD	0	10	20	30	40	50	60	70	80	90	100
ENERGY	KCAL	220.00	1.00	11	EEEEEEEE
VITAMIN A	IU	0.00	0.00	0	-
VITAMIN C	MG	0.00	0.00	0	-
THIAMIN	MG	0.04	0.36	4	TTT
RIBOFLAVN	MG	0.03	0.23	3	RR
NIACIN	MG	0.60	0.39	4	NNN
IRON	MG	0.40	0.23	3	II
CALCIUM	MG	14.00	0.14	2	K
PHOSPHRUS	MG	40.00	0.40	4	XXXX
POTASSIUM	MG	33.00	0.06	1	Y
PROTEIN	G	6.00	1.09	12	PPPPPPPP P
CARBOHYDT	G	26.00	0.86	9	HHHHHHHH
FAT	G	11.00	1.28	14	FFFFFFFFFF IFF
OLEIC A	G	6.30	2.34	26	OOOOOOOOOIOOOOOOOOOOOO
LINOL A	G	0.90	0.41	5	LLLL
SAT FAT A	G	2.70	0.86	9	SSSSSSSSI

450 BUCKWHEAT PANCAKES MADE FROM MIX
ANALYSIS OF 27 GRAMS WHICH IS 1 CAKE 4-IN DIAM

NUTRIENT	UNIT	AMOUNT	INQ	% STD	0	10	20	30	40	50	60	70	80	90	100
ENERGY	KCAL	55.00	1.00	3	EE
VITAMIN A	IU	60.00	0.55	2	AI
VITAMIN C	MG	0.00	0.00	0	-I
THIAMIN	MG	0.04	1.45	4	TIT
RIBOFLAVN	MG	0.05	1.52	4	RIR
NIACIN	MG	0.20	0.52	1	NI
IRON	MG	0.40	0.91	3	II
CALCIUM	MG	59.00	2.38	7	KIKKK
PHOSPHRUS	MG	91.00	3.68	10	XIXXXXXX
POTASSIUM	MG	66.00	0.48	1	YI
PROTEIN	G	2.00	1.45	4	PIP
CARBOHYDT	G	6.00	0.79	2	HH
FAT	G	2.00	0.93	3	FF
OLEIC A	G	0.90	1.34	4	OIO
LINOL A	G	0.40	0.73	2	LL
SAT FAT A	G	0.80	1.02	3	SS

451   PANCAKE MADE FROM HOME RECIPE
ANALYSIS OF 27 GRAMS WHICH IS 1 CAKE 4-IN DIAM

NUTRIENT	UNIT	AMOUNT	INQ	% STD	0
ENERGY	KCAL	60.00	1.00	3	EE
VITAMIN A	IU	30.00	0.25	1	AI
VITAMIN C	MG	0.00	0.00	0	-I
THIAMIN	MG	0.06	2.00	6	TITTT
RIBOFLAVN	MG	0.07	1.94	6	RIRRR
NIACIN	MG	0.50	1.19	4	NIN
IRON	MG	0.40	0.83	3	II
CALCIUM	MG	27.00	1.00	3	KK
PHOSPHRUS	MG	38.00	1.41	4	XIX
POTASSIUM	MG	33.00	0.22	1	YI
PROTEIN	G	2.00	1.33	4	PIP
CARBOHYDT	G	9.00	1.09	3	HIH
FAT	G	2.00	0.85	3	FF
OLEIC A	G	0.80	1.09	3	OIO
LINOL A	G	0.50	0.83	2	LL
SAT FAT A	G	0.50	0.58	2	SI

452   PANCAKE MADE FROM MIX
ANALYSIS OF 27 GRAMS WHICH IS 1 CAKE 4-IN DIAM

NUTRIENT	UNIT	AMOUNT	INQ	% STD	0
ENERGY	KCAL	60.00	1.00	3	EE
VITAMIN A	IU	70.00	0.58	2	AI
VITAMIN C	MG	0.00	0.00	0	-I
THIAMIN	MG	0.04	1.33	4	TIT
RIBOFLAVN	MG	0.06	1.67	5	RIRR
NIACIN	MG	0.20	0.48	1	NI
IRON	MG	0.30	0.63	2	II
CALCIUM	MG	58.00	2.15	6	KIKKK
PHOSPHRUS	MG	70.00	2.59	8	XIXXXX
POTASSIUM	MG	42.00	0.28	1	YI
PROTEIN	G	2.00	1.33	4	PIP
CARBOHYDT	G	9.00	1.09	3	HIH
FAT	G	2.00	0.85	3	FF
OLEIC A	G	0.70	0.95	3	OO
LINOL A	G	0.30	0.50	2	LI
SAT FAT A	G	0.70	0.82	2	SS

453 APPLE PIE
ANALYSIS OF 945 GRAMS WHICH IS 1 PIE 9-IN DIAM

```
                                    0    10   20   30   40   50   60   70   80   90   100
NUTRIENT  UNIT  AMOUNT   INQ  % STD
ENERGY    KCAL  2420.00  1.00  121  EEEEEEEEEEEEEEEEEEEEEEEEEEEEEEEEEEEEEEEEEEEEEEEEEEEEEEEEEEEE  *121
VITAMIN A IU     280.00  0.06    7  AAAAAA                                                         *
VITAMIN C MG       9.00  0.12   15  CCCCCCCCCCCC                                                   *
THIAMIN   MG       1.06  0.88  106  TTTTTTTTTTTTTTTTTTTTTTTTTTTTTTTTTTTTTTTTTTTTTTTTTTTTT       *106
RIBOFLAVN MG       0.79  0.54   66  RRRRRRRRRRRRRRRRRRRRRRRRRRRRRRRRR                               *
NIACIN    MG       9.30  0.55   66  NNNNNNNNNNNNNNNNNNNNNNNNNNNNNNNNN                               *
IRON      MG       6.60  0.34   41  IIIIIIIIIIIIIIIIIIII                                           *
CALCIUM   MG      76.00  0.07    8  KKKKKKK                                                        *
PHOSPHRUS MG     208.00  0.19   23  XXXXXXXXXXX                                                    *
POTASSIUM MG     756.00  0.12   15  YYYYYYYY                                                       *
PROTEIN   G       21.00  0.35   42  PPPPPPPPPPPPPPPPPPPPP                                           *
CARBOHYDT G      360.00  1.08  131  HHHHHHHHHHHHHHHHHHHHHHHHHHHHHHHHHHHHHHHHHHHHHHHHHHHHHHHHHHHHHHHHHHH  *131
FAT       G      105.00  1.11  135  FFFFFFFFFFFFFFFFFFFFFFFFFFFFFFFFFFFFFFFFFFFFFFFFFFFFFFFFFFFFFFFFFFFFF  *135
OLEIC A   G       44.50  1.50  182  OOOOOOOOOOOOOOOOOOOOOOOOOOOOOOOOOOOOOOOOOOOOOOOOOOOOOOOOOOOOOOOOOOOOOOOOOOOOOOOOOOOOOOOOOOOOOO  *182
LINOL A   G       25.20  1.04  126  LLLLLLLLLLLLLLLLLLLLLLLLLLLLLLLLLLLLLLLLLLLLLLLLLLLLLLLLLLLLLLLLL  *126
SAT FAT A G       27.00  0.78   95  SSSSSSSSSSSSSSSSSSSSSSSSSSSSSSSSSSSSSSSSSSSSSSSSS               *
**********************************
```

454 APPLE PIE
ANALYSIS OF 135 GRAMS WHICH IS SECTOR, 1/7 OF PIE

```
                                    0    10   20   30   40   50   60   70   80   90   100
NUTRIENT  UNIT  AMOUNT   INQ  % STD
ENERGY    KCAL  345.00  1.00   17  EEEEEEEEEEE                                                     *
VITAMIN A IU     40.00  0.06    1  A                                                               *
VITAMIN C MG      2.00  0.19    3  CCC                                                             *
THIAMIN   MG      0.15  0.87   15  TTTTTTTTTTT                                                     *
RIBOFLAVN MG      0.11  0.53    9  RRRRRR                                                          *
NIACIN    MG      1.30  0.54    9  NNNNNN                                                          *
IRON      MG      0.90  0.33    6  IIIII                                                           *
CALCIUM   MG     11.00  0.07    1  K                                                               *
PHOSPHRUS MG     30.00  0.19    3  XXX                                                             *
POTASSIUM MG    108.00  0.13    2  YY                                                              *
PROTEIN   G       3.00  0.35    6  PPPP                                                            *
CARBOHYDT G      51.00  1.08   19  HHHHHHHHHHHHHIH                                                 *
FAT       G      15.00  1.11   19  FFFFFFFFFFFFFIF                                                 *
OLEIC A   G       6.40  1.51   26  OOOOOOOOOOOOOOIOOOOOOO                                          *
LINOL A   G       3.60  1.04   18  LLLLLLLLLLLLL                                                   *
SAT FAT A G       3.90  0.79   14  SSSSSSSSSS                                                      *
**********************************
```

455 BANANA CREAM PIE
ANALYSIS OF 910 GRAMS WHICH IS 1 PIE 9-IN DIAM

NUTRIENT	UNIT	AMOUNT	INQ	% STD
ENERGY	KCAL	2010.00	1.00	101
VITAMIN A	IU	2280.00	0.57	57
VITAMIN C	MG	9.00	0.15	15
THIAMIN	MG	0.77	0.77	77
RIBOFLAVN	MG	1.51	1.25	126
NIACIN	MG	7.00	0.50	50
IRON	MG	7.30	0.45	46
CALCIUM	MG	601.00	0.66	67
PHOSPHRUS	MG	746.00	0.82	83
POTASSIUM	MG	1847.00	0.37	37
PROTEIN	MG	41.00	0.82	82
CARBOHYDT	G	279.00	1.01	101
FAT	G	85.00	1.08	109
OLEIC A	G	33.20	1.35	136
LINOL A	G	16.20	0.81	81
SAT FAT A	G	26.70	0.93	94

456 BANANA CREAM PIE
ANALYSIS OF 130 GRAMS WHICH IS 1 SECTOR, 1/7 OF PIE

NUTRIENT	UNIT	AMOUNT	INQ	% STD
ENERGY	KCAL	285.00	1.00	14
VITAMIN A	IU	330.00	0.58	8
VITAMIN C	MG	0.12	0.12	2
THIAMIN	MG	0.11	0.77	11
RIBOFLAVN	MG	0.22	1.29	18
NIACIN	MG	1.00	0.50	7
IRON	MG	1.00	0.44	6
CALCIUM	MG	86.00	0.67	10
PHOSPHRUS	MG	107.00	0.83	12
POTASSIUM	MG	264.00	0.37	5
PROTEIN	G	6.00	0.84	12
CARBOHYDT	G	40.00	1.02	15
FAT	G	12.00	1.08	15
OLEIC A	G	4.70	1.35	19
LINOL A	G	2.30	0.81	12
SAT FAT A	G	3.80	0.94	13

457   BLUEBERRY PIE
ANALYSIS OF 945 GRAMS WHICH IS 1 PIE 9-IN DIAM

NUTRIENT	UNIT	AMOUNT	INQ	% STD
ENERGY	KCAL	2285.00	1.00	114
VITAMIN A	IU	280.00	0.06	7
VITAMIN C	MG	28.00	0.41	47
THIAMIN	MG	1.03	0.90	103
RIBOFLAVN	MG	0.80	0.58	67
NIACIN	MG	10.00	0.63	71
IRON	MG	9.50	0.52	59
CALCIUM	MG	104.00	0.10	12
PHOSPHRUS	MG	217.00	0.21	24
POTASSIUM	MG	614.00	0.11	12
PROTEIN	G	23.00	0.40	46
CARBOHYDT	G	330.00	1.05	120
FAT	G	102.00	1.14	131
OLEIC A	G	43.70	1.56	178
LINOL A	G	25.10	1.10	126
SAT FAT A	G	24.80	0.76	87

458   BLUEBERRY PIE
ANALYSIS OF 135 GRAMS WHICH IS 1 SECTOR, 1/7 OF PIE

NUTRIENT	UNIT	AMOUNT	INQ	% STD
ENERGY	KCAL	325.00	1.00	16
VITAMIN A	IU	40.00	0.06	1
VITAMIN C	MG	4.00	0.41	7
THIAMIN	MG	0.15	0.92	15
RIBOFLAVN	MG	0.11	0.56	9
NIACIN	MG	1.40	0.62	10
IRON	MG	1.40	0.54	9
CALCIUM	MG	15.00	0.10	2
PHOSPHRUS	MG	31.00	0.21	3
POTASSIUM	MG	88.00	0.11	2
PROTEIN	G	3.00	0.37	6
CARBOHYDT	G	47.00	1.05	17
FAT	G	15.00	1.18	19
OLEIC A	G	6.20	1.56	25
LINOL A	G	3.60	1.11	18
SAT FAT A	G	3.50	0.76	12

459 CHERRY PIE
ANALYSIS OF 945 GRAMS WHICH IS 1 PIE 9-IN DIAM

NUTRIENT	UNIT	AMOUNT	INQ	% STD
ENERGY	KCAL	2465.00	1.00	123
VITAMIN A	IU	4160.00	0.84	104
VITAMIN C	MG	0.00	0.00	0
THIAMIN	MG	1.09	0.88	109
RIBOFLAVN	MG	0.84	0.57	70
NIACIN	MG	9.80	0.57	70
IRON	MG	6.60	0.33	41
CALCIUM	MG	132.00	0.12	15
PHOSPHRUS	MG	236.00	0.21	26
POTASSIUM	MG	992.00	0.16	20
PROTEIN	G	25.00	0.41	50
CARBOHYDT	G	363.00	1.07	132
FAT	G	107.00	1.11	137
OLEIC A	G	45.00	1.49	184
LINOL A	G	25.30	1.03	127
SAT FAT A	G	28.20	0.80	99

460 CHERRY PIE
ANALYSIS OF 135 GRAMS WHICH IS 1 SECTOR, 1/7 OF PIE

NUTRIENT	UNIT	AMOUNT	INQ	% STD
ENERGY	KCAL	350.00	1.00	17
VITAMIN A	IU	590.00	0.84	15
VITAMIN C	MG	0.00	0.00	0
THIAMIN	MG	0.16	0.91	16
RIBOFLAVN	MG	0.12	0.57	10
NIACIN	MG	1.40	0.57	10
IRON	MG	0.90	0.32	6
CALCIUM	MG	19.00	0.12	2
PHOSPHRUS	MG	34.00	0.22	4
POTASSIUM	MG	142.00	0.16	3
PROTEIN	G	4.00	0.46	8
CARBOHYDT	G	52.00	1.08	19
FAT	G	15.00	1.10	19
OLEIC A	G	6.40	1.49	26
LINOL A	G	3.60	1.03	18
SAT FAT A	G	4.00	0.80	14

461 CUSTARD PIE
ANALYSIS OF 910 GRAMS WHICH IS 1 PIE 9-IN DIAM

NUTRIENT	UNIT	AMOUNT	INQ	% STD
ENERGY	KCAL	1985.00	1.00	99
VITAMIN A	IU	2090.00	0.53	52
VITAMIN C	MG	0.00	0.00	0
THIAMIN	MG	0.79	0.80	79
RIBOFLAVN	MG	1.92	1.61	160
NIACIN	MG	5.60	0.40	40
IRON	MG	8.20	0.52	51
CALCIUM	MG	874.00	0.98	97
PHOSPHRUS	MG	1028.00	1.15	114
POTASSIUM	MG	1247.00	0.25	25
PROTEIN	G	56.00	1.13	112
CARBOHYDT	G	213.00	0.78	77
FAT	G	101.00	1.30	129
OLEIC A	G	38.50	1.58	157
LINOL A	G	17.50	0.88	88
SAT FAT A	G	33.90	1.20	119

462 CUSTARD PIE
ANALYSIS OF 130 GRAMS WHICH IS 1 SECTOR, 1/7 OF PIE

NUTRIENT	UNIT	AMOUNT	INQ	% STD
ENERGY	KCAL	285.00	1.00	14
VITAMIN A	IU	300.00	0.53	8
VITAMIN C	MG	0.00	0.00	0
THIAMIN	MG	0.11	0.77	11
RIBOFLAVN	MG	0.27	1.58	23
NIACIN	MG	0.80	0.40	6
IRON	MG	1.20	0.53	7
CALCIUM	MG	125.00	0.97	14
PHOSPHRUS	MG	147.00	1.15	16
POTASSIUM	MG	178.00	0.25	4
PROTEIN	G	8.00	1.12	16
CARBOHYDT	G	30.00	0.77	11
FAT	G	14.00	1.26	18
OLEIC A	G	5.50	1.58	22
LINOL A	G	2.50	0.88	13
SAT FAT A	G	4.80	1.18	17

463 LEMON MERINGUE PIE
ANALYSIS OF 840 GRAMS WHICH IS 1 PIE 9-IN DIAM

NUTRIENT	UNIT	AMOUNT	INQ	% STD
ENERGY	KCAL	2140.00	1.00	107
VITAMIN A	IU	1430.00	0.33	36
VITAMIN C	MG	25.00	0.39	42
THIAMIN	MG	0.61	0.57	61
RIBOFLAVN	MG	0.84	0.65	70
NIACIN	MG	5.20	0.35	37
IRON	MG	6.70	0.39	42
CALCIUM	MG	118.00	0.12	13
PHOSPHRUS	MG	412.00	0.43	46
POTASSIUM	MG	420.00	0.08	8
PROTEIN	G	31.00	0.58	62
CARBOHYDT	G	317.00	1.08	115
FAT	G	86.00	1.03	110
OLEIC A	G	33.80	1.29	138
LINOL A	G	16.40	0.77	82
SAT FAT A	G	26.10	0.86	92

```
        0    10   20   30   40   50   60   70   80   90   100
ENERGY  EEEEEEEEEEEEEEEEEEEEEEEEEEEEEEEEEEEEEEEEEEEEEEEEEEEEE *107
VIT A   AAAAAAAAAAAAAAAAAAAA                                  *
VIT C   CCCCCCCCCCCCCCCCCCCCC                                 *
THIAMIN TTTTTTTTTTTTTTTTTTTTTTTTTTTTTT                        *
RIBOFL  RRRRRRRRRRRRRRRRRRRRRRRRRRRRRRRRRRR                   *
NIACIN  NNNNNNNNNNNNNNNNNN                                    *
IRON    IIIIIIIIIIIIIIIIIIIII                                 *
CALCIUM KKKKKK                                                *
PHOSPH  XXXXXXXXXXXXXXXXXXXXXXX                               *
POTASS  YYYYY                                                 *
PROTEIN PPPPPPPPPPPPPPPPPPPPPPPPPPPPPP                        *
CARBOHY HHHHHHHHHHHHHHHHHHHHHHHHHHHHHHHHHHHHHHHHHHHHHHHHHHHHHHHHHH *115
FAT     FFFFFFFFFFFFFFFFFFFFFFFFFFFFFFFFFFFFFFFFFFFFFFFFFFFFFFF *110
OLEIC A OOOOOOOOOOOOOOOOOOOOOOOOOOOOOOOOOOOOOOOOOOOOOOOOOOOOOOOOOOOOOOO *138
LINOL A LLLLLLLLLLLLLLLLLLLLLLLLLLLLLLLLLLLLLLLLLL            *
SAT FAT SSSSSSSSSSSSSSSSSSSSSSSSSSSSSSSSSSSSSSSSSSSSSS        *
**********************************************************************
```

464 LEMON MERINGUE PIE
ANALYSIS OF 120 GRAMS WHICH IS 1 SECTOR, 1/7 OF PIE

NUTRIENT	UNIT	AMOUNT	INQ	% STD
ENERGY	KCAL	305.00	1.00	15
VITAMIN A	IU	200.00	0.33	5
VITAMIN C	MG	4.00	0.44	7
THIAMIN	MG	0.09	0.59	9
RIBOFLAVN	MG	0.12	0.66	10
NIACIN	MG	0.70	0.33	5
IRON	MG	1.00	0.41	6
CALCIUM	MG	17.00	0.12	2
PHOSPHRUS	MG	59.00	0.43	7
POTASSIUM	MG	60.00	0.08	1
PROTEIN	G	4.00	0.52	8
CARBOHYDT	G	45.00	1.07	16
FAT	G	12.00	1.01	15
OLEIC A	G	4.80	1.28	20
LINOL A	G	2.30	0.75	12
SAT FAT A	G	3.70	0.85	13

```
        0    10   20   30   40   50   60   70   80   90   100
ENERGY  EEEEEEEEEE |                                          *
VIT A   AAAA       |                                          *
VIT C   CCCCC      |                                          *
THIAMIN TTTTTTT    |                                          *
RIBOFL  RRRRRRRR   |                                          *
NIACIN  NNNN       |                                          *
IRON    IIIII      |                                          *
CALCIUM KK         |                                          *
PHOSPH  XXXXX      |                                          *
POTASS  Y          |                                          *
PROTEIN PPPPPP     |                                          *
CARBOHY HHHHHHHHHHHH|H                                        *
FAT     FFFFFFFFFFF |                                         *
OLEIC A OOOOOOOOOOOO|OOOO                                     *
LINOL A LLLLLLLLL   |                                         *
SAT FAT SSSSSSSSSS  |                                         *
**********************************************************************
```

465 MINCE PIE
ANALYSIS OF 945 GRAMS WHICH IS 1 PIE 9-IN DIAM

NUTRIENT	UNIT	AMOUNT	INQ	% STD
ENERGY	KCAL	2560.00	1.00	128
VITAMIN A	IU	20.00	0.00	1
VITAMIN C	MG	9.00	0.12	15
THIAMIN	MG	0.96	0.75	96
RIBOFLAVN	MG	0.86	0.56	72
NIACIN	MG	9.80	0.55	70
IRON	MG	13.30	0.65	83
CALCIUM	MG	265.00	0.23	29
PHOSPHRUS	MG	359.00	0.31	40
POTASSIUM	MG	1682.00	0.26	34
PROTEIN	G	24.00	0.38	48
CARBOHYDT	G	389.00	1.11	141
FAT	G	109.00	1.09	140
OLEIC A	G	45.90	1.46	187
LINOL A	G	25.20	0.98	126
SAT FAT A	G	28.00	0.77	98

```
                  0    10   20   30   40   50   60   70   80   90   100
ENERGY     KCAL   EEEEEEEEEEEEEEEEEEEEEEEEEEEEEEEEEEEEEEEEEEEEEEEEEE * 128
VITAMIN A  IU     -                                                    *
VITAMIN C  MG     CCCCCCCCCC                                           *
THIAMIN    MG     TTTTTTTTTTTTTTTTTTTTTTTTTTTTTTTTTTTTTTTTTTTTTTTT     *
RIBOFLAVN  MG     RRRRRRRRRRRRRRRRRRRRRRRRRRRRRRRRRRRR                 *
NIACIN     MG     NNNNNNNNNNNNNNNNNNNNNNNNNNNNNNNNNNN                  *
IRON       MG     IIIIIIIIIIIIIIIIIIIIIIIIIIIIIIIIIIIIIIIII           *
CALCIUM    MG     KKKKKKKKKKKKKK                                       *
PHOSPHRUS  MG     XXXXXXXXXXXXXXXXXXXX                                 *
POTASSIUM  MG     YYYYYYYYYYYYYYYYY                                    *
PROTEIN    G      PPPPPPPPPPPPPPPPPPPPPPPP                             *
CARBOHYDT  G      HHHHHHHHHHHHHHHHHHHHHHHHHHHHHHHHHHHHHHHHHHHHHHHHHHH *141
FAT        G      FFFFFFFFFFFFFFFFFFFFFFFFFFFFFFFFFFFFFFFFFFFFFFFFFFF *140
OLEIC A    G      OOOOOOOOOOOOOOOOOOOOOOOOOOOOOOOOOOOOOOOOOOOOOOOOOOO *187
LINOL A    G      LLLLLLLLLLLLLLLLLLLLLLLLLLLLLLLLLLLLLLLLLLLLLLLLLLL *126
SAT FAT A  G      SSSSSSSSSSSSSSSSSSSSSSSSSSSSSSSSSSSSSSSSSSSSSSSSSSS*
                  *************************************************
```

466 MINCE PIE
ANALYSIS OF 135 GRAMS WHICH IS 1 SECTOR, 1/7 OF PIE

NUTRIENT	UNIT	AMOUNT	INQ	% STD
ENERGY	KCAL	365.00	1.00	18
VITAMIN A	IU	0.00	0.00	0
VITAMIN C	MG	1.00	0.09	2
THIAMIN	MG	0.14	0.77	14
RIBOFLAVN	MG	0.12	0.55	10
NIACIN	MG	1.40	0.55	10
IRON	MG	1.90	0.65	12
CALCIUM	MG	38.00	0.23	4
PHOSPHRUS	MG	51.00	0.31	6
POTASSIUM	MG	240.00	0.26	5
PROTEIN	G	3.00	0.33	6
CARBOHYDT	G	56.00	1.12	20
FAT	G	16.00	1.12	21
OLEIC A	G	6.60	1.48	27
LINOL A	G	3.60	0.99	18
SAT FAT A	G	4.00	0.77	14

```
                  0    10   20   30   40   50   60   70   80   90   100
ENERGY     KCAL   EEEEEEEEEEEEEEEE                                     *
VITAMIN A  IU     -                                                    *
VITAMIN C  MG     C                                                    *
THIAMIN    MG     TTTTTTTTTTTT                                         *
RIBOFLAVN  MG     RRRRRRRR                                             *
NIACIN     MG     NNNNNNNN                                             *
IRON       MG     IIIIIIIIII                                           *
CALCIUM    MG     KKK                                                  *
PHOSPHRUS  MG     XXXXX                                                *
POTASSIUM  MG     YYYY                                                 *
PROTEIN    G      PPPPP                                                *
CARBOHYDT  G      HHHHHHHHHHHHHHHHHH                                   *
FAT        G      FFFFFFFFFFFFFFFFFFF                                  *
OLEIC A    G      OOOOOOOOOOOOOOOOOOOOOOOOO                            *
LINOL A    G      LLLLLLLLLLLLLLLL                                     *
SAT FAT A  G      SSSSSSSSSSSSS                                        *
                  *************************************************
```

467 PEACH PIE
ANALYSIS OF 945 GRAMS WHICH IS 1 PIE 9-IN DIAM

NUTRIENT	UNIT	AMOUNT	INQ	%STD
ENERGY	KCAL	2410.00	1.00	121
VITAMIN A	IU	6900.00	1.43	173
VITAMIN C	MG	28.00	0.39	47
THIAMIN	MG	1.04	0.86	104
RIBOFLAVN	MG	0.97	0.67	81
NIACIN	MG	14.00	0.83	100
IRON	MG	8.50	0.44	53
CALCIUM	MG	95.00	0.09	11
PHOSPHRUS	MG	274.00	0.25	30
POTASSIUM	MG	1408.00	0.23	28
PROTEIN	G	24.00	0.40	48
CARBOHYDT	G	361.00	1.09	131
FAT	G	101.00	1.07	129
OLEIC A	G	43.70	1.48	178
LINOL A	G	25.10	1.04	126
SAT FAT A	G	24.80	0.72	87

468 PEACH PIE
ANALYSIS OF 135 GRAMS WHICH IS 1 SECTOR, 1/7 OF PIE

NUTRIENT	UNIT	AMOUNT	INQ	%STD
ENERGY	KCAL	345.00	1.00	17
VITAMIN A	IU	990.00	1.43	25
VITAMIN C	MG	4.00	0.39	7
THIAMIN	MG	0.15	0.87	15
RIBOFLAVN	MG	0.14	0.68	12
NIACIN	MG	2.00	0.83	14
IRON	MG	1.20	0.43	7
CALCIUM	MG	14.00	0.09	2
PHOSPHRUS	MG	39.00	0.25	4
POTASSIUM	MG	201.00	0.23	4
PROTEIN	G	3.00	0.35	6
CARBOHYDT	G	52.00	1.10	19
FAT	G	14.00	1.04	18
OLEIC A	G	6.20	1.47	25
LINOL A	G	3.60	1.04	18
SAT FAT A	G	3.50	0.71	12

469 PECAN PIE
ANALYSIS OF 825 GRAMS WHICH IS 1 PIE 9-IN DIAM

NUTRIENT	UNIT	AMOUNT	INQ	% STD
ENERGY	KCAL	3450.00	1.00	173
VITAMIN A	IU	1320.00	0.19	33
VITAMIN C	MG	0.00	0.00	0
THIAMIN	MG	1.80	1.04	180
RIBOFLAVN	MG	0.95	0.46	79
NIACIN	MG	6.90	0.29	49
IRON	MG	25.60	0.93	160
CALCIUM	MG	388.00	0.25	43
PHOSPHRUS	MG	850.00	0.55	94
POTASSIUM	MG	1015.00	0.12	20
PROTEIN	G	42.00	0.49	84
CARBOHYDT	G	423.00	0.89	154
FAT	G	189.00	1.40	242
OLEIC A	G	10.10	0.24	41
LINOL A	G	44.20	1.28	221
SAT FAT A	G	27.80	0.57	98

470 PECAN PIE
ANALYSIS OF 118 GRAMS WHICH IS 1 SECTOR, 1/7 OF PIE

NUTRIENT	UNIT	AMOUNT	INQ	% STD
ENERGY	KCAL	495.00	1.00	25
VITAMIN A	IU	190.00	0.19	5
VITAMIN C	MG	0.00	0.00	0
THIAMIN	MG	0.26	1.05	26
RIBOFLAVN	MG	0.14	0.47	12
NIACIN	MG	1.00	0.29	7
IRON	MG	3.70	0.93	23
CALCIUM	MG	55.00	0.25	6
PHOSPHRUS	MG	122.00	0.55	14
POTASSIUM	MG	145.00	0.12	3
PROTEIN	G	6.00	0.48	12
CARBOHYDT	G	61.00	0.90	22
FAT	G	27.00	1.40	35
OLEIC A	G	14.40	2.37	59
LINOL A	G	6.30	1.27	32
SAT FAT A	G	4.00	0.57	14

471 PUMPKIN PIE
ANALYSIS OF 910 GRAMS WHICH IS 1 PIE 9-IN DIAM

```
                          0        10        20        30        40        50        60        70        80        90       100
NUTRIENT  UNIT  AMOUNT     INQ  % STD
ENERGY    KCAL  1920.00   1.00   96   EEEEEEEEEEEEEEEEEEEEEEEEEEEEEEEEEEEEEEEEEEEEEEEEEEEEEEEEEEEEEEEEEEEEEEEEEEEEEEEEEEEEEEEEE *
VITAMIN A IU   22480.00   5.85  562   AAAAAAAAAAAAAAAAAAAAAAAAAAAAAAAAAAAAAAAAAAAAAAAAAAAAAAAAAAAAAAAAAAAAAAAAAAAAAAAAAAAAAAAAAAAAA|AAA *562
VITAMIN C MG       0.00   0.00    0   - *
THIAMIN   MG       0.78   0.81   78   TTTTTTTTTTTTTTTTTTTTTTTTTTTTTTTTTTTTTTTTTTTTTTTTTTTTTTTTTTTTTTTTTTTTTTTTTTTTTT|         *
RIBOFLAVN MG       1.27   1.10  106   RRRRRRRRRRRRRRRRRRRRRRRRRRRRRRRRRRRRRRRRRRRRRRRRRRRRRRRRRRRRRRRRRRRRRRRRRRRRRRRRRRRRRRRRRRR|RRR *106
NIACIN    MG       7.00   0.52   50   NNNNNNNNNNNNNNNNNNNNNNNNNNNNNNNNNNNNNNNNNNNNNNNNNNN|         *
IRON      MG       7.30   0.48   46   IIIIIIIIIIIIIIIIIIIIIIIIIIIIIIIIIIIIIIIIIIIIIII *
CALCIUM   MG     464.00   0.54   52   KKKKKKKKKKKKKKKKKKKKKKKKKKKKKKKKKKKKKKKKKKKKKKKKKKKKK *
PHOSPHRUS MG     628.00   0.73   70   XXXXXXXXXXXXXXXXXXXXXXXXXXXXXXXXXXXXXXXXXXXXXXXXXXXXXXXXXXXXXXXXXXXXXXXX *
POTASSIUM MG    1450.00   0.30   29   YYYYYYYYYYYYYYYYYYYYYYYYYYYYY *
PROTEIN   G       36.00   0.75   72   PPPPPPPPPPPPPPPPPPPPPPPPPPPPPPPPPPPPPPPPPPPPPPPPPPPPPPPPPPPPPPPPPPPPPPPPP *
CARBOHYDT G      223.00   0.84   81   HHHHHHHHHHHHHHHHHHHHHHHHHHHHHHHHHHHHHHHHHHHHHHHHHHHHHHHHHHHHHHHHHHHHHHHHHHHHHHHHHHH *
FAT       G      102.00   1.36  131   FFFFFFFFFFFFFFFFFFFFFFFFFFFFFFFFFFFFFFFFFFFFFFFFFFFFFFFFFFFFFFFFFFFFFFFFFFFFFFFFFFFFFFFFFFFFFFFFFFFFFFFFFFFFFFFFFFFFFFFFFFFFFFFFFFFFFFIFFF *131
OLEIC A   G       37.50   1.59  153   OOOOOOOOOOOOOOOOOOOOOOOOOOOOOOOOOOOOOOOOOOOOOOOOOOOOOOOOOOOOOOOOOOOOOOOOOOOOOOOOOOOOOOOOOOOOOOOOOOOOOOOOOOOOOOOOOOOOOOOOOOOOOOOOOOOOOOOOO|OOO *153
LINOL A   G       16.60   0.86   83   LLLLLLLLLLLLLLLLLLLLLLLLLLLLLLLLLLLLLLLLLLLLLLLLLLLLLLLLLLLLLLLLLLLLLLLLLLLLLLLLLLLLL *
SAT FAT A G       37.40   1.37  131   SSSSSSSSSSSSSSSSSSSSSSSSSSSSSSSSSSSSSSSSSSSSSSSSSSSSSSSSSSSSSSSSSSSSSSSSSSSSSSSSSSSSSSSSSSSSSSSSSSSSSSSSSSSSSSSSSSSSSSSSSSSSSSSSS|SSS *131
********************************************************
```

472 PUMPKIN PIE
ANALYSIS OF 130 GRAMS WHICH IS 1 SECTOR, 1/7 OF PIE

```
                          0        10        20        30        40        50        60        70        80        90       100
NUTRIENT  UNIT  AMOUNT     INQ  % STD
ENERGY    KCAL   275.00   1.00   14   EEEEEEEEEE *
VITAMIN A IU    3210.00   5.84   80   AAAAAAAAAA|AAAAAAAAAAAAAAAAAAAAAAAAAAAAAAAAAAAAAAAAAAAAAAAAAAAAAAAAAAAAAAAAAA *
VITAMIN C MG       0.00   0.00    0   - *
THIAMIN   MG       0.11   0.80   11   TTTTTTTTTT| *
RIBOFLAVN MG       0.18   1.09   15   RRRRRRRRRRRRRRR|R *
NIACIN    MG       1.00   0.45    7   NNNNNNN *
IRON      MG       1.00   0.53    6   IIIII *
CALCIUM   MG      66.00   0.53    7   KKKKKKK *
PHOSPHRUS MG      90.00   0.73   10   XXXXXXXXX| *
POTASSIUM MG     208.00   0.30    4   YYY *
PROTEIN   G        5.00   0.73   10   HHHHHHHHHH| *
CARBOHYDT G       32.00   0.85   12   FFFFFFFFFFFIFFFF *
FAT       G       15.00   1.40   19   OOOOOOOOOOOIOOOOOOOO *
OLEIC A   G        5.40   1.60   22   OOOOOOOOOOOOOIOOOOOOOO *
LINOL A   G        2.40   0.87   12   LLLLLLLLLLLL| *
SAT FAT A G        5.40   1.38   19   SSSSSSSSSSSISSS *
********************************************************
```

473 PIECRUST (HOME RECIPE) MADE WITH VEGETABLE SHORTENING,BAKED
ANALYSIS OF 180 GRAMS WHICH IS 1 PIE SHELL, 9-IN DIAM

```
NUTRIENT  UNIT  AMOUNT   INQ   % STD   0        10        20        30        40        50        60        70        80        90       100
ENERGY    KCAL  900.00   1.00    45    EEEEEEEEEEEEEEEEEEEEEEEEEEEEE                                                                          *
VITAMIN A IU      0.00   0.00     0    -                                                                                                     *
VITAMIN C MG      0.00   0.00     0    -                                                                                                     *
THIAMIN   MG      0.47   1.04    47    TTTTTTTTTTTTTTTTTTTTTTTTTTTTTT                                                                         *
RIBOFLAVN MG      0.40   0.74    33    RRRRRRRRRRRRRRRRRRRRR                                                                                  *
NIACIN    MG      5.00   0.79    36    NNNNNNNNNNNNNNNNNNNNNN                                                                                 *
IRON      MG      3.10   0.43    19    IIIIIIIIIIIIII                                                                                        *
CALCIUM   MG     25.00   0.06     3    KK                                                                                                    *
PHOSPHRUS MG     90.00   0.22    10    XXXXXXX                                                                                               *
POTASSIUM MG     89.00   0.02     2    Y                                                                                                     *
PROTEIN   G      11.00   0.49    22    PPPPPPPPPPPPPP                                                                                        *
CARBOHYDT G      79.00   0.64    29    HHHHHHHHHHHHHHHHHHH                                                                                   *
FAT       G      60.00   1.71    77    FFFFFFFFFFFFFFFFFFFFFFFFFFFFFFFFFFFFFFFFFFFFFFFFFF                                                    *
OLEIC A   G      26.10   2.37   107    OOOOOOOOOOOOOOOOOOOOOOOOOOOOOOOOOOOOOOOOOOOOOOOOOOOOOOOOOOOOOOOOOOOOOOOOO  *107
LINOL A   G      14.90   1.66    75    LLLLLLLLLLLLLLLLLLLLLLLLLLLLLLLLLLLLLLLLLLLLLLLLL                                                     *
SAT FAT A G      14.80   1.15    52    SSSSSSSSSSSSSSSSSSSSSSSSSSSSSSSSSS                                                                    *
***********************************************************************
```

474 PIECRUST MIX MADE WITH VEGETABLE SHORTENING,
ANALYSIS OF 320 GRAMS WHICH IS 10 OZ PKG, CRUST FOR 2-CRUST PIE 9-IN DIAM

```
NUTRIENT  UNIT  AMOUNT   INQ   % STD   0        10        20        30        40        50        60        70        80        90       100
ENERGY    KCAL 1485.00   1.00    74    EEEEEEEEEEEEEEEEEEEEEEEEEEEEEEEEEEEEEEEEEEEEEEEE                                                       *
VITAMIN A IU      0.00   0.00     0    -                                                                                                     *
VITAMIN C MG      0.00   0.00     0    -                                                                                                     *
THIAMIN   MG      1.07   1.44   107    TTTTTTTTTTTTTTTTTTTTTTTTTTTTTTTTTTTTTTTTTTTTTTTTTTTTTTTTTTTTTTTTTTTTTT  *107
RIBOFLAVN MG      0.79   0.89    66    RRRRRRRRRRRRRRRRRRRRRRRRRRRRRRRRRRRRRRRRRR                                                            *
NIACIN    MG      9.90   0.95    71    NNNNNNNNNNNNNNNNNNNNNNNNNNNNNNNNNNNNNNNNNNNNNN                                                        *
IRON      MG      6.10   0.51    38    IIIIIIIIIIIIIIIIIIIIIIIII                                                                             *
CALCIUM   MG    131.00   0.20    15    KKKKKKKKKK                                                                                            *
PHOSPHRUS MG    272.00   0.41    30    XXXXXXXXXXXXXXXXXXXX                                                                                  *
POTASSIUM MG    179.00   0.05     4    YYY                                                                                                   *
PROTEIN   G      20.00   0.54    40    PPPPPPPPPPPPPPPPPPPPPPPPPP                                                                            *
CARBOHYDT G     141.00   0.69    51    HHHHHHHHHHHHHHHHHHHHHHHHHHHHHHHHHH                                                                    *
FAT       G      93.00   1.61   119    FFFFFFFFFFFFFFFFFFFFFFFFFFFFFFFFFFFFFFFFFFFFFFFFFFFFFFFFFFFFFFFFFFFFFFFFFFFFFFFF  *119
OLEIC A   G      39.70   2.18   162    OOOOOOOOOOOOOOOOOOOOOOOOOOOOOOOOOOOOOOOOOOOOOOOOOOOOOOOOOOOOOOOOOOOOOOOOOOOOOOOOOO  *162
LINOL A   G      23.40   1.58   117    LLLLLLLLLLLLLLLLLLLLLLLLLLLLLLLLLLLLLLLLLLLLLLLLLLLLLLLLLLLLLLLLLLLLLLLLLLLLLL  *117
SAT FAT A G      22.70   1.07    80    SSSSSSSSSSSSSSSSSSSSSSSSSSSSSSSSSSSSSSSSSSSSSSSSSSSSSS                                                 *
***********************************************************************
```

475 PIZZA(CHEESE), BAKED
ANALYSIS OF 60 GRAMS WHICH IS 1 SECTOR, 1/8 OF 12-IN DIAM PIE

NUTRIENT	UNIT	AMOUNT	INQ	% STD
ENERGY	KCAL	145.00	1.00	7
VITAMIN A	IU	230.00	0.79	6
VITAMIN C	MG	4.00	0.92	7
THIAMIN	MG	0.18	2.21	16
RIBOFLAVN	MG	0.18	2.07	15
NIACIN	MG	1.60	1.58	11
IRON	MG	1.10	0.95	7
CALCIUM	MG	86.00	1.32	10
PHOSPHRUS	MG	89.00	1.36	10
POTASSIUM	MG	67.00	0.18	1
PROTEIN	G	6.00	1.66	12
CARBOHYDT	G	22.00	1.10	8
FAT	G	4.00	0.71	5
OLEIC A	G	1.50	0.84	6
LINOL A	G	0.60	0.41	3
SAT FAT A	G	1.70	0.82	6

476 POPCORN, PLAIN-LARGE KERNEL, POPPED
ANALYSIS OF 6 GRAMS WHICH IS 1 CUP

NUTRIENT	UNIT	AMOUNT	INQ	% STD
ENERGY	KCAL	25.00	1.00	1
VITAMIN A	IU	0.00	0.00	0
VITAMIN C	MG	0.00	0.00	0
THIAMIN	MG	0.02	1.60	2
RIBOFLAVN	MG	0.01	0.67	1
NIACIN	MG	0.10	0.57	1
IRON	MG	0.20	1.00	1
CALCIUM	MG	1.00	0.09	0
PHOSPHRUS	MG	17.00	1.51	2
POTASSIUM	MG	15.00	0.24	0
PROTEIN	G	1.00	1.60	2
CARBOHYDT	G	5.00	1.45	2
FAT	G	0.00	0.00	0
OLEIC A	G	0.10	0.33	0
LINOL A	G	0.20	0.80	1
SAT FAT A	G	0.00	0.00	0

477 POPCORN, WITH COCONUT OIL AND SALT
ANALYSIS OF 9 GRAMS WHICH IS 1 CUP

NUTRIENT	UNIT	AMOUNT	INQ	% STD
ENERGY	KCAL	40.00	1.00	2
VITAMIN A	IU	0.00	0.00	0
VITAMIN C	MG	0.00	0.00	0
THIAMIN	MG	0.03	1.50	3
RIBOFLAVN	MG	0.01	0.42	1
NIACIN	MG	0.20	0.71	1
IRON	MG	0.20	0.63	1
CALCIUM	MG	1.00	0.06	0
PHOSPHRUS	MG	19.00	1.06	2
POTASSIUM	MG	23.00	0.23	0
PROTEIN	G	1.00	1.00	2
CARBOHYDT	G	5.00	0.91	2
FAT	G	2.00	1.28	3
OLEIC A	G	2.00	0.41	1
LINOL A	G	0.20	0.50	1
SAT FAT A	G	1.50	2.63	5

478 POPCORN, SUGAR COATED
ANALYSIS OF 35 GRAMS WHICH IS 1 CUP

NUTRIENT	UNIT	AMOUNT	INQ	% STD
ENERGY	KCAL	135.00	1.00	7
VITAMIN A	IU	0.00	0.00	0
VITAMIN C	MG	0.00	0.00	0
THIAMIN	MG	0.13	1.93	13
RIBOFLAVN	MG	0.02	0.25	2
NIACIN	MG	0.40	0.42	3
IRON	MG	0.50	0.46	3
CALCIUM	MG	2.00	0.03	0
PHOSPHRUS	MG	47.00	0.77	5
POTASSIUM	MG	90.00	0.27	2
PROTEIN	G	2.00	0.59	4
CARBOHYDT	G	30.00	1.62	11
FAT	G	1.00	0.19	1
OLEIC A	G	0.20	0.12	1
LINOL A	G	0.40	0.30	2
SAT FAT A	G	0.50	0.26	2

479 PRETZELS,DUTCH TWISTED
ANALYSIS OF 16 GRAMS WHICH IS 1 PRETZEL 2 3/4 BY 2 5/8-IN

NUTRIENT	UNIT	AMOUNT	INQ	% STD	0	10	20	30	40	50	60	70	80	90	100
ENERGY	KCAL	60.00	1.00	3	EE										
VITAMIN A	IU	0.00	0.00	0	-I										
VITAMIN C	MG	0.00	0.00	0	-I										
THIAMIN	MG	0.05	1.67	5	TITT										
RIBOFLAVN	MG	0.04	1.11	3	RIR										
NIACIN	MG	0.70	1.67	5	NINN										
IRON	MG	0.20	0.42	1	II										
CALCIUM	MG	4.00	0.15	0	XX										
PHOSPHRUS	MG	21.00	0.78	2	XX										
POTASSIUM	MG	21.00	0.14	0	-I										
PROTEIN	G	2.00	1.33	4	PIP										
CARBOHYDT	G	12.00	1.45	4	HIH										
FAT	G	1.00	0.43	1	FI										
OLEIC A	G	0.50	0.68	2	OO										
LINOL A	G	0.00	0.00	0	-I										
SAT FAT A	G	0.20	0.23	1	SI										

****

480 PRETZELS,THIN TWISTED
ANALYSIS OF 60 GRAMS WHICH IS 10 PRETZEL 3 1/4 BY 2 1/4 BY 1/4-IN.

NUTRIENT	UNIT	AMOUNT	INQ	% STD	0	10	20	30	40	50	60	70	80	90	100
ENERGY	KCAL	235.00	1.00	12	EEEEEEEE										
VITAMIN A	IU	0.00	0.00	0	-I										
VITAMIN C	MG	0.00	0.00	0	-I										
THIAMIN	MG	0.20	1.70	20	TTTTTTTITTTTTTT										
RIBOFLAVN	MG	0.15	1.06	13	RRRRRRRIR										
NIACIN	MG	2.50	1.52	18	NNNNNNNINNNNN										
IRON	MG	0.90	0.48	6	IIIII										
CALCIUM	MG	13.00	0.12	1	K										
PHOSPHRUS	MG	79.00	0.75	9	XXXXXX										
POTASSIUM	MG	78.00	0.13	2	Y										
PROTEIN	G	6.00	1.02	12	PPPPPPPIP										
CARBOHYDT	G	46.00	1.42	17	HHHHHHHIHHHH										
FAT	G	3.00	0.33	4	FFF										
OLEIC A	G	1.80	0.63	7	OOOOOO										
LINOL A	G	0.00	0.00	0	-I										
SAT FAT A	G	0.60	0.18	2	SS										

****

481 PRETZELS,STICK
ANALYSIS OF 3 GRAMS WHICH IS 10 PRETZELS 2 1/4-IN LONG

NUTRIENT	UNIT	AMOUNT	INQ	% STD	0	10	20	30	40	50	60	70	80	90	100
ENERGY	KCAL	10.00	1.00	1	-										*****************
VITAMIN A	IU	0.00	0.00	0	-										
VITAMIN C	MG	0.00	0.00	0	-										
THIAMIN	MG	0.01	2.00	1	T										
RIBOFLAVN	MG	0.01	1.67	1	R										
NIACIN	MG	0.10	1.43	1	N										
IRON	MG	0.00	0.00	0	-										
CALCIUM	MG	1.00	0.22	0	-										
PHOSPHRUS	MG	4.00	0.89	0	-										
POTASSIUM	MG	4.00	0.16	0	-										
PROTEIN	G	0.00	0.00	0	-										
CARBOHYDT	G	2.00	1.45	1	H										
FAT	G	0.00	0.00	0	-										
OLEIC A	G	0.10	0.82	0	-										
LINOL A	G	0.00	0.00	0	-										
SAT FAT A	G	0.00	0.00	0	-										

****

482 RICE,INSTANT, ENRICHED, COOKED
ANALYSIS OF 165 GRAMS WHICH IS 1 CUP

NUTRIENT	UNIT	AMOUNT	INQ	% STD	0	10	20	30	40	50	60	70	80	90	100
ENERGY	KCAL	180.00	1.00	9	EEEEEE										*****************
VITAMIN A	IU	0.00	0.00	0	-										
VITAMIN C	MG	0.00	0.00	0	-										
THIAMIN	MG	0.21	2.33	21	TTTTTTTTTTTTTTTTT										
RIBOFLAVN	MG	0.00	0.00	0	-										
NIACIN	MG	1.70	1.35	12	NNNNNNNNNNNN										
IRON	MG	1.30	0.90	8	IIIIIIII										
CALCIUM	MG	5.00	0.06	1	-										
PHOSPHRUS	MG	31.00	0.38	3	XXX										
POTASSIUM	MG	0.00	0.00	0	-										
PROTEIN	G	4.00	0.89	8	PPPPPPPP										
CARBOHYDT	G	40.00	1.62	15	HHHHHHHHHHHHHHH										
FAT	G	0.00	0.00	0	-										
OLEIC A	G	0.00	0.00	0	-										
LINOL A	G	0.00	0.00	0	-										
SAT FAT A	G	0.00	0.00	0	-										

****

483 RICE,LONG GRAIN, ENRICHED, RAW
ANALYSIS OF 185 GRAMS WHICH IS 1 CUP

NUTRIENT	UNIT	AMOUNT	INQ	% STD
ENERGY	KCAL	670.00	1.00	33
VITAMIN A	IU	0.00	0.00	0
VITAMIN C	MG	0.00	0.00	0
THIAMIN	MG	0.81	2.42	81
RIBOFLAVN	MG	0.06	0.15	5
NIACIN	MG	6.50	1.39	46
IRON	MG	5.40	1.01	34
CALCIUM	MG	44.00	0.15	5
PHOSPHRUS	MG	174.00	0.58	19
POTASSIUM	MG	170.00	0.10	3
PROTEIN	G	12.00	0.72	24
CARBOHYDT	G	149.00	1.62	54
FAT	G	1.00	0.04	1
OLEIC A	G	0.20	0.02	1
LINOL A	G	0.20	0.03	1
SAT FAT A	G	0.20	0.02	1

484 RICE,LONG GRAIN, ENRICHED, COOKED
ANALYSIS OF 205 GRAMS WHICH IS 1 CUP

NUTRIENT	UNIT	AMOUNT	INQ	% STD
ENERGY	KCAL	225.00	1.00	11
VITAMIN A	IU	0.00	0.00	0
VITAMIN C	MG	0.00	0.00	0
THIAMIN	MG	0.23	2.04	23
RIBOFLAVN	MG	0.02	0.15	2
NIACIN	MG	2.10	1.33	15
IRON	MG	1.80	1.00	11
CALCIUM	MG	21.00	0.21	2
PHOSPHRUS	MG	57.00	0.56	6
POTASSIUM	MG	57.00	0.10	1
PROTEIN	G	4.00	0.71	8
CARBOHYDT	G	50.00	1.62	18
FAT	G	0.00	0.04	0
OLEIC A	G	0.10	0.04	0
LINOL A	G	0.10	0.04	0
SAT FAT A	G	0.10	0.03	0

485 RICE,PARBOILED, ENRICHED, RAW
ANALYSIS OF 185 GRAMS WHICH IS 1 CUP

NUTRIENT	UNIT	AMOUNT	INQ	% STD
ENERGY	KCAL	685.00	1.00	34
VITAMIN A	IU	0.00	0.00	0
VITAMIN C	MG	0.00	0.00	0
THIAMIN	MG	0.81	2.36	81
RIBOFLAVN	MG	0.07	0.17	6
NIACIN	MG	6.50	1.36	46
IRON	MG	5.40	0.99	34
CALCIUM	MG	111.00	0.36	12
PHOSPHRUS	MG	370.00	1.20	41
POTASSIUM	MG	278.00	0.16	6
PROTEIN	G	14.00	0.82	28
CARBOHYDT	G	150.00	1.59	55
FAT	G	1.00	0.04	1
OLEIC A	G	0.10	0.01	0
LINOL A	G	0.20	0.03	1
SAT FAT A	G	0.20	0.02	1

486 RICE,PARBOILED, ENRICHED, COOKED
ANALYSIS OF 175 GRAMS WHICH IS 1 CUP

NUTRIENT	UNIT	AMOUNT	INQ	% STD
ENERGY	KCAL	185.00	1.00	9
VITAMIN A	IU	0.00	0.00	0
VITAMIN C	MG	0.00	0.00	0
THIAMIN	MG	0.19	2.05	19
RIBOFLAVN	MG	0.02	0.18	2
NIACIN	MG	2.10	1.62	15
IRON	MG	1.40	0.95	9
CALCIUM	MG	33.00	0.40	4
PHOSPHRUS	MG	100.00	1.20	11
POTASSIUM	MG	75.00	0.16	2
PROTEIN	G	4.00	0.86	8
CARBOHYDT	G	41.00	1.61	15
FAT	G	0.00	0.00	0
OLEIC A	G	0.10	0.04	0
LINOL A	G	0.10	0.05	1
SAT FAT A	G	0.10	0.04	0

487 ROLLS,BROWN AND SERVE, BROWNED
ANALYSIS OF 26 GRAMS WHICH IS 1 ROLL

NUTRIENT	UNIT	AMOUNT	INQ	% STD	0	10	20	30	40	50	60	70	80	90	100
ENERGY	KCAL	85.00	1.00	4	EEE										
VITAMIN A	IU	0.00	0.00	0	-I										
VITAMIN C	MG	0.00	0.00	0	-I										
THIAMIN	MG	0.10	2.35	10	TTITTTT										
RIBOFLAVN	MG	0.06	1.18	5	RRIR										
NIACIN	MG	0.90	1.51	6	NNINN										
IRON	MG	0.50	0.74	3	III										
CALCIUM	MG	20.00	0.52	2	KKI										
PHOSPHRUS	MG	23.00	0.60	3	XXI										
POTASSIUM	MG	25.00	0.12	1	-I										
PROTEIN	G	2.00	0.94	4	PPP										
CARBOHYDT	G	14.00	1.20	5	HHIH										
FAT	G	2.00	0.60	3	FFI										
OLEIC A	G	0.70	0.67	3	OOI										
LINOL A	G	0.50	0.59	3	LLI										
SAT FAT A	G	0.40	0.33	1	SI										

488 ROLLS,CLOVERLEAF OR PAN
ANALYSIS OF 28 GRAMS WHICH IS 1 ROLL 2 1/2-IN DIAM, 2-IN HIGH

NUTRIENT	UNIT	AMOUNT	INQ	% STD	0	10	20	30	40	50	60	70	80	90	100
ENERGY	KCAL	85.00	1.00	4	EEE										
VITAMIN A	IU	0.00	0.00	0	-I										
VITAMIN C	MG	0.00	0.00	0	-I										
THIAMIN	MG	0.11	2.59	11	TTITTTT										
RIBOFLAVN	MG	0.07	1.37	6	RRIRR										
NIACIN	MG	0.90	1.51	6	NNINN										
IRON	MG	0.50	0.74	3	III										
CALCIUM	MG	21.00	0.55	2	KKI										
PHOSPHRUS	MG	24.00	0.63	3	XXI										
POTASSIUM	MG	27.00	0.13	1	-I										
PROTEIN	G	2.00	0.94	4	PPP										
CARBOHYDT	G	15.00	1.28	5	HHIH										
FAT	G	2.00	0.60	3	FFI										
OLEIC A	G	0.60	0.58	2	OOI										
LINOL A	G	0.40	0.47	2	LLI										
SAT FAT A	G	0.40	0.33	1	SI										

489 HAMBURGER OR FRANKFURTER BUN
ANALYSIS OF 40 GRAMS WHICH IS 1 ROLL (8 PER 11 1/2-OZ PKG)

NUTRIENT	UNIT	AMOUNT	INQ	% STD	0 ... 10 ... 20
ENERGY	KCAL	120.00	1.00	6	EEEEE
VITAMIN A	IU	0.00	0.00	0	-
VITAMIN C	MG	0.00	0.00	0	-
THIAMIN	MG	0.16	2.67	16	TITI|TTTTTTT
RIBOFLAVN	MG	0.10	1.39	8	RRRRIRR
NIACIN	MG	1.30	1.55	9	NNNNINN
IRON	MG	0.80	0.83	5	IIIII
CALCIUM	MG	30.00	0.56	3	KKK
PHOSPHRUS	MG	34.00	0.63	4	XXX
POTASSIUM	MG	38.00	0.13	1	Y
PROTEIN	G	3.00	1.00	6	PPPPP
CARBOHYDT	G	21.00	1.27	8	HHHHIH
FAT	G	2.00	0.43	3	FF
OLEIC A	G	0.80	0.54	3	OOO
LINOL A	G	0.60	0.50	3	LL
SAT FAT A	G	0.50	0.29	2	S

490 HARD ROLLS
ANALYSIS OF 50 GRAMS WHICH IS 1 ROLL 3 3/4-IN DIAM, 2-IN HIGH

NUTRIENT	UNIT	AMOUNT	INQ	% STD	0 ... 10 ... 20
ENERGY	KCAL	155.00	1.00	8	EEEEE
VITAMIN A	IU	0.00	0.00	0	-
VITAMIN C	MG	0.00	0.00	0	-
THIAMIN	MG	0.20	2.58	20	TTTTI|TTTTTTTT
RIBOFLAVN	MG	0.12	1.29	10	RRRRIRR
NIACIN	MG	1.70	1.57	12	NNNNNINNN
IRON	MG	1.20	0.97	7	IIIII
CALCIUM	MG	24.00	0.34	3	KK
PHOSPHRUS	MG	46.00	0.66	5	XXX
POTASSIUM	MG	49.00	0.13	1	Y
PROTEIN	G	5.00	1.29	10	PPPPPIPP
CARBOHYDT	G	30.00	1.41	11	HHHHHIHHH
FAT	G	2.00	0.33	3	FF
OLEIC A	G	0.60	0.32	2	OO
LINOL A	G	0.50	0.32	3	LL
SAT FAT A	G	0.40	0.18	1	S

491 HOAGIE OR SUBMARINE BUNS
ANALYSIS OF 135 GRAMS WHICH IS 1 BUN (11 1/2 BY 3 BY 2 1/2 IN.)

NUTRIENT	UNIT	AMOUNT	INQ	% STD
ENERGY	KCAL	390.00	1.00	20
VITAMIN A	IU	0.00	0.00	0
VITAMIN C	MG	0.00	0.00	0
THIAMIN	MG	0.54	2.77	54
RIBOFLAVN	MG	0.32	1.37	27
NIACIN	MG	4.50	1.65	32
IRON	MG	3.00	0.96	19
CALCIUM	MG	58.00	0.33	6
PHOSPHRUS	MG	115.00	0.66	13
POTASSIUM	MG	122.00	0.13	2
PROTEIN	G	12.00	1.23	24
CARBOHYDT	G	75.00	1.40	27
FAT	G	4.00	0.26	5
OLEIC A	G	1.40	0.29	6
LINOL A	G	1.40	0.36	7
SAT FAT A	G	0.90	0.16	3

492 CLOVERLEAF ROLLS FROM HOME RECIPE
ANALYSIS OF 35 GRAMS WHICH IS 1 ROLL (2 1/2-IN DIAM.,2-IN HIGH

NUTRIENT	UNIT	AMOUNT	INQ	% STD
ENERGY	KCAL	120.00	1.00	6
VITAMIN A	IU	30.00	0.13	1
VITAMIN C	MG	0.00	0.00	0
THIAMIN	MG	0.12	2.00	12
RIBOFLAVN	MG	0.12	1.67	10
NIACIN	MG	1.20	1.43	9
IRON	MG	0.70	0.73	4
CALCIUM	MG	16.00	0.30	2
PHOSPHRUS	MG	36.00	0.67	4
POTASSIUM	MG	41.00	0.14	1
PROTEIN	G	3.00	1.00	6
CARBOHYDT	G	20.00	1.21	7
FAT	G	3.00	0.64	4
OLEIC A	G	1.10	0.75	4
LINOL A	G	0.70	0.58	4
SAT FAT A	G	0.80	0.47	3

493 SPAGHETTI,ENRICHED,COOKED,FIRM STAGE
ANALYSIS OF 130 GRAMS WHICH IS 1 CUP

NUTRIENT	UNIT	AMOUNT	INQ	% STD	0 10 20 30 40 50 60 70 80 90 100
ENERGY	KCAL	190.00	1.00	10	EEEEEEE
VITAMIN A	IU	0.00	0.00	0	-
VITAMIN C	MG	0.00	0.00	0	-
THIAMIN	MG	0.23	2.42	23	TTTTTTTTITTTTTTTT
RIBOFLAVN	MG	0.13	1.14	11	RRRRRRR R
NIACIN	MG	1.80	1.35	13	NNNNNNN NN
IRON	MG	1.40	0.92	9	IIIIIII
CALCIUM	MG	14.00	0.16	2	X
PHOSPHRUS	MG	85.00	0.99	9	XXXXXXX
POTASSIUM	MG	103.00	0.22	2	K
PROTEIN	G	7.00	1.47	14	YY
CARBOHYDT	G	39.00	1.49	14	PPPPPP PPP
FAT	G	1.00	0.13	1	HHHHHH HHH
OLEIC A	G	0.00	0.00	0	F
LINOL A	G	0.00	0.00	0	-
SAT FAT A	G	0.00	0.00	0	-

494 SPAGHETTI,ENRICHED,COOKED,TENDER STAGE
ANALYSIS OF 140 GRAMS WHICH IS 1 CUP

NUTRIENT	UNIT	AMOUNT	INQ	% STD	0 10 20 30 40 50 60 70 80 90 100
ENERGY	KCAL	155.00	1.00	8	EEEEE
VITAMIN A	IU	0.00	0.00	0	-
VITAMIN C	MG	0.00	0.00	0	-
THIAMIN	MG	0.20	2.58	20	TTTTTIITTTTTTTT
RIBOFLAVN	MG	0.11	1.18	9	RRRRRIR
NIACIN	MG	1.50	1.38	11	NNNNN INNN
IRON	MG	1.30	1.05	8	IIIIII I
CALCIUM	MG	11.00	0.16	1	X
PHOSPHRUS	MG	70.00	1.00	8	XXXXX
POTASSIUM	MG	85.00	0.22	2	Y
PROTEIN	G	5.00	1.29	10	PPPPPIPP
CARBOHYDT	G	32.00	1.50	12	HHHHIHHH
FAT	G	1.00	0.17	1	F
OLEIC A	G	0.00	0.00	0	-
LINOL A	G	0.00	0.00	0	-
SAT FAT A	G	0.00	0.00	0	-

495 SPAGHETTI, ENRICHED, IN TOMATO SAUCE WITH CHEESE, HOME RECIPE
ANALYSIS OF 250 GRAMS WHICH IS 1 CUP

```
                                    0        10        20        30        40        50        60        70        80        90       100
NUTRIENT  UNIT  AMOUNT   INQ   % STD
ENERGY    KCAL  260.00   1.00   13  EEEEEEEE
VITAMIN A IU   1080.00   2.08   27  AAAAAAAAIAAAAAAAAAA
VITAMIN C MG     13.00   1.67   22  CCCCCCCCICCCCCC
THIAMIN   MG      0.25   1.92   25  TTTTTTTTITTTTTTTTT
RIBOFLAVN MG      0.18   1.15   15  RRRRRRRRIRR
NIACIN    MG      2.30   1.26   16  NNNNNNNNINNN
IRON      MG      2.30   1.11   14  IIIIIIIIII
CALCIUM   MG     80.00   0.68    9  KKKKKKK
PHOSPHRUS MG    135.00   1.15   15  XXXXXXXXIXx
POTASSIUM MG    408.00   0.63    8  YYYYYYY
PROTEIN   G       9.00   1.38   18  PPPPPPPPIPPPP
CARBOHYDT G      37.00   1.03   13  HHHHHHHHIH
FAT       G       9.00   0.89   12  FFFFFFFFFI
OLEIC A   G       5.40   1.70   22  OOOOOOOOOIOOOOOOOO
LINOL A   G       0.70   0.27    4  LLL
SAT FAT A G       2.00   0.54    7  SSSSSS
*************************************************
```

496 SPAGHETTI, ENRICHED, IN TOMATO SAUCE WITH CHEESE, CANNED
ANALYSIS OF 250 GRAMS WHICH IS 1 CUP

```
                                    0        10        20        30        40        50        60        70        80        90       100
NUTRIENT  UNIT  AMOUNT   INQ   % STD
ENERGY    KCAL  190.00   1.00   10  EEEEEEE
VITAMIN A IU    930.00   2.45   23  AAAAAAAIAAAAAAAAA
VITAMIN C MG     10.00   1.75   17  CCCCCCCICCCCC
THIAMIN   MG      0.35   3.68   35  TTTTTTTITTTTTTTTTTTTTTTT
RIBOFLAVN MG      0.28   2.46   23  RRRRRRRIRRRRRRRRR
NIACIN    MG      4.50   3.38   32  NNNNNNNINNNNNNNNNNNNN
IRON      MG      2.80   1.84   18  IIIIIIIIIIIIII
CALCIUM   MG     40.00   0.47    4  KKKK
PHOSPHRUS MG     88.00   1.03   10  XXXXXXX
POTASSIUM MG    303.00   0.64    6  YYYYY
PROTEIN   G       6.00   1.26   12  PPPPPPIPP
CARBOHYDT G      39.00   1.49   14  HHHHHHIHHH
FAT       G       2.00   0.27    3  FF
OLEIC A   G       0.30   0.13    1  O
LINOL A   G       0.40   0.21    2  LL
SAT FAT A G       0.50   0.18    2  S
*************************************************
```

497 SPAGHETTI, ENRICHED, WITH MEAT BALLS IN TOMATO SAUCE, HOME RECIPE
ANALYSIS OF 248 GRAMS WHICH IS 1 CUP

NUTRIENT	UNIT	AMOUNT	INQ	% STD	0 10 20 30 40 50 60 70 80 90 100
ENERGY	KCAL	330.00	1.00	17	EEEEEEEEEE
VITAMIN A	IU	1590.00	2.41	40	AAAAAAAAAAI AAAAAAAAAAAAAAAAAAA
VITAMIN C	MG	22.00	2.22	37	CCCCCCCCCCI CCCCCCCCCCCCCCCC
THIAMIN	MG	0.25	1.52	25	TTTTTTTTTTTTTTT
RIBOFLAVN	MG	0.30	1.52	25	RRRRRRRRRRRRRR I RRRRRR
NIACIN	MG	4.00	1.73	29	NNNNNNNNNNNNNNI NNNNNNNNN
IRON	MG	3.70	1.40	23	IIIIIIIIIIIIII I IIIIIII
CALCIUM	MG	124.00	0.84	14	KKKKKKKKKKK I
PHOSPHRUS	MG	236.00	1.59	26	XXXXXXXXXXXXXX IXXXXXXX I
POTASSIUM	MG	665.00	0.81	13	YYYYYYYYYY I
PROTEIN	G	19.00	2.30	38	PPPPPPPPPPPPPP IPPPPPPPPPPPPP
CARBOHYDT	G	39.00	0.86	14	HHHHHHHHHHH I
FAT	G	12.00	0.93	15	FFFFFFFFFFFFFFF I
OLEIC A	G	6.30	1.56	26	OOOOOOOOOOOOO IOOOOOOOO
LINOL A	G	0.90	0.27	5	LLLL I
SAT FAT A	G	3.30	0.70	12	SSSSSSSSS I

****

498 SPAGHETTI, ENRICHED, WITH MEAT BALLS IN TOMATO SAUCE, CANNED
ANALYSIS OF 250 GRAMS WHICH IS 1 CUP

NUTRIENT	UNIT	AMOUNT	INQ	% STD	0 10 20 30 40 50 60 70 80 90 100
ENERGY	KCAL	260.00	1.00	13	EEEEEEEEE
VITAMIN A	IU	1000.00	1.92	25	AAAAAAAAAI AAAAAAAA
VITAMIN C	MG	5.00	0.64	8	CCCCCCC I
THIAMIN	MG	0.15	1.15	15	TTTTTTTTTTIT
RIBOFLAVN	MG	0.18	1.15	15	RRRRRRRRRRIRR
NIACIN	MG	2.30	1.26	16	NNNNNNNNNNINNN
IRON	MG	3.30	1.59	21	IIIIIIIIIIIIIIII
CALCIUM	MG	53.00	0.45	6	KKKKK I
PHOSPHRUS	MG	113.00	0.97	13	XXXXXXXXXX
POTASSIUM	MG	245.00	0.38	5	YYYY I
PROTEIN	G	12.00	1.85	24	PPPPPPPPPPIPPPPPPPP
CARBOHYDT	G	29.00	0.81	11	HHHHHHHH I
FAT	G	10.00	0.99	13	FFFFFFFFFFF
OLEIC A	G	3.30	1.04	13	OOOOOOOOOOIO
LINOL A	G	3.90	1.50	20	LLLLLLLLLLILLLLL
SAT FAT A	G	2.20	0.59	8	SSSSS I

****

499 TOASTER PASTRIES
ANALYSIS OF 50 GRAMS WHICH IS 1 PASTRY

```
                                    0        10        20        30        40        50        60        70        80        90       100
                                                                                                                                       **************
NUTRIENT    UNIT  AMOUNT   INQ  % STD
ENERGY      KCAL  200.00   1.00   10  EEEEEEE
VITAMIN A   IU    500.00   1.25   13  AAAAAAIAA
VITAMIN C   MG      0.00   0.00    0  -
THIAMIN     MG      0.16   0.60   16  TTTTTTITTTTT
RIBOFLAVN   MG      0.17   1.42   14  RRRRRRIRRR
NIACIN      MG      2.10   1.50   15  NNNNNNINNNN
IRON        MG      1.90   1.19   12  IIIIIIIII
CALCIUM     MG     54.00   0.60    6  KKKKK
PHOSPHRUS   MG     67.00   0.74    7  XXXXX
POTASSIUM   MG     74.00   0.15    1  Y
PROTEIN     G       3.00   0.60    6  PPPP
CARBOHYDT   G      36.00   1.31   13  HHHHHHIHH
FAT         G       6.00   0.77    8  FFFFF
OLEIC A     G       2.60   1.06   11  OOOOOOO
LINOL A     G       0.80   0.80    8  LLLLLL
SAT FAT A   G       1.50   0.53    5  SSSS
*****************************************
```

500 WAFFLES FROM HOME RECIPE
ANALYSIS OF 75 GRAMS WHICH IS 1 WAFFLE 7-IN DIAM

```
                                    0        10        20        30        40        50        60        70        80        90       100
                                                                                                                                       **************
NUTRIENT    UNIT  AMOUNT   INQ  % STD
ENERGY      KCAL  210.00   1.00   11  EEEEEEE
VITAMIN A   IU    250.00   0.60    6  AAAA
VITAMIN C   MG      0.00   0.00    0  -
THIAMIN     MG      0.17   1.62   17  TTTTTTITTTTTT
RIBOFLAVN   MG      0.23   1.83   19  RRRRRRIRRRRRR
NIACIN      MG      1.40   0.95   10  NNNNNNNN
IRON        MG      1.30   0.77    8  IIIIIII
CALCIUM     MG     85.00   0.90    9  KKKKKKK
PHOSPHRUS   MG    130.00   1.38   14  XXXXXXXIXXXX
POTASSIUM   MG    109.00   0.21    2  YY
PROTEIN     G       7.00   1.33   14  PPPPPPIPPP
CARBOHYDT   G      28.00   0.97   10  HHHHHHH
FAT         G       7.00   0.85    9  FFFFFFFI
OLEIC A     G       2.80   1.09   11  OOOOOOOIO
LINOL A     G       1.40   0.67    7  LLLLL
SAT FAT A   G       2.30   0.77    8  SSSSS
*****************************************
```

501 WAFFLES FROM MIX, EGG AND MILK ADDED
ANALYSIS OF 75 GRAMS WHICH IS 1 WAFFLE 7-IN. DIAM

```
                                              0    10   20   30   40   50   60   70   80   90  100
NUTRIENT   UNIT  AMOUNT  INQ    % STD
ENERGY     KCAL  205.00  1.00   10    EEEEEE
VITAMIN A  IU    170.00  0.41    4    AAA
VITAMIN C  MG      0.00  0.00    0    -
THIAMIN    MG      0.14  1.37   14    TTTTTTT|TTT
RIBOFLAVN  MG      0.22  1.79   18    RRRRRRR|RRRRRR
NIACIN     MG      0.90  0.63    6    NNNN
IRON       MG      1.00  0.61    6    IIIII |
CALCIUM    MG    179.00  1.94   20    KKKKKKK|KKKKKKK
PHOSPHRUS  MG    257.00  2.79   29    XXXXXXX|XXXXXXXXXXXXXX
POTASSIUM  MG    146.00  0.28    3    YY
PROTEIN    G      7.00   1.37   14    PPPPPPP|PPP
CARBOHYDT  G     27.00   0.96   10    HHHHHHH
FAT        G      8.00   1.00   10    FFFFFFF
OLEIC A    G      2.90   1.15   12    OOOOOOO|O
LINOL A    G      1.20   0.59    6    LLLLL |
SAT FAT A  G      2.80   0.96   10    SSSSSSS
```

502 WHEAT FLOUR, ENRICHED, ALL PURPOSE, SIFTED, SPOONED
ANALYSIS OF 115 GRAMS WHICH IS 1 CUP

```
                                              0    10   20   30   40   50   60   70   80   90  100
NUTRIENT   UNIT  AMOUNT  INQ    % STD
ENERGY     KCAL  420.00  1.00   21    EEEEEEEEEEEEE
VITAMIN A  IU      0.00  0.00    0    -
VITAMIN C  MG      0.00  0.00    0    -
THIAMIN    MG      0.74  3.52   74    TTTTTTTTTTTTTTTTTTTTTTTTTTTTTTTTTTTTT
RIBOFLAVN  MG      0.46  1.83   38    RRRRRRRRR|RRRRRRRRR
NIACIN     MG      6.10  2.07   44    NNNNNNNNN|NNNNNNNNNNNNNNNNNNNN
IRON       MG      3.30  0.98   21    IIIIIIIII|IIIIIIIII
CALCIUM    MG     18.00  0.10    2    KK
PHOSPHRUS  MG    100.00  0.53   11    XXXXXXXXX
POTASSIUM  MG    109.00  0.10    2    YY
PROTEIN    G     12.00   1.14   24    PPPPPPPPP|PPPP
CARBOHYDT  G     88.00   1.52   32    HHHHHHHHH|HHHHHHHHH
FAT        G      1.00   0.06    1    F
OLEIC A    G      0.10   0.02    0    -
LINOL A    G      0.50   0.12    3    LL
SAT FAT A  G      0.20   0.03    1    S
```

503 WHEAT FLOUR,ENRICHED, ALL PURPOSE, UNSIFTED, SPOONED
ANALYSIS OF 125 GRAMS WHICH IS 1 CUP

NUTRIENT	UNIT	AMOUNT	INQ	% STD
ENERGY	KCAL	455.00	1.00	23
VITAMIN A	IU	0.00	0.00	0
VITAMIN C	MG	0.00	0.00	0
THIAMIN	MG	0.80	3.52	80
RIBOFLAVN	MG	0.50	1.83	42
NIACIN	MG	6.60	2.07	47
IRON	MG	3.60	0.99	23
CALCIUM	MG	20.00	0.10	2
PHOSPHRUS	MG	109.00	0.53	12
POTASSIUM	MG	119.00	0.10	2
PROTEIN	G	13.00	1.14	26
CARBOHYDT	G	95.00	1.52	35
FAT	G	1.00	0.06	1
OLEIC A	G	0.10	0.02	0
LINOL A	G	0.50	0.11	3
SAT FAT A	G	0.20	0.03	1

504 CAKE OR PASTRY FLOUR, ENRICHED, SIFTED, SPOONED
ANALYSIS OF 96 GRAMS WHICH IS 1 CUP

NUTRIENT	UNIT	AMOUNT	INQ	% STD
ENERGY	KCAL	350.00	1.00	17
VITAMIN A	IU	0.00	0.00	0
VITAMIN C	MG	0.00	0.00	0
THIAMIN	MG	0.61	3.49	61
RIBOFLAVN	MG	0.38	1.81	32
NIACIN	MG	5.10	2.08	36
IRON	MG	2.80	1.00	18
CALCIUM	MG	16.00	0.10	2
PHOSPHRUS	MG	70.00	0.44	8
POTASSIUM	MG	91.00	0.10	2
PROTEIN	G	7.00	0.80	14
CARBOHYDT	G	76.00	1.58	28
FAT	G	1.00	0.07	1
OLEIC A	G	0.10	0.02	0
LINOL A	G	0.30	0.09	2
SAT FAT A	G	0.10	0.02	0

505 SELF-RISING FLOUR, ENRICHED, UNSIFTED, SPOONED
ANALYSIS OF 125 GRAMS WHICH IS 1 CUP

NUTRIENT	UNIT	AMOUNT	INQ	% STD
ENERGY	KCAL	440.00	1.00	22
VITAMIN A	IU	0.00	0.00	0
VITAMIN C	MG	0.00	0.00	0
THIAMIN	MG	0.80	3.64	80
RIBOFLAVN	MG	0.50	1.89	42
NIACIN	MG	6.60	2.14	47
IRON	MG	3.60	1.02	23
CALCIUM	MG	331.00	1.67	37
PHOSPHRUS	MG	583.00	2.94	65
POTASSIUM	MG	112.00	0.10	2
PROTEIN	G	12.00	1.09	24
CARBOHYDT	G	93.00	1.54	34
FAT	G	1.00	0.06	1
OLEIC A	G	0.10	0.02	0
LINOL A	G	0.50	0.11	3
SAT FAT A	G	0.20	0.03	1

506 WHOLE WHEAT FLOUR
ANALYSIS OF 120 GRAMS WHICH IS 1 CUP

NUTRIENT	UNIT	AMOUNT	INQ	% STD
ENERGY	KCAL	400.00	1.00	20
VITAMIN A	IU	0.00	0.00	0
VITAMIN C	MG	0.00	0.00	0
THIAMIN	MG	0.66	3.30	66
RIBOFLAVN	MG	0.14	0.58	12
NIACIN	MG	5.20	1.86	37
IRON	MG	4.00	1.25	25
CALCIUM	MG	49.00	0.27	5
PHOSPHRUS	MG	446.00	2.48	50
POTASSIUM	MG	444.00	0.44	9
PROTEIN	G	16.00	1.60	32
CARBOHYDT	G	85.00	1.55	31
FAT	G	2.00	0.13	1
OLEIC A	G	0.20	0.04	1
LINOL A	G	1.00	0.25	5
SAT FAT A	G	0.40	0.07	1

507 ALMONDS, CHOPPED
ANALYSIS OF 130 GRAMS WHICH IS 1 CUP (130 ALMONDS)

NUTRIENT	UNIT	AMOUNT	INQ	% STD
ENERGY	KCAL	775.00	1.00	39
VITAMIN A	IU	0.00	0.00	0
VITAMIN C	MG	0.00	0.00	0
THIAMIN	MG	0.31	0.80	31
RIBOFLAVN	MG	1.20	2.58	100
NIACIN	MG	4.60	0.85	33
IRON	MG	6.10	0.98	38
CALCIUM	MG	304.00	0.87	34
PHOSPHRUS	MG	655.00	1.88	73
POTASSIUM	MG	1005.00	0.52	20
PROTEIN	G	24.00	1.24	48
CARBOHYDT	G	25.00	0.23	9
FAT	G	70.00	2.32	90
OLEIC A	G	47.70	5.02	195
LINOL A	G	12.80	1.65	64
SAT FAT A	G	5.60	0.51	20

508 ALMONDS, SLIVERED
ANALYSIS OF 115 GRAMS WHICH IS 1 CUP (115 NUTS)

NUTRIENT	UNIT	AMOUNT	INQ	% STD
ENERGY	KCAL	690.00	1.00	34
VITAMIN A	IU	0.00	0.00	0
VITAMIN C	MG	0.00	0.00	0
THIAMIN	MG	0.28	0.81	28
RIBOFLAVN	MG	1.06	2.56	88
NIACIN	MG	4.00	0.83	29
IRON	MG	5.40	0.98	34
CALCIUM	MG	269.00	0.87	30
PHOSPHRUS	MG	580.00	1.87	64
POTASSIUM	MG	889.00	0.52	18
PROTEIN	G	21.00	1.22	42
CARBOHYDT	G	22.00	0.23	8
FAT	G	62.00	2.30	79
OLEIC A	G	42.20	4.99	172
LINOL A	G	11.30	1.64	57
SAT FAT A	G	5.00	0.51	18

509 DRY BEANS, GREAT NORTHERN COOKED, DRAINED
ANALYSIS OF 180 GRAMS WHICH IS 1 CUP

NUTRIENT	UNIT	AMOUNT	INQ	% STD
ENERGY	KCAL	210.00	1.00	11
VITAMIN A	IU	0.00	0.00	0
VITAMIN C	MG	0.00	0.00	0
THIAMIN	MG	0.25	2.38	25
RIBOFLAVN	MG	0.13	1.03	11
NIACIN	MG	1.30	0.88	9
IRON	MG	4.90	2.92	31
CALCIUM	MG	90.00	0.95	10
PHOSPHRUS	MG	266.00	2.81	30
POTASSIUM	MG	749.00	1.43	15
PROTEIN	G	14.00	2.67	28
CARBOHYDT	G	38.00	1.32	14
FAT	G	1.00	0.12	1
OLEIC A	G	0.00	0.00	0
LINOL A	G	0.00	0.00	0
SAT FAT A	G	0.00	0.00	0

510 DRY BEANS, NAVY, COOKED, DRAINED
ANALYSIS OF 190 GRAMS WHICH IS 1 CUP

NUTRIENT	UNIT	AMOUNT	INQ	% STD
ENERGY	KCAL	225.00	1.00	11
VITAMIN A	IU	0.00	0.00	0
VITAMIN C	MG	0.00	0.00	0
THIAMIN	MG	0.27	2.40	27
RIBOFLAVN	MG	0.13	0.96	11
NIACIN	MG	1.30	0.83	9
IRON	MG	5.10	2.83	32
CALCIUM	MG	95.00	0.94	11
PHOSPHRUS	MG	281.00	2.78	31
POTASSIUM	MG	790.00	1.40	16
PROTEIN	G	15.00	2.67	30
CARBOHYDT	G	40.00	1.29	15
FAT	G	1.00	0.11	1
OLEIC A	G	0.00	0.00	0
LINOL A	G	0.00	0.00	0
SAT FAT A	G	0.00	0.00	0

```
                                                                   0    10    20    30    40    50    60    70    80    90   100
511  BEANS WITH FRANKFURTERS,CANNED                                * * * * * * * * * * * * * * * * * * * *
ANALYSIS OF 255 GRAMS WHICH IS 1 CUP

NUTRIENT   UNIT   AMOUNT   INQ   % STD
ENERGY     KCAL   365.00   1.00    18    EEEEEEEEEEEEEE
VITAMIN A  IU     330.00   0.45     8    AAAAAAA
VITAMIN C  MG       0.00   0.00     0    -
THIAMIN    MG       0.18   0.99    18    TTTTTTTTTTTTT
RIBOFLAVN  MG       0.15   0.68    13    RRRRRRRRRR
NIACIN     MG       3.30   1.29    24    NNNNNNNNNNNNNNNN|NNNN
IRON       MG       4.80   1.64    30    IIIIIIIIIIIII|IIIIIIII
CALCIUM    MG      94.00   0.57    10    KKKKKKK
PHOSPHRUS  MG     303.00   1.84    34    XXXXXXXXXXXXX|XXXXXXXXXXX
POTASSIUM  MG     668.00   0.73    13    YYYYYYYYY
PROTEIN    G       19.00   2.08    38    PPPPPPPPPPPPP|PPPPPPPPPPP
CARBOHYDT  G       32.00   0.64    12    HHHHHHHH
FAT        G       18.00   1.26    23    FFFFFFFFFFFF|FFF
OLEIC A    G        7.60   1.70    31    OOOOOOOOOOOOO|OOOOOOOOO
LINOL A    G        0.00   0.00     0    -
SAT FAT A  G        7.60   1.46    27    SSSSSSSSSSSSSS|SSSSS
*******************************************
```

```
                                                                   0    10    20    30    40    50    60    70    80    90   100
512  PORK AND BEANS IN TOMATO SAUCE                                * * * * * * * * * * * * * * * * * * * *
ANALYSIS OF 255 GRAMS WHICH IS 1 CUP

NUTRIENT   UNIT   AMOUNT   INQ   % STD
ENERGY     KCAL   310.00   1.00    16    EEEEEEEEEEEE
VITAMIN A  IU     330.00   0.53     8    AAAAAAA
VITAMIN C  MG       5.00   0.54     8    CCCCCCC
THIAMIN    MG       0.20   1.29    20    TTTTTTTTTTT|TTTT
RIBOFLAVN  MG       0.08   0.43     7    RRRRR
NIACIN     MG       1.50   0.69    11    NNNNNNNNN
IRON       MG       4.60   1.85    29    IIIIIIIIIII|IIIIIIIIIII
CALCIUM    MG     138.00   0.99    15    KKKKKKKKKKKK|K
PHOSPHRUS  MG     235.00   1.68    26    XXXXXXXXXXX|XXXXXXXX
POTASSIUM  MG     536.00   0.69    11    YYYYYYYYY
PROTEIN    G       16.00   2.06    32    PPPPPPPPPPP|PPPPPPPPPPPP
CARBOHYDT  G       48.00   1.13    17    HHHHHHHHHHHH|HH
FAT        G        7.00   0.58     9    FFFFFFF
OLEIC A    G        2.80   0.74    11    OOOOOOOOO
LINOL A    G        0.60   0.19     3    LL
SAT FAT A  G        2.40   0.54     8    SSSSSSS
*******************************************
```

513 PORK AND BEANS IN SWEET SAUCE
ANALYSIS OF 255 GRAMS WHICH IS 1 CUP

```
                                        0        10        20        30        40        50        60        70        80        90       100
NUTRIENT   UNIT   AMOUNT    INQ   % STD
ENERGY     KCAL   385.00    1.00   19   EEEEEEEEEEEEE                                                                                       *
VITAMIN A  IU     330.00    0.43    8   AAAAAAA                                                                                             *
VITAMIN C  MG       0.00    0.00    0   -                                                                                                   *
THIAMIN    MG       0.15    0.78   15   TTTTTTTTTTT                                                                                         *
RIBOFLAVN  MG       0.10    0.43    8   RRRRRRR |                                                                                           *
NIACIN     MG       1.30    0.48    9   NNNNNNN                                                                                             *
IRON       MG       5.90    1.92   37   IIIIIIIIIIIIIIII|IIIIIIIIIIIIIIIII                                                                  *
CALCIUM    MG     161.00    0.93   18   KKKKKKKKKKKKK|                                                                                      *
PHOSPHRUS  MG     291.00    1.68   32   XXXXXXXXXXXXX|XXXXXXXXXXX                                                                           *
POTASSIUM  MG     536.00    0.56   11   YYYYYYYY                                                                                            *
PROTEIN    G       16.00    1.66   32   PPPPPPPPPPPPP|PPPPPPPPPP                                                                            *
CARBOHYDT  G       54.00    1.02   20   HHHHHHHHHHHHHH|H                                                                                    *
FAT        G       12.00    0.80   15   FFFFFFFFFFF                                                                                         *
OLEIC A    G        5.00    1.06   20   OOOOOOOOOOOOOO|O                                                                                    *
LINOL A    G        1.10    0.29    6   LLL                                                                                                 *
SAT FAT A  G        4.30    0.78   15   SSSSSSSSSSS                                                                                         *
*******************************************************************************************************************
```

514 RED KIDNEY BEANS, CANNED
ANALYSIS OF 255 GRAMS WHICH IS 1 CUP

```
                                        0        10        20        30        40        50        60        70        80        90       100
NUTRIENT   UNIT   AMOUNT    INQ   % STD
ENERGY     KCAL   230.00    1.00   12   EEEEEEEE                                                                                            *
VITAMIN A  IU      10.00    0.02    0   -                                                                                                   *
VITAMIN C  MG       0.00    0.00    0                                                                                                       *
THIAMIN    MG       0.13    1.13   13   TTTTTTTTT                                                                                           *
RIBOFLAVN  MG       0.10    0.72    8   RRRRRR |                                                                                            *
NIACIN     MG       1.50    0.93   11   NNNNNNNNN                                                                                           *
IRON       MG       4.60    2.50   29   IIIIIIIII|IIIIIIIIIIIIIII                                                                           *
CALCIUM    MG      74.00    0.71    8   KKKKKKK |                                                                                           *
PHOSPHRUS  MG     278.00    2.69   31   XXXXXXXX|XXXXXXXXXXXXXXXX                                                                           *
POTASSIUM  MG     667.00    1.17   13   YYYYYYYY|Y                                                                                          *
PROTEIN    G       15.00    2.61   30   PPPPPPP|PPPPPPPPPPPPPPPP                                                                            *
CARBOHYDT  G       42.00    1.33   15   HHHHHHHH|HHH                                                                                        *
FAT        G        1.00    0.11    1   F                                                                                                   *
OLEIC A    G        0.00    0.00    0   -                                                                                                   *
LINOL A    G        0.00    0.00    0   -                                                                                                   *
SAT FAT A  G        0.00    0.00    0   -                                                                                                   *
*******************************************************************************************************************
```

```
                                        100 * * * * * * * * * * * * * * * * *                    100 * * * * * * * * * * * * * * * *


                                         90                                                       90


                                         80                                                       80


                                         70                                                       70


                                         60                                                       60


                                         50                                                       50


                                         40                                                       40


                                         30                                                       30


                                         20                                                       20


515  DRY LIMA BEANS, COOKED, DRAINED      10                             516  BLACKEYE PEAS,DRY,COOKED     10
ANALYSIS OF 190 GRAMS WHICH IS 1 CUP                                     ANALYSIS OF 250 GRAMS WHICH IS 1 CUP

NUTRIENT   UNIT  AMOUNT   INQ   % STD  0        10                       NUTRIENT   UNIT  AMOUNT   INQ   % STD  0        10
ENERGY     KCAL  260.00   1.00    13   EEEEEEEEE                         ENERGY     KCAL  190.00   1.00    10   EEEEEEE
VITAMIN A  IU      0.00   0.00     0   -                                 VITAMIN A  IU     30.00   0.08     1   A
VITAMIN C  MG      0.00   0.00     0   -                                 VITAMIN C  MG      0.00   0.00     0   -
THIAMIN    MG      0.25   1.92    25   TTTTTTTTT|TTTTTTTTT               THIAMIN    MG      0.40   4.21    40   TTTTTTT|TTTTTTTTTTTTTTTTTTTTTTTTTT
RIBOFLAVN  MG      0.11   0.71     9   RRRRRRR |                         RIBOFLAVN  MG      0.10   0.88     8   RRRRRRR|
NIACIN     MG      1.30   0.71     9   NNNNNNN |                         NIACIN     MG      1.00   0.75     7   NNNNNN |
IRON       MG      5.90   2.84    37   IIIIIIIII|IIIIIIIIIIIIIIIIIIIIIII  IRON      MG      3.30   2.17    21   IIIIIII|IIIIIIIII
CALCIUM    MG     55.00   0.47     6   KKKKK  |                          CALCIUM    MG     43.00   0.50     5   KKKK   |
PHOSPHRUS  MG    293.00   2.50    33   XXXXXXXXX|XXXXXXXXXXXXXXXX         PHOSPHRUS  MG    238.00   2.78    26   XXXXXXX|XXXXXXXXXXXXXXXX
POTASSIUM  MG   1163.00   1.79    23   YYYYYYYYY|YYYYYY                   POTASSIUM  MG    573.00   1.21    11   YYYYYYY|Y
PROTEIN    G      16.00   2.46    32   PPPPPPPPP|PPPPPPPPPPPPPPP          PROTEIN    G      13.00   2.74    26   PPPPPPP|PPPPPPPPP
CARBOHYDT  G      49.00   1.37    18   HHHHHHHH|HHHH                      CARBOHYDT  G      35.00   1.34    13   HHHHHH |HH
FAT        G       1.00   0.10     1   F                                 FAT        G       1.00   0.13     1   F
OLEIC A    G       0.00   0.00     0   -                                 OLEIC A    G       0.00   0.00     0   -
LINOL A    G       0.00   0.00     0   -                                 LINOL A    G       0.00   0.00     0   -
SAT FAT A  G       0.00   0.00     0   -                                 SAT FAT A  G       0.00   0.00     0   -
*********************************                                        *********************************
```

517 BRAZIL NUTS
ANALYSIS OF 28 GRAMS WHICH IS 1 OZ. (6-8 LARGE KERNALS)

NUTRIENT	UNIT	AMOUNT	INQ	% STD	0 10 20 30 40 50 60 70 80 90 100
ENERGY	KCAL	185.00	1.00	9	EEEEEE
VITAMIN A	IU	0.00	0.00	0	-
VITAMIN C	MG	0.00	0.00	0	-
THIAMIN	MG	0.27	2.92	27	TTTTT|TTTTTTTTTTTT
RIBOFLAVN	MG	0.03	0.27	3	RR
NIACIN	MG	0.50	0.39	4	NNN
IRON	MG	1.00	0.68	6	IIIII
CALCIUM	MG	53.00	0.64	6	KKKKK
PHOSPHRUS	MG	196.00	2.35	22	XXXXXX|XXXXXXXXXX
POTASSIUM	MG	203.00	0.44	4	YYY
PROTEIN	G	4.00	0.86	8	PPPPPP
CARBOHYDT	G	3.00	0.12	1	H
FAT	G	19.00	2.63	24	FFFFFF|FFFFFFFFFF
OLEIC A	G	6.20	2.74	25	OOOOOO|OOOOOOOOOOOO
LINOL A	G	7.10	3.84	36	LLLLLL|LLLLLLLLLLLLLLLLLLL
SAT FAT A	G	4.80	1.82	17	SSSSSS|SSSSSS

518 CASHEW NUTS, ROASTED IN OIL
ANALYSIS OF 140 GRAMS WHICH IS 1 CUP

NUTRIENT	UNIT	AMOUNT	INQ	% STD	0 10 20 30 40 50 60 70 80 90 100
ENERGY	KCAL	785.00	1.00	39	EEEEEEEEEEEEEEEEEEEEEEEEEE
VITAMIN A	IU	140.00	0.09	4	AAA
VITAMIN C	MG	0.00	0.00	0	-
THIAMIN	MG	0.60	1.53	60	TTTTTTTTTTTTTTTTTTTTTTTT|TTTTTTTTTTTTTTTTTT
RIBOFLAVN	MG	0.35	0.74	29	RRRRRRRRRRRRRRRRRRR
NIACIN	MG	2.50	0.45	18	NNNNNNNNNNNNN
IRON	MG	5.30	0.84	33	IIIIIIIIIIIIIIIIIIIIII
CALCIUM	MG	53.00	0.15	6	KKKKK
PHOSPHRUS	MG	522.00	1.48	58	XXXXXXXXXXXXXXXXXXXXXXXX|XXXXXXXXXXXXXXXXX
POTASSIUM	MG	650.00	0.33	13	YYYYYYYYY
PROTEIN	G	24.00	1.22	48	PPPPPPPPPPPPPPPPPPPPP|PPPPPPP
CARBOHYDT	G	41.00	0.38	15	HHHHHHHHHH
FAT	G	64.00	2.09	82	FFFFFFFFFFFFFFFFFFFFFFF|FFFFFFFFFFFFFFFFFFFFFFFFFFFFFFFFFF
OLEIC A	G	36.80	3.83	150	OOOOOO|OOOOOOOOOOOOOOOOOOOOOOOOOOOOOOOOOOOOOO *150
LINOL A	G	10.20	1.30	51	LLLLLL|LLLLLLLLLLLLLLLLLLL
SAT FAT A	G	12.90	1.15	45	SSSSSSSSSSSSSSSSSS|SSS

519 COCONUT,FRESH
ANALYSIS OF 45 GRAMS WHICH IS 1 PIECE 2 BY 2 BY 1/2-IN

NUTRIENT	UNIT	AMOUNT	INQ	% STD
ENERGY	KCAL	155.00	1.00	8
VITAMIN A	IU	0.00	0.00	0
VITAMIN C	MG	1.00	0.22	2
THIAMIN	MG	0.02	0.26	2
RIBOFLAVN	MG	0.01	0.11	1
NIACIN	MG	0.20	0.18	1
IRON	MG	0.80	0.65	5
CALCIUM	MG	6.00	0.09	1
PHOSPHRUS	MG	43.00	0.62	5
POTASSIUM	MG	115.00	0.30	2
PROTEIN	G	2.00	0.52	4
CARBOHYDT	G	4.00	0.19	1
FAT	G	16.00	2.65	21
OLEIC A	G	0.90	0.47	4
LINOL A	G	0.30	0.19	2
SAT FAT A	G	14.00	6.34	49

520 COCONUT SHREDDED OR GRATED
ANALYSIS OF 80 GRAMS WHICH IS 1 CUP, NOT PRESSED DOWN,

NUTRIENT	UNIT	AMOUNT	INQ	% STD
ENERGY	KCAL	275.00	1.00	14
VITAMIN A	IU	0.00	0.00	0
VITAMIN C	MG	2.00	0.24	3
THIAMIN	MG	0.04	0.29	4
RIBOFLAVN	MG	0.02	0.12	2
NIACIN	MG	0.40	0.21	3
IRON	MG	1.40	0.64	9
CALCIUM	MG	10.00	0.08	1
PHOSPHRUS	MG	76.00	0.61	8
POTASSIUM	MG	205.00	0.30	4
PROTEIN	G	3.00	0.44	6
CARBOHYDT	G	8.00	0.21	3
FAT	G	28.00	2.61	36
OLEIC A	G	1.60	0.47	7
LINOL A	G	0.50	0.18	3
SAT FAT A	G	24.80	6.33	87

521 FILBERTS (HAZELNUTS), CHOPPED
ANALYSIS OF 115 GRAMS WHICH IS 1 CUP (80 KERNELS)

NUTRIENT	UNIT	AMOUNT	INQ	% STD										
					0	10	20	30	40	50	60	70	80	90	100
ENERGY	KCAL	730.00	1.00	37	EEEEEEEEEEEEEEEEEEEEEEEEEEE									
VITAMIN A	IU	0.00	0.00	0										
VITAMIN C	MG	0.00	0.00	0										
THIAMIN	MG	0.53	1.45	53	TTTTTTTTTTTTTTTTTTTTTTTTTTTTTTTTTTTTTTTTTTTTTTTTTTTT									
RIBOFLAVN	MG	0.00	0.00	0										
NIACIN	MG	1.00	0.20	7	NNNNNN									
IRON	MG	3.90	0.67	24	IIIIIIIIIIIIIIIIIIIIIIII									
CALCIUM	MG	240.00	0.73	27	KKKKKKKKKKKKKKKKKKKKKKKKKKK									
PHOSPHRUS	MG	388.00	1.18	43	XXXXXXXXXXXXXXXXXXXXXXXXXXXXXXXXXXXXXXXXXXX									
POTASSIUM	MG	810.00	0.44	16	YYYYYYYYYYYYYYYY									
PROTEIN	G	14.00	0.77	28	PPPPPPPPPPPPPPPPPPPPPPPPPPPP									
CARBOHYDT	G	19.00	0.19	7	HHHHHHH									
FAT	G	72.00	2.53	92	FFFFFFFFFFFFFFFFFFFFFFFFFFFFFFFFFFFFFFFFFFFFFFFFFFFFFFFFFFFFFFFFFFFFFFFFFFFFFFFFFFFFFFFFFFFFFF									
OLEIC A	G	55.20	6.17	225	OOOOOOOOOOOOOOOOOOOOOOOOOOOOOOOOOOOOOOOOOOOOOOOOOOOOOOOOOOOOOOOOOOOOOOOOOOOOOOOOOOOOOOOOOOOOOOOOOOO * 225									
LINOL A	G	7.30	1.00	37	LLLLLLLLLLLLLLLLLLLLLLLLLLLLLLLLLLLLL									
SAT FAT A	G	5.10	0.49	18	SSSSSSSSSSSSSS									

522 LENTILS, WHOLE, COOKED
ANALYSIS OF 200 GRAMS WHICH IS 1 CUP

NUTRIENT	UNIT	AMOUNT	INQ	% STD										
					0	10	20	30	40	50	60	70	80	90	100
ENERGY	KCAL	210.00	1.00	11	EEEEEEEE									
VITAMIN A	IU	40.00	0.10	1	A									
VITAMIN C	MG	0.00	0.00	1										
THIAMIN	MG	0.14	1.33	14	TTTTTTTTTTTTTT									
RIBOFLAVN	MG	0.12	0.95	10	RRRRRRRRR									
NIACIN	MG	1.20	0.82	9	NNNNNNNN									
IRON	MG	4.20	2.50	26	IIIIIIIIIIIIIIIIIIIIIIIIII									
CALCIUM	MG	50.00	0.53	6	KKKK									
PHOSPHRUS	MG	238.00	2.52	26	XXXXXXXXXXXXXXXXXXXXXXXXXX									
POTASSIUM	MG	498.00	0.95	10	YYYYYYYYY									
PROTEIN	G	16.00	3.05	32	PPPPPPPPPPPPPPPPPPPPPPPPPPPPPPPP									
CARBOHYDT	G	39.00	1.35	14	HHHHHHHHHHHHHH									
FAT	G	0.00	0.00	0										
OLEIC A	G	0.00	0.00	0										
LINOL A	G	0.00	0.00	0										
SAT FAT A	G	0.00	0.00	0										

523 PEANUTS, ROASTED IN OIL, SALTED
ANALYSIS OF 144 GRAMS WHICH IS 1 CUP (WHOLE, HALVES, CHOPPED)

NUTRIENT	UNIT	AMOUNT	INQ	% STD
ENERGY	KCAL	840.00	1.00	42
VITAMIN A	IU	0.00	0.00	0
VITAMIN C	MG	0.00	0.00	0
THIAMIN	MG	0.46	1.10	46
RIBOFLAVN	MG	0.19	0.38	16
NIACIN	MG	24.80	4.22	177
IRON	MG	3.00	0.45	19
CALCIUM	MG	107.00	0.28	12
PHOSPHRUS	MG	577.00	1.53	64
POTASSIUM	MG	971.00	0.46	19
PROTEIN	G	37.00	1.76	74
CARBOHYDT	G	27.00	0.23	10
FAT	G	72.00	2.20	92
OLEIC A	G	33.00	3.21	135
LINOL A	G	20.70	2.46	104
SAT FAT A	G	13.70	1.14	48

524 PEANUT BUTTER
ANALYSIS OF 16 GRAMS WHICH IS 1 TBSP

NUTRIENT	UNIT	AMOUNT	INQ	% STD
ENERGY	KCAL	95.00	1.00	5
VITAMIN A	IU	0.00	0.00	0
VITAMIN C	MG	0.00	0.00	0
THIAMIN	MG	0.02	0.42	2
RIBOFLAVN	MG	0.02	0.35	2
NIACIN	MG	2.40	3.61	17
IRON	MG	0.30	0.39	2
CALCIUM	MG	9.00	0.21	1
PHOSPHRUS	MG	61.00	1.43	7
POTASSIUM	MG	100.00	0.42	2
PROTEIN	G	4.00	1.68	8
CARBOHYDT	G	3.00	0.23	1
FAT	G	8.00	2.16	10
OLEIC A	G	3.70	3.18	15
LINOL A	G	2.30	2.42	12
SAT FAT A	G	1.50	1.11	5

525 SPLIT PEAS, DRY,COOKED
ANALYSIS OF 200 GRAMS WHICH IS 1 CUP

NUTRIENT	UNIT	AMOUNT	INQ	% STD	0 10 20 30 40 50 60 70 80 90 100
ENERGY	KCAL	230.00	1.00	12	EEEEEEE
VITAMIN A	IU	80.00	0.17	2	AA
VITAMIN C	MG	0.00	0.00	0	-
THIAMIN	MG	0.30	2.61	30	TTTTTTTTTTTTTTTTTTTTTTTTTTTT
RIBOFLAVN	MG	0.18	1.30	15	RRRRRRRIRRR
NIACIN	MG	1.80	1.12	13	NNNNNNNIN
IRON	MG	3.40	1.85	21	IIIIIIIIIIIIIIIIIIIII
CALCIUM	MG	22.00	0.21	2	KK
PHOSPHRUS	MG	178.00	1.72	20	XXXXXXXXIXXXXXXX
POTASSIUM	MG	592.00	1.03	12	YYYYYYY
PROTEIN	G	16.00	2.78	32	PPPPPPPIPPPPPPPPPPPPPP
CARBOHYDT	G	42.00	1.33	15	HHHHHHHIHHH
FAT	G	1.00	0.11	1	F
OLEIC A	G	0.00	0.00	0	-
LINOL A	G	0.00	0.00	0	-
SAT FAT A	G	0.00	0.00	0	-

526 PECANS, CHOPPED OR PIECES
ANALYSIS OF 118 GRAMS WHICH IS 1 CUP (120 LARGE HALVES)

NUTRIENT	UNIT	AMOUNT	INQ	% STD	0 10 20 30 40 50 60 70 80 90 100
ENERGY	KCAL	810.00	1.00	41	EEEEEEEEEEEEEEEEEEEEEEEEEEEEEEEEEEEEEEEEE
VITAMIN A	IU	150.00	0.09	4	AAA
VITAMIN C	MG	2.00	0.08	3	CCC
THIAMIN	MG	1.01	2.49	101	TTTTTTTTTTTTTTTTTTTTTTTTTTTTTTTTTTTTTTTTTTTTTTTTTTTTTTTTTTTTTTTTTTTTTTTTTTTTTTTTTTTTTTTTTTTTTTTTTTTTTTTTTTTTTTTTTTTTTTTTTT * 101
RIBOFLAVN	MG	0.15	0.31	13	RRRRRRRRR
NIACIN	MG	1.10	0.19	8	NNNNN
IRON	MG	2.80	0.43	18	IIIIIIIIIIIIIIIII
CALCIUM	MG	86.00	0.24	10	KKKKKKK
PHOSPHRUS	MG	341.00	0.94	38	XXXXXXXXXXXXXXXXXXXXXXXXXXXXXXXXXXXXXX
POTASSIUM	MG	712.00	0.35	14	YYYYYYYYYY
PROTEIN	G	11.00	0.54	22	PPPPPPPPPPPPPPPPPPPPP
CARBOHYDT	G	17.00	0.15	6	HHHHH
FAT	G	84.00	2.66	108	FFFFFFFFFFFFFFFFFFFFFFFFFFFFFFFFFFFFFFFFFFFFFFFFFFFFFFFFFFFFFFFFFFFFFFFFFFFFFFFFFFFFFFFFFFFFFFFFFFFFFFFFFFFFFFFFFFFFFFF * 108
OLEIC A	G	50.50	5.09	206	OOOOOOOOOOOOOOOOOOOOOOOOOOOOOOOOOOOOOOOOOOOOOOOOOOOOOOOOOOOOOOOOOOOOOOOOOOOOOOOOOOOOOOOOOOOOOOOOOOOOOOOOOOOOOOOOOOOOOOOOOO * 206
LINOL A	G	20.00	2.47	100	LLLLLLLLLLLLLLLLLLLLLLLLLLLLLLLLLLLLLLLLLLLLLLLLLLLLLLLLLLLLLLLLLLLLLLLLLLLLLLLLLLLLLLLLLLLLLLLLLLLLLLLLLLLLLLLLLLLLLLL
SAT FAT A	G	7.20	0.62	25	SSSSSSSSSSSSSSSSSSSSSSSSS

527 PUMPKIN AND SQUASH SEEDS, DRY, HULLED
ANALYSIS OF 140 GRAMS WHICH IS 1 CUP

NUTRIENT	UNIT	AMOUNT	INQ	% STD
ENERGY	KCAL	775.00	1.00	39
VITAMIN A	IU	100.00	0.06	3
VITAMIN C	MG	0.00	0.00	0
THIAMIN	MG	0.34	0.88	34
RIBOFLAVN	MG	0.27	0.58	23
NIACIN	MG	3.40	0.63	24
IRON	MG	15.70	2.53	98
CALCIUM	MG	71.00	0.20	8
PHOSPHRUS	MG	1602.00	4.59	178
POTASSIUM	MG	1386.00	0.72	28
PROTEIN	G	41.00	2.12	82
CARBOHYDT	G	21.00	0.20	8
FAT	G	65.00	2.15	83
OLEIC A	G	23.50	2.48	96
LINOL A	G	27.50	3.55	138
SAT FAT A	G	11.80	1.07	41

528 SUNFLOWER SEEDS, DRY, HULLED
ANALYSIS OF 145 GRAMS WHICH IS 1 CUP

NUTRIENT	UNIT	AMOUNT	INQ	% STD
ENERGY	KCAL	810.00	1.00	41
VITAMIN A	IU	70.00	0.04	2
VITAMIN C	MG	0.00	0.00	0
THIAMIN	MG	2.84	7.01	284
RIBOFLAVN	MG	0.33	0.68	28
NIACIN	MG	7.80	1.38	56
IRON	MG	10.50	1.59	64
CALCIUM	MG	174.00	0.48	19
PHOSPHRUS	MG	1214.00	3.33	135
POTASSIUM	MG	1334.00	0.66	27
PROTEIN	G	35.00	1.73	70
CARBOHYDT	G	29.00	0.26	11
FAT	G	69.00	2.18	88
OLEIC A	G	13.70	1.38	56
LINOL A	G	43.20	5.33	216
SAT FAT A	G	8.20	0.71	29

```
529  BLACK WALNUTS, CHOPPED
ANALYSIS OF 125 GRAMS WHICH IS 1 CUP

NUTRIENT   UNIT   AMOUNT   INQ    % STD   0        10        20        30        40        50        60        70        80        90        100
ENERGY     KCAL   785.06   1.00     39    EEEEEEEEEEEEEEEEEEEEEEEEEEE                                                                          *
VITAMIN A  IU     380.00   0.24     10    AAAAAAA                                                                                             *
VITAMIN C  MG       0.00   0.00      0    -                                                                                                   *
THIAMIN    MG       0.28   0.71     28    TTTTTTTTTTTTTTTTTTTTT                                                                               *
RIBOFLAVN  MG       0.14   0.30     12    RRRRRRRR                                                                                            *
NIACIN     MG       0.90   0.16      6    NNNNN                                                                                               *
IRON       MG       7.50   1.19     47    IIIIIIIIIIIIIIIIIIIIIIIIIIIIIIIIIII                                                                 *
CALCIUM    MG       0.00   0.00      0    -                                                                                                   *
PHOSPHRUS  MG     713.00   2.02     79    XXXXXXXXXXXXXXXXXXXXXXXXXXXXXXXXXXXXXXXXXXXXXXXXXXXXXXXXXXXXX                                       *
POTASSIUM  MG     575.00   0.29     12    YYYYYYYY                                                                                            *
PROTEIN    G      26.00    1.32     52    PPPPPPPPPPPPPPPPPPPPPPPPPPPPPPPPPPPPPPPP                                                            *
CARBOHYDT  G      19.00    0.18      7    HHHHH                                                                                               *
FAT        G      74.00    2.42     95    FFFFFFFFFFFFFFFFFFFFFFFFFFFFFFFFFFFFFFFFFFFFFFFFFFFFFFFFFFFFFFFFFFFFFFFFFF                          *
OLEIC A    G      13.30    1.38     54    OOOOOOOOOOOOOOOOOOOOOOOOOOOOOOOOOOOOOOOOOO                                                          *
LINOL A    G      45.70    5.82    229    LLLLLLLLLLLLLLLLLLLLLLLLLLLLLLLLLLLLLLLLLLLLLLLLLLLLLLLLLLLLLLLLLLLLLLLLLLLLLLLLLLLLLLLLLLLLLL   *229
SAT FAT A  G       6.30    0.56     22    SSSSSSSSSSSSSSSSS                                                                                   *
*********************************************************************************************************************
```

```
530  BLACK WALNUTS, GROUND
ANALYSIS OF 80 GRAMS WHICH IS 1 CUP

NUTRIENT   UNIT   AMOUNT   INQ    % STD   0        10        20        30        40        50        60        70        80        90        100
ENERGY     KCAL   500.00   1.00     25    EEEEEEEEEEEEEEEEEE                                                                                  *
VITAMIN A  IU     240.00   0.24      6    AAAAA                                                                                               *
VITAMIN C  MG       0.00   0.00      0    -                                                                                                   *
THIAMIN    MG       0.18   0.72     18    TTTTTTTTTTTTT                                                                                       *
RIBOFLAVN  MG       0.09   0.30      8    RRRRR                                                                                               *
NIACIN     MG       0.60   0.17      4    NNN                                                                                                 *
IRON       MG       4.80   1.20     30    IIIIIIIIIIIIIIIIIIIIII                                                                              *
CALCIUM    MG       0.00   0.00      0    -                                                                                                   *
PHOSPHRUS  MG     456.00   2.03     51    XXXXXXXXXXXXXXXXXXXXXXXXXXXXXXXXXXXXXXX                                                             *
POTASSIUM  MG     368.00   0.29      7    YYYYY                                                                                               *
PROTEIN    G      16.00    1.28     32    PPPPPPPPPPPPPPPPPPPPPPPP                                                                            *
CARBOHYDT  G      12.00    0.17      4    HHH                                                                                                 *
FAT        G      47.00    2.41     60    FFFFFFFFFFFFFFFFFFFFFFFFFFFFFFFFFFFFFFFFFFFFFF                                                      *
OLEIC A    G       8.50    1.39     35    OOOOOOOOOOOOOOOOOOOOOOOOOO                                                                          *
LINOL A    G      29.20    5.84    146    LLLLLLLLLLLLLLLLLLLLLLLLLLLLLLLLLLLLLLLLLLLLLLLLLLLLLLLLLLLLLLLLLLLLLLLLLLLLLLLLLLLLLLLLLLLLLL   *146
SAT FAT A  G       4.00    0.56     14    SSSSSSSSSS                                                                                          *
*********************************************************************************************************************
```

531 PERSIAN OR ENGLISH WALNUTS, CHOPPED
ANALYSIS OF 120 GRAMS WHICH IS 1 CUP (60 HALVES)

```
NUTRIENT    UNIT   AMOUNT    INQ   % STD    0        10        20        30        40        50        60        70        80        90       100
ENERGY      KCAL   780.00   1.00    39      EEEEEEEEEEEEEEEEEEEEEEEEEEEEE                                                                        *
VITAMIN A   IU      40.00   0.03     1      A                                                                                                   *
VITAMIN C   MG       2.00   0.09     3      CCC                                                                                                 *
THIAMIN     MG       0.40   1.03    40      TTTTTTTTTTTTTTTTTTTTTTTTTTTTTTTTTTTTTTT|T                                                           *
RIBOFLAVN   MG       0.16   0.34    13      RRRRRRRRRRRR                                                                                        *
NIACIN      MG       1.10   0.20     8      NNNNN                                                                                               *
IRON        MG       3.70   0.59    23      IIIIIIIIIIIIIIIIIIII                                                                                *
CALCIUM     MG     119.00   0.34    13      KKKKKKKKKK                                                                                          *
PHOSPHRUS   MG     456.00   1.30    51      XXXXXXXXXXXXXXXXXXXXXXXXXXXXXX|XXXXXXXXXX                                                            *
POTASSIUM   MG     540.00   0.28    11      PPPPPPPPPP                                                                                          *
PROTEIN     G       18.00   0.92    36      YYYYYYYY                                                                                            *
CARBOHYDT   G       19.00   0.18     7      HHHHHH                                                                                              *
FAT         G       77.00   2.53    99      FFFFFFFFFFFFFFFFFFFFFFFFFFFFFFFFFFFFFFFF|FFFFFFFFFFFFFFFFFFFFFFFFFFFFFFFFFFFFFFFFFFFFFFFFFFFFFFF*
OLEIC A     G       11.80   1.23    48      OOOOOOOOOOOOOOOOOOOOOOOOOOOOOOOOOOOOOOO|OOOOOOO                                                      *
LINOL A     G       42.20   5.41   211      LLLLLLLLLLLLLLLLLLLLLLLLLLLLLLLLLLLLLLLL|LLLLLLLLLLLLLLLLLLLLLLLLLLLLLLLLLLLLLLLLLLLLLLLLLLLLLLL* 211
SAT FAT A   G        8.40   0.76    29      SSSSSSSSSSSSSSSSSSSSSSSSSSS
```
****

532 BOILED WHITE ICING, PLAIN
ANALYSIS OF 94 GRAMS WHICH IS 1 CUP

```
NUTRIENT    UNIT   AMOUNT    INQ   % STD    0        10        20        30        40        50        60        70        80        90       100
ENERGY      KCAL   295.00   1.00    15      EEEEEEEEEE                                                                                          *
VITAMIN A   IU       0.00   0.00     0      |                                                                                                  *
VITAMIN C   MG       0.00   0.00     0      |                                                                                                  *
THIAMIN     MG       0.00   0.00     0      |                                                                                                  *
RIBOFLAVN   MG       0.03   0.17     3      RR                                                                                                  *
NIACIN      MG       0.00   0.00     0      |                                                                                                  *
IRON        MG       0.00   0.00     0      |                                                                                                  *
CALCIUM     MG       2.00   0.02     0      |                                                                                                  *
PHOSPHRUS   MG       2.00   0.02     0      |                                                                                                  *
POTASSIUM   MG      17.00   0.02     0      |                                                                                                  *
PROTEIN     G        1.00   0.14     2      PP                                                                                                  *
CARBOHYDT   G       75.00   1.85    27      HHHHHHHHHHHHH|HHHHHHHHHHHH                                                                           *
FAT         G        0.00   0.00     0      |                                                                                                  *
OLEIC A     G        0.00   0.00     0      |                                                                                                  *
LINOL A     G        0.00   0.00     0      |                                                                                                  *
SAT FAT A   G        0.00   0.00     0      |
```
****

533 BOILED WHITE ICING WITH COCONUT
ANALYSIS OF 166 GRAMS WHICH IS 1 CUP

NUTRIENT	UNIT	AMOUNT	INQ	% STD
ENERGY	KCAL	605.00	1.00	30
VITAMIN A	IU	0.00	0.00	0
VITAMIN C	MG	0.00	0.00	0
THIAMIN	MG	0.02	0.07	2
RIBOFLAVN	MG	0.07	0.19	6
NIACIN	MG	0.30	0.07	2
IRON	MG	0.80	0.17	5
CALCIUM	MG	10.00	0.04	1
PHOSPHRUS	MG	50.00	0.18	6
POTASSIUM	MG	277.00	0.18	6
PROTEIN	G	3.00	0.20	6
CARBOHYDT	G	124.00	1.49	45
FAT	G	13.00	0.55	17
OLEIC A	G	0.90	0.12	4
LINOL A	G	0.00	0.00	0
SAT FAT A	G	11.00	1.28	39

534 UNCOOKED CHOCOLATE ICING (MADE WITH MILK AND BUTTER)
ANALYSIS OF 275 GRAMS WHICH IS 1 CUP

NUTRIENT	UNIT	AMOUNT	INQ	% STD
ENERGY	KCAL	1035.00	1.00	52
VITAMIN A	IU	580.00	0.28	15
VITAMIN C	MG	1.00	0.03	2
THIAMIN	MG	0.06	0.12	6
RIBOFLAVN	MG	0.28	0.45	23
NIACIN	MG	0.60	0.08	4
IRON	MG	3.30	0.40	21
CALCIUM	MG	165.00	0.35	18
PHOSPHRUS	MG	305.00	0.65	34
POTASSIUM	MG	536.00	0.21	11
PROTEIN	G	9.00	0.35	18
CARBOHYDT	G	185.00	1.30	67
FAT	G	38.00	0.94	48
OLEIC A	G	11.70	0.92	5
LINOL A	G	1.00	0.10	5
SAT FAT A	G	23.40	1.59	82

535 UNCOOKED CREAMY FUDGE FROM A MIX
ANALYSIS OF 245 GRAMS WHICH IS 1 CUP

NUTRIENT	UNIT	AMOUNT	INQ	% STD
ENERGY	KCAL	830.00	1.00	42
VITAMIN A	IU	0.00	0.00	0
VITAMIN C	MG	0.00	0.00	0
THIAMIN	MG	0.05	0.12	5
RIBOFLAVN	MG	0.20	0.40	17
NIACIN	MG	0.70	0.12	5
IRON	MG	2.70	0.41	17
CALCIUM	MG	96.00	0.26	11
PHOSPHRUS	MG	218.00	0.58	24
POTASSIUM	MG	236.00	0.11	5
PROTEIN	G	7.00	0.34	14
CARBOHYDT	G	183.00	1.60	67
FAT	G	16.00	0.49	21
OLEIC A	G	6.70	0.66	27
LINOL A	G	3.10	0.37	16
SAT FAT A	G	5.10	0.43	18

536 UNCOOKED WHITE ICING
ANALYSIS OF 319 GRAMS WHICH IS 1 CUP

NUTRIENT	UNIT	AMOUNT	INQ	% STD
ENERGY	KCAL	1200.00	1.00	60
VITAMIN A	IU	860.00	0.36	22
VITAMIN C	MG	0.00	0.00	0
THIAMIN	MG	0.00	0.00	0
RIBOFLAVN	MG	0.06	0.08	5
NIACIN	MG	0.00	0.00	0
IRON	MG	0.00	0.00	0
CALCIUM	MG	48.00	0.09	5
PHOSPHRUS	MG	38.00	0.07	4
POTASSIUM	MG	57.00	0.02	1
PROTEIN	G	2.00	0.07	4
CARBOHYDT	G	260.00	1.58	95
FAT	G	21.00	0.45	27
OLEIC A	G	5.10	0.35	21
LINOL A	G	0.50	0.04	3
SAT FAT A	G	12.70	0.74	45

537 CARMELS, PLAIN OR CHOCOLATE
ANALYSIS OF 28 GRAMS WHICH IS 1 OZ.

NUTRIENT	UNIT	AMOUNT	INQ	% STD	0 10 20 ... 100
ENERGY	KCAL	115.00	1.00	6	EEEEE
VITAMIN A	IU	0.00	0.00	0	-
VITAMIN C	MG	0.00	0.00	0	-
THIAMIN	MG	0.01	0.17	1	T
RIBOFLAVN	MG	0.05	0.72	4	RRR
NIACIN	MG	0.10	0.12	1	N
IRON	MG	0.40	0.43	3	II
CALCIUM	MG	42.00	0.81	5	KKKK
PHOSPHRUS	MG	35.00	0.68	4	XXX
POTASSIUM	MG	54.00	0.19	1	Y
PROTEIN	G	1.00	0.35	2	PP
CARBOHYDT	G	22.00	1.39	8	HHHHH
FAT	G	3.00	0.67	4	FFF
OLEIC A	G	1.10	0.78	4	OOOO
LINOL A	G	0.10	0.09	1	-
SAT FAT A	G	1.60	0.98	6	SSSS

538 MILK CHOCOLATE, PLAIN
ANALYSIS OF 28 GRAMS WHICH IS 1 OZ.

NUTRIENT	UNIT	AMOUNT	INQ	% STD	0 10 20 ... 100
ENERGY	KCAL	145.00	1.00	7	EEEEE
VITAMIN A	IU	80.00	0.28	2	AA
VITAMIN C	MG	0.00	0.00	0	-
THIAMIN	MG	0.02	0.28	2	TT
RIBOFLAVN	MG	0.10	1.15	8	RRRRR
NIACIN	MG	0.10	0.10	1	N
IRON	MG	0.30	0.26	2	II
CALCIUM	MG	65.00	1.00	7	KKKKK
PHOSPHRUS	MG	65.00	1.00	7	XXXXX
POTASSIUM	MG	109.00	0.30	2	YY
PROTEIN	G	2.00	0.55	4	PPP
CARBOHYDT	G	16.00	0.80	6	HHHHH
FAT	G	9.00	1.59	12	FFFFFIFFF
OLEIC A	G	3.00	1.69	12	OOOOOIOOOO
LINOL A	G	0.30	0.21	2	L
SAT FAT A	G	5.50	2.66	19	SSSSSISSSSSSSSSS

539 SEMISWEET CHOCOLATE SMALL PIECES
ANALYSIS OF 170 GRAMS WHICH IS 1 CUP (6 OZ PKG.)

```
                                    0      10      20      30      40      50      60      70      80      90     100
NUTRIENT   UNIT   AMOUNT    INQ  % STD
ENERGY     KCAL   860.00   1.00   43    EEEEEEEEEEEEEEEEEEEEEEEE                                                   *
VITAMIN A  IU      30.00   0.02    1    A                                                                         *
VITAMIN C  MG       0.00   0.00    0    -                                                                         *
THIAMIN    MG       0.02   0.05    2    TT                                                                        *
RIBOFLAVN  MG       0.14   0.27   12    RRRRRRRR                                                                  *
NIACIN     MG       0.90   0.15    6    NNNNN                                                                     *
IRON       MG       4.40   0.64   28    IIIIIIIIIIIIIIIIIIIII                                                     *
CALCIUM    MG      51.00   0.13    6    KKKKK                                                                     *
PHOSPHRUS  MG     255.00   0.66   28    XXXXXXXXXXXXXXXXXXXXXX                                                    *
POTASSIUM  MG     553.00   0.26   11    YYYYYYYY                                                                  *
PROTEIN    G        7.00   0.33   14    PPPPPPPPPP                                                                *
CARBOHYDT  G       97.00   0.82   35    HHHHHHHHHHHHHHHHHHHHHHHHHHH                                               *
FAT        G       61.00   1.82   78    FFFFFFFFFFFFFFFFFFFFFFFFFFFFFFFFFFFFFFFFFFFFFFFFFFFFFFFFFFFF               *
OLEIC A    G       19.80   1.88   81    OOOOOOOOOOOOOOOOOOOOOOOOOOOOOOOOOOOOOOOOOOOOOOOOOOOOOOOOOOOOOO             *
LINOL A    G        1.70   0.20    9    LLLLLL                                                                    *
SAT FAT A  G       36.20   2.95  127    SSSSSSSSSSSSSSSSSSSSSSSSSSSSSSSSSSSSSSSSSSSSSSSSSSSSSSSSSSSSSSSSSSSSS *127
********************************************
```

540 CHOCOLATE COATED PEANUTS
ANALYSIS OF 28 GRAMS WHICH IS 1 OZ

```
                                    0      10      20      30      40      50      60      70      80      90     100
NUTRIENT   UNIT   AMOUNT    INQ  % STD
ENERGY     KCAL   160.00   1.00    8    EEEEE                                                                     *
VITAMIN A  IU       0.00   0.00    0    -                                                                         *
VITAMIN C  MG       0.00   0.00    0    -                                                                         *
THIAMIN    MG       0.10   1.25   10    TTTTTTT                                                                   *
RIBOFLAVN  MG       0.05   0.52    4    RRR                                                                       *
NIACIN     MG       2.10   1.88   15    NNNNNINNNNN                                                               *
IRON       MG       0.40   0.31    3    II                                                                        *
CALCIUM    MG      33.00   0.46    4    KKK                                                                       *
PHOSPHRUS  MG      84.00   1.17    9    XXXXXIX                                                                   *
POTASSIUM  MG     143.00   0.36    3    YY                                                                        *
PROTEIN    G        5.00   1.25   10    PPPPPIPP                                                                  *
CARBOHYDT  G       11.00   0.50    4    HHH                                                                       *
FAT        G       12.00   1.92   15    FFFFPIFFFFFF                                                              *
OLEIC A    G        4.70   2.40   19    OOOOIOOOOOOOOO                                                            *
LINOL A    G        2.10   1.31   11    LLLLILL                                                                   *
SAT FAT A  G        4.00   1.75   14    SSSSSISSSS                                                                *
********************************************
```

541 FONDANT, UNCOATED (MINTS, CANDY CORN ETC)
ANALYSIS OF 28 GRAMS WHICH IS 1 OZ.

NUTRIENT	UNIT	AMOUNT	INQ	% STD	0	10	20	30	40	50	60	70	80	90	100
ENERGY	KCAL	105.00	1.00	5	EEEE										
VITAMIN A	IU	0.00	0.00	0	-										
VITAMIN C	MG	0.00	0.00	0	-										
THIAMIN	MG	0.00	0.00	0	-										
RIBOFLAVN	MG	0.00	0.00	0	-										
NIACIN	MG	0.00	0.00	0	-										
IRON	MG	0.30	0.36	2	II										
CALCIUM	MG	4.00	0.08	0	-										
PHOSPHRUS	MG	2.00	0.04	0	-										
POTASSIUM	MG	1.00	0.00	0	-										
PROTEIN	G	0.00	0.00	0	-										
CARBOHYDT	G	25.00	1.73	9	HHH|HHH										
FAT	G	1.00	0.24	1	F										
OLEIC A	G	0.30	0.23	1	O										
LINOL A	G	0.10	0.10	1	-										
SAT FAT A	G	0.10	0.07	0	-										

****

542 FUDGE,PLAIN, CHOCOLATE
ANALYSIS OF 28 GRAMS WHICH IS 1 OZ.

NUTRIENT	UNIT	AMOUNT	INQ	% STD	0	10	20	30	40	50	60	70	80	90	100
ENERGY	KCAL	115.00	1.00	6	EEEEE										
VITAMIN A	IU	0.00	0.00	0	-										
VITAMIN C	MG	0.00	0.00	0	-										
THIAMIN	MG	0.01	0.17	1	T										
RIBOFLAVN	MG	0.03	0.43	3	RR										
NIACIN	MG	0.10	0.12	1	N										
IRON	MG	0.30	0.33	2	II										
CALCIUM	MG	22.00	0.43	2	KK										
PHOSPHRUS	MG	24.00	0.46	3	XX										
POTASSIUM	MG	42.00	0.15	1	Y										
PROTEIN	G	1.00	0.35	2	PP										
CARBOHYDT	G	21.00	1.33	8	HHHH|H										
FAT	G	3.00	0.67	4	FFF|										
OLEIC A	G	1.40	0.99	6	OOOOO										
LINOL A	G	0.60	0.52	3	LL										
SAT FAT A	G	1.30	0.79	5	SSSS|										

****

543 GUM DROPS
ANALYSIS OF 28 GRAMS WHICH IS 1 OZ.

NUTRIENT	UNIT	AMOUNT	INQ	% STD	0	10	20	30	40	50	60	70	80	90	100
ENERGY	KCAL	100.00	1.00	5	EEEE										
VITAMIN A	IU	0.00	0.00	0	-										
VITAMIN C	MG	0.00	0.00	0	-										
THIAMIN	MG	0.00	0.00	0	-										
RIBOFLAVN	MG	0.00	0.00	0	-										
NIACIN	MG	0.00	0.00	0	-										
IRON	MG	0.10	0.13	1	I										
CALCIUM	MG	2.00	0.04	0	-										
PHOSPHRUS	MG	0.00	0.00	0	-										
POTASSIUM	MG	1.00	0.00	0	-										
PROTEIN	G	0.00	0.00	0	-										
CARBOHYDT	G	25.00	1.82	9	HHHIHHHH										
FAT	G	0.00	0.00	0	-										
OLEIC A	G	0.00	0.00	0	-										
LINOL A	G	0.00	0.00	0	-										
SAT FAT A	G	0.00	0.00	0	-										

544 HARD CANDY
ANALYSIS OF 28 GRAMS WHICH IS 1 OZ.

NUTRIENT	UNIT	AMOUNT	INQ	% STD	0	10	20	30	40	50	60	70	80	90	100
ENERGY	KCAL	110.00	1.00	6	EEEE										
VITAMIN A	IU	0.00	0.00	0	-										
VITAMIN C	MG	0.00	0.00	0	-										
THIAMIN	MG	0.00	0.00	0	-										
RIBOFLAVN	MG	0.00	0.00	0	-										
NIACIN	MG	0.00	0.00	0	-										
IRON	MG	0.50	0.57	3	III										
CALCIUM	MG	6.00	0.12	1	K										
PHOSPHRUS	MG	2.00	0.04	0	-										
POTASSIUM	MG	1.00	0.00	0	-										
PROTEIN	G	0.00	0.00	0	-										
CARBOHYDT	G	28.00	1.85	10	HHHIHHHH										
FAT	G	0.00	0.00	0	-										
OLEIC A	G	0.00	0.00	0	-										
LINOL A	G	0.00	0.00	0	-										
SAT FAT A	G	0.00	0.00	0	-										

```
                                    0    10    20    30    40    50    60    70    80    90   100
                                    *********************************************************
```

545 MARSHMALLOWS
ANALYSIS OF 28 GRAMS WHICH IS 1 OZ.

NUTRIENT	UNIT	AMOUNT	INQ	% STD	0
ENERGY	KCAL	90.00	1.00	5	EEEE
VITAMIN A	IU	0.00	0.00	0	-
VITAMIN C	MG	0.00	0.00	0	-
THIAMIN	MG	0.00	0.00	0	-
RIBOFLAVN	MG	0.00	0.00	0	-
NIACIN	MG	0.00	0.00	0	III
IRON	MG	0.50	0.69	3	III
CALCIUM	MG	5.00	0.12	1	-
PHOSPHRUS	MG	2.00	0.05	0	-
POTASSIUM	MG	2.00	0.01	0	-
PROTEIN	G	1.00	0.44	2	PP
CARBOHYDT	G	23.00	1.86	8	HHHIHHH
FAT	G	0.00	0.00	0	-
OLEIC A	G	0.00	0.00	0	-
LINOL A	G	0.00	0.00	0	-
SAT FAT A	G	0.00	0.00	0	-

```
*************************************************************
```

546 CHOCOLATE FLAVORED BEVERAGE POWDER WITH NONFAT DRY MILK
ANALYSIS OF 28 GRAMS WHICH IS 1 OZ (4 HEAPING TSP)

NUTRIENT	UNIT	AMOUNT	INQ	% STD	0
ENERGY	KCAL	100.00	1.00	5	EEEE
VITAMIN A	IU	10.00	0.05	0	-
VITAMIN C	MG	1.00	0.33	2	C
THIAMIN	MG	0.04	0.80	4	TTTI
RIBOFLAVN	MG	0.21	3.50	17	RRRIRRRRRRRR
NIACIN	MG	0.20	0.29	1	N
IRON	MG	0.50	0.63	3	III
CALCIUM	MG	167.00	3.71	19	KKKIKKKKKKKKKK
PHOSPHRUS	MG	155.00	3.44	17	XXXIXXXXXXXXX
POTASSIUM	MG	227.00	0.91	5	YYYY
PROTEIN	G	5.00	2.00	10	PPPIPPPP
CARBOHYDT	G	20.00	1.45	7	HHHIHH
FAT	G	1.00	0.26	1	F
OLEIC A	G	0.30	0.24	1	O
LINOL A	G	0.00	0.00	0	-
SAT FAT A	G	0.50	0.35	2	S

```
*************************************************************
```

547   CHOCOLATE FLAVORED BEVERAGE POWDER WITHOUT MILK
ANALYSIS OF 28 GRAMS WHICH IS 1 OZ. (4 HEAPING TSP)

NUTRIENT	UNIT	AMOUNT	INQ	% STD	0 10 20 30 40 50 60 70 80 90 100
ENERGY	KCAL	100.00	1.00	5	EEEE
VITAMIN A	IU	0.00	0.00	0	-
VITAMIN C	MG	0.00	0.00	0	-
THIAMIN	MG	0.01	0.20	1	T
RIBOFLAVN	MG	0.03	0.50	3	RR
NIACIN	MG	0.10	0.14	1	N
IRON	MG	0.60	0.75	4	III
CALCIUM	MG	9.00	0.20	1	K
PHOSPHRUS	MG	48.00	1.07	5	XXXX
POTASSIUM	MG	142.00	0.57	3	YY
PROTEIN	G	1.00	0.40	2	PP
CARBOHYDT	G	25.00	1.82	9	HHHIHHH
FAT	G	1.00	0.26	1	F
OLEIC A	G	0.20	0.16	1	O
LINOL A	G	0.00	0.00	0	-
SAT FAT A	G	0.40	0.28	1	S

548   HONEY
ANALYSIS OF 21 GRAMS WHICH IS 1 TBSP

NUTRIENT	UNIT	AMOUNT	INQ	% STD	0 10 20 30 40 50 60 70 80 90 100
ENERGY	KCAL	65.00	1.00	3	EEE
VITAMIN A	IU	0.00	0.00	0	-
VITAMIN C	MG	0.00	0.00	0	-
THIAMIN	MG	0.00	0.00	0	-
RIBOFLAVN	MG	0.01	0.26	1	R
NIACIN	MG	0.10	0.22	1	N
IRON	MG	0.10	0.19	1	I
CALCIUM	MG	1.00	0.03	0	-
PHOSPHRUS	MG	1.00	0.03	0	-
POTASSIUM	MG	11.00	0.07	0	-
PROTEIN	G	0.00	0.00	0	-
CARBOHYDT	G	17.00	1.90	6	HHHIHH
FAT	G	0.00	0.00	0	-
OLEIC A	G	0.00	0.00	0	-
LINOL A	G	0.00	0.00	0	-
SAT FAT A	G	0.00	0.00	0	-

549 JAMS AND PRESERVES
ANALYSIS OF 20 GRAMS WHICH IS 1 TBSP

NUTRIENT	UNIT	AMOUNT	INQ	% STD
ENERGY	KCAL	55.00	1.00	3
VITAMIN A	IU	0.00	0.00	0
VITAMIN C	MG	0.00	0.00	0
THIAMIN	MG	0.00	0.00	0
RIBOFLAVN	MG	0.01	0.30	1
NIACIN	MG	0.00	0.45	0
IRON	MG	0.20	0.45	1
CALCIUM	MG	4.00	0.16	0
PHOSPHRUS	MG	2.00	0.08	0
POTASSIUM	MG	18.00	0.13	0
PROTEIN	G	0.00	0.00	0
CARBOHYDT	G	14.00	1.85	5
FAT	G	0.00	0.00	0
OLEIC A	G	0.00	0.00	0
LINOL A	G	0.00	0.00	0
SAT FAT A	G	0.00	0.00	0

550 JAMS AND PRESERVES
ANALYSIS OF 14 GRAMS WHICH IS 1 PACKET

NUTRIENT	UNIT	AMOUNT	INQ	% STD
ENERGY	KCAL	40.00	1.00	2
VITAMIN A	IU	0.00	0.00	0
VITAMIN C	MG	0.00	0.00	0
THIAMIN	MG	0.00	0.00	0
RIBOFLAVN	MG	0.00	0.00	0
NIACIN	MG	0.00	0.31	0
IRON	MG	0.10	0.17	1
CALCIUM	MG	3.00	0.06	0
PHOSPHRUS	MG	1.00	0.12	0
POTASSIUM	MG	12.00	0.00	0
PROTEIN	G	0.00	0.00	0
CARBOHYDT	G	10.00	1.82	4
FAT	G	0.00	0.00	0
OLEIC A	G	0.00	0.00	0
LINOL A	G	0.00	0.00	0
SAT FAT A	G	0.00	0.00	0

551 JELLIES
ANALYSIS OF 18 GRAMS WHICH IS 1 TBSP

NUTRIENT	UNIT	AMOUNT	INQ	% STD	0
ENERGY	KCAL	50.00	1.00	3	EE
VITAMIN A	IU	0.00	0.00	0	I
VITAMIN C	MG	1.00	0.67	2	CI
THIAMIN	MG	0.00	0.00	0	I
RIBOFLAVN	MG	0.01	0.33	1	RI
NIACIN	MG	0.00	0.00	0	I
IRON	MG	0.30	0.75	2	II
CALCIUM	MG	4.00	0.18	0	I
PHOSPHRUS	MG	1.00	0.04	0	I
POTASSIUM	MG	14.00	0.11	0	I
PROTEIN	G	0.00	0.00	0	I
CARBOHYDT	G	13.00	1.89	5	HIHH
FAT	G	0.00	0.00	0	I
OLEIC A	G	0.00	0.00	0	I
LINOL A	G	0.00	0.00	0	I
SAT FAT A	G	0.00	0.00	0	I

552 JELLIES
ANALYSIS OF 14 GRAMS WHICH IS 1 PACKET

NUTRIENT	UNIT	AMOUNT	INQ	% STD	0
ENERGY	KCAL	40.00	1.00	2	EE
VITAMIN A	IU	0.00	0.00	0	I
VITAMIN C	MG	1.00	0.83	2	CI
THIAMIN	MG	0.00	0.00	0	I
RIBOFLAVN	MG	0.00	0.00	0	I
NIACIN	MG	0.00	0.00	0	I
IRON	MG	0.20	0.63	1	II
CALCIUM	MG	3.00	0.17	0	I
PHOSPHRUS	MG	1.00	0.06	0	I
POTASSIUM	MG	11.00	0.11	0	I
PROTEIN	G	0.00	0.00	0	I
CARBOHYDT	G	10.00	1.82	4	HIH
FAT	G	0.00	0.00	0	I
OLEIC A	G	0.00	0.00	0	I
LINOL A	G	0.00	0.00	0	I
SAT FAT A	G	0.00	0.00	0	I

553 CHOCOLATE FLAVORED SYRUP, THIN TYPE
ANALYSIS OF 38 GRAMS WHICH IS 1 FL. OZ.OR 2 TBSP.

```
                                              10        20        30        40        50        60        70        80        90       100
NUTRIENT   UNIT   AMOUNT    INQ   % STD  0                                                                                                 *** ***** ******** ******
ENERGY     KCAL    90.00   1.00    5    EEEE
VITAMIN A  IU       0.00   0.00    0    -
VITAMIN C  MG       0.00   0.00    0    -
THIAMIN    MG       0.01   0.22    0    T
RIBOFLAVN  MG       0.03   0.56    3    RR
NIACIN     MG       0.20   0.32    1    N
IRON       MG       0.60   0.83    4    III
CALCIUM    MG       6.00   0.15    1    K
PHOSPHRUS  MG      35.00   0.86    4    XXX
POTASSIUM  MG     106.00   0.47    2    YY
PROTEIN    G        1.00   0.44    2    PP
CARBOHYDT  G       24.00   1.94    9    HHH|HHH
FAT        G        1.00   0.28    1    F
OLEIC A    G        0.30   0.27    1    O
LINOL A    G        0.00   0.00    0    -
SAT FAT A  G        0.50   0.39    2    S
***********************************************
```

554 CHOCOLATE FLAVORED TOPPING, FUDGE TYPE
ANALYSIS OF 38 GRAMS WHICH IS 1 FL OZ OR 2 TBSP

```
                                              10        20        30        40        50        60        70        80        90       100
NUTRIENT   UNIT   AMOUNT    INQ   % STD  0                                                                                                 *** ***** ********* *****
ENERGY     KCAL   125.00   1.00    6    EEEEE
VITAMIN A  IU      60.00   0.24    2    A
VITAMIN C  MG       0.00   0.00    0    -
THIAMIN    MG       0.02   0.32    2    TT
RIBOFLAVN  MG       0.08   1.07    7    RRRR
NIACIN     MG       0.20   0.23    1    N
IRON       MG       0.50   0.50    3    III
CALCIUM    MG      48.00   0.85    5    KKKK
PHOSPHRUS  MG      60.00   1.07    7    XXXXX
POTASSIUM  MG     107.00   0.34    2    YY
PROTEIN    G        2.00   0.64    4    PPP
CARBOHYDT  G       20.00   1.16    7    HHHH|H
FAT        G        5.00   1.03    6    FFFF
OLEIC A    G        1.60   1.04    7    OOOOO
LINOL A    G        0.10   0.08    1    -
SAT FAT A  G        3.10   1.74   11    SSSS|SSSS
***********************************************
```

555 MOLASSES, LIGHT CANE
ANALYSIS OF 20 GRAMS WHICH IS 1 TBSP.

NUTRIENT	UNIT	AMOUNT	INQ	% STD	0											
						10	20	30	40	50	60	70	80	90	100	
ENERGY	KCAL	50.00	1.00	3	EE											*
VITAMIN A	IU	0.00	0.00	0	-I											*
VITAMIN C	MG	0.00	0.00	0	-I											*
THIAMIN	MG	0.01	0.40	1	TI											*
RIBOFLAVN	MG	0.01	0.33	1	RI											*
NIACIN	MG	0.00	0.00	0	-I											*
IRON	MG	0.90	2.25	6	IIIII											*
CALCIUM	MG	33.00	1.47	4	KIK											*
PHOSPHRUS	MG	9.00	0.40	1	XI											*
POTASSIUM	MG	183.00	1.46	4	YIY											*
PROTEIN	G	0.00	0.00	0	-IY											*
CARBOHYDT	G	13.00	1.89	5	HIHH											*
FAT	G	0.00	0.00	0	-I											*
OLEIC A	G	0.00	0.00	0	-I											*
LINOL A	G	0.00	0.00	0	-I											*
SAT FAT A	G	0.00	0.00	0	-I											*

556 BLACKSTRAP MOLASSES
ANALYSIS OF 20 GRAMS WHICH IS 1 TBSP.

NUTRIENT	UNIT	AMOUNT	INQ	% STD	0											
						10	20	30	40	50	60	70	80	90	100	
ENERGY	KCAL	45.00	1.00	2	EE											*
VITAMIN A	IU	0.00	0.00	0	-I											*
VITAMIN C	MG	0.00	0.00	0	-I											*
THIAMIN	MG	0.02	0.89	2	TT											*
RIBOFLAVN	MG	0.04	1.48	3	RIR											*
NIACIN	MG	0.40	1.27	3	NN											*
IRON	MG	3.20	8.89	20	IIIIIIIIIIIII											*
CALCIUM	MG	137.00	6.77	15	KIKKKKKKKKK											*
PHOSPHRUS	MG	17.00	0.84	2	XX											*
POTASSIUM	MG	585.00	5.20	12	YIYYYYYY											*
PROTEIN	G	0.00	0.00	0	-I											*
CARBOHYDT	G	11.00	1.78	4	HIH											*
FAT	G	0.00	0.00	0	-I											*
OLEIC A	G	0.00	0.00	0	-I											*
LINOL A	G	0.00	0.00	0	-I											*
SAT FAT A	G	0.00	0.00	0	-I											*

557 SORGHUM
ANALYSIS OF 21 GRAMS WHICH IS 1 TBSP

```
                                    100        90        80        70        60        50        40        30        20        10
                                    * * * * * * * * * * * * * * * *
```

NUTRIENT	UNIT	AMOUNT	INQ	% STD	0	10
ENERGY	KCAL	55.00	1.00	3	EE	
VITAMIN A	IU	0.00	0.00	0	-I	
VITAMIN C	MG	0.00	0.00	0	-I	
THIAMIN	MG	0.03	1.09	3	TT	
RIBOFLAVN	MG	0.02	0.61	2	RI	
NIACIN	MG	0.00	0.00	0	RI	
IRON	MG	2.60	5.91	16	I IIIIIIIIIII	
CALCIUM	MG	35.00	1.41	4	K|K	
PHOSPHRUS	MG	5.00	0.20	1	-I	
POTASSIUM	MG	37.00	0.27	1	-Y	
PROTEIN	G	0.00	0.00	0	-I	
CARBOHYDT	G	14.00	1.85	5	HIHH	
FAT	G	0.00	0.00	0	-I	
OLEIC A	G	0.00	0.00	0	-I	
LINOL A	G	0.00	0.00	0	-I	
SAT FAT A	G	0.00	0.00	0	-I	

```
*******************************************
```

558 TABLE BLEND SYRUPS (CHIEFLY CORN) LIGHT AND DARK
ANALYSIS OF 21 GRAMS WHICH IS 1 TBSP

```
                                    100        90        80        70        60        50        40        30        20        10
                                    * * * * * * * * * * * * * * * *
```

NUTRIENT	UNIT	AMOUNT	INQ	% STD	0	10
ENERGY	KCAL	60.00	1.00	3	EE	
VITAMIN A	IU	0.00	0.00	0	-I	
VITAMIN C	MG	0.00	0.00	0	-I	
THIAMIN	MG	0.00	0.00	0	-I	
RIBOFLAVN	MG	0.00	0.00	0	-I	
NIACIN	MG	0.00	0.00	0	-I	
IRON	MG	0.80	1.67	5	I II	
CALCIUM	MG	9.00	0.33	1	-K	
PHOSPHRUS	MG	3.00	0.11	0	-I	
POTASSIUM	MG	1.00	0.01	0	-I	
PROTEIN	G	0.00	0.00	0	-I	
CARBOHYDT	G	15.00	1.82	5	HIHH	
FAT	G	0.00	0.00	0	-I	
OLEIC A	G	0.00	0.00	0	-I	
LINOL A	G	0.00	0.00	0	-I	
SAT FAT A	G	0.00	0.00	0	-I	

```
*******************************************
```

559 BROWN SUGAR
ANALYSIS OF 220 GRAMS WHICH IS 1 CUP, PRESSED DOWN

NUTRIENT	UNIT	AMOUNT	INQ	% STD
ENERGY	KCAL	820.00	1.00	41
VITAMIN A	IU	0.00	0.00	0
VITAMIN C	MG	0.00	0.00	0
THIAMIN	MG	0.02	0.05	2
RIBOFLAVN	MG	0.07	0.14	6
NIACIN	MG	0.40	0.07	3
IRON	MG	7.50	1.14	47
CALCIUM	MG	187.00	0.51	21
PHOSPHRUS	MG	42.00	0.11	5
POTASSIUM	MG	757.00	0.37	15
PROTEIN	G	0.00	0.00	0
CARBOHYDT	G	212.00	1.88	77
FAT	G	0.00	0.00	0
OLEIC A	G	0.00	0.00	0
LINOL A	G	0.00	0.00	0
SAT FAT A	G	0.00	0.00	0

560 WHITE SUGAR, GRANULATED
ANALYSIS OF 200 GRAMS WHICH IS 1 CUP

NUTRIENT	UNIT	AMOUNT	INQ	% STD
ENERGY	KCAL	770.00	1.00	39
VITAMIN A	IU	0.00	0.00	0
VITAMIN C	MG	0.00	0.00	0
THIAMIN	MG	0.00	0.00	0
RIBOFLAVN	MG	0.00	0.00	0
NIACIN	MG	0.00	0.00	0
IRON	MG	0.20	0.03	1
CALCIUM	MG	0.00	0.00	0
PHOSPHRUS	MG	0.00	0.00	0
POTASSIUM	MG	6.00	0.00	0
PROTEIN	G	0.00	0.00	0
CARBOHYDT	G	199.00	1.88	72
FAT	G	0.00	0.00	0
OLEIC A	G	0.00	0.00	0
LINOL A	G	0.00	0.00	0
SAT FAT A	G	0.00	0.00	0

100 * * * * * * * * * * * * * *

561 WHITE SUGAR, GRANULATED
ANALYSIS OF 12 GRAMS WHICH IS 1 TBSP

NUTRIENT	UNIT	AMOUNT	INQ	% STD	0
ENERGY	KCAL	45.00	1.00	2	EE
VITAMIN A	IU	0.00	0.00	0	-
VITAMIN C	MG	0.00	0.00	0	-
THIAMIN	MG	0.00	0.00	0	-
RIBOFLAVN	MG	0.00	0.00	0	-
NIACIN	MG	0.00	0.00	0	-
IRON	MG	0.00	0.00	0	-
CALCIUM	MG	0.00	0.00	0	-
PHOSPHRUS	MG	0.00	0.00	0	-
POTASSIUM	MG	0.00	0.00	0	-
PROTEIN	G	0.00	0.00	4	HIH
CARBOHYDT	G	12.00	1.94	4	-
FAT	G	0.00	0.00	0	-
OLEIC A	G	0.00	0.00	0	-
LINOL A	G	0.00	0.00	0	-
SAT FAT A	G	0.00	0.00	0	

100 * * * * * * * * * * * * * * *

562 WHITE SUGAR, GRANULATED
ANALYSIS OF 6 GRAMS WHICH IS 1 PACKET

NUTRIENT	UNIT	AMOUNT	INQ	% STD	0
ENERGY	KCAL	23.00	1.00	1	E
VITAMIN A	IU	0.00	0.00	0	-
VITAMIN C	MG	0.00	0.00	0	-
THIAMIN	MG	0.00	0.00	0	-
RIBOFLAVN	MG	0.00	0.00	0	-
NIACIN	MG	0.00	0.00	0	-
IRON	MG	0.00	0.00	0	-
CALCIUM	MG	0.00	0.00	0	-
PHOSPHRUS	MG	0.00	0.00	0	-
POTASSIUM	MG	0.00	0.00	0	-
PROTEIN	G	0.00	0.00	2	IH
CARBOHYDT	G	6.00	1.90	0	-
FAT	G	0.00	0.00	0	-
OLEIC A	G	0.00	0.00	0	-
LINOL A	G	0.00	0.00	0	-
SAT FAT A	G	0.00	0.00	0	

563 POWDERED SUGAR, SIFTED, SPOONED
ANALYSIS OF 100 GRAMS WHICH IS 1 CUP

```
                                        0        10       20       30       40       50       60       70       80       90      100
                                        *  *  *  *  *  *  *  *  *  *  *  *  *  *  *  *  *  *
NUTRIENT   UNIT  AMOUNT   INQ   % STD
ENERGY     KCAL  385.00   1.00   19     EEEEEEEEEEE
VITAMIN A  IU      0.00   0.00    0     I
VITAMIN C  MG      0.00   0.00    0     I
THIAMIN    MG      0.00   0.00    0     I
RIBOFLAVN  MG      0.00   0.00    0     I
NIACIN     MG      0.00   0.00    0     I
IRON       MG      0.10   0.03    1     I
CALCIUM    MG      0.00   0.00    0     I
PHOSPHRUS  MG      0.00   0.00    0     I
POTASSIUM  MG      3.00   0.00    0     I
PROTEIN    G       0.00   0.00    0     I
CARBOHYDT  G     100.00   1.89   36     HHHHHHHHHHHHHH I HHHHHHHHHHHHH
FAT        G       0.00   0.00    0     I
OLEIC A    G       0.00   0.00    0     I
LINOL A    G       0.00   0.00    0     I
SAT FAT A  G       0.00   0.00    0     I
*********************************************************
```

564 ASPARAGUS, COOKED,DRAINED,FROM RAW (CUTS AND TIPS, 1 1/2 TO 2-IN LENGTHS)
ANALYSIS OF 145 GRAMS WHICH IS 1 CUP

```
                                         0        10       20       30       40       50       60       70       80       90      100
                                         *  *  *  *  *  *  *  *  *  *  *  *  *  *  *  *  *  *  *  *
NUTRIENT   UNIT  AMOUNT    INQ    % STD
ENERGY     KCAL    30.00    1.00    2    E
VITAMIN A  IU    1310.00   21.83   33    I AAAAAAAAAAAAAAAAAAAAAA
VITAMIN C  MG      38.00   42.22   63    I CCCCCCCCCCCCCCCCCCCCCCCCCCCCCCCCCCCCCCCCCCCC
THIAMIN    MG       0.23   15.33   23    I TTTTTTTTTTTTTTTT
RIBOFLAVN  MG       0.26   14.44   22    I RRRRRRRRRRRRRRR
NIACIN     MG       2.00    9.52   14    I NNNNNNNNNN
IRON       MG       0.90    3.75    6    I IIII
CALCIUM    MG      30.00    2.22    3    I KK
PHOSPHRUS  MG      73.00    5.41    8    I XXXXX
POTASSIUM  MG     265.00    3.53    5    I YYY
PROTEIN    G        3.00    4.00    6    I PPPP
CARBOHYDT  G        5.00    1.21    2    I H
FAT        G        0.00    0.00    0    I
OLEIC A    G        0.00    0.00    0    I
LINOL A    G        0.00    0.00    0    I
SAT FAT A  G        0.00    0.00    0    I
*********************************************************
```

565 ASPARAGUS, COOKED,DRAINED,FROM FROZEN
ANALYSIS OF 180 GRAMS WHICH IS 1 CUP (CUTS AND TIPS, 1 1/2 TO 2-IN LENGTHS)

NUTRIENT	UNIT	AMOUNT	INQ	% STD	0 10 20 30 40 50 60 70 80 90 100
ENERGY	KCAL	40.00	1.00	2	EE
VITAMIN A	IU	1530.00	19.13	38	A|AAAAAAAAAAAAAAAAAAAAAA
VITAMIN C	MG	41.00	34.17	68	C|CCCCCCCCCCCCCCCCCCCCCCCCCCCCCCCCCCCCCCCCC
THIAMIN	MG	0.25	12.50	25	T|TTTTTTTTTTTTTTT
RIBOFLAVN	MG	0.23	9.58	19	R|RRRRRRRRRRR
NIACIN	MG	1.80	6.43	13	N|NNNNNNNN
IRON	MG	2.20	6.88	14	I|IIIIIIIII
CALCIUM	MG	40.00	2.22	4	K|KK
PHOSPHRUS	MG	115.00	6.39	13	X|XXXXXXX
POTASSIUM	MG	396.00	3.96	8	Y|YYYY
PROTEIN	G	6.00	6.00	12	P|PPPPPPP
CARBOHYDT	G	6.00	1.09	2	HH
FAT	G	0.00	0.00	0	-|
OLEIC A	G	0.00	0.00	0	-|
LINOL A	G	0.00	0.00	0	-|
SAT FAT A	G	0.00	0.00	0	-|

566 ASPARAGUS, SPEARS 1/2-IN DIAM AT BASE FROM RAW
ANALYSIS OF 60 GRAMS WHICH IS 4 SPEARS

NUTRIENT	UNIT	AMOUNT	INQ	% STD	0 10 20 30 40 50 60 70 80 90 100
ENERGY	KCAL	10.00	1.00	1	-
VITAMIN A	IU	540.00	27.00	14	AAAAAAAA
VITAMIN C	MG	16.00	53.33	27	CCCCCCCCCCCCCCCCCC
THIAMIN	MG	0.10	20.00	10	TTTTTTT
RIBOFLAVN	MG	0.11	18.33	9	RRRRRR
NIACIN	MG	0.80	11.43	6	NNNN
IRON	MG	0.40	5.00	3	II
CALCIUM	MG	13.00	2.89	1	K
PHOSPHRUS	MG	30.00	6.67	3	XXX
POTASSIUM	MG	110.00	4.40	2	YY
PROTEIN	G	1.00	4.00	2	PP
CARBOHYDT	G	2.00	1.45	1	H
FAT	G	0.00	0.00	0	-
OLEIC A	G	0.00	0.00	0	-
LINOL A	G	0.00	0.00	0	-
SAT FAT A	G	0.00	0.00	0	-

567 ASPARAGUS, SPEARS 1/2-IN DIAM AT BASE FROM FROZEN
ANALYSIS OF 60 GRAMS WHICH IS 4 SPEARS

```
                                    0    10    20    30    40    50    60    70    80    90   100
NUTRIENT    UNIT    AMOUNT    INQ   % STD
ENERGY      KCAL     15.00    1.00     1   E
VITAMIN A   IU      470.00   15.67    12   IAAAAAAA
VITAMIN C   MG       16.00   35.56    27   ICCCCCCCCCCCCCCCCCCC
THIAMIN     MG        0.10   13.33    10   ITTTTTTT
RIBOFLAVN   MG        0.08    8.89     7   IRRRR
NIACIN      MG        0.70    6.67     5   INNN
IRON        MG        0.70    5.83     4   IIII
CALCIUM     MG       13.00    1.93     1   K
PHOSPHRUS   MG       40.00    5.93     4   IXXX
POTASSIUM   MG      143.00    3.81     3   IY
PROTEIN     G         2.00    5.33     4   IPP
CARBOHYDT   G         2.00    0.97     1   H
FAT         G         0.00    0.00     0   I
OLEIC A     G         0.00    0.00     0   I
LINOL A     G         0.00    0.00     0   I
SAT FAT A   G         0.00    0.00     0   I
*****************************************************
```

568 ASPARAGUS, CANNED SPEARS
ANALYSIS OF 80 GRAMS WHICH IS 4 SPEARS

```
                                    0    10    20    30    40    50    60    70    80    90   100
NUTRIENT    UNIT    AMOUNT    INQ   % STD
ENERGY      KCAL     15.00    1.00     1   E
VITAMIN A   IU      640.00   21.33    16   IAAAAAAAAAA
VITAMIN C   MG       12.00   26.67    20   ICCCCCCCCCCCC
THIAMIN     MG        0.05    6.67     5   ITTT
RIBOFLAVN   MG        0.08    8.89     7   IRRRR
NIACIN      MG        0.60    5.71     4   INN
IRON        MG        1.50   12.50     9   IIIIIIII
CALCIUM     MG       15.00    2.22     2   K
PHOSPHRUS   MG       42.00    6.22     5   IXXX
POTASSIUM   MG      133.00    3.55     3   IY
PROTEIN     G         2.00    5.33     4   IPP
CARBOHYDT   G         3.00    1.45     1   H
FAT         G         0.00    0.00     0   I
OLEIC A     G         0.00    0.00     0   I
LINOL A     G         0.00    0.00     0   I
SAT FAT A   G         0.00    0.00     0   I
*****************************************************
```

569 LIMA BEANS,(FORDHOOKS),FROZEN,COOKED,DRAINED
ANALYSIS OF 170 GRAMS WHICH IS 1 CUP

NUTRIENT	UNIT	AMOUNT	INQ	% STD	0 10 20 30 40 50 60 70 80 90 100
ENERGY	KCAL	170.00	1.00	9	EEEEEE
VITAMIN A	IU	390.00	1.15	10	AAAAAA|A
VITAMIN C	MG	29.00	5.69	48	CCCCC|CCCCCCCCCCCCCCCCCCCCCCCCCCCCCCCCCCC
THIAMIN	MG	0.12	1.41	12	TTTTT|TTT
RIBOFLAVN	MG	0.09	0.88	8	RRRRR|R
NIACIN	MG	1.70	1.43	12	NNNNN|NNN
IRON	MG	2.90	2.13	18	IIIII|IIIIIIIII
CALCIUM	MG	34.00	0.44	4	KKK
PHOSPHRUS	MG	153.00	2.00	17	XXXXX|XXXXXXX
POTASSIUM	MG	724.00	1.70	14	YYYYY|YYYYY
PROTEIN	G	10.00	2.35	20	PPPPP|PPPPPPPPPP
CARBOHYDT	G	32.00	1.37	12	HHHHH|HH
FAT	G	0.00	0.00	0	-
OLEIC A	G	0.00	0.00	0	-
LINOL A	G	0.00	0.00	0	-
SAT FAT A	G	0.00	0.00	0	-

570 LIMA BEANS. (BABY LIMAS), FROZEN, COOKED, DRAINED
ANALYSIS OF 180 GRAMS WHICH IS 1 CUP

NUTRIENT	UNIT	AMOUNT	INQ	% STD	0 10 20 30 40 50 60 70 80 90 100
ENERGY	KCAL	210.00	1.00	11	EEEEEEE
VITAMIN A	IU	400.00	0.95	10	AAAAAAAA
VITAMIN C	MG	22.00	3.49	37	CCCCCC|CCCCCCCCCCCCCCCCCCCCCCCCC
THIAMIN	MG	0.16	1.52	16	TTTTTT|TTTT
RIBOFLAVN	MG	0.09	0.71	8	RRRRR|R
NIACIN	MG	2.20	1.50	16	NNNNN|NNNNN
IRON	MG	4.70	2.80	29	IIIIII|IIIIIIIIIIIIIIII
CALCIUM	MG	63.00	0.67	7	KKKKK|K
PHOSPHRUS	MG	227.00	2.40	25	XXXXX|XXXXXXXXXXXXXXX
POTASSIUM	MG	709.00	1.35	14	YYYYY|YYYYY
PROTEIN	G	13.00	2.48	26	PPPPP|PPPPPPPPPPPPPPPPPPPPP
CARBOHYDT	G	40.00	1.59	15	HHHHH|HHHH
FAT	G	0.00	0.00	0	-
OLEIC A	G	0.00	0.00	0	-
LINOL A	G	0.00	0.00	0	-
SAT FAT A	G	0.00	0.00	0	-

571 GREEN SNAP BEANS, COOKED, DRAINED, FROM RAW
ANALYSIS OF 125 GRAMS WHICH IS 1 CUP

NUTRIENT	UNIT	AMOUNT	INQ	% STD	0 10 20
ENERGY	KCAL	30.00	1.00	2	E
VITAMIN A	IU	680.00	11.33	17	|AAAAAAAAAA
VITAMIN C	MG	15.00	16.67	25	|CCCCCCCCCCCCCCC
THIAMIN	MG	0.09	6.00	9	|TTTTTT
RIBOFLAVN	MG	0.11	6.11	9	|RRRRR
NIACIN	MG	0.60	2.86	4	|NN
IRON	MG	0.80	3.33	5	|III
CALCIUM	MG	63.00	4.67	7	|KKKKK
PHOSPHRUS	MG	46.00	3.41	5	|XXX
POTASSIUM	MG	189.00	2.52	4	|YY
PROTEIN	G	2.00	2.67	4	|PP
CARBOHYDT	G	7.00	1.70	3	|H
FAT	G	0.00	0.00	0	I
OLEIC A	G	0.00	0.00	0	I
LINOL A	G	0.00	0.00	0	I
SAT FAT A	G	0.00	0.00	0	I

572 GREEN SNAP BEANS, COOKED, DRAINED,CUTS FROM FROZEN
ANALYSIS OF 135 GRAMS WHICH IS 1 CUP

NUTRIENT	UNIT	AMOUNT	INQ	% STD	0 10 20
ENERGY	KCAL	35.00	1.00	2	E
VITAMIN A	IU	780.00	11.14	20	|AAAAAAAAAAA
VITAMIN C	MG	7.00	6.67	12	|CCCCCCC
THIAMIN	MG	0.09	5.14	9	|TTTTT
RIBOFLAVN	MG	0.12	5.71	10	|RRRRRR
NIACIN	MG	0.50	2.04	4	|NN
IRON	MG	0.90	3.21	6	|IIII
CALCIUM	MG	54.00	3.43	6	|KKKK
PHOSPHRUS	MG	43.00	2.73	5	|XXX
POTASSIUM	MG	205.00	2.34	4	|YY
PROTEIN	G	2.00	2.29	4	|PP
CARBOHYDT	G	8.00	1.66	3	|H
FAT	G	0.00	0.00	0	I
OLEIC A	G	0.00	0.00	0	I
LINOL A	G	0.00	0.00	0	I
SAT FAT A	G	0.00	0.00	0	I

573 GREEN SNAP BEANS, COOKED, DRAINED,FRENCH CUTS FROM FROZEN
ANALYSIS OF 130 GRAMS WHICH IS 1 CUP

```
                                  0        10        20        30        40        50        60        70        80        90       100
NUTRIENT   UNIT  AMOUNT   INQ  % STD
ENERGY     KCAL   35.00   1.00    2    E
VITAMIN A  IU    690.00   9.86   17    IAAAAAAAAAAA
VITAMIN C  MG      9.00   8.57   15    ICCCCCCCCCC
THIAMIN    MG      0.08   4.57    8    ITTTTT
RIBOFLAVN  MG      0.10   4.76    8    IRRRRR
NIACIN     MG      0.40   1.63    3    IN
IRON       MG      1.20   4.29    7    IIIIII
CALCIUM    MG     49.00   3.11    5    IKKK
PHOSPHRUS  MG     39.00   2.48    4    IXX
POTASSIUM  MG    177.00   2.02    4    IYY
PROTEIN    G       2.00   2.29    4    IPP
CARBOHYDT  G       8.00   1.66    3    IH
FAT        G       0.00   0.00    0    I
OLEIC A    G       0.00   0.00    0    I
LINOL A    G       0.00   0.00    0    I
SAT FAT A  G       0.00   0.00    0    I
***********************************************************
```

574 GREEN SNAP BEANS, CANNED, DRAINED SOLIDS (CUTS)
ANALYSIS OF 135 GRAMS WHICH IS 1 CUP

```
                                  0        10        20        30        40        50        60        70        80        90       100
NUTRIENT   UNIT  AMOUNT   INQ  % STD
ENERGY     KCAL   30.00   1.00    2    E
VITAMIN A  IU    630.00  10.50   16    IAAAAAAAAAA
VITAMIN C  MG      5.00   5.56    8    ICCCCCC
THIAMIN    MG      0.04   2.67    4    ITT
RIBOFLAVN  MG      0.07   3.89    6    IRRR
NIACIN     MG      0.40   1.90    3    IN
IRON       MG      2.00   8.33   13    IIIIIIIII
CALCIUM    MG     61.00   4.52    7    IKKKK
PHOSPHRUS  MG     34.00   2.52    4    IXX
POTASSIUM  MG    128.00   1.71    3    IY
PROTEIN    G       2.00   2.67    4    IPP
CARBOHYDT  G       7.00   1.70    3    IH
FAT        G       0.00   0.00    0    I
OLEIC A    G       0.00   0.00    0    I
LINOL A    G       0.00   0.00    0    I
SAT FAT A  G       0.00   0.00    0    I
***********************************************************
```

```
                              0   10   20   30   40   50   60   70   80   90  100
                              *********************************************  *
```

575 YELLOW OR WAX BEANS, COOKED, DRAINED, FROM RAW
ANALYSIS OF 125 GRAMS WHICH IS 1 CUP

NUTRIENT	UNIT	AMOUNT	INQ	% STD	
ENERGY	KCAL	30.00	1.00	2	E
VITAMIN A	IU	290.00	4.83	7	AAAAA
VITAMIN C	MG	16.00	17.78	27	CCCCCCCCCCCCCCCCCC
THIAMIN	MG	0.09	6.00	9	TTTTTT
RIBOFLAVN	MG	0.11	6.11	9	RRRRRR
NIACIN	MG	0.60	2.86	4	NN
IRON	MG	0.80	3.33	5	III
CALCIUM	MG	63.00	4.67	7	KKKKK
PHOSPHRUS	MG	46.00	3.41	5	XXX
POTASSIUM	MG	189.00	2.52	4	YY
PROTEIN	G	2.00	2.67	4	PP
CARBOHYDT	G	6.00	1.45	2	H
FAT	G	0.00	0.00	0	
OLEIC A	G	0.00	0.00	0	
LINOL A	G	0.00	0.00	0	
SAT FAT A	G	0.00	0.00	0	

```
                              0   10   20   30   40   50   60   70   80   90  100
                              *********************************************  *
```

576 YELLOW OR WAX BEANS, COOKED, DRAINED CUTS FROM FROZEN
ANALYSIS OF 135 GRAMS WHICH IS 1 CUP

NUTRIENT	UNIT	AMOUNT	INQ	% STD	
ENERGY	KCAL	35.00	1.00	2	E
VITAMIN A	IU	140.00	2.00	4	AA
VITAMIN C	MG	8.00	7.62	13	CCCCCCCCC
THIAMIN	MG	0.09	5.14	9	TTTTT
RIBOFLAVN	MG	0.11	5.24	9	RRRRR
NIACIN	MG	0.50	2.04	4	NN
IRON	MG	0.90	3.21	6	IIII
CALCIUM	MG	47.00	2.98	5	KKK
PHOSPHRUS	MG	42.00	2.67	5	XXX
POTASSIUM	MG	221.00	2.53	4	YYY
PROTEIN	G	2.00	2.29	4	PP
CARBOHYDT	G	8.00	1.66	3	H
FAT	G	0.00	0.00	0	
OLEIC A	G	0.00	0.00	0	
LINOL A	G	0.00	0.00	0	
SAT FAT A	G	0.00	0.00	0	

577 YELLOW OR WAX BEANS, CANNED, DRAINED SOLIDS (CUTS)
ANALYSIS OF 135 GRAMS WHICH IS 1 CUP

NUTRIENT	UNIT	AMOUNT	INQ	% STD	0 10 20 30 ... 100
ENERGY	KCAL	30.00	1.00	2	E
VITAMIN A	IU	140.00	2.33	4	IAA
VITAMIN C	MG	7.00	7.78	12	ICCCCCCC
THIAMIN	MG	0.04	2.67	4	ITT
RIBOFLAVN	MG	0.07	3.89	6	IRRRR
NIACIN	MG	0.40	1.90	3	IN
IRON	MG	2.00	8.33	13	IIIIIIIII
CALCIUM	MG	61.00	4.52	7	IKKKK
PHOSPHRUS	MG	34.00	2.52	4	IXX
POTASSIUM	MG	128.00	1.71	3	IY
PROTEIN	G	2.00	2.67	4	IPP
CARBOHYDT	G	7.00	1.70	3	IH
FAT	G	0.00	0.00	0	I
OLEIC A	G	0.00	0.00	0	I
LINOL A	G	0.00	0.00	0	I
SAT FAT A	G	0.00	0.00	0	I

578 BEAN SPROUTS,(MUNG),RAW
ANALYSIS OF 105 GRAMS WHICH IS 1 CUP

NUTRIENT	UNIT	AMOUNT	INQ	% STD	0 10 20 30 ... 100
ENERGY	KCAL	35.00	1.00	2	E
VITAMIN A	IU	20.00	0.29	1	E
VITAMIN C	MG	20.00	19.05	33	ICCCCCCCCCCCCCCCCCCCCCCCCCCCCCCCC
THIAMIN	MG	0.14	8.00	14	ITTTTTTTT
RIBOFLAVN	MG	0.14	6.67	12	IRRRRRRR
NIACIN	MG	0.80	3.27	6	INNNN
IRON	MG	1.40	5.00	9	IIIIII
CALCIUM	MG	20.00	1.27	2	IK
PHOSPHRUS	MG	67.00	4.25	7	IXXXX
POTASSIUM	MG	234.00	2.67	5	IYYY
PROTEIN	G	4.00	4.57	8	IPPPP
CARBOHYDT	G	7.00	1.45	3	IH
FAT	G	0.00	0.00	0	I
OLEIC A	G	0.00	0.00	0	I
LINOL A	G	0.00	0.00	0	I
SAT FAT A	G	0.00	0.00	0	I

579 BEAN SPROUTS,(MUNG),COOKED, DRAINED
ANALYSIS OF 125 GRAMS WHICH IS 1 CUP

NUTRIENT	UNIT	AMOUNT	INQ	% STD	0 10 20 30 40 50 60 70 80 90 100
ENERGY	KCAL	35.00	1.00	2	E
VITAMIN A	IU	30.00	0.43	1	A
VITAMIN C	MG	8.00	7.62	13	CCCCCCCCC
THIAMIN	MG	0.11	6.29	11	TTTTTTT
RIBOFLAVN	MG	0.13	6.19	11	RRRRRRR
NIACIN	MG	0.90	3.67	6	NNNN
IRON	MG	1.10	3.93	7	IIIII
CALCIUM	MG	21.00	1.33	2	K
PHOSPHRUS	MG	60.00	3.81	7	XXXX
POTASSIUM	MG	195.00	2.23	4	YY
PROTEIN	G	4.00	4.57	8	PPPPP
CARBOHYDT	G	7.00	1.45	3	H
FAT	G	0.00	0.00	0	-
OLEIC A	G	0.00	0.00	0	-
LINOL A	G	0.00	0.00	0	-
SAT FAT A	G	0.00	0.00	0	-

580 BEETS, COOKED DRAINED, PEELED
ANALYSIS OF 100 GRAMS WHICH IS 2 WHOLE BEETS, 2-IN DIAM.

NUTRIENT	UNIT	AMOUNT	INQ	% STD	0 10 20 30 40 50 60 70 80 90 100
ENERGY	KCAL	30.00	1.00	2	E
VITAMIN A	IU	20.00	0.33	1	A
VITAMIN C	MG	6.00	6.67	10	CCCCCCC
THIAMIN	MG	0.03	2.00	3	T
RIBOFLAVN	MG	0.04	2.22	3	RR
NIACIN	MG	0.30	1.43	2	N
IRON	MG	0.50	2.08	3	II
CALCIUM	MG	14.00	1.04	2	K
PHOSPHRUS	MG	23.00	1.70	3	X
POTASSIUM	MG	208.00	2.77	4	YY
PROTEIN	G	1.00	1.33	2	P
CARBOHYDT	G	7.00	1.70	3	H
FAT	G	0.00	0.00	0	-
OLEIC A	G	0.00	0.00	0	-
LINOL A	G	0.00	0.00	0	-
SAT FAT A	G	0.00	0.00	0	-

581 BEETS, COOKED DRAINED,DICED OR SLICED
ANALYSIS OF 170 GRAMS WHICH IS 1 CUP

NUTRIENT	UNIT	AMOUNT	INQ	% STD	0	10	20	30	40	50	60	70	80	90	100
ENERGY	KCAL	55.00	1.00	3	EE										************
VITAMIN A	IU	30.00	0.27	1	AI										
VITAMIN C	MG	10.00	6.06	17	CICCCCCCCCCC										
THIAMIN	MG	0.05	1.82	5	TITT										
RIBOFLAVN	MG	0.07	2.12	6	RIRRR										
NIACIN	MG	0.50	1.30	4	NIN										
IRON	MG	0.90	2.05	6	IIIII										
CALCIUM	MG	24.00	0.97	3	KK										
PHOSPHRUS	MG	39.00	1.58	4	XIX										
POTASSIUM	MG	354.00	2.57	7	YIYYYY										
PROTEIN	G	2.00	1.45	4	PIP										
CARBOHYDT	G	12.00	1.59	4	HIH										
FAT	G	0.00	0.00	0	-I										
OLEIC A	G	0.00	0.00	0	-I										
LINOL A	G	0.00	0.00	0	-I										
SAT FAT A	G	0.00	0.00	0	-I										

582 BEETS, CANNED, DRAINED SOLIDS, WHOLE SMALL BEETS
ANALYSIS OF 160 GRAMS WHICH IS 1 CUP

NUTRIENT	UNIT	AMOUNT	INQ	% STD	0	10	20	30	40	50	60	70	80	90	100
ENERGY	KCAL	60.00	1.00	3	EE										************
VITAMIN A	IU	30.00	0.25	1	AI										
VITAMIN C	MG	5.00	2.78	8	CICCCCC										
THIAMIN	MG	0.02	0.67	2	TT										
RIBOFLAVN	MG	0.05	1.39	4	RIR										
NIACIN	MG	0.20	0.48	1	NI										
IRON	MG	1.10	2.29	7	IIIII										
CALCIUM	MG	30.00	1.11	3	KIK										
PHOSPHRUS	MG	29.00	1.07	3	XIX										
POTASSIUM	MG	267.00	1.78	5	YIYY										
PROTEIN	G	2.00	1.33	4	PIP										
CARBOHYDT	G	14.00	1.70	5	HIHH										
FAT	G	0.00	0.00	0	-I										
OLEIC A	G	0.00	0.00	0	-I										
LINOL A	G	0.00	0.00	0	-I										
SAT FAT A	G	0.00	0.00	0	-I										

583 BEETS, CANNED, DRAINED SOLIDS, DICED OR SLICED
ANALYSIS OF 170 GRAMS WHICH IS 1 CUP

NUTRIENT	UNIT	AMOUNT	INQ	% STD
ENERGY	KCAL	65.00	1.00	3
VITAMIN A	IU	30.00	0.23	1
VITAMIN C	MG	5.00	2.56	8
THIAMIN	MG	0.02	0.62	2
RIBOFLAVN	MG	0.05	1.28	4
NIACIN	MG	0.20	0.44	1
IRON	MG	1.20	2.31	7
CALCIUM	MG	32.00	1.09	4
PHOSPHRUS	MG	31.00	1.06	3
POTASSIUM	MG	284.00	1.75	6
PROTEIN	G	2.00	1.23	4
CARBOHYDT	G	15.00	1.68	5
FAT	G	0.00	0.00	0
OLEIC A	G	0.00	0.00	0
LINOL A	G	0.00	0.00	0
SAT FAT A	G	0.00	0.00	0

584 BEET GREENS, COOKED, DRAINED
ANALYSIS OF 145 GRAMS WHICH IS 1 CUP

NUTRIENT	UNIT	AMOUNT	INQ	% STD
ENERGY	KCAL	25.00	1.00	1
VITAMIN A	IU	7400.00	146.00	185
VITAMIN C	MG	22.00	29.33	37
THIAMIN	MG	0.10	8.00	10
RIBOFLAVN	MG	0.22	14.67	18
NIACIN	MG	0.40	2.29	3
IRON	MG	2.80	14.00	18
CALCIUM	MG	144.00	12.80	16
PHOSPHRUS	MG	36.00	3.20	4
POTASSIUM	MG	481.00	7.70	10
PROTEIN	G	2.00	3.20	4
CARBOHYDT	G	5.00	1.45	2
FAT	G	0.00	0.00	0
OLEIC A	G	0.00	0.00	0
LINOL A	G	0.00	0.00	0
SAT FAT A	G	0.00	0.00	0

VITAMIN A *185

585 BLACKEYE PEAS, COOKED, DRAINED, FROM RAW
ANALYSIS OF 165 GRAMS WHICH IS 1 CUP

NUTRIENT	UNIT	AMOUNT	INQ	% STD
ENERGY	KCAL	180.00	1.00	9
VITAMIN A	IU	580.00	1.61	15
VITAMIN C	MG	28.00	5.19	47
THIAMIN	MG	0.50	5.56	50
RIBOFLAVN	MG	0.18	1.67	15
NIACIN	MG	2.30	1.83	16
IRON	MG	3.50	2.43	22
CALCIUM	MG	40.00	0.49	4
PHOSPHRUS	MG	241.00	2.98	27
POTASSIUM	MG	625.00	1.39	13
PROTEIN	G	13.00	2.89	26
CARBOHYDT	G	30.00	1.21	11
FAT	G	1.00	0.14	1
OLEIC A	G	0.00	0.00	0
LINOL A	G	0.00	0.00	0
SAT FAT A	G	0.00	0.00	0

586 BLACKEYE PEAS, COOKED, DRAINED, FROM FROZEN
ANALYSIS OF 170 GRAMS WHICH IS 1 CUP

NUTRIENT	UNIT	AMOUNT	INQ	% STD
ENERGY	KCAL	220.00	1.00	11
VITAMIN A	IU	290.00	0.66	7
VITAMIN C	MG	15.00	2.27	25
THIAMIN	MG	0.68	6.18	68
RIBOFLAVN	MG	0.19	1.44	16
NIACIN	MG	2.40	1.56	17
IRON	MG	4.80	2.73	30
CALCIUM	MG	43.00	0.43	5
PHOSPHRUS	MG	286.00	2.89	32
POTASSIUM	MG	573.00	1.04	11
PROTEIN	G	15.00	2.73	30
CARBOHYDT	G	40.00	1.32	15
FAT	G	1.00	0.12	1
OLEIC A	G	0.00	0.00	0
LINOL A	G	0.00	0.00	0
SAT FAT A	G	0.00	0.00	0

587 BROCCOLI, COOKED, DRAINED, FROM RAW
ANALYSIS OF 187 GRAMS WHICH IS 1 WHOLE MEDIUM STALK

NUTRIENT	UNIT	AMOUNT	INQ	% STD
ENERGY	KCAL	45.00	1.00	2
VITAMIN A	IU	450.00	50.00	113
VITAMIN C	MG	162.00	120.00	270
THIAMIN	MG	0.16	7.11	16
RIBOFLAVN	MG	0.36	13.33	30
NIACIN	MG	1.40	4.44	10
IRON	MG	1.40	3.89	9
CALCIUM	MG	158.00	7.80	18
PHOSPHRUS	MG	112.00	5.53	12
POTASSIUM	MG	481.00	4.28	10
PROTEIN	G	6.00	5.33	12
CARBOHYDT	G	8.00	1.29	3
FAT	G	1.00	0.57	1
OLEIC A	G	0.00	0.00	0
LINOL A	G	0.00	0.00	0
SAT FAT A	G	0.00	0.00	0

588 BROCCOLI, COOKED, DRAINED, FROM RAW
ANALYSIS OF 155 GRAMS WHICH IS 1 CUP (STALKS CUT INTO 1/2-IN PIECES)

NUTRIENT	UNIT	AMOUNT	INQ	% STD
ENERGY	KCAL	40.00	1.00	2
VITAMIN A	IU	3880.00	48.50	97
VITAMIN C	MG	140.00	116.67	233
THIAMIN	MG	0.14	7.00	14
RIBOFLAVN	MG	0.31	12.92	26
NIACIN	MG	1.20	4.29	9
IRON	MG	1.20	3.75	7
CALCIUM	MG	136.00	7.56	15
PHOSPHRUS	MG	96.00	5.33	11
POTASSIUM	MG	414.00	4.14	8
PROTEIN	G	5.00	5.00	10
CARBOHYDT	G	7.00	1.27	3
FAT	G	0.00	0.00	0
OLEIC A	G	0.00	0.00	0
LINOL A	G	0.00	0.00	0
SAT FAT A	G	0.00	0.00	0

589 BROCCOLI, FROM FROZEN, COOKED, DRAINED
ANALYSIS OF 30 GRAMS WHICH IS 1 PIECE, 4 1/2 TO 5 IN LONG

NUTRIENT	UNIT	AMOUNT	INQ	% STD	0 10 20 30 40 50 60 70 80 90 100
ENERGY	KCAL	10.00	1.00	1	-
VITAMIN A	IU	570.00	28.50	14	AAAAAAAAA
VITAMIN C	MG	22.00	73.33	37	CCCCCCCCCCCCCCCCCCCCCCCCCCCCCCCCCCCCC
THIAMIN	MG	0.02	4.00	2	TT
RIBOFLAVN	MG	0.03	5.00	3	RR
NIACIN	MG	0.20	2.86	1	N
IRON	MG	0.20	2.50	1	I
CALCIUM	MG	12.00	2.67	1	K
PHOSPHRUS	MG	17.00	3.78	2	XX
POTASSIUM	MG	66.00	2.64	1	Y
PROTEIN	G	1.00	4.00	2	PP
CARBOHYDT	G	1.00	0.73	0	-
FAT	G	0.00	0.00	0	-
OLEIC A	G	0.00	0.00	0	-
LINOL A	G	0.00	0.00	0	-
SAT FAT A	G	0.00	0.00	0	-

590 BROCCOLI, FROM FROZEN, CHOPPED, COOKED, DRAINED
ANALYSIS OF 185 GRAMS WHICH IS 1 CUP

NUTRIENT	UNIT	AMOUNT	INQ	% STD	0 10 20 30 40 50 60 70 80 90 100
ENERGY	KCAL	50.00	1.00	3	EE
VITAMIN A	IU	4810.00	48.10	120	AIAAAAAAAAAAAAAAAAAAAAAAAAAAAAAAAAAAAAAAAAAAAAAAAAAAAAAAAAAAAAAAAAAAAAAAAAAAAAAAAAAAAAAAAAAAAAAAAA *120
VITAMIN C	MG	105.00	70.00	175	CICCCCCCCCCCCCCCCCCCCCCCCCCCCCCCCCCCCCCCCCCCCCCCCCCCCCCCCCCCCCCCCCCCCCCCCCCCCCCCCCCCCCCCCCCCCCC *175
THIAMIN	MG	0.11	4.40	11	TITTTTTTT
RIBOFLAVN	MG	0.22	7.33	18	RIRRRRRRRRRRRRRRR
NIACIN	MG	0.90	2.57	6	NINNN
IRON	MG	1.30	3.25	8	IIIIIII
CALCIUM	MG	100.00	4.44	11	KIKKKKKK
PHOSPHRUS	MG	104.00	4.62	12	XIXXXXXXX
POTASSIUM	MG	392.00	3.14	8	YIYYYYY
PROTEIN	G	5.00	4.00	10	PIPPPPPP
CARBOHYDT	G	1.00	0.51	1	HIH
FAT	G	0.00	0.00	0	FI
OLEIC A	G	0.00	0.00	0	-I
LINOL A	G	0.00	0.00	0	-I
SAT FAT A	G	0.00	0.00	0	-I

591 BRUSSELS SPROUTS, COOKED, DRAINED, FROM RAW
ANALYSIS OF 155 GRAMS WHICH IS 7-8 SPROUTS (1 1/4 TO 1 1/2-IN DIAM) 1 CUP

```
NUTRIENT   UNIT   AMOUNT   INQ   % STD   0      10      20      30      40      50      60      70      80      90     100
ENERGY     KCAL    55.00   1.00     3    EE                                                                          *
VITAMIN A  IU     810.00   7.36    20    AIAAAAAAAAAAAA                                                              *
VITAMIN C  MG     135.00  81.82   225    CICCCCCCCCCCCCCCCCCCCCCCCCCCCCCCCCCCCCCCCCCCCCCCCCCCCCCCCCCC  * 225
THIAMIN    MG       0.12   4.36    12    TITTTTTTT                                                                   *
RIBOFLAVN  MG       0.22   6.67    18    RIRRRRRRRRRRR                                                               *
NIACIN     MG       1.20   3.12     9    NINNNN                                                                      *
IRON       MG       1.70   3.86    11    IIIIIIII                                                                    *
CALCIUM    MG      50.00   2.02     6    KIKK                                                                        *
PHOSPHRUS  MG     112.00   4.53    12    XIXXXXXXX                                                                   *
POTASSIUM  MG     423.00   3.08     8    YIYYYYY                                                                     *
PROTEIN    G        7.00   5.09    14    PIPPPPPPPP                                                                  *
CARBOHYDT  G       10.00   1.32     4    HIH                                                                         *
FAT        G        1.00   0.47     1    FI                                                                          *
OLEIC A    G        0.00   0.00     0    -I                                                                         *
LINOL A    G        0.00   0.00     0    -I                                                                         *
SAT FAT A  G        0.00   0.00     0    -I                                                                          *
***************************************
```

592 BRUSSELS SPROUTS, COOKED, DRAINED, FROM FROZEN
ANALYSIS OF 155 GRAMS WHICH IS 1 CUP

```
NUTRIENT   UNIT   AMOUNT   INQ   % STD   0      10      20      30      40      50      60      70      80      90     100
ENERGY     KCAL    50.00   1.00     3    EE                                                                          *
VITAMIN A  IU     880.00   8.80    22    AIAAAAAAAAAAAAA                                                             *
VITAMIN C  MG     126.00  84.00   210    CICCCCCCCCCCCCCCCCCCCCCCCCCCCCCCCCCCCCCCCCCCCCCCCCCCCCCCCCC  * 210
THIAMIN    MG       0.12   4.80    12    TITTTTTTT                                                                   *
RIBOFLAVN  MG       0.16   5.33    13    RIRRRRRRRR                                                                  *
NIACIN     MG       0.90   2.57     6    NINNN                                                                       *
IRON       MG       1.20   3.00     7    IIIIII                                                                      *
CALCIUM    MG      33.00   1.47     4    KIK                                                                         *
PHOSPHRUS  MG      95.00   4.22    11    XIXXXXX                                                                     *
POTASSIUM  MG     457.00   3.66     9    YIYYYY                                                                      *
PROTEIN    G        5.00   4.00    10    PIPPPPP                                                                     *
CARBOHYDT  G       10.00   1.45     4    HIH                                                                         *
FAT        G        0.00   0.00     0    -I                                                                         *
OLEIC A    G        0.00   0.00     0    --I                                                                         *
LINOL A    G        0.00   0.00     0    -I                                                                         *
SAT FAT A  G        0.00   0.00     0    -I                                                                          *
***************************************
```

593 CABBAGE, RAW, COARSLY SHREDDED OR CHOPPED
ANALYSIS OF 70 GRAMS WHICH IS 1 CUP

NUTRIENT	UNIT	AMOUNT	INQ	% STD	0	10	20	30	40	50	60	70	80	90	100
ENERGY	KCAL	15.00	1.00	1	E										*****
VITAMIN A	IU	90.00	3.00	2	A										*
VITAMIN C	MG	33.00	73.33	55	CCCCCCCCCCCCCCCCCCCCCCCCCCCCCCCCCCCCCCCCCCCCCCCCCCCCCCC										**************
THIAMIN	MG	0.04	5.33	4	TT										*
RIBOFLAVN	MG	0.04	4.44	3	RR										********
NIACIN	MG	0.20	1.90	1	N										*
IRON	MG	0.30	2.50	2	II										****
CALCIUM	MG	34.00	5.04	4	KK										*
PHOSPHRUS	MG	20.00	2.96	2	X										**
POTASSIUM	MG	163.00	4.35	3	YY										**
PROTEIN	G	1.00	2.67	2	P										**
CARBOHYDT	G	4.00	1.94	1	H										*
FAT	G	0.00	0.00	0	I										
OLEIC A	G	0.00	0.00	0	I										
LINOL A	G	0.00	0.00	0	I										
SAT FAT A	G	0.00	0.00	0											

594 CABBAGE,RAW, FINELY SHREDDED
ANALYSIS OF 90 GRAMS WHICH IS 1 CUP

NUTRIENT	UNIT	AMOUNT	INQ	% STD	0	10	20	30	40	50	60	70	80	90	100
ENERGY	KCAL	20.00	1.00	1	E										******
VITAMIN A	IU	120.00	3.00	3	A										**
VITAMIN C	MG	42.00	70.00	70	CCCCCCCCCCCCCCCCCCCCCCCCCCCCCCCCCCCCCCCCCCCCCCCCCCCCCCCCCCCCCCCCCCCCCC										***********
THIAMIN	MG	0.05	5.00	5	TTT										*
RIBOFLAVN	MG	0.05	4.17	4	RR										********
NIACIN	MG	0.30	2.14	2	N										*
IRON	MG	0.40	2.50	3	II										****
CALCIUM	MG	44.00	4.89	5	KKK										*
PHOSPHRUS	MG	26.00	2.89	3	X										**
POTASSIUM	MG	210.00	4.20	4	YY										**
PROTEIN	G	1.00	2.00	2	P										**
CARBOHYDT	G	5.00	1.82	2	H										*
FAT	G	0.00	0.00	0	I										
OLEIC A	G	0.00	0.00	0	I										
LINOL A	G	0.00	0.00	0	I										
SAT FAT A	G	0.00	0.00	0											

595 CABBAGE, COOKED, DRAINED
ANALYSIS OF 145 GRAMS WHICH IS 1 CUP

NUTRIENT	UNIT	AMOUNT	INQ	% STD	Chart
ENERGY	KCAL	30.00	1.00	2	E
VITAMIN A	IU	190.00	3.17	5	AAA
VITAMIN C	MG	48.00	53.33	80	CCCCCCCCCCCCCCCCCCCCCCCCCCCCCCCCCCCCCCCCCCCCCCCCCCCCCCCCCCCCCCCCCCCCCCCCCCCCCCCC
THIAMIN	MG	0.06	4.00	6	TTTT
RIBOFLAVN	MG	0.06	3.33	5	RRR
NIACIN	MG	0.40	1.90	3	N
IRON	MG	0.40	1.67	3	I
CALCIUM	MG	64.00	4.74	7	KKKKK
PHOSPHRUS	MG	29.00	2.15	3	XX
POTASSIUM	MG	236.00	3.15	5	YYY
PROTEIN	G	2.00	2.67	4	PP
CARBOHYDT	G	6.00	1.45	2	H
FAT	G	0.00	0.00	0	
OLEIC A	G	0.00	0.00	0	
LINOL A	G	0.00	0.00	0	
SAT FAT A	G	0.00	0.00	0	

596 RED CABBAGE, RAW, COARSELY SHREDDED
ANALYSIS OF 70 GRAMS WHICH IS 1 CUP

NUTRIENT	UNIT	AMOUNT	INQ	% STD	Chart
ENERGY	KCAL	20.00	1.00	1	E
VITAMIN A	IU	30.00	0.75	1	A
VITAMIN C	MG	43.00	71.67	72	CCCCCCCCCCCCCCCCCCCCCCCCCCCCCCCCCCCCCCCCCCCCCCCCCCCCCCCCCCCCCCCCCCCCCCCCCC
THIAMIN	MG	0.06	6.00	6	TTTT
RIBOFLAVN	MG	0.04	3.33	3	RR
NIACIN	MG	0.30	2.14	2	N
IRON	MG	0.60	3.75	4	III
CALCIUM	MG	29.00	3.22	3	KK
PHOSPHRUS	MG	25.00	2.78	3	X
POTASSIUM	MG	188.00	3.76	4	YY
PROTEIN	G	1.00	2.00	2	P
CARBOHYDT	G	5.00	1.82	2	H
FAT	G	0.00	0.00	0	
OLEIC A	G	0.00	0.00	0	
LINOL A	G	0.00	0.00	0	
SAT FAT A	G	0.00	0.00	0	

597 SAVOY CABBAGE, RAW, COARSELY SHREDDED
ANALYSIS OF 70 GRAMS WHICH IS 1 CUP

NUTRIENT	UNIT	AMOUNT	INQ	% STD	0 10 20 30 40 50 60 70 80 90 100
ENERGY	KCAL	15.00	1.00	1	E
VITAMIN A	IU	140.00	4.67	4	IAA
VITAMIN C	MG	39.00	86.67	65	ICCCCCCCCCCCCCCCCCCCCCCCCCCCCCCCCCCCCCCCCCCC
THIAMIN	MG	0.04	5.33	4	ITT
RIBOFLAVN	MG	0.06	6.67	5	IRRR
NIACIN	MG	0.20	1.90	1	N
IRON	MG	0.60	5.00	4	III
CALCIUM	MG	47.00	6.96	5	IKKK
PHOSPHRUS	MG	38.00	5.63	4	IXX
POTASSIUM	MG	188.00	5.01	4	IYY
PROTEIN	G	2.00	5.33	4	IPP
CARBOHYDT	G	3.00	1.45	1	H
FAT	G	0.00	0.00	0	I
OLEIC A	G	0.00	0.00	0	I
LINOL A	G	0.00	0.00	0	I
SAT FAT A	G	0.00	0.00	0	I

598 CELERY CABBAGE (WONGBOK), RAW
ANALYSIS OF 75 GRAMS WHICH IS 1 CUP (1-IN PIECES)

NUTRIENT	UNIT	AMOUNT	INQ	% STD	0 10 20 30 40 50 60 70 80 90 100
ENERGY	KCAL	10.00	1.00	1	-
VITAMIN A	IU	110.00	5.50	3	AA
VITAMIN C	MG	19.00	63.33	32	CCCCCCCCCCCCCCCCCCCCCCCCCCCC
THIAMIN	MG	0.04	8.00	4	TTT
RIBOFLAVN	MG	0.03	5.00	3	RR
NIACIN	MG	0.50	7.14	4	NNN
IRON	MG	0.50	6.25	3	III
CALCIUM	MG	32.00	7.11	4	KKK
PHOSPHRUS	MG	30.00	6.67	3	XXX
POTASSIUM	MG	190.00	7.60	4	YYY
PROTEIN	G	1.00	4.00	2	PP
CARBOHYDT	G	2.00	1.45	1	H
FAT	G	0.00	0.00	0	-
OLEIC A	G	0.00	0.00	0	-
LINOL A	G	0.00	0.00	0	-
SAT FAT A	G	0.00	0.00	0	-

599 WHITE MUSTARD CABBAGE, COOKED, DRAINED
ANALYSIS OF 170 GRAMS WHICH IS 1 CUP

NUTRIENT	UNIT	AMOUNT	INQ	% STD
ENERGY	KCAL	25.00	1.00	1
VITAMIN A	IU	5270.00	105.40	132
VITAMIN C	MG	26.00	34.67	43
THIAMIN	MG	0.07	5.60	7
RIBOFLAVN	MG	0.14	9.33	12
NIACIN	MG	1.20	6.86	9
IRON	MG	1.00	5.00	6
CALCIUM	MG	252.00	42.40	28
PHOSPHRUS	MG	56.00	4.98	6
POTASSIUM	MG	364.00	5.82	7
PROTEIN	G	2.00	3.20	4
CARBOHYDT	G	4.00	1.16	1
FAT	G	0.00	0.00	0
OLEIC A	G	0.00	0.00	0
LINOL A	G	0.00	0.00	0
SAT FAT A	G	0.00	0.00	0

600 CARROTS, RAW, PEELED
ANALYSIS OF 72 GRAMS WHICH IS 1 CARROT OR 18 STRIPS 2 1/2 TO 3-IN LONG

NUTRIENT	UNIT	AMOUNT	INQ	% STD
ENERGY	KCAL	30.00	1.00	2
VITAMIN A	IU	7930.00	132.17	198
VITAMIN C	MG	6.00	6.67	10
THIAMIN	MG	0.04	2.67	4
RIBOFLAVN	MG	0.04	2.22	3
NIACIN	MG	0.40	1.90	3
IRON	MG	0.50	2.08	3
CALCIUM	MG	27.00	2.00	3
PHOSPHRUS	MG	26.00	1.93	3
POTASSIUM	MG	246.00	3.28	5
PROTEIN	G	1.00	1.33	2
CARBOHYDT	G	7.00	1.70	3
FAT	G	0.00	0.00	0
OLEIC A	G	0.00	0.00	0
LINOL A	G	0.00	0.00	0
SAT FAT A	G	0.00	0.00	0

601 CARROTS, RAW, PEELED, GRATED
ANALYSIS OF 110 GRAMS WHICH IS 1 CUP

NUTRIENT	UNIT	AMOUNT	INQ	% STD		0	10	20	30	40	50	60	70	80	90	100
ENERGY	KCAL	45.00	1.00	2	EE											
VITAMIN A	IU	12100.00	134.44	302	AIAAAAAAAAAAAAAAAAAAAAAAAAAAAAAAAAAAAAAAAAAAAAAAAAAAAAAAAAAAAAAAAAAAAAAAAAAAAAAAAAAAAA *302
VITAMIN C	MG	9.00	6.67	15	CICCCCCCCCC
THIAMIN	MG	0.07	3.11	7	TITTTT
RIBOFLAVN	MG	0.06	2.22	5	RIRR
NIACIN	MG	0.70	2.22	5	NINN
IRON	MG	0.80	2.02	5	IIII
CALCIUM	MG	41.00	2.02	5	KIKK
PHOSPHRUS	MG	40.00	1.98	4	XIXX
POTASSIUM	MG	375.00	3.33	8	YIYYYY
PROTEIN	G	1.00	0.89	2	PP
CARBOHYDT	G	11.00	1.78	4	HIH
FAT	G	0.00	0.00	0	-I
OLEIC A	G	0.00	0.00	0	-I
LINOL A	G	0.00	0.00	0	-I
SAT FAT A	G	0.00	0.00	0	-I

****

602 CARROTS (CROSSWISE CUTS) COOKED, DRAINED
ANALYSIS OF 155 GRAMS WHICH IS 1 CUP

NUTRIENT	UNIT	AMOUNT	INQ	% STD		0	10	20	30	40	50	60	70	80	90	100
ENERGY	KCAL	50.00	1.00	3	EE											
VITAMIN A	IU	16280.00	162.80	407	AIAAAAAAAAAAAAAAAAAAAAAAAAAAAAAAAAAAAAAAAAAAAAAAAAAAAAAAAAAAAAAAAAAAAAAAAAAAAAAAAAAAAA *407
VITAMIN C	MG	9.00	6.00	15	CICCCCCCCCC
THIAMIN	MG	0.08	3.20	8	TITTTT
RIBOFLAVN	MG	0.08	2.67	7	RIRRR
NIACIN	MG	0.80	2.29	6	NINNN
IRON	MG	0.90	2.25	6	IIIII
CALCIUM	MG	51.00	2.27	6	KIKKK
PHOSPHRUS	MG	48.00	2.13	5	XIXX
POTASSIUM	MG	344.00	2.75	7	YIYYYY
PROTEIN	G	1.00	0.80	2	PP
CARBOHYDT	G	11.00	1.60	4	HIH
FAT	G	0.00	0.00	0	-I
OLEIC A	G	0.00	0.00	0	-I
LINOL A	G	0.00	0.00	0	-I
SAT FAT A	G	0.00	0.00	0	-I

****

603 CARROTS, CANNED, SLICED, DRAINED SOLIDS
ANALYSIS OF 155 GRAMS WHICH IS 1 CUP

NUTRIENT	UNIT	AMOUNT	INQ	% STD
ENERGY	KCAL	45.00	1.00	2
VITAMIN A	IU	23250.00	258.33	581
VITAMIN C	MG	3.00	2.22	5
THIAMIN	MG	0.03	1.33	3
RIBOFLAVN	MG	0.05	1.85	4
NIACIN	MG	0.60	1.90	4
IRON	MG	1.10	3.06	7
CALCIUM	MG	47.00	2.32	5
PHOSPHRUS	MG	34.00	1.68	4
POTASSIUM	MG	186.00	1.65	4
PROTEIN	G	1.00	0.89	2
CARBOHYDT	G	10.00	1.62	4
FAT	G	0.00	0.00	0
OLEIC A	G	0.00	0.00	0
LINOL A	G	0.00	0.00	0
SAT FAT A	G	0.00	0.00	0

604 CARROTS,STRAINED OR BABY FOOD
ANALYSIS OF 28 GRAMS WHICH IS 1 OZ (1 3/4 TO 2 TBSP)

NUTRIENT	UNIT	AMOUNT	INQ	% STD
ENERGY	KCAL	10.00	1.00	1
VITAMIN A	IU	3690.00	184.50	92
VITAMIN C	MG	1.00	3.33	2
THIAMIN	MG	0.01	1.00	1
RIBOFLAVN	MG	0.01	1.67	1
NIACIN	MG	0.10	1.43	1
IRON	MG	0.10	1.25	1
CALCIUM	MG	7.00	1.56	1
PHOSPHRUS	MG	6.00	1.33	1
POTASSIUM	MG	51.00	2.04	1
PROTEIN	G	0.00	0.00	0
CARBOHYDT	G	2.00	1.45	1
FAT	G	0.00	0.00	0
OLEIC A	G	0.00	0.00	0
LINOL A	G	0.00	0.00	0
SAT FAT A	G	0.00	0.00	0

605 CAULIFLOWER, RAW, CHOPPED
ANALYSIS OF 115 GRAMS WHICH IS 1 CUP

NUTRIENT	UNIT	AMOUNT	INQ	% STD	0 10 20 30 40 50 60 70 80 90 100
ENERGY	KCAL	31.00	1.00	2	E
VITAMIN A	IU	70.00	1.13	2	A
VITAMIN C	MG	90.00	96.77	150	CCCCCCCCCCCCCCCCCCCCCCCCCCCCCCCCCCCCCCCCCCCCCCCCCCCCCCCCCCCCCCCCCCCCCCCCCCCCCCCCCCCCCCCCCCCCCC *150
THIAMIN	MG	0.13	8.39	13	TTTTTTTT
RIBOFLAVN	MG	0.12	6.45	10	RRRRRR
NIACIN	MG	0.80	3.69	6	NNNN
IRON	MG	1.30	5.24	8	IIIIII
CALCIUM	MG	29.00	2.08	3	KK
PHOSPHRUS	MG	64.00	4.59	7	XXXXX
POTASSIUM	MG	339.00	4.37	7	YYYY
PROTEIN	G	3.00	3.87	6	PPPP
CARBOHYDT	G	6.00	1.41	2	H
FAT	G	0.00	0.00	0	-
OLEIC A	G	0.00	0.00	0	I
LINOL A	G	0.00	0.00	0	I
SAT FAT A	G	0.00	0.00	0	I

606 CAULIFLOWER, COOKED, DRAINED FROM RAW
ANALYSIS OF 125 GRAMS WHICH IS 1 CUP

NUTRIENT	UNIT	AMOUNT	INQ	% STD	0 10 20 30 40 50 60 70 80 90 100
ENERGY	KCAL	30.00	1.00	2	E
VITAMIN A	IU	80.00	1.33	2	A
VITAMIN C	MG	69.00	76.67	115	CCCCCCCCCCCCCCCCCCCCCCCCCCCCCCCCCCCCCCCCCCCCCCCCCCCCCCCCCCCCCCCCCCCCCCCCCCCCCCCCCCCCCCCCCCCCCC *115
THIAMIN	MG	0.11	7.33	11	TTTTTTT
RIBOFLAVN	MG	0.10	5.56	8	RRRRR
NIACIN	MG	0.80	3.81	6	NNNN
IRON	MG	0.90	3.75	6	IIII
CALCIUM	MG	26.00	1.93	3	K
PHOSPHRUS	MG	53.00	3.93	6	XXXX
POTASSIUM	MG	258.00	3.44	5	YYY
PROTEIN	G	3.00	4.00	6	PPPP
CARBOHYDT	G	5.00	1.21	2	H
FAT	G	0.00	0.00	0	-
OLEIC A	G	0.00	0.00	0	I
LINOL A	G	0.00	0.00	0	I
SAT FAT A	G	0.00	0.00	0	I

607 CAULIFLOWER, COOKED, DRAINED FROM FROZEN
ANALYSIS OF 180 GRAMS WHICH IS 1 CUP

NUTRIENT	UNIT	AMOUNT	INQ	% STD										
					0	10	20	30	40	50	60	70	80	90 100
ENERGY	KCAL	30.00	1.00	2	E									
VITAMIN A	IU	50.00	0.83	1	A									
VITAMIN C	MG	74.00	82.22	123	CCCCCCCCCCCCCCCCCCCCCCCCCCCCCCCCCCCCCCCCCCCCCCCCCCCCCCCCCCCC *123
THIAMIN	MG	0.07	4.67	7	TTTTT									
RIBOFLAVN	MG	0.09	5.00	8	RRRRR									
NIACIN	MG	0.70	3.33	5	NNN									
IRON	MG	0.90	3.75	6	IIII									
CALCIUM	MG	31.00	2.30	3	KK									
PHOSPHRUS	MG	68.00	5.04	8	XXXXX									
POTASSIUM	MG	373.00	4.97	7	YYYYY									
PROTEIN	G	3.00	1.45	2	PPPP									
CARBOHYDT	G	6.00	0.00	0	H									
FAT	G	0.00	0.00	0	I									
OLEIC A	G	0.00	0.00	0	I									
LINOL A	G	0.00	0.00	0	I									
SAT FAT A	G	0.00	0.00	0	I									

608 CELERY (PASCAL) RAW
ANALYSIS OF 40 GRAMS WHICH IS 1 STALK, 8 BY 1 1/2 IN

NUTRIENT	UNIT	AMOUNT	INQ	% STD										
					0	10	20	30	40	50	60	70	80	90 100
ENERGY	KCAL	5.00	1.00	1	-									
VITAMIN A	IU	110.00	11.00	3	AA									
VITAMIN C	MG	4.00	26.67	7	CCCCC									
THIAMIN	MG	0.01	4.00	1	T									
RIBOFLAVN	MG	0.01	3.33	1	R									
NIACIN	MG	0.10	2.86	1	N									
IRON	MG	0.10	2.50	1	I									
CALCIUM	MG	16.00	7.11	2	X									
PHOSPHRUS	MG	11.00	4.89	1	X									
POTASSIUM	MG	136.00	10.88	3	YY									
PROTEIN	G	0.00	0.00	1	I									
CARBOHYDT	G	2.00	2.91	1	H									
FAT	G	0.00	0.00	0	I									
OLEIC A	G	0.00	0.00	0	I									
LINOL A	G	0.00	0.00	0	I									
SAT FAT A	G	0.00	0.00	0	I									

609 CELERY, RAW DICED
ANALYSIS OF 120 GRAMS WHICH IS 1 CUP

NUTRIENT	UNIT	AMOUNT	INQ	% STD
ENERGY	KCAL	20.00	1.00	1
VITAMIN A	IU	320.00	8.00	8
VITAMIN C	MG	11.00	18.33	18
THIAMIN	MG	0.04	4.00	4
RIBOFLAVN	MG	0.04	3.33	3
NIACIN	MG	0.40	2.86	3
IRON	MG	0.40	2.50	3
CALCIUM	MG	47.00	5.22	5
PHOSPHRUS	MG	34.00	3.78	4
POTASSIUM	MG	409.00	8.18	8
PROTEIN	G	1.00	2.00	2
CARBOHYDT	G	5.00	1.82	2
FAT	G	0.00	0.00	0
OLEIC A	G	0.00	0.00	0
LINOL A	G	0.00	0.00	0
SAT FAT A	G	0.00	0.00	0

610 COLLARDS, COOKED, DRAINED, FROM RAW
ANALYSIS OF 190 GRAMS WHICH IS 1 CUP

NUTRIENT	UNIT	AMOUNT	INQ	% STD
ENERGY	KCAL	65.00	1.00	3
VITAMIN A	IU	14820.00	114.00	371
VITAMIN C	MG	144.00	73.85	240
THIAMIN	MG	0.21	6.46	21
RIBOFLAVN	MG	0.38	9.74	32
NIACIN	MG	2.30	5.05	16
IRON	MG	1.50	2.88	9
CALCIUM	MG	357.00	12.21	40
PHOSPHRUS	MG	99.00	3.38	11
POTASSIUM	MG	498.00	3.06	10
PROTEIN	G	7.00	4.31	14
CARBOHYDT	G	10.00	1.12	4
FAT	G	1.00	0.39	1
OLEIC A	G	0.00	0.00	0
LINOL A	G	0.00	0.00	0
SAT FAT A	G	0.00	0.00	0

611 COLLARDS, COOKED DRAINED, FROM FROZEN
ANALYSIS OF 170 GRAMS WHICH IS 1 CUP

NUTRIENT	UNIT	AMOUNT	INQ	% STD
ENERGY	KCAL	50.00	1.00	3
VITAMIN A	IU	11560.00	115.60	289
VITAMIN C	MG	56.00	37.33	93
THIAMIN	MG	0.10	4.00	10
RIBOFLAVN	MG	0.24	8.00	20
NIACIN	MG	1.00	2.86	7
IRON	MG	1.70	4.25	11
CALCIUM	MG	299.00	13.29	33
PHOSPHRUS	MG	87.00	3.87	10
POTASSIUM	MG	401.00	3.21	8
PROTEIN	G	5.00	4.00	10
CARBOHYDT	G	10.00	1.45	4
FAT	G	1.00	0.51	1
OLEIC A	G	0.00	0.00	0
LINOL A	G	0.00	0.00	0
SAT FAT A	G	0.00	0.00	0

612 CORN, COOKED, DRAINED FROM RAW, WT WITHOUT COB
ANALYSIS OF 77 GRAMS WHICH IS 1 EAR (5 BY 1 3/4-IN)

NUTRIENT	UNIT	AMOUNT	INQ	% STD
ENERGY	KCAL	70.00	1.00	4
VITAMIN A	IU	310.00	2.21	8
VITAMIN C	MG	7.00	3.33	12
THIAMIN	MG	0.09	2.57	9
RIBOFLAVN	MG	0.08	1.90	7
NIACIN	MG	1.10	2.24	8
IRON	MG	0.50	0.89	3
CALCIUM	MG	2.00	0.06	0
PHOSPHRUS	MG	69.00	2.19	8
POTASSIUM	MG	151.00	0.86	3
PROTEIN	G	2.00	1.14	4
CARBOHYDT	G	16.00	1.66	6
FAT	G	1.00	0.37	1
OLEIC A	G	0.00	0.00	0
LINOL A	G	0.00	0.00	0
SAT FAT A	G	0.00	0.00	0

613 CORN, COOKED, DRAINED FROM FROZEN, WT WITHOUT COB
ANALYSIS OF 126 GRAMS WHICH IS 1 EAR (5-IN LONG)

```
                                      0        10        20        30        40        50        60        70        80        90       100
                                                                                                                                         * * * * * * * * * * * * * * * * *
NUTRIENT    UNIT    AMOUNT    INQ    % STD
ENERGY      KCAL    120.00    1.00    6     EEEE
VITAMIN A   IU      440.00    1.83   11     AAAAIAAAA
VITAMIN C   MG        9.00    2.50   15     CCCCICCCCCCC
THIAMIN     MG        0.18    3.00   18     TTTTITTTTTTTTT
RIBOFLAVN   MG        0.10    1.39    8     RRRRIRR
NIACIN      MG        2.10    2.50   15     NNNNINNNNNNN
IRON        MG        1.00    1.04    6     IIIII
CALCIUM     MG        4.00    0.07    0     -  I
PHOSPHRUS   MG      121.00    2.24   13     XXXXIXXXXXX
POTASSIUM   MG      291.00    0.97    6     YYYY
PROTEIN     G         4.00    1.33    8     PPPPIP
CARBOHYDT   G        27.00    1.64   10     HHHHIHHH
FAT         G         1.00    0.21    1     F
OLEIC A     G         0.00    0.00    0     -  I
LINUL A     G         0.00    0.00    0     -  I
SAT FAT A   G         0.00    0.00    0     -  I
```
****

614 CORN, COOKED, DRAINED FROM FROZEN
ANALYSIS OF 165 GRAMS WHICH IS 1 CUP KERNELS

```
                                      0        10        20        30        40        50        60        70        80        90       100
                                                                                                                                         * * * * * * * * * * * * * * * * *
NUTRIENT    UNIT    AMOUNT    INQ    % STD
ENERGY      KCAL    130.00    1.00    7     EEEEE
VITAMIN A   IU      580.00    2.23   15     AAAAIAAAAAA
VITAMIN C   MG        8.00    2.05   13     CCCCICCCCC
THIAMIN     MG        0.15    2.31   15     TTTTITTTTTT
RIBOFLAVN   MG        0.10    1.28    8     RRRRIRR
NIACIN      MG        2.50    2.75   18     NNNNINNNNNNNN
IRON        MG        1.30    1.25    8     IIIIIII
CALCIUM     MG        5.00    0.09    1     -  I
PHOSPHRUS   MG      120.00    2.05   13     XXXXIXXXXX
POTASSIUM   MG      304.00    0.94    6     YYYYY
PROTEIN     G         5.00    1.54   10     PPPPIPPP
CARBOHYDT   G        31.00    1.73   11     HHHHIHHHH
FAT         G         1.00    0.20    1     F
OLEIC A     G         0.00    0.00    0     -  I
LINUL A     G         0.00    0.00    0     -  I
SAT FAT A   G         0.00    0.00    0     -  I
```
****

615 CORN, CANNED CREAM STYLE
ANALYSIS OF 256 GRAMS WHICH IS 1 CUP

NUTRIENT	UNIT	AMOUNT	INQ	% STD
ENERGY	KCAL	210.00	1.00	11
VITAMIN A	IU	840.00	2.00	21
VITAMIN C	MG	13.00	2.06	22
THIAMIN	MG	0.08	0.76	8
RIBOFLAVN	MG	0.13	1.03	11
NIACIN	MG	2.60	1.77	19
IRON	MG	1.50	0.89	9
CALCIUM	MG	8.00	0.08	1
PHOSPHRUS	MG	143.00	1.51	16
POTASSIUM	MG	248.00	0.47	5
PROTEIN	G	5.00	0.95	10
CARBOHYDT	G	51.00	1.77	19
FAT	G	2.00	0.24	3
OLEIC A	G	0.00	0.00	0
LINOL A	G	0.00	0.00	0
SAT FAT A	G	0.00	0.00	0

616 CORN, CANNED, WHOLE KERNAL, VACUUM PACK
ANALYSIS OF 210 GRAMS WHICH IS 1 CUP

NUTRIENT	UNIT	AMOUNT	INQ	% STD
ENERGY	KCAL	175.00	1.00	9
VITAMIN A	IU	740.00	2.11	19
VITAMIN C	MG	11.00	2.10	18
THIAMIN	MG	0.06	0.69	6
RIBOFLAVN	MG	0.13	1.24	11
NIACIN	MG	2.30	1.88	16
IRON	MG	1.10	0.79	7
CALCIUM	MG	6.00	0.08	1
PHOSPHRUS	MG	153.00	1.94	17
POTASSIUM	MG	204.00	0.47	4
PROTEIN	G	5.00	1.14	10
CARBOHYDT	G	43.00	1.79	16
FAT	G	1.00	0.15	1
OLEIC A	G	0.00	0.00	0
LINOL A	G	0.00	0.00	0
SAT FAT A	G	0.00	0.00	0

617 CORN, CANNED, WET PACK, DRAINED SOLIDS
ANALYSIS OF 165 GRAMS WHICH IS 1 CUP

NUTRIENT	UNIT	AMOUNT	INQ	% STD	0 10 20 30 40 50 60 70 80 90 100
ENERGY	KCAL	140.00	1.00	7	EEEEE
VITAMIN A	IU	580.00	2.07	15	AAAAA|AAAAAA
VITAMIN C	MG	7.00	1.67	12	CCCC|CCC
THIAMIN	MG	0.05	0.71	5	TTT|
RIBOFLAVN	MG	0.08	0.95	7	RRRR|
NIACIN	MG	1.50	1.53	11	NNNNN|NNN
IRON	MG	0.80	0.71	5	IIII|
CALCIUM	MG	8.00	0.13	1	K
PHOSPHRUS	MG	81.00	1.29	9	XXXXX|X
POTASSIUM	MG	160.00	0.46	3	YYY|
PROTEIN	G	4.00	1.14	8	PPPPP
CARBOHYDT	G	33.00	1.71	12	HHHHH|HHHH
FAT	G	1.00	0.18	1	F
OLEIC A	G	0.00	0.00	0	-
LINOL A	G	0.00	0.00	0	-
SAT FAT A	G	0.00	0.00	0	-

****

618 CUCUMBER, WITH PEEL
ANALYSIS OF 28 GRAMS WHICH IS 6 LARGE OR 8 SMALL SLICES

NUTRIENT	UNIT	AMOUNT	INQ	% STD	0 10 20 30 40 50 60 70 80 90 100
ENERGY	KCAL	5.00	1.00	0	
VITAMIN A	IU	70.00	7.00	2	A
VITAMIN C	MG	3.00	20.00	5	CCCC
THIAMIN	MG	0.01	4.00	1	T
RIBOFLAVN	MG	0.01	3.33	1	R
NIACIN	MG	0.10	2.86	1	N
IRON	MG	0.30	7.50	2	II
CALCIUM	MG	7.00	3.11	1	X
PHOSPHRUS	MG	8.00	3.56	1	K
POTASSIUM	MG	45.00	3.60	1	Y
PROTEIN	G	0.00	0.00	0	-
CARBOHYDT	G	1.00	1.45	0	-
FAT	G	0.00	0.00	0	-
OLEIC A	G	0.00	0.00	0	-
LINOL A	G	0.00	0.00	0	-
SAT FAT A	G	0.00	0.00	0	-

****

619 CUCUMBER, WITHOUT PEEL
ANALYSIS OF 28 GRAMS WHICH IS 6 1/2 LARGE OR 9 SMALL SLICES

```
                                0    10   20   30   40   50   60   70   80   90   100
NUTRIENT    UNIT  AMOUNT   INQ    % STD
ENERGY      KCAL    5.00   1.00     0   I
VITAMIN A   IU      0.00   0.00     0   I
VITAMIN C   MG      3.00  20.00     5   CCCC
THIAMIN     MG      0.01   4.00     1   T
RIBOFLAVN   MG      0.01   3.33     1   R
NIACIN      MG      0.10   2.86     1   N
IRON        MG      0.10   2.50     1   I
CALCIUM     MG      5.00   2.22     1   I
PHOSPHRUS   MG      5.00   2.22     1   I
POTASSIUM   MG     45.00   3.60     1   Y
PROTEIN     G       0.00   0.00     0   I
CARBOHYDT   G       1.00   1.45     0   I
FAT         G       0.00   0.00     0   I
OLEIC A     G       0.00   0.00     0   I
LINOL A     G       0.00   0.00     0   I
SAT FAT A   G       0.00   0.00     0   I
*************************************************************
```

620 DANDELION GREENS, COOKED, DRAINED
ANALYSIS OF 105 GRAMS WHICH IS 1 CUP

```
                                    0    10   20   30   40   50   60   70   80   90   100
NUTRIENT    UNIT  AMOUNT      INQ     % STD
ENERGY      KCAL    35.00     1.00      2   E
VITAMIN A   IU   12290.00   175.57    307   AAAAAAAAAAAAAAAAAAAAAAAAAAAAAAAAAAAAAAAAAAAAAAAAAAAAAAAAAAAAAAAA * 307
VITAMIN C   MG      19.00    18.10     32   CCCCCCCCCCCCCCCCCCCCCC
THIAMIN     MG       0.14     8.00     14   TTTTTTTTT
RIBOFLAVN   MG       0.17     8.10     14   RRRRRRRRR
NIACIN      MG       0.00     0.00      0
IRON        MG       1.90     6.79     12   IIIIIIIII
CALCIUM     MG     147.00     9.33     16   KKKKKKKKKKK
PHOSPHRUS   MG      44.00     2.79      5   XXX
POTASSIUM   MG     244.00     2.79      5   YYY
PROTEIN     G        2.00     2.29      4   PP
CARBOHYDT   G        7.00     1.45      3   H
FAT         G        1.00     0.73      1   F
OLEIC A     G        0.00     0.00      0   I
LINOL A     G        0.00     0.00      0   I
SAT FAT A   G        0.00     0.00      0   I
*************************************************************
```

621 ENDIVE,CURLY,RAW SMALL PIECES
ANALYSIS OF 50 GRAMS WHICH IS 1 CUP

NUTRIENT	UNIT	AMOUNT	INQ	% STD	0 10 20 30 40 50 60 70 80 90 100
ENERGY	KCAL	10.00	1.00	1	-
VITAMIN A	IU	1650.00	82.50	41	AAAAAAAAAAAAAAAAAAAAAAAAAAAAAAAAAAAAAAAAA
VITAMIN C	MG	5.00	16.67	8	CCCCCCC
THIAMIN	MG	0.04	8.00	4	TTT
RIBOFLAVN	MG	0.07	11.67	6	RRRR
NIACIN	MG	0.30	4.29	2	NN
IRON	MG	0.90	11.25	6	IIIII
CALCIUM	MG	41.00	9.11	5	KKKK
PHOSPHRUS	MG	27.00	6.00	3	XX
POTASSIUM	MG	147.00	5.88	3	YY
PROTEIN	G	1.00	4.00	2	PP
CARBOHYDT	G	2.00	1.45	1	H
FAT	G	0.00	0.00	0	-
OLEIC A	G	0.00	0.00	0	-
LINOL A	G	0.00	0.00	0	-
SAT FAT A	G	0.00	0.00	0	-

622 KALE, COOKED, DRAINED, FROM RAW, LEAVES WITHOUT STEMS
ANALYSIS OF 110 GRAMS WHICH IS 1 CUP

NUTRIENT	UNIT	AMOUNT	INQ	% STD	0 10 20 30 40 50 60 70 80 90 100
ENERGY	KCAL	45.00	1.00	2	EE
VITAMIN A	IU	9130.00	101.44	228	AIAAAAAAAAAAAAAAAAAAAAAAAAAAAAAAAAAAAAAAAAAAAAAAAAAAAAAAAAAAAAAAAAAAAAAAAAAAAAAAAAAAAAAAAAAAA * 228
VITAMIN C	MG	102.00	75.56	170	CICCCCCCCCCCCCCCCCCCCCCCCCCCCCCCCCCCCCCCCCCCCCCCCCCCCCCCCCCCCCCCCCCCCCCCC * 170
THIAMIN	MG	0.11	4.89	11	TITTTTTT
RIBOFLAVN	MG	0.20	7.41	17	RIRRRRRRRRR
NIACIN	MG	1.80	5.71	13	NINNNNNNN
IRON	MG	1.80	5.00	11	IIIIIIII
CALCIUM	MG	206.00	10.17	23	KIKKKKKKKKKKKKK
PHOSPHRUS	MG	64.00	3.16	7	XIXXXX
POTASSIUM	MG	243.00	2.16	5	YIYY
PROTEIN	G	7.00	4.44	10	PIPPPPP
CARBOHYDT	G	7.00	1.13	3	HH
FAT	G	1.00	0.57	1	FI
OLEIC A	G	0.00	0.00	0	-I
LINOL A	G	0.00	0.00	0	-I
SAT FAT A	G	0.00	0.00	0	-I

623 KALE, COOKED, DRAINED, FROM FROZEN, LEAF STYLE
ANALYSIS OF 130 GRAMS WHICH IS 1 CUP

```
NUTRIENT   UNIT  AMOUNT      INQ    % STD    0        10        20        30        40        50        60        70        80        90       100
ENERGY     KCAL   40.00     1.00        2    EE                                                                                                    *
VITAMIN A  IU  10660.00  133.25      266    AIAAAAAAAAAAAAAAAAAAAAAAAAAAAAAAAAAAAAAAAAAAAAAAAAAAAAAAAAAAAAAAAAAAAAAAAAAAAAAAAAAAA * 266
VITAMIN C  MG     49.00    40.83       82    CICCCCCCCCCCCCCCCCCCCCCCCCCCCCCCCCCCCCCCCCCCCCCCCCCCCCCCCCCCCCCCCCCCCCCCCCCCCCCCCC *
THIAMIN    MG      0.08     4.00        8    TITTTT                                                                                              *
RIBOFLAVN  MG      0.20     8.33       17    RIRRRRRRRRRR                                                                                        *
NIACIN     MG      0.90     3.21        6    NINNN                                                                                               *
IRON       MG      1.30     4.06        8    IIIIIII                                                                                             *
CALCIUM    MG    157.00     8.72       17    KIKKKKKKKKKKK                                                                                       *
PHOSPHRUS  MG     62.00     3.44        7    XIXXXX                                                                                              *
POTASSIUM  MG    251.00     2.51        5    YIYY                                                                                                *
PROTEIN    G       4.00     4.00        8    PIPPPP                                                                                              *
CARBOHYDT  G       7.00     1.27        3    HH                                                                                                  *
FAT        G       1.00     0.64        1    FI                                                                                                  *
OLEIC A    G       0.00     0.00        0    -I                                                                                                  *
LINOL A    G       0.00     0.00        0    -I                                                                                                  *
SAT FAT A  G       0.00     0.00        0    -I                                                                                                  *
*******************************************************************************************************************************
```

624 BUTTERHEAD LETTUCE, RAW
ANALYSIS OF 220 GRAMS WHICH IS 1 HEAD, 5-IN DIAM.

```
NUTRIENT   UNIT  AMOUNT     INQ    % STD    0        10        20        30        40        50        60        70        80        90       100
ENERGY     KCAL   25.00    1.00        1    E                                                                                                    *
VITAMIN A  IU  1580.00   31.60       40    IAAAAAAAAAAAAAAAAAAAAAAAAAAAAAAAAA                                                                    *
VITAMIN C  MG     13.00   17.33       22    ICCCCCCCCCCCCCCCCCC                                                                                  *
THIAMIN    MG      0.10    8.00       10    ITTTTTT                                                                                              *
RIBOFLAVN  MG      0.10    6.67        8    IRRRRR                                                                                               *
NIACIN     MG      0.50    2.86        4    INN                                                                                                  *
IRON       MG      3.30   16.50       21    IIIIIIIIIIIIIIII                                                                                     *
CALCIUM    MG     57.00    5.07        6    IKKK                                                                                                 *
PHOSPHRUS  MG     42.00    3.73        5    IXXX                                                                                                 *
POTASSIUM  MG    430.00    6.88        9    IYYYYY                                                                                               *
PROTEIN    G       2.00    3.20        4    IPP                                                                                                  *
CARBOHYDT  G       4.00    1.16        1    H                                                                                                    *
FAT        G       0.00    0.00        0    I                                                                                                    *
OLEIC A    G       0.00    0.00        0    I                                                                                                    *
LINOL A    G       0.00    0.00        0    I                                                                                                    *
SAT FAT A  G       0.00    0.00        0    -                                                                                                    *
*******************************************************************************************************************************
```

625 BUTTERHEAD LETTUCE, RAW
ANALYSIS OF 15 GRAMS WHICH IS 1 OUTER OR 2 INNER OR 3 HEART LEAVES

NUTRIENT	UNIT	AMOUNT	INQ	% STD	0	10	20	30	40	50	60	70	80	90	100
ENERGY	KCAL	0.00	0.00	0	-										*********************
VITAMIN A	IU	150.00	1.00*********	4	AAA										
VITAMIN C	MG	1.00*********		2	C										
THIAMIN	MG	0.01*********		1	T										
RIBOFLAVN	MG	0.01*********		1	R										
NIACIN	MG	0.00	0.00	0	-										
IRON	MG	0.30*********		2	II										
CALCIUM	MG	5.00*********		1	-										
PHOSPHRUS	MG	4.00*********		0	-										
POTASSIUM	MG	40.00*********		1	Y										
PROTEIN	G	0.00	0.00	0	-										
CARBOHYDT	G	0.00	0.00	0	-										
FAT	G	0.00	0.00	0	-										
OLEIC A	G	0.00	0.00	0	-										
LINOL A	G	0.00	0.00	0	-										
SAT FAT A	G	0.00	0.00	0	-										

****

626 ICEBERG LETTUCE (CRISPHEAD)
ANALYSIS OF 567 GRAMS WHICH IS 1 HEAD, 6-IN DIAM

NUTRIENT	UNIT	AMOUNT	INQ	% STD	0	10	20	30	40	50	60	70	80	90	100
ENERGY	KCAL	70.00	1.00	4	EEE										*********************
VITAMIN A	IU	1780.00	12.71	45	AA	AAAAAAAAAAAAAAAAAAAAAAAAAAA									
VITAMIN C	MG	32.00	15.24	53	CC	CCCCCCCCCCCCCCCCCCCCCCCCCCCCCCCC								
THIAMIN	MG	0.32	9.14	32	TT	TTTTTTTTTTTTTTTTTTT									
RIBOFLAVN	MG	0.32	7.62	27	RR	RRRRRRRRRRRRRR									
NIACIN	MG	1.60	3.27	11	NN	NNNNN									
IRON	MG	2.70	4.82	17	II	IIIIIIIII									
CALCIUM	MG	108.00	3.43	12	KK	KKKKKK									
PHOSPHRUS	MG	118.00	3.75	13	XX	XXXXX									
POTASSIUM	MG	943.00	5.39	19	YY	YYYYYYY									
PROTEIN	G	5.00	2.86	10	PP	PPPP									
CARBOHYDT	G	16.00	1.66	6	HH	HH									
FAT	G	1.00	0.37	1	F										
OLEIC A	G	0.00	0.00	0	-										
LINOL A	G	0.00	0.00	0	-										
SAT FAT A	G	0.00	0.00	0	-										

****

627 ICEBERG LETTUCE (CRISPHEAD)
ANALYSIS OF 135 GRAMS WHICH IS 1 WEDGE (1/4 HEAD)

```
                                      0   10   20   30   40   50   60   70   80   90  100
                                      **************************************************
NUTRIENT    UNIT   AMOUNT    INQ  % STD
ENERGY      KCAL    20.00   1.00    1   E
VITAMIN A   IU     450.00  11.25   11   AAAAAAA
VITAMIN C   MG       8.00  13.33   13   CCCCCCCCC
THIAMIN     MG       0.08   8.00    8   TTTTT
RIBOFLAVN   MG       0.08   6.67    7   RRRR
NIACIN      MG       0.40   2.86    3   N
IRON        MG       0.70   4.38    4   IIII
CALCIUM     MG      27.00   3.00    3   IK
PHOSPHRUS   MG      30.00   3.33    3   Ixx
POTASSIUM   MG     236.00   4.72    5   IYYY
PROTEIN     G        1.00   2.00    2   IP
CARBOHYDT   G        4.00   1.45    1   H
FAT         G        0.00   0.00    0   I
OLEIC A     G        0.00   0.00    0   I
LINOL A     G        0.00   0.00    0   I
SAT FAT A   G        0.00   0.00    0
                                      **************************************************
```

628 ICEBERG LETTUCE, (CRISPHEAD), PIECES, CHOPPED OR SHREDDED
ANALYSIS OF 55 GRAMS WHICH IS 1 CUP

```
                                      0   10   20   30   40   50   60   70   80   90  100
                                      **************************************************
NUTRIENT    UNIT   AMOUNT    INQ  % STD
ENERGY      KCAL     5.00   1.00    0   E
VITAMIN A   IU     180.00  18.00    5   AAAA
VITAMIN C   MG       3.00  20.00    5   CCCC
THIAMIN     MG       0.03  12.00    3   TT
RIBOFLAVN   MG       0.03  10.00    3   RR
NIACIN      MG       0.20   5.71    1   N
IRON        MG       0.30   7.50    2   II
CALCIUM     MG      11.00   4.89    1   K
PHOSPHRUS   MG      12.00   5.33    1   X
POTASSIUM   MG      96.00   7.68    2   YY
PROTEIN     G        0.00   0.00    0   I
CARBOHYDT   G        2.00   2.91    1   H
FAT         G        0.00   0.00    0   I
OLEIC A     G        0.00   0.00    0   I
LINOL A     G        0.00   0.00    0   I
SAT FAT A   G        0.00   0.00    0
                                      **************************************************
```

629 LOOSELEAF LETTUCE, CHOPPED OR SHREDDED
ANALYSIS OF 55 GRAMS WHICH IS 1 CUP

NUTRIENT	UNIT	AMOUNT	INQ	% STD	Chart
ENERGY	KCAL	10.00	1.00	1	-
VITAMIN A	IU	1050.00	52.50	26	AAAAAAAAAAAAAAAAAAAAAAAAAA
VITAMIN C	MG	10.00	33.33	17	CCCCCCCCCCCCCCCCC
THIAMIN	MG	0.03	6.00	3	TT
RIBOFLAVN	MG	0.04	6.67	3	RRR
NIACIN	MG	0.20	2.86	1	N
IRON	MG	0.80	10.00	5	IIIII
CALCIUM	MG	37.00	8.22	4	KKKK
PHOSPHRUS	MG	14.00	3.11	2	X
POTASSIUM	MG	145.00	5.80	3	YY
PROTEIN	G	1.00	4.00	2	PP
CARBOHYDT	G	2.00	1.45	1	H
FAT	G	0.00	0.00	0	-
OLEIC A	G	0.00	0.00	0	-
LINOL A	G	0.00	0.00	0	-
SAT FAT A	G	0.00	0.00	0	-

630 MUSHROOMS, RAW, SLICED OR CHOPPED
ANALYSIS OF 70 GRAMS WHICH IS 1 CUP

NUTRIENT	UNIT	AMOUNT	INQ	% STD	Chart
ENERGY	KCAL	20.00	1.00	1	E
VITAMIN A	IU	0.00	0.00	1	
VITAMIN C	MG	2.00	3.33	3	ICC
THIAMIN	MG	0.07	7.00	7	ITTTTT
RIBOFLAVN	MG	0.32	26.67	27	IRRRRRRRRRRRRRRRRRRRRRRRRRR
NIACIN	MG	2.90	20.71	21	INNNNNNNNNNNNNNNNNNN
IRON	MG	0.60	3.75	4	III
CALCIUM	MG	4.00	0.44	0	I
PHOSPHRUS	MG	81.00	9.00	9	IXXXXXX
POTASSIUM	MG	290.00	5.80	6	IYYYY
PROTEIN	G	4.00	4.00	4	IPP
CARBOHYDT	G	3.00	1.09	1	H
FAT	G	0.00	0.00	0	-
OLEIC A	G	0.00	0.00	0	-
LINOL A	G	0.00	0.00	0	-
SAT FAT A	G	0.00	0.00	0	-

631 MUSTARD GREENS, COOKED, DRAINED, WITHOUT STEMS
ANALYSIS OF 140 GRAMS WHICH IS 1 CUP

NUTRIENT	UNIT	AMOUNT	INQ	% STD	Chart
ENERGY	KCAL	30.00	1.00	2	E
VITAMIN A	IU	8120.00	135.33	203	AAAAAAAAAAAAAAAAAAAAAAAAAAAAAAAAAAAAAAAA * 203
VITAMIN C	MG	67.00	74.44	112	CCCCCCCCCCCCCCCCCCCCCCCC * 112
THIAMIN	MG	0.11	7.33	11	TTTTTTT
RIBOFLAVN	MG	0.20	11.11	17	RRRRRRRRRR
NIACIN	MG	0.80	3.81	6	NNNN
IRON	MG	2.50	10.42	16	IIIIIIIIIII
CALCIUM	MG	193.00	14.30	21	KKKKKKKKKKKKK
PHOSPHRUS	MG	45.00	3.33	5	XXX
POTASSIUM	MG	308.00	4.11	6	YYYY
PROTEIN	G	3.00	4.00	6	PPPP
CARBOHYDT	G	6.00	1.45	2	IH
FAT	G	1.00	0.85	1	F
OLEIC A	G	0.00	0.00	0	
LINOL A	G	0.00	0.00	0	
SAT FAT A	G	0.00	0.00	0	

632 OKRA PODS, COOKED
ANALYSIS OF 106 GRAMS WHICH IS 10 PODS 3 BY 5/8 IN

NUTRIENT	UNIT	AMOUNT	INQ	% STD	Chart
ENERGY	KCAL	30.00	1.00	2	E
VITAMIN A	IU	520.00	8.67	13	AAAAAAAA
VITAMIN C	MG	21.00	23.33	35	CCCCCCCCCCCCCCCCCCCCCCCC
THIAMIN	MG	0.14	9.33	14	TTTTTTTT
RIBOFLAVN	MG	0.19	10.56	16	RRRRRRRRRR
NIACIN	MG	1.00	4.76	7	NNNNN
IRON	MG	0.50	2.08	3	II
CALCIUM	MG	98.00	7.26	11	KKKKKKK
PHOSPHRUS	MG	43.00	3.19	5	XXX
POTASSIUM	MG	184.00	2.45	4	YY
PROTEIN	G	2.45	2.67	4	PP
CARBOHYDT	G	6.00	1.45	2	IH
FAT	G	0.00	0.00	0	
OLEIC A	G	0.00	0.00	0	
LINOL A	G	0.00	0.00	0	
SAT FAT A	G	0.00	0.00	0	

```
                                          100 * * * * * * * * * * * * * * * * * *

                                           90

                                           80

                                           70

                                           60

                                           50

                                           40

                                           30

                                           20

                                           10

633  ONIONS, MATURE, RAW, CHOPPED
ANALYSIS OF 170 GRAMS WHICH IS 1 CUP

NUTRIENT   UNIT   AMOUNT   INQ    % STD   0
ENERGY     KCAL    65.00   1.00      3    EEE
VITAMIN A  IU       0.00   0.00      0    I
VITAMIN C  MG      17.00   8.72     28    CC|CCCCCCCCCCCCCCCCCCC
THIAMIN    MG       0.05   1.54      5    T|T
RIBOFLAVN  MG       0.07   1.79      6    RR|RR
NIACIN     MG       0.30   0.66      2    NN|
IRON       MG       0.90   1.73      6    II|II
CALCIUM    MG      46.00   1.57      5    KK|K
PHOSPHRUS  MG      61.00   2.09      7    XX|XX
POTASSIUM  MG     267.00   1.64      5    YY|Y
PROTEIN    G         3.00   1.85      6    PP|PP
CARBOHYDT  G       15.00   1.68      5    HH|H
FAT        G         0.00   0.00      0    - |
OLEIC A    G         0.00   0.00      0    - |
LINOL A    G         0.00   0.00      0    - |
SAT FAT A  G         0.00   0.00      0    - |
*************************************************
```

```
                                          100 * * * * * * * * * * * * * * * * *

                                           90

                                           80

                                           70

                                           60

                                           50

                                           40

                                           30

                                           20

                                           10

634  ONIONS, MATURE, RAW SLICED
ANALYSIS OF 115 GRAMS WHICH IS 1 CUP

NUTRIENT   UNIT   AMOUNT   INQ    % STD   0
ENERGY     KCAL    45.00   1.00      2    EE
VITAMIN A  IU       0.00   0.00      0    I
VITAMIN C  MG      12.00   8.89     20    C|CCCCCCCCCCC
THIAMIN    MG       0.03   1.33      3    TT
RIBOFLAVN  MG       0.05   1.85      4    R|R
NIACIN     MG       0.20   0.63      1    N|
IRON       MG       0.60   1.67      4    II|I
CALCIUM    MG      31.00   1.53      3    K|K
PHOSPHRUS  MG      41.00   2.02      5    X|XX
POTASSIUM  MG     181.00   1.61      4    Y|Y
PROTEIN    G         2.00   1.78      4    P|P
CARBOHYDT  G       10.00   1.62      4    H|H
FAT        G         0.00   0.00      0    - |
OLEIC A    G         0.00   0.00      0    - |
LINOL A    G         0.00   0.00      0    - |
SAT FAT A  G         0.00   0.00      0    - |
*************************************************
```

```
                                              0    10   20   30   40   50   60   70   80   90   100
                                                                                                 * * * * * * * * * * * * * * * * * *
```

635 ONIONS, MATURE, COOKED, DRAINED, WHOLE OR SLICED
ANALYSIS OF 210 GRAMS WHICH IS 1 CUP

NUTRIENT	UNIT	AMOUNT	INQ	% STD	0	10	20
ENERGY	KCAL	60.00	1.00	3	E		
VITAMIN A	IU	0.00	0.00	0	I		
VITAMIN C	MG	15.00	8.33	25	CICCCCCCCCCCCCCCCCCC		
THIAMIN	MG	0.06	2.00	6	TITTT		
RIBOFLAVN	MG	0.06	1.67	5	RIRR		
NIACIN	MG	0.40	0.95	3	NN		
IRON	MG	0.80	1.67	5	IIII		
CALCIUM	MG	50.00	1.85	6	KIKK		
PHOSPHRUS	MG	61.00	2.26	7	XIXXX		
POTASSIUM	MG	231.00	1.54	5	YIYY		
PROTEIN	G	3.00	2.00	6	PIPPP		
CARBOHYDT	G	14.00	1.70	5	HIHH		
FAT	G	0.00	0.00	0	I		
OLEIC A	G	0.00	0.00	0	I		
LINOL A	G	0.00	0.00	0	I		
SAT FAT A	G	0.00	0.00	0	I		

```
************************************************
```

```
                                              0    10   20   30   40   50   60   70   80   90   100
                                                                                                 * * * * * * * * * * * * * * * * * *
```

636 GREEN ONION
ANALYSIS OF 30 GRAMS WHICH IS 6 ONIONS (3/8-IN DIAM BULB)

NUTRIENT	UNIT	AMOUNT	INQ	% STD	0	10	20
ENERGY	KCAL	15.00	1.00	1	E		
VITAMIN A	IU	0.00	0.00	0	I		
VITAMIN C	MG	8.00	17.78	13	ICCCCCCCC		
THIAMIN	MG	0.02	2.67	2	IT		
RIBOFLAVN	MG	0.01	1.11	1	R		
NIACIN	MG	0.10	0.95	1	N		
IRON	MG	0.20	1.67	1	I		
CALCIUM	MG	12.00	1.78	1	K		
PHOSPHRUS	MG	12.00	1.78	1	X		
POTASSIUM	MG	69.00	1.84	1	Y		
PROTEIN	G	0.00	0.00	0	I		
CARBOHYDT	G	3.00	1.45	1	H		
FAT	G	0.00	0.00	0	I		
OLEIC A	G	0.00	0.00	0	I		
LINOL A	G	0.00	0.00	0	I		
SAT FAT A	G	0.00	0.00	0	I		

```
************************************************
```

637 PARSLEY, RAW, CHOPPED
ANALYSIS OF 4 GRAMS WHICH IS 1 TBSP

```
                                   0    10   20   30   40   50   60   70   80   90  100
                                   * * * * * * * * * * * * * * * * * * * *
NUTRIENT   UNIT  AMOUNT    INQ  % STD
ENERGY     KCAL      0.00  0.00   0   -
VITAMIN A  IU    300.00******** 8   AAAAAA
VITAMIN C  MG      6.00******** 10  CCCCCCC
THIAMIN    MG      0.00  0.00   0   -
RIBOFLAVN  MG      0.01******** 1   R
NIACIN     MG      0.00  0.00   0   -
IRON       MG      0.20******** 1   I
CALCIUM    MG      7.00******** 1   K
PHOSPHRUS  MG      2.00******** 0   -
POTASSIUM  MG     25.00******** 1   -
PROTEIN    G       0.00  0.00   0   -
CARBOHYDT  G       0.00  0.00   0   -
FAT        G       0.00  0.00   0   -
OLEIC A    G       0.00  0.00   0   -
LINOL A    G       0.00  0.00   0   -
SAT FAT A  G       0.00  0.00   0   -
*****************************************
```

638 PARSNIPS, COOKED, DICED
ANALYSIS OF 155 GRAMS WHICH IS 1 CUP

```
                                   0    10   20   30   40   50   60   70   80   90  100
                                   * * * * * * * * * * * * * * * * * * * *
NUTRIENT   UNIT  AMOUNT    INQ  % STD
ENERGY     KCAL   100.00   1.00   5   EEEE
VITAMIN A  IU      50.00   0.25   1   A
VITAMIN C  MG      16.00   5.33  27   CCC|CCCCCCCCCCCCCCC
THIAMIN    MG       0.11   2.20  11   TTT|TTTTT
RIBOFLAVN  MG       0.12   2.00  10   RRR|RRRR
NIACIN     MG       0.20   0.29   1   N
IRON       MG       0.90   1.13   6   III|II
CALCIUM    MG      70.00   1.56   8   KKK|KK
PHOSPHRUS  MG      96.00   2.13  11   XXX|XXXXX
POTASSIUM  MG     587.00   2.35  12   YYY|YYYYY
PROTEIN    G        2.00   0.80   4   PPP|
CARBOHYDT  G       23.00   1.67   8   HHH|HHH
FAT        G        1.00   0.26   1   F|
OLEIC A    G        0.00   0.00   0   -
LINOL A    G        0.00   0.00   0   -
SAT FAT A  G        0.00   0.00   0   -
*****************************************
```

639 GREEN PEAS, CANNED, DRAINED SOLIDS
ANALYSIS OF 170 GRAMS WHICH IS 1 CUP

NUTRIENT	UNIT	AMOUNT	INQ	% STD
ENERGY	KCAL	150.00	1.00	8
VITAMIN A	IU	1170.00	3.90	29
VITAMIN C	MG	14.00	3.11	23
THIAMIN	MG	0.15	2.00	15
RIBOFLAVN	MG	0.10	1.11	8
NIACIN	MG	1.40	1.33	10
IRON	MG	3.20	2.67	20
CALCIUM	MG	44.00	0.65	5
PHOSPHRUS	MG	129.00	1.91	14
POTASSIUM	MG	163.00	0.43	3
PROTEIN	G	8.00	2.13	16
CARBOHYDT	G	29.00	1.41	11
FAT	G	1.00	0.17	1
OLEIC A	G	0.00	0.00	0
LINOL A	G	0.00	0.00	0
SAT FAT A	G	0.00	0.00	0

640 GREEN PEAS, STRAINED (BABY FOOD)
ANALYSIS OF 28 GRAMS WHICH IS 1 OZ (1 3/4 TO 2 TBSP)

NUTRIENT	UNIT	AMOUNT	INQ	% STD
ENERGY	KCAL	15.00	1.00	1
VITAMIN A	IU	140.00	4.67	4
VITAMIN C	MG	3.00	6.67	5
THIAMIN	MG	0.02	2.67	2
RIBOFLAVN	MG	0.03	3.33	3
NIACIN	MG	0.30	2.86	2
IRON	MG	0.30	2.50	2
CALCIUM	MG	3.00	0.44	0
PHOSPHRUS	MG	18.00	2.67	2
POTASSIUM	MG	28.00	0.75	1
PROTEIN	G	1.00	1.45	1
CARBOHYDT	G	3.00	0.00	0
FAT	G	0.00	0.00	0
OLEIC A	G	0.00	0.00	0
LINOL A	G	0.00	0.00	0
SAT FAT A	G	0.00	0.00	0

641 GREEN PEAS, FROZEN, COOKED, DRAINED
ANALYSIS OF 160 GRAMS WHICH IS 1 CUP

```
                                          0    10   20   30   40   50   60   70   80   90  100
NUTRIENT    UNIT   AMOUNT    INQ   % STD
ENERGY      KCAL   110.00    1.00     6    EEEE
VITAMIN A   IU     960.00    4.36    24    AAAIAAAAAAAAAAAAA
VITAMIN C   MG      21.00    6.36    35    CCCICCCCCCCCCCCCCCCCCCCCCC
THIAMIN     MG       0.43    7.82    43    TTTITTTTTTTTTTTTTTTTTTTTTTTTTTTTT
RIBOFLAVN   MG       0.14    2.12    12    RRRIRRRRR
NIACIN      MG       2.70    3.51    19    NNNINNNNNNNNNNN
IRON        MG       3.00    3.41    19    IIIIIIIIIIIIII
CALCIUM     MG      30.00    0.61     3    KKKI
PHOSPHRUS   MG     138.00    2.79    15    XXXIXXXXXXX
POTASSIUM   MG     216.00    0.79     4    YYYI
PROTEIN     G        8.00    2.91    16    PPPIPPPPPPP
CARBOHYDT   G       19.00    1.26     7    HHHIHH
FAT         G        0.00    0.00     0    - I
OLEIC A     G        0.00    0.00     0    - I
LINOL A     G        0.00    0.00     0    - I
SAT FAT A   G        0.00    0.00     0    -
**********************************************************
```

642 PEPPERS, HOT, RED, WITHOUT SEEDS, DRIED (GROUND CHILI PWDR ADDED SEASONING)
ANALYSIS OF 2 GRAMS WHICH IS 1 TSP

```
                                          0    10   20   30   40   50   60   70   80   90  100
NUTRIENT    UNIT   AMOUNT    INQ   % STD
ENERGY      KCAL     5.00    1.00     0    -
VITAMIN A   IU    1300.00  130.00    33    AAAAAAAAAAAAAAAAAAAAAAAAAAA
VITAMIN C   MG       0.00    0.00     0    -
THIAMIN     MG       0.02    6.67     2    R
RIBOFLAVN   MG       0.20    5.71     1    N
NIACIN      MG       0.30    7.50     2    II
IRON        MG       5.00    2.22     1    -
CALCIUM     MG       4.00    1.78     0    -
PHOSPHRUS   MG      20.00    1.60     0    -
POTASSIUM   G        1.00    1.45     0    -
PROTEIN     G        0.00    0.00     0    -
CARBOHYDT   G        0.00    0.00     0    -
FAT         G        0.00    0.00     0    -
OLEIC A     G        0.00    0.00     0    -
LINOL A     G        0.00    0.00     0    -
SAT FAT A   G        0.00    0.00     0
**********************************************************
```

643 SWEET PEPPERS, RAW
ANALYSIS OF 74 GRAMS WHICH IS 1 POD (5 PER LB)

NUTRIENT	UNIT	AMOUNT	INQ	% STD
ENERGY	KCAL	15.00	1.00	1
VITAMIN A	IU	310.00	10.33	8
VITAMIN C	MG	94.00	208.89	157
THIAMIN	MG	0.06	8.00	6
RIBOFLAVN	MG	0.06	6.67	5
NIACIN	MG	0.40	3.81	3
IRON	MG	0.50	4.17	3
CALCIUM	MG	7.00	1.04	1
PHOSPHRUS	MG	16.00	2.37	2
POTASSIUM	MG	157.00	4.19	3
PROTEIN	G	1.00	2.67	2
CARBOHYDT	G	4.00	1.94	1
FAT	G	0.00	0.00	0
OLEIC A	G	0.00	0.00	0
LINOL A	G	0.00	0.00	0
SAT FAT A	G	0.00	0.00	0

644 SWEET PEPPERS, COOKED, DRAINED
ANALYSIS OF 73 GRAMS WHICH IS 1 POD

NUTRIENT	UNIT	AMOUNT	INQ	% STD
ENERGY	KCAL	15.00	1.00	1
VITAMIN A	IU	310.00	10.33	8
VITAMIN C	MG	70.00	155.56	117
THIAMIN	MG	0.05	6.67	5
RIBOFLAVN	MG	0.05	5.56	4
NIACIN	MG	0.40	3.81	3
IRON	MG	0.40	3.33	3
CALCIUM	MG	7.00	1.04	1
PHOSPHRUS	MG	12.00	1.78	1
POTASSIUM	MG	109.00	2.91	2
PROTEIN	G	1.00	2.67	2
CARBOHYDT	G	3.00	1.45	1
FAT	G	0.00	0.00	0
OLEIC A	G	0.00	0.00	0
LINOL A	G	0.00	0.00	0
SAT FAT A	G	0.00	0.00	0

```
                                                        0        10        20        30        40        50        60        70        80        90        100
```

645   BAKED POTATO, PEELED AFTER BAKING
ANALYSIS OF 156 GRAMS WHICH IS 1 POTATO (2 PER LB)

NUTRIENT	UNIT	AMOUNT	INQ	% STD	
ENERGY	KCAL	145.00	1.00	7	EEEEE
VITAMIN A	IU	0.00	0.00	0	-
VITAMIN C	MG	31.00	7.13	52	CCCCICCCCCCCCCCCCCCCCCCCCCCCCCC
THIAMIN	MG	0.15	2.07	15	TTTTIITTTTT
RIBOFLAVN	MG	0.07	0.80	6	RRRRI
NIACIN	MG	2.70	2.66	19	NNNNININNNNNNNNN
IRON	MG	1.10	0.95	7	IIIIII
CALCIUM	MG	14.00	0.21	2	K
PHOSPHRUS	MG	101.00	1.55	11	XXXXXIXXX
POTASSIUM	MG	782.00	2.16	16	YYYYYIYYYYYYY
PROTEIN	G	4.00	1.10	8	PPPPPP
CARBOHYDT	G	33.00	1.66	12	HHHHHIHHHH
FAT	G	0.00	0.00	0	-
OLEIC A	G	0.00	0.00	0	-
LINOL A	G	0.00	0.00	0	-
SAT FAT A	G	0.00	0.00	0	-

646   BOILED POTATO, PEELED AFTER BOILING
ANALYSIS OF 137 GRAMS WHICH IS 1 POTATO (3 PER LB)

NUTRIENT	UNIT	AMOUNT	INQ	% STD	
ENERGY	KCAL	105.00	1.00	5	EEEE
VITAMIN A	IU	0.00	0.00	0	-
VITAMIN C	MG	22.00	6.98	37	CCCICCCCCCCCCCCCCCCCCCCCCCC
THIAMIN	MG	0.12	2.29	12	TTTITTTTTTT
RIBOFLAVN	MG	0.05	0.79	4	RRRI
NIACIN	MG	2.00	2.72	14	NNNINNNNNNNN
IRON	MG	0.80	0.95	5	IIII
CALCIUM	MG	10.00	0.21	1	K
PHOSPHRUS	MG	72.00	1.52	8	XXXIXX
POTASSIUM	MG	556.00	2.12	11	YYYIYYYYY
PROTEIN	G	3.00	1.14	6	PPPIP
CARBOHYDT	G	23.00	1.59	8	HHHIHHH
FAT	G	0.00	0.00	0	-
OLEIC A	G	0.00	0.00	0	-
LINOL A	G	0.00	0.00	0	-
SAT FAT A	G	0.00	0.00	0	-

647 BOILED POTATOES, PEELED BEFORE BOILING
ANALYSIS OF 135 GRAMS WHICH IS 1 POTATO (3 PER LB)

```
                                                        0    10   20   30   40   50   60   70   80   90   100
```

NUTRIENT	UNIT	AMOUNT	INQ	% STD											
ENERGY	KCAL	90.00	1.00	5	EEEE
VITAMIN A	IU	0.00	0.00	0	-
VITAMIN C	MG	22.00	8.15	37	CCCICCCCCCCCCCCCCCCCCCCCCCC
THIAMIN	MG	0.12	2.67	12	TTTITTTTT
RIBOFLAVN	MG	0.05	0.93	4	RRRI
NIACIN	MG	1.60	2.54	11	NNNINNNNN
IRON	MG	0.70	0.97	4	IIII
CALCIUM	MG	8.00	0.20	1	K
PHOSPHRUS	MG	57.00	1.41	6	XXXIX
POTASSIUM	MG	385.00	1.71	8	YYYIYY
PROTEIN	G	3.00	1.33	6	PPPIP
CARBOHYDT	G	20.00	1.62	7	HHHIHH
FAT	G	0.00	0.00	0	-
OLEIC A	G	0.00	0.00	0	-
LINOL A	G	0.00	0.00	0	-
SAT FAT A	G	0.00	0.00	0	-

****

648 FRENCH FRIED POTATOES, PREPARED FROM RAW
ANALYSIS OF 50 GRAMS WHICH IS 10 STRIPS 2 TO 3 1/2 IN LONG

```
                                                        0    10   20   30   40   50   60   70   80   90   100
```

NUTRIENT	UNIT	AMOUNT	INQ	% STD											
ENERGY	KCAL	135.00	1.00	7	EEEEE
VITAMIN A	IU	0.00	0.00	0	-
VITAMIN C	MG	11.00	2.72	18	CCCICCCCCCCCC
THIAMIN	MG	0.07	1.04	7	TITTIT
RIBOFLAVN	MG	0.04	0.49	3	RRRI
NIACIN	MG	1.60	1.69	11	NNNINNNN
IRON	MG	0.70	0.65	4	IIII
CALCIUM	MG	8.00	0.13	1	K
PHOSPHRUS	MG	56.00	0.92	6	XXXXX
POTASSIUM	MG	427.00	1.27	9	YYYYIYY
PROTEIN	G	2.00	0.59	4	PPPI
CARBOHYDT	G	18.00	0.97	7	HHHHH
FAT	G	7.00	1.33	9	FFFFIFF
OLEIC A	G	1.20	0.73	5	OOOOI
LINOL A	G	3.30	2.44	17	LLLLILLLLLLLLL
SAT FAT A	G	1.70	0.88	6	SSSSS

****

649 FRENCH FRIED POTATOES, FROZEN, OVEN HEATED
ANALYSIS OF 50 GRAMS WHICH IS 10 STRIPS

```
NUTRIENT   UNIT  AMOUNT  INQ   % STD  0        10        20        30   40   50   60   70   80   90   100
ENERGY     KCAL  110.00  1.00    6    EEEE
VITAMIN A  IU      0.00  0.00    0    -
VITAMIN C  MG     11.00  3.33   18    CCCICCCCCCCCCCC
THIAMIN    MG      0.07  1.27    7    TTTITT
RIBOFLAVN  MG      0.01  0.15    1    R
NIACIN     MG      1.30  1.69    9    NNNINNN
IRON       MG      0.90  1.02    6    IIIII
CALCIUM    MG      5.00  0.10    1    -
PHOSPHRUS  MG     43.00  0.87    5    XXXX
POTASSIUM  MG    326.00  1.19    7    YYYIY
PROTEIN    G       2.00  0.73    4    PPPI
CARBOHYDT  G      17.00  1.12    6    HHHIH
FAT        G       4.00  0.93    5    FFFF
OLEIC A    G       0.80  0.59    3    OOOI
LINOL A    G       2.10  1.91   11    LLLILLLL
SAT FAT A  G       1.10  0.70    4    SSSI
*****************************************************
```

650 HASHBROWN POTATOES, PREPARED FROM FROZEN
ANALYSIS OF 155 GRAMS WHICH IS 1 CUP

```
NUTRIENT   UNIT  AMOUNT  INQ   % STD  0        10        20        30   40   50   60   70   80   90   100
ENERGY     KCAL  345.00  1.00   17    EEEEEEEEEEEE
VITAMIN A  IU      0.00  0.00    0    -
VITAMIN C  MG     12.00  1.16   20    CCCCCCCCCCCCICC
THIAMIN    MG      0.11  0.64   11    TTTTTTTT
RIBOFLAVN  MG      0.03  0.14    3    RR
NIACIN     MG      1.60  0.66   11    NNNNNNNN
IRON       MG      1.90  0.69   12    IIIIIIIII
CALCIUM    MG     26.00  0.18    3    KK
PHOSPHRUS  MG     78.00  0.50    9    XXXXXXX
POTASSIUM  MG    439.00  0.51    9    YYYYYY
PROTEIN    G       3.00  0.35    6    PPPPP
CARBOHYDT  G      45.00  0.95   16    HHHHHHHHHHHHH
FAT        G      18.00  1.34   23    FFFFFFFFFFFFFIFFFF
OLEIC A    G       3.20  0.76   13    OOOOOOOOOO
LINOL A    G       9.00  2.61   45    LLLLLLLLLLLLLLLLLLLLLLLLLLLLLLLLLL
SAT FAT A  G       4.60  0.94   16    SSSSSSSSSSSSI
*****************************************************
```

651 MASHED POTATOES, PREPARED FROM RAW, MILK ADDED
ANALYSIS OF 210 GRAMS WHICH IS 1 CUP

NUTRIENT	UNIT	AMOUNT	INQ	% STD	0	10	20	30	40	50	60	70	80	90	100
ENERGY	KCAL	135.00	1.00	7	EEEEE										
VITAMIN A	IU	40.00	0.15	1	A										
VITAMIN C	MG	21.00	5.19	35	CCCCICCCCCCCCCCCCCCCCCCC										
THIAMIN	MG	0.17	2.52	17	TTTTITTTTTTTT										
RIBOFLAVN	MG	0.11	1.36	9	RRRRIRR										
NIACIN	MG	2.10	2.22	15	NNNNINNNNNNN										
IRON	MG	0.80	0.74	5	IIIII										
CALCIUM	MG	50.00	0.82	6	KKKKI										
PHOSPHRUS	MG	103.00	1.70	11	XXXXIXXXX										
POTASSIUM	MG	548.00	1.62	11	YYYYIYYYY										
PROTEIN	G	4.00	1.19	8	PPPPIP										
CARBOHYDT	G	27.00	1.45	10	HHHHIHHH										
FAT	G	2.00	0.38	3	FFI										
OLEIC A	G	0.40	0.24	2	OI										
LINOL A	G	0.00	0.00	0	-I										
SAT FAT A	G	0.70	0.36	2	SSI										

652 MASHED POTATOES, PREPARED FROM RAW, MILK AND BUTTER ADDED
ANALYSIS OF 210 GRAMS WHICH IS 1 CUP

NUTRIENT	UNIT	AMOUNT	INQ	% STD	0	10	20	30	40	50	60	70	80	90	100
ENERGY	KCAL	195.00	1.00	10	EEEEEE										
VITAMIN A	IU	360.00	0.92	9	AAAAAAI										
VITAMIN C	MG	19.00	3.25	32	CCCCCCICCCCCCCCCCCCCCCC										
THIAMIN	MG	0.17	1.74	17	TTTTTITTTTT										
RIBOFLAVN	MG	0.11	0.94	9	RRRRRRI										
NIACIN	MG	2.10	1.54	15	NNNNNNNINNNN										
IRON	MG	0.80	0.51	5	IIII I										
CALCIUM	MG	50.00	0.57	6	KKKK I										
PHOSPHRUS	MG	101.00	1.15	11	XXXXXXIX										
POTASSIUM	MG	525.00	1.08	11	YYYYYYY										
PROTEIN	G	4.00	0.82	8	PPPPPP I										
CARBOHYDT	G	26.00	0.97	9	HHHHHHH										
FAT	G	9.00	1.18	12	FFFFFFFIF										
OLEIC A	G	2.30	0.96	9	OOOUOOOO										
LINOL A	G	0.20	0.10	1	L I										
SAT FAT A	G	5.60	2.02	20	SSSSSSISSSSSSS										

653 POTATOES, DEHYDRATED FLAKES, WATER, MILK, BUTTER, SALT ADDED
ANALYSIS OF 210 GRAMS WHICH IS 1 CUP

```
                                    0        10        20        30        40        50        60        70        80        90       100
NUTRIENT   UNIT  AMOUNT   INQ  % STD
ENERGY     KCAL  195.00  1.00   10  EEEEEEE
VITAMIN A  IU    270.00  0.69    7  AAAAA
VITAMIN C  MG     11.00  1.88   18  CCCCCCCICCCCCCC
THIAMIN    MG      0.08  0.82    8  TTTTT
RIBOFLAVN  MG      0.08  0.68    7  RRRRR
NIACIN     MG      1.90  1.39   14  NNNNNNNINNN
IRON       MG      0.60  0.38    4  III
CALCIUM    MG     65.00  0.74    7  KKKKKK
PHOSPHRUS  MG     99.00  1.13   11  XXXXXXXIX
POTASSIUM  MG    601.00  1.23   12  YYYYYYYIYY
PROTEIN    G       4.00  0.82    8  PPPPP
CARBOHYDT  G      30.00  1.12   11  HHHHHHHIH
FAT        G       7.00  0.92    9  FFFFFFFI
OLEIC A    G       2.10  0.88    9  OOOOOOOI
LINOL A    G       0.20  0.10    1  L
SAT FAT A  G       3.60  1.30   13  SSSSSSSISS
*******************************************
```

654 POTATO CHIPS
ANALYSIS OF 20 GRAMS WHICH IS 10 CHIPS 1 3/4 BY 2 1/2-IN

```
                                    0        10        20        30        40        50        60        70        80        90       100
NUTRIENT   UNIT  AMOUNT   INQ  % STD
ENERGY     KCAL  115.00  1.00    6  EEEEE
VITAMIN A  IU      0.00  0.00    0  -
VITAMIN C  MG      3.00  0.87    5  CCCCI
THIAMIN    MG      0.04  0.70    4  TTT
RIBOFLAVN  MG      0.01  0.14    1  R
NIACIN     MG      1.00  1.24    7  NNNNIN
IRON       MG      0.40  0.43    3  II
CALCIUM    MG      8.00  0.15    1  K
PHOSPHRUS  MG     28.00  0.54    3  XX
POTASSIUM  MG    226.00  0.79    5  YYYY
PROTEIN    G       1.00  0.35    2  PP
CARBOHYDT  G      10.00  0.63    4  HHH
FAT        G       8.00  1.78   10  FFFFIFFF
OLEIC A    G       1.40  0.99    6  OOOOO
LINOL A    G       4.00  3.48   20  LLLLILLLLLLLLLLL
SAT FAT A  G       2.10  1.28    7  SSSSIS
*******************************************
```

655 POTATO SALAD MADE WITH COOKED SALAD DRESSING
ANALYSIS OF 250 GRAMS WHICH IS 1 CUP

NUTRIENT	UNIT	AMOUNT	INQ	% STD	0 10 20 30 40 50 60 70 80 90 100
ENERGY	KCAL	250.00	1.00	13	EEEEEEEE
VITAMIN A	IU	350.00	0.70	9	AAAAAAA
VITAMIN C	MG	28.00	3.73	47	CCCCCCC|CCCCCCCCCCCCCCCCCCCCCCCCCCCCCCCCCCCCCC
THIAMIN	MG	0.20	1.60	20	TTTTTTTT|TTTTTTTT
RIBOFLAVN	MG	0.18	1.20	15	RRRRRRRR|RR
NIACIN	MG	2.80	1.60	20	NNNNNNNNN|NNNNNNN
IRON	MG	1.50	0.75	9	IIIIIIII
CALCIUM	MG	80.00	0.71	9	KKKKKKK
PHOSPHRUS	MG	160.00	1.42	18	XXXXXXXXXX|XXXX
POTASSIUM	MG	798.00	1.28	16	YYYYYYYYY|YYY
PROTEIN	G	7.00	1.12	14	PPPPPPPP|P
CARBOHYDT	G	41.00	1.19	15	HHHHHHHHH|HH
FAT	G	7.00	0.72	9	FFFFFF
OLEIC A	G	2.70	0.88	11	OOOOOOOOO|
LINOL A	G	1.30	0.52	7	LLLL
SAT FAT A	G	2.00	0.56	7	SSSSS

656 PUMPKIN, CANNED
ANALYSIS OF 245 GRAMS WHICH IS 1 CUP

NUTRIENT	UNIT	AMOUNT	INQ	% STD	0 10 20 30 40 50 60 70 80 90 100
ENERGY	KCAL	80.00	1.00	4	EEE
VITAMIN A	IU	15680.00	98.00	392	AA|AAAAAAAAAAAAAAAAAAAAAAAAAAAAAAAAAAAAAAAAAAAAAAAAAAAAAAAAAAAAAAAAAAAAAAAAAAAAAAAAAAAAAA * 392
VITAMIN C	MG	12.00	5.00	20	CC|CCCCCCCCCCCCC
THIAMIN	MG	0.07	1.75	7	TT|TTT
RIBOFLAVN	MG	0.12	2.50	10	RR|RRRRR
NIACIN	MG	1.50	2.68	11	NN|NNNNN
IRON	MG	1.00	1.56	6	II|III
CALCIUM	MG	61.00	1.69	7	KK|KK
PHOSPHRUS	MG	64.00	1.78	7	XX|XXX
POTASSIUM	MG	588.00	2.94	12	YY|YYYYY
PROTEIN	G	2.00	1.00	4	PPP
CARBOHYDT	G	19.00	1.73	7	HH|HHH
FAT	G	1.00	0.32	1	F
OLEIC A	G	0.00	0.00	0	-
LINOL A	G	0.00	0.00	0	-
SAT FAT A	G	0.00	0.00	0	-

657 RADISHES,RAW
ANALYSIS OF 18 GRAMS WHICH IS 4 RADISHES

```
                                              0    10   20   30   40   50   60   70   80   90  100
NUTRIENT   UNIT   AMOUNT   INQ    % STD
ENERGY     KCAL     5.00   1.00      0        -                                                  *
VITAMIN A  IU       0.00   0.00      0        -                                                  *
VITAMIN C  MG       5.00  33.33      8        CCCCCC                                             *
THIAMIN    MG       0.01   4.00      1        T                                                  *
RIBOFLAVN  MG       0.01   3.33      1        R                                                  *
NIACIN     MG       0.10   2.86      1        N                                                  *
IRON       MG       0.20   5.00      1        I                                                  *
CALCIUM    MG       5.00   2.22      1        X                                                  *
PHOSPHRUS  MG       6.00   2.67      1        Y                                                  *
POTASSIUM  MG      58.00   4.64      1        -                                                  *
PROTEIN    G        0.00   0.00      0        -                                                  *
CARBOHYDT  G        1.00   1.45      0        -                                                  *
FAT        G        0.00   0.00      0        -                                                  *
OLEIC A    G        0.00   0.00      0        -                                                  *
LINOL A    G        0.00   0.00      0        -                                                  *
SAT FAT A  G        0.00   0.00      0        -                                                  *
*******************************************************************************************
```

658 SAUERKRAUT, CANNED,SOLIDS AND LIQUIDS
ANALYSIS OF 235 GRAMS WHICH IS 1 CUP

```
                                              0    10   20   30   40   50   60   70   80   90  100
NUTRIENT   UNIT   AMOUNT   INQ    % STD
ENERGY     KCAL    40.00   1.00      2        EE                                                 *
VITAMIN A  IU     120.00   1.50      3        AA                                                 *
VITAMIN C  MG      33.00  27.50     55        CICCCCCCCCCCCCCCCCCCCCCCCCCCCCCCCCCCCCCC          *
THIAMIN    MG       0.07   3.50      7        TITTTT                                             *
RIBOFLAVN  MG       0.09   3.75      8        RIRRRR                                             *
NIACIN     MG       0.50   1.79      4        NIN                                                *
IRON       MG       1.20   3.75      7        IIIIII                                             *
CALCIUM    MG      85.00   4.72      9        KIKKKKKK                                           *
PHOSPHRUS  MG      42.00   2.33      5        XIXX                                               *
POTASSIUM  MG     329.00   3.29      7        YIYYY                                              *
PROTEIN    G        2.00   2.00      4        PIP                                                *
CARBOHYDT  G        9.00   1.64      3        HIH                                                *
FAT        G        0.00   0.00      0        -I                                                 *
OLEIC A    G        0.00   0.00      0        -I                                                 *
LINOL A    G        0.00   0.00      0        -I                                                 *
SAT FAT A  G        0.00   0.00      0        -I                                                 *
*******************************************************************************************
```

659 SPINACH, RAW, CHOPPED
ANALYSIS OF 55 GRAMS WHICH IS 1 CUP

NUTRIENT	UNIT	AMOUNT	INQ	% STD
ENERGY	KCAL	15.00	1.00	1
VITAMIN A	IU	4460.00	148.67	112
VITAMIN C	MG	28.00	62.22	47
THIAMIN	MG	0.06	8.00	6
RIBOFLAVN	MG	0.11	12.22	9
NIACIN	MG	0.30	2.86	2
IRON	MG	1.70	14.17	11
CALCIUM	MG	51.00	7.56	6
PHOSPHRUS	MG	28.00	4.15	3
POTASSIUM	MG	259.00	6.91	5
PROTEIN	G	2.00	5.33	4
CARBOHYDT	G	2.00	0.97	1
FAT	G	0.00	0.00	0
OLEIC A	G	0.00	0.00	0
LINOL A	G	0.00	0.00	0
SAT FAT A	G	0.00	0.00	0

660 SPINACH, COOKED, DRAINED FROM RAW
ANALYSIS OF 180 GRAMS WHICH IS 1 CUP

NUTRIENT	UNIT	AMOUNT	INQ	% STD
ENERGY	KCAL	40.00	1.00	2
VITAMIN A	IU	14580.00	182.25	365
VITAMIN C	MG	50.00	41.67	83
THIAMIN	MG	0.13	6.50	13
RIBOFLAVN	MG	0.25	10.42	21
NIACIN	MG	0.90	3.21	6
IRON	MG	4.00	12.50	25
CALCIUM	MG	167.00	9.28	19
PHOSPHRUS	MG	68.00	3.78	8
POTASSIUM	MG	583.00	5.83	12
PROTEIN	G	5.00	5.00	10
CARBOHYDT	G	6.00	1.09	2
FAT	G	1.00	0.64	1
OLEIC A	G	0.00	0.00	0
LINOL A	G	0.00	0.00	0
SAT FAT A	G	0.00	0.00	0

661 SPINACH, COOKED, DRAINED FROM FROZEN, CHOPPED
ANALYSIS OF 205 GRAMS WHICH IS 1 CUP

```
NUTRIENT   UNIT  AMOUNT     INQ    % STD   0      10      20      30      40      50      60      70      80      90      100
ENERGY     KCAL    45.00    1.00     2     EE
VITAMIN A  IU   16200.00  180.00   405     AIAAAAAAAAAAAAAAAAAAAAAAAAAAAAAAAAAAAAAAAAAAAAAAAAAAAAAAAAAAAAAAAAAAAAAAAAAAAAAAAAAAAAAAAAA * 405
VITAMIN C  MG      39.00   28.89    65     CICCCCCCCCCCCCCCCCCCCCCCCCCCCC
THIAMIN    MG       0.14    6.22    14     TITTTTTTTT
RIBOFLAVN  MG       0.31   11.48    26     RIRRRRRRRRRRRRR
NIACIN     MG       0.80    2.54     6     NINNN
IRON       MG       4.30   11.94    27     IIIIIIIIIIIIIIIIIIIIIIII
CALCIUM    MG     232.00   11.46    26     KIKKKKKKKKKKKKK
PHOSPHRUS  MG      90.00    4.44    10     XIXXXXX
POTASSIUM  MG     683.00    6.07    14     YIYYYYYYY
PROTEIN    G        6.00    5.33    12     PIPPPPPP
CARBOHYDT  G        8.00    1.29     3     HH
FAT        G        1.00    0.57     1     FI
OLEIC A    G        0.00    0.00     0     -I
LINOL A    G        0.00    0.00     0     -I
SAT FAT A  G        0.00    0.00     0     -I
*****************************************************
```

662 SPINACH, COOKED, DRAINED FROM FROZEN, LEAF
ANALYSIS OF 190 GRAMS WHICH IS 1 CUP

```
NUTRIENT   UNIT  AMOUNT     INQ    % STD   0      10      20      30      40      50      60      70      80      90      100
ENERGY     KCAL    45.00    1.00     2     EE
VITAMIN A  IU   15390.00  171.00   385     AIAAAAAAAAAAAAAAAAAAAAAAAAAAAAAAAAAAAAAAAAAAAAAAAAAAAAAAAAAAAAAAAAAAAAAAAAAAAAAAAAAAAAAAAAA * 385
VITAMIN C  MG      53.00   39.26    88     CICCCCCCCCCCCCCCCCCCCCCCCCCCCCCCCCCCCCCC
THIAMIN    MG       0.15    6.67    15     TITTTTTTTTT
RIBOFLAVN  MG       0.27   10.00    23     RIRRRRRRRRRRRR
NIACIN     MG       1.00    3.17     7     NINNNN
IRON       MG       4.80   13.33    30     IIIIIIIIIIIIIIIIIIIIIIIIIII
CALCIUM    MG     200.00    9.88    22     KIKKKKKKKKKKKK
PHOSPHRUS  MG      84.00    4.15     9     XIXXXXX
POTASSIUM  MG     688.00    6.12    14     YIYYYYYYY
PROTEIN    G        6.00    5.33    12     PIPPPPPP
CARBOHYDT  G        7.00    1.13     3     HH
FAT        G        1.00    0.57     1     FI
OLEIC A    G        0.00    0.00     0     -I
LINOL A    G        0.00    0.00     0     -I
SAT FAT A  G        0.00    0.00     0     -I
*****************************************************
```

663 SPINACH, CANNED, DRAINED SOLIDS
ANALYSIS OF 205 GRAMS WHICH IS 1 CUP

NUTRIENT	UNIT	AMOUNT	INQ	% STD
ENERGY	KCAL	50.00	1.00	3
VITAMIN A	IU	16400.00	164.00	410
VITAMIN C	MG	29.00	19.33	48
THIAMIN	MG	0.04	1.60	4
RIBOFLAVN	MG	0.25	8.33	21
NIACIN	MG	0.60	1.71	4
IRON	MG	5.30	13.25	33
CALCIUM	MG	242.00	10.76	27
PHOSPHRUS	MG	53.00	2.36	6
POTASSIUM	MG	513.00	4.10	10
PROTEIN	G	6.00	4.80	12
CARBOHYDT	G	7.00	1.02	3
FAT	G	1.00	0.51	1
OLEIC A	G	0.00	0.00	0
LINOL A	G	0.00	0.00	0
SAT FAT A	G	0.00	0.00	0

664 SUMMER SQUASH, COOKED, DICED, DRAINED
ANALYSIS OF 210 GRAMS WHICH IS 1 CUP

NUTRIENT	UNIT	AMOUNT	INQ	% STD
ENERGY	KCAL	30.00	1.00	2
VITAMIN A	IU	820.00	13.67	21
VITAMIN C	MG	21.00	23.33	35
THIAMIN	MG	0.11	7.33	11
RIBOFLAVN	MG	0.17	9.44	14
NIACIN	MG	1.70	6.10	12
IRON	MG	0.80	3.33	5
CALCIUM	MG	53.00	3.93	6
PHOSPHRUS	MG	53.00	3.93	6
POTASSIUM	MG	296.00	3.95	6
PROTEIN	G	2.00	2.67	4
CARBOHYDT	G	7.00	1.70	3
FAT	G	0.00	0.00	0
OLEIC A	G	0.00	0.00	0
LINOL A	G	0.00	0.00	0
SAT FAT A	G	0.00	0.00	0

665 WINTER SQUASH, BAKED, MASHED
ANALYSIS OF 205 GRAMS WHICH IS 1 CUP

NUTRIENT	UNIT	AMOUNT	ING	% STD
ENERGY	KCAL	130.00	1.00	7
VITAMIN A	IU	8610.00	53.12	215
VITAMIN C	MG	27.00	0.92	45
THIAMIN	MG	0.16	1.54	10
RIBOFLAVN	MG	0.27	3.46	23
NIACIN	MG	1.40	1.54	10
IRON	MG	1.60	1.54	10
CALCIUM	MG	57.00	0.97	6
PHOSPHRUS	MG	98.00	1.68	11
POTASSIUM	MG	945.00	2.91	19
PROTEIN	G	4.00	1.23	8
CARBOHYDT	G	32.00	1.79	12
FAT	G	1.00	0.20	1
OLEIC A	G	0.00	0.00	0
LINOL A	G	0.00	0.00	0
SAT FAT A	G	0.00	0.00	0

666 SWEETPOTATOES COOKED BAKED IN SKIN, PEELED
ANALYSIS OF 114 GRAMS WHICH IS 1 POTATO (2 1/2 PER LB)

NUTRIENT	UNIT	AMOUNT	ING	% STD
ENERGY	KCAL	160.00	1.00	8
VITAMIN A	IU	9230.00	28.84	231
VITAMIN C	MG	25.00	5.21	42
THIAMIN	MG	0.10	1.25	10
RIBOFLAVN	MG	0.08	0.83	7
NIACIN	MG	0.80	0.71	6
IRON	MG	1.00	0.78	6
CALCIUM	MG	46.00	0.64	5
PHOSPHRUS	MG	66.00	0.92	7
POTASSIUM	MG	342.00	0.86	7
PROTEIN	G	2.00	0.50	4
CARBOHYDT	G	37.00	1.68	13
FAT	G	1.00	0.16	1
OLEIC A	G	0.00	0.00	0
LINOL A	G	0.00	0.00	0
SAT FAT A	G	0.00	0.00	0

667 SWEETPOTATOES COOKED, BOILED IN SKIN, PEELED
ANALYSIS OF 151 GRAMS WHICH IS 1 POTATO (2 1/2 PER LB)

NUTRIENT	UNIT	AMOUNT	INQ	% STD
ENERGY	KCAL	170.00	1.00	9
VITAMIN A	IU	11940.00	35.12	299
VITAMIN C	MG	26.00	5.10	43
THIAMIN	MG	0.14	1.65	14
RIBOFLAVN	MG	0.09	0.88	8
NIACIN	MG	0.90	0.76	6
IRON	MG	1.10	0.81	7
CALCIUM	MG	48.00	0.63	5
PHOSPHRUS	MG	71.00	0.93	8
POTASSIUM	MG	367.00	0.86	7
PROTEIN	G	3.00	0.71	6
CARBOHYDT	G	40.00	1.71	15
FAT	G	1.00	0.15	1
OLEIC A	G	0.00	0.00	0
LINOL A	G	0.00	0.00	0
SAT FAT A	G	0.00	0.00	0

668 SWEETPOTATOES, CANDIED
ANALYSIS OF 105 GRAMS WHICH IS 1 PIECE (2 1/2 BY 2-IN)

NUTRIENT	UNIT	AMOUNT	INQ	% STD
ENERGY	KCAL	175.00	1.00	9
VITAMIN A	IU	6620.00	18.91	166
VITAMIN C	MG	11.00	2.10	18
THIAMIN	MG	0.06	0.69	6
RIBOFLAVN	MG	0.04	0.38	3
NIACIN	MG	0.40	0.33	3
IRON	MG	0.90	0.64	6
CALCIUM	MG	39.00	0.50	4
PHOSPHRUS	MG	45.00	0.57	5
POTASSIUM	MG	200.00	0.46	4
PROTEIN	G	1.00	0.23	2
CARBOHYDT	G	36.00	1.50	13
FAT	G	3.00	0.44	4
OLEIC A	G	0.80	0.37	3
LINOL A	G	0.10	0.06	1
SAT FAT A	G	2.00	0.80	7

669 SWEETPOTATOES, CANNED SOLID PACK, MASHED
ANALYSIS OF 255 GRAMS WHICH IS 1 CUP

NUTRIENT	UNIT	AMOUNT	1NG	% STD
ENERGY	KCAL	275.00	1.00	14
VITAMIN A	IU	19890.00	50.16	497
VITAMIN C	MG	36.00	4.36	60
THIAMIN	MG	0.10	0.13	13
RIBOFLAVN	MG	0.61	0.78	8
NIACIN	MG	1.50	0.78	11
IRON	MG	2.00	0.91	13
CALCIUM	MG	64.00	0.52	7
PHOSPHRUS	MG	105.00	0.85	12
POTASSIUM	MG	510.00	0.74	10
PROTEIN	G	5.00	0.73	10
CARBOHYDT	G	63.00	1.67	23
FAT	G	1.00	0.09	1
OLEIC A	G	0.00	0.00	0
LINOL A	G	0.00	0.00	0
SAT FAT A	G	0.00	0.00	0

Scale: 0 10 20 30 40 50 60 70 80 90 100

670 SWEETPOTATOES, CANNED, VACUUM PACK
ANALYSIS OF 40 GRAMS WHICH IS 1 PIECE 2 3/4 BY 1-IN

NUTRIENT	UNIT	AMOUNT	1NG	% STD
ENERGY	KCAL	45.00	1.00	2
VITAMIN A	IU	3120.00	34.67	78
VITAMIN C	MG	6.00	4.44	10
THIAMIN	MG	0.02	0.89	2
RIBOFLAVN	MG	0.02	0.74	2
NIACIN	MG	0.20	0.63	1
IRON	MG	0.30	0.83	2
CALCIUM	MG	10.00	0.49	1
PHOSPHRUS	MG	16.00	0.79	2
POTASSIUM	MG	80.00	0.71	2
PROTEIN	G	1.00	0.89	2
CARBOHYDT	G	10.00	1.62	4
FAT	G	0.00	0.00	0
OLEIC A	G	0.00	0.00	0
LINOL A	G	0.00	0.00	0
SAT FAT A	G	0.00	0.00	0

Scale: 0 10 20 30 40 50 60 70 80 90 100

```
                                    0    10    20    30    40    50    60    70    80    90    100
                                    * * * * * * * * * * * * * * * * * *
```

671   TOMATOES, RAW
ANALYSIS OF 135 GRAMS WHICH IS 1 TOMATO 2 3/5-IN DIAM

NUTRIENT	UNIT	AMOUNT	INQ	% STD	
ENERGY	KCAL	25.00	1.00	1	E
VITAMIN A	IU	1110.00	22.20	28	IAAAAAAAAAAAAAAAAAA
VITAMIN C	MG	28.00	37.33	47	ICCCCCCCCCCCCCCCCCCCCCCCCCC
THIAMIN	MG	0.07	5.60	7	ITTTT
RIBOFLAVN	MG	0.05	3.33	4	IRR
NIACIN	MG	0.90	5.14	6	INNNN
IRON	MG	0.60	3.00	4	III
CALCIUM	MG	16.00	1.42	2	K
PHOSPHRUS	MG	33.00	2.93	4	IXX
POTASSIUM	MG	300.00	4.80	6	IYYY
PROTEIN	G	1.00	1.60	2	IP
CARBOHYDT	G	6.00	1.75	2	IH
FAT	G	0.00	0.00	0	I
OLEIC A	G	0.00	0.00	0	I
LINOL A	G	0.00	0.00	0	I
SAT FAT A	G	0.00	0.00	0	I

```
                                    0    10    20    30    40    50    60    70    80    90    100
                                    * * * * * * * * * * * * * * * * * *
```

672   TOMATOES, CANNED,SOLIDS AND LIQUIDS
ANALYSIS OF 241 GRAMS WHICH IS 1 CUP

NUTRIENT	UNIT	AMOUNT	INQ	% STD	
ENERGY	KCAL	50.00	1.00	3	EE
VITAMIN A	IU	2170.00	21.70	54	AIAAAAAAAAAAAAAAAAAAAAAAAAAAAAAAAAAAAAAAAAAAA
VITAMIN C	MG	41.00	27.33	68	CICCCCCCCCCCCCCCCCCCCCCCCCCCCCCCCCCCCCCCCCCCCCCCCCCCCCCC
THIAMIN	MG	0.12	4.80	12	TITTTTTTTT
RIBOFLAVN	MG	0.07	2.33	6	RIRRR
NIACIN	MG	1.70	4.86	12	NINNNNNNNN
IRON	MG	1.20	3.00	7	IIIIII
CALCIUM	MG	14.00	0.62	2	KI
PHOSPHRUS	MG	46.00	2.04	5	XIXX
POTASSIUM	MG	523.00	4.18	10	YIYYYYY
PROTEIN	G	2.00	1.60	4	PIP
CARBOHYDT	G	10.00	1.45	4	HIH
FAT	G	0.00	0.00	0	I
OLEIC A	G	0.00	0.00	0	I
LINOL A	G	0.00	0.00	0	I
SAT FAT A	G	0.00	0.00	0	I

673 TOMATO CATSUP
ANALYSIS OF 273 GRAMS WHICH IS 1 CUP

NUTRIENT	UNIT	AMOUNT	INQ	% STD
ENERGY	KCAL	290.00	1.00	15
VITAMIN A	IU	3820.00	6.59	96
VITAMIN C	MG	41.00	4.71	68
THIAMIN	MG	0.25	1.72	25
RIBOFLAVN	MG	0.19	1.09	16
NIACIN	MG	4.40	2.17	31
IRON	MG	2.20	0.95	14
CALCIUM	MG	60.00	0.46	7
PHOSPHRUS	MG	137.00	1.05	15
POTASSIUM	MG	991.00	1.37	20
PROTEIN	G	5.00	0.69	10
CARBOHYDT	G	69.00	1.73	25
FAT	G	1.00	0.09	1
OLEIC A	G	0.00	0.00	0
LINOL A	G	0.00	0.00	0
SAT FAT A	G	0.00	0.00	0

674 TOMATO CATSUP
ANALYSIS OF 15 GRAMS WHICH IS 1 TBSP

NUTRIENT	UNIT	AMOUNT	INQ	% STD
ENERGY	KCAL	15.00	1.00	1
VITAMIN A	IU	210.00	7.00	5
VITAMIN C	MG	2.00	4.44	3
THIAMIN	MG	0.01	1.33	1
RIBOFLAVN	MG	0.01	1.11	1
NIACIN	MG	0.20	1.90	1
IRON	MG	0.10	0.83	1
CALCIUM	MG	3.00	0.44	0
PHOSPHRUS	MG	8.00	1.19	1
POTASSIUM	MG	54.00	1.44	1
PROTEIN	G	0.00	0.00	0
CARBOHYDT	G	4.00	1.94	1
FAT	G	0.00	0.00	0
OLEIC A	G	0.00	0.00	0
LINOL A	G	0.00	0.00	0
SAT FAT A	G	0.00	0.00	0

675 TOMATO JUICE, CANNED
ANALYSIS OF 243 GRAMS WHICH IS 1 CUP

NUTRIENT	UNIT	AMOUNT	INQ	% STD
ENERGY	KCAL	45.00	1.00	2
VITAMIN A	IU	1940.00	21.56	49
VITAMIN C	MG	39.00	28.89	65
THIAMIN	MG	0.12	5.33	12
RIBOFLAVN	MG	0.07	2.59	6
NIACIN	MG	1.90	6.03	14
IRON	MG	2.20	6.11	14
CALCIUM	MG	17.00	0.84	2
PHOSPHRUS	MG	44.00	2.17	5
POTASSIUM	MG	552.00	4.91	11
PROTEIN	G	2.00	1.78	4
CARBOHYDT	G	10.00	1.62	4
FAT	G	0.00	0.00	0
OLEIC A	G	0.00	0.00	0
LINOL A	G	0.00	0.00	0
SAT FAT A	G	0.00	0.00	0

676 TOMATO JUICE, CANNED
ANALYSIS OF 182 GRAMS WHICH IS 1 GLASS 6 FL OZ

NUTRIENT	UNIT	AMOUNT	INQ	% STD
ENERGY	KCAL	35.00	1.00	2
VITAMIN A	IU	1460.00	20.86	37
VITAMIN C	MG	29.00	27.62	48
THIAMIN	MG	0.09	5.14	9
RIBOFLAVN	MG	0.05	2.36	4
NIACIN	MG	1.50	6.12	11
IRON	MG	1.60	5.71	10
CALCIUM	MG	13.00	0.83	1
PHOSPHRUS	MG	33.00	2.10	4
POTASSIUM	MG	413.00	4.72	8
PROTEIN	G	2.00	2.29	4
CARBOHYDT	G	8.00	1.66	3
FAT	G	0.00	0.00	0
OLEIC A	G	0.00	0.00	0
LINOL A	G	0.00	0.00	0
SAT FAT A	G	0.00	0.00	0

677 TURNIPS, COOKED, DICED
ANALYSIS OF 155 GRAMS WHICH IS 1 CUP

NUTRIENT	UNIT	AMOUNT	INQ	% STD	0 10 20 30 40 50 60 70 80 90 100
ENERGY	KCAL	35.00	1.00	2	E
VITAMIN A	IU	0.00	0.00	0	-
VITAMIN C	MG	34.00	32.38	57	CCCCCCCCCCCCCCCCCCCCCCCCCCCCCC
THIAMIN	MG	0.08	3.43	6	TTTT
RIBOFLAVN	MG	0.06	3.81	7	RRRR
NIACIN	MG	0.50	2.04	4	NN
IRON	MG	0.60	2.14	4	II
CALCIUM	MG	54.00	3.43	6	KKKK
PHOSPHRUS	MG	37.00	2.35	4	XX
POTASSIUM	MG	291.00	3.53	6	YYYY
PROTEIN	G	1.00	1.14	2	P
CARBOHYDT	G	8.00	1.66	3	H
FAT	G	0.00	0.00	0	-
OLEIC A	G	0.00	0.00	0	-
LINOL A	G	0.00	0.00	0	-
SAT FAT A	G	0.00	0.00	0	-

****

678 TURNIP GREENS, COOKED, DRAINED, FROM RAW (LEAVES AND STEMS)
ANALYSIS OF 145 GRAMS WHICH IS 1 CUP

NUTRIENT	UNIT	AMOUNT	INQ	% STD	0 10 20 30 40 50 60 70 80 90 100
ENERGY	KCAL	30.00	1.00	2	E
VITAMIN A	IU	8270.00	157.83	207	AAAAAAAAAAAAAAAAAAAAAAAAAAAAAAAAAAAAAAAAAAAAAAAAAAAAAAAAAAAAAAAAAAAAAAAAAAAAAAAAAAAAAAAAAAAAAAAAAA * 207
VITAMIN C	MG	66.00	75.56	113	CCCCCCCCCCCCCCCCCCCCCCCCCCCCCCCCCCCCCCCCCCCCCCCCCCCCCCCCCCCCCCCCCCCCCCCCC * 113
THIAMIN	MG	0.15	10.00	15	TTTTTTTTTT
RIBOFLAVN	MG	0.33	18.33	26	RRRRRRRRRRRRRRRRRR
NIACIN	MG	0.70	3.33	5	NNN
IRON	MG	1.50	6.25	9	IIIIII
CALCIUM	MG	252.00	18.67	28	KKKKKKKKKKKKKKKKKK
PHOSPHRUS	MG	49.00	3.63	5	XXX
POTASSIUM	MG	470.00	6.27	9	YYYYYY
PROTEIN	G	3.00	4.00	6	PPPP
CARBOHYDT	G	5.00	1.21	2	H
FAT	G	0.00	0.00	0	-
OLEIC A	G	0.00	0.00	0	-
LINOL A	G	0.00	0.00	0	-
SAT FAT A	G	0.00	0.00	0	-

****

679 TURNIP GREENS, COOKED, DRAINED, FROM FROZEN,CHOPPED
ANALYSIS OF 165 GRAMS WHICH IS 1 CUP

NUTRIENT	UNIT	AMOUNT	INQ	% STD										
					0	10	20	30	40	50	60	70	80	90	100
ENERGY	KCAL	40.00	1.00	2	EE									
VITAMIN A	IU	11390.00	142.38	285	AIAAAAAAAAAAAAAAAAAAAAAAAAAAAAAAAAAAAAAAAAAAAAAAAAAAAAAAAAAAAAAAAAAAAAAAAAAAAAAAAAAAAAAAAA * 285
VITAMIN C	MG	31.00	25.83	52	CICCCCCCCCCCCCCCCCCCCCCCCCCCCCCCCCCCCCCCCCCCCCCCCC
THIAMIN	MG	0.08	4.00	8	TITTTT
RIBOFLAVN	MG	0.15	6.25	13	RIRRRRRRR
NIACIN	MG	0.70	2.50	5	NINN
IRON	MG	2.60	8.13	16	IIIIIIIIIIII
CALCIUM	MG	195.00	10.83	22	KIKKKKKKKKKKKKKKK
PHOSPHRUS	MG	64.00	3.56	7	XIXXXX
POTASSIUM	MG	246.00	2.46	5	YIYY
PROTEIN	G	4.00	4.00	8	PIPPPP
CARBOHYDT	G	6.00	1.09	2	HH
FAT	G	0.00	0.00	0	-I
OLEIC A	G	0.00	0.00	0	-I
LINOL A	G	0.00	0.00	0	-I
SAT FAT A	G	0.00	0.00	0	-I

680 VEGETABLES, MIXED, FROZEN, COOKED, DRAINED
ANALYSIS OF 182 GRAMS WHICH IS 1 CUP

NUTRIENT	UNIT	AMOUNT	INQ	% STD										
					0	10	20	30	40	50	60	70	80	90	100
ENERGY	KCAL	115.00	1.00	6	EEEEE									
VITAMIN A	IU	9010.00	39.17	225	AAAAIAAAAAAAAAAAAAAAAAAAAAAAAAAAAAAAAAAAAAAAAAAAAAAAAAAAAAAAAAAAAAAAAAAAAAAAAAAAAAAAAAAAA * 225
VITAMIN C	MG	15.00	4.35	25	CCCCICCCCCCCCCCCCCC
THIAMIN	MG	0.22	3.83	22	TITIITTTTTTTTTTTTTTT
RIBOFLAVN	MG	0.13	1.88	11	RRRRIRRRR
NIACIN	MG	2.00	2.48	14	NNNNINNNNNN
IRON	MG	2.40	2.61	15	IIIIIIIIIIIII
CALCIUM	MG	46.00	0.89	5	KKKKI
PHOSPHRUS	MG	115.00	2.22	13	XXXXIXXXXX
POTASSIUM	MG	348.00	1.21	7	YYYYIY
PROTEIN	G	6.00	2.09	12	PPPPIPPPPP
CARBOHYDT	G	24.00	1.52	9	HHHHIHH
FAT	G	1.00	0.22	1	F
OLEIC A	G	0.00	0.00	0	-I
LINOL A	G	0.00	0.00	0	-I
SAT FAT A	G	0.00	0.00	0	-I

681 BAKING POWDERS, SODIUM ALUMINUM SULFATE w/ MONO CALCIUM PHOSPHATE
ANALYSIS OF 3 GRAMS WHICH IS 1 TSP

NUTRIENT	UNIT	AMOUNT	ING	% STD	0	10	20	30	40	50	60	70	80	90	100
ENERGY	KCAL	5.00	1.00	0	-										
VITAMIN A	IU	0.00	0.00	0	-										
VITAMIN C	MG	0.00	0.00	0	-										
THIAMIN	MG	0.00	0.00	0	-										
RIBOFLAVN	MG	0.00	0.00	0	-										
NIACIN	MG	0.00	0.00	0	-										
IRON	MG	0.00	0.00	0	-										
CALCIUM	MG	58.00	25.78	6	KKKK										
PHOSPHRUS	MG	87.00	38.67	10	XXXXXXXX										
POTASSIUM	MG	5.00	0.40	0	-										
PROTEIN	G	0.00	0.00	0	-										
CARBOHYDT	G	1.00	1.45	0	-										
FAT	G	0.00	0.00	0	-										
OLEIC A	G	0.00	0.00	0	-										
LINOL A	G	0.00	0.00	0	-										
SAT FAT A	G	0.00	0.00	0	-										

682 BAKING POWDERS, SODIUM ALUMINUM SULFATE w/ CALCIUM PHOSPHATE, CA SO4
ANALYSIS OF 3 GRAMS WHICH IS 1 TSP

NUTRIENT	UNIT	AMOUNT	ING	% STD	0	10	20	30	40	50	60	70	80	90	100
ENERGY	KCAL	5.00	1.00	0	-										
VITAMIN A	IU	0.00	0.00	0	-										
VITAMIN C	MG	0.00	0.00	0	-										
THIAMIN	MG	0.00	0.00	0	-										
RIBOFLAVN	MG	0.00	0.00	0	-										
NIACIN	MG	0.00	0.00	0	-										
IRON	MG	0.00	0.00	0	-										
CALCIUM	MG	183.00	81.33	20	KKKKKKKKKKKKK										
PHOSPHRUS	MG	45.00	20.00	5	XXXX										
POTASSIUM	MG	4.00	0.32	0	-										
PROTEIN	G	0.00	0.00	0	-										
CARBOHYDT	G	1.00	1.45	0	-										
FAT	G	0.00	0.00	0	-										
OLEIC A	G	0.00	0.00	0	-										
LINOL A	G	0.00	0.00	0	-										
SAT FAT A	G	0.00	0.00	0	-										

683 BAKING POWDERS, STRAIGHT PHOSPHATE
ANALYSIS OF 4 GRAMS WHICH IS 1 TSP

NUTRIENT	UNIT	AMOUNT	INQ	% STD
ENERGY	KCAL	5.00	1.00	0
VITAMIN A	IU	0.00	0.00	0
VITAMIN C	MG	0.00	0.00	0
THIAMIN	MG	0.00	0.00	0
RIBOFLAVN	MG	0.00	0.00	0
NIACIN	MG	0.00	0.00	0
IRON	MG	0.00	0.00	0
CALCIUM	MG	239.00	106.22	27
PHOSPHRUS	MG	359.00	159.56	40
POTASSIUM	MG	0.00	0.48	0
PROTEIN	G	0.00	1.45	0
CARBOHYDT	G	1.00	0.00	0
FAT	G	0.00	0.00	0
OLEIC A	G	0.00	0.00	0
LINOL A	G	0.00	0.00	0
SAT FAT A	G	0.00	0.00	0

684 BAKING POWDERS, LOW SODIUM
ANALYSIS OF 4 GRAMS WHICH IS 1 TSP

NUTRIENT	UNIT	AMOUNT	INQ	% STD
ENERGY	KCAL	5.00	1.00	0
VITAMIN A	IU	0.00	0.00	0
VITAMIN C	MG	0.00	0.00	0
THIAMIN	MG	0.00	0.00	0
RIBOFLAVN	MG	0.00	0.00	0
NIACIN	MG	0.00	0.00	0
IRON	MG	0.00	0.00	0
CALCIUM	MG	207.00	92.00	23
PHOSPHRUS	MG	314.00	139.56	35
POTASSIUM	MG	471.00	37.68	9
PROTEIN	G	0.00	0.00	0
CARBOHYDT	G	2.00	2.91	1
FAT	G	0.00	0.00	0
OLEIC A	G	0.00	0.00	0
LINOL A	G	0.00	0.00	0
SAT FAT A	G	0.00	0.00	0

685 BARBECUE SAUCE
ANALYSIS OF 250 GRAMS WHICH IS 1 CUP

```
                                  0        10        20        30        40        50        60        70        80        90        100
```

NUTRIENT	UNIT	AMOUNT	INQ	% STD	
ENERGY	KCAL	230.00	1.00	12	EEEEEEE
VITAMIN A	IU	900.00	1.96	23	AAAAAAAAIAAAAAAAAA
VITAMIN C	MG	13.00	1.88	22	CCCCCCCCICCCCCCCC
THIAMIN	MG	0.03	0.26	3	TT
RIBOFLAVN	MG	0.03	0.22	3	RR
NIACIN	MG	0.80	0.50	6	NNNNN
IRON	MG	2.00	1.09	13	IIIIIIIII
CALCIUM	MG	53.00	0.51	6	KKKKK
PHOSPHRUS	MG	50.00	0.48	6	XXXX
POTASSIUM	MG	435.00	0.76	9	YYYYYYY
PROTEIN	G	4.00	0.70	8	PPPPP
CARBOHYDT	G	20.00	0.63	7	HHHHH
FAT	G	17.00	1.90	22	FFFFFFFFIFFFFFFF
OLEIC A	G	4.30	1.53	18	OOOOOOOOIOOOOO
LINOL A	G	10.00	4.35	50	LLLLLLLLILLLLLLLLLLLLLLLLLLLLLLLL
SAT FAT A	G	2.20	0.67	8	SSSSS

686 BEER
ANALYSIS OF 360 GRAMS WHICH IS 12 FL OZ

```
                                  0        10        20        30        40        50        60        70        80        90        100
```

NUTRIENT	UNIT	AMOUNT	INQ	% STD	
ENERGY	KCAL	150.00	1.00	8	EEEEE
VITAMIN A	IU	0.00	0.00	0	-
VITAMIN C	MG	0.00	0.00	0	-
THIAMIN	MG	0.01	0.13	1	T
RIBOFLAVN	MG	0.11	1.22	9	RRRRRIR
NIACIN	MG	2.20	2.10	16	NNNNNINNNNNNN
IRON	MG	0.00	0.00	0	-
CALCIUM	MG	18.00	0.27	2	KK
PHOSPHRUS	MG	108.00	1.60	12	XXXXXIXXXX
POTASSIUM	MG	90.00	0.24	2	Y
PROTEIN	G	1.00	0.27	2	PP
CARBOHYDT	G	14.00	0.68	5	HHHH
FAT	G	0.00	0.00	0	-
OLEIC A	G	0.00	0.00	0	-
LINOL A	G	0.00	0.00	0	-
SAT FAT A	G	0.00	0.00	0	-

687 GIN, RUM, VODKA, WHISKY, 80-PROOF
ANALYSIS OF 42 GRAMS WHICH IS 1 1/2-FL OZ JIGGER

NUTRIENT	UNIT	AMOUNT	INQ	% STD	0
ENERGY	KCAL	95.00	1.00	5	EEEE
VITAMIN A	IU	0.00	0.00	0	-
VITAMIN C	MG	0.00	0.00	0	-
THIAMIN	MG	0.00	0.00	0	-
RIBOFLAVN	MG	0.00	0.00	0	-
NIACIN	MG	0.00	0.00	0	-
IRON	MG	0.00	0.00	0	-
CALCIUM	MG	0.00	0.00	0	-
PHOSPHRUS	MG	0.00	0.00	0	-
POTASSIUM	MG	1.00	0.00	0	-
PROTEIN	G	0.00	0.00	0	-
CARBOHYDT	G	0.00	0.00	0	-
FAT	G	0.00	0.00	0	-
OLEIC A	G	0.00	0.00	0	-
LINOL A	G	0.00	0.00	0	-
SAT FAT A	G	0.00	0.00	0	-

688 GIN, RUM, VODKA, WHISKY, 86-PROOF
ANALYSIS OF 42 GRAMS WHICH IS 1 1/2-FL OZ JIGGER

NUTRIENT	UNIT	AMOUNT	INQ	% STD	0
ENERGY	KCAL	105.00	1.00	5	EEEE
VITAMIN A	IU	0.00	0.00	0	-
VITAMIN C	MG	0.00	0.00	0	-
THIAMIN	MG	0.00	0.00	0	-
RIBOFLAVN	MG	0.00	0.00	0	-
NIACIN	MG	0.00	0.00	0	-
IRON	MG	0.00	0.00	0	-
CALCIUM	MG	0.00	0.00	0	-
PHOSPHRUS	MG	0.00	0.00	0	-
POTASSIUM	MG	1.00	0.00	0	-
PROTEIN	G	0.00	0.00	0	-
CARBOHYDT	G	0.00	0.00	0	-
FAT	G	0.00	0.00	0	-
OLEIC A	G	0.00	0.00	0	-
LINOL A	G	0.00	0.00	0	-
SAT FAT A	G	0.00	0.00	0	-

689 GIN, RUM, VODKA, WHISKY, 90-PROOF
ANALYSIS OF 42 GRAMS WHICH IS 1 1/2-FL OZ JIGGER

NUTRIENT	UNIT	AMOUNT	INQ	% STD	0	10	20	30	40	50	60	70	80	90	100
ENERGY	KCAL	110.00	1.00	6	EEEE										* * * * * * * * * * * * * * * * * *
VITAMIN A	IU	0.00	0.00	0	-										
VITAMIN C	MG	0.00	0.00	0	-										
THIAMIN	MG	0.00	0.00	0	I										
RIBOFLAVN	MG	0.00	0.00	0	-										
NIACIN	MG	0.00	0.00	0	I										
IRON	MG	0.00	0.00	0	I										
CALCIUM	MG	0.00	0.00	0	I										
PHOSPHRUS	MG	0.00	0.00	0	I										
POTASSIUM	MG	1.00	0.00	0	I										
PROTEIN	G	0.00	0.00	0	I										
CARBOHYDT	G	0.00	0.00	0	I										
FAT	G	0.00	0.00	0	I										
OLEIC A	G	0.00	0.00	0	I										
LINOL A	G	0.00	0.00	0	I										
SAT FAT A	G	0.00	0.00	0	I										

690 DESSERT WINE
ANALYSIS OF 103 GRAMS WHICH IS 3 1/2-FL OZ GLASS

NUTRIENT	UNIT	AMOUNT	INQ	% STD	0	10	20	30	40	50	60	70	80	90	100
ENERGY	KCAL	140.00	1.00	7	EEEEE										* * * * * * * * * * * * * * * *
VITAMIN A	IU	0.00	0.00	0	-										
VITAMIN C	MG	0.00	0.00	0	-										
THIAMIN	MG	0.01	0.14	1	T										
RIBOFLAVN	MG	0.02	0.24	2	R										
NIACIN	MG	0.20	0.20	1	N										
IRON	MG	0.00	0.00	0	-										
CALCIUM	MG	8.00	0.13	1	K										
PHOSPHRUS	MG	0.00	0.00	0	-										
POTASSIUM	MG	77.00	0.22	2	Y										
PROTEIN	G	0.00	0.00	0	-										
CARBOHYDT	G	8.00	0.42	3	HH										
FAT	G	0.00	0.00	0	I										
OLEIC A	G	0.00	0.00	0	I										
LINOL A	G	0.00	0.00	0	I										
SAT FAT A	G	0.00	0.00	0	I										

```
                0    10   20   30   40   50   60   70   80   90   100
                *******************************                    *****************
```

691   TABLE WINE
ANALYSIS OF 102 GRAMS WHICH IS 3 1/2-FL OZ GLASS

NUTRIENT	UNIT	AMOUNT	INQ	% STD
ENERGY	KCAL	85.00	1.00	4
VITAMIN A	IU	0.00	0.00	0
VITAMIN C	MG	0.00	0.00	0
THIAMIN	MG	0.01	0.20	1
RIBOFLAVN	MG	0.10	0.17	1
NIACIN	MG	0.40	0.59	3
IRON	MG	0.40	0.24	1
CALCIUM	MG	9.00	0.24	1
PHOSPHRUS	MG	10.00	0.26	1
POTASSIUM	MG	94.00	0.44	2
PROTEIN	G	0.00	0.00	0
CARBOHYDT	G	4.00	0.34	1
FAT	G	0.00	0.00	0
OLEIC A	G	0.00	0.00	0
LINOL A	G	0.00	0.00	0
SAT FAT A	G	0.00	0.00	0

692   CARBONATED WATER
ANALYSIS OF 366 GRAMS WHICH IS 12-FL OZ

NUTRIENT	UNIT	AMOUNT	INQ	% STD
ENERGY	KCAL	115.00	1.00	6
VITAMIN A	IU	0.00	0.00	0
VITAMIN C	MG	0.00	0.00	0
THIAMIN	MG	0.00	0.00	0
RIBOFLAVN	MG	0.00	0.00	0
NIACIN	MG	0.00	0.00	0
IRON	MG	0.00	0.00	0
CALCIUM	MG	0.00	0.00	0
PHOSPHRUS	MG	0.00	0.00	0
POTASSIUM	MG	0.00	0.00	0
PROTEIN	G	0.00	0.00	0
CARBOHYDT	G	29.00	1.83	11
FAT	G	0.00	0.00	0
OLEIC A	G	0.00	0.00	0
LINOL A	G	0.00	0.00	0
SAT FAT A	G	0.00	0.00	0

693 COLA TYPE SOFT DRINK
ANALYSIS OF 369 GRAMS WHICH IS 12-FL OZ

```
NUTRIENT   UNIT   AMOUNT    INQ   % STD   0         10        20        30        40        50        60        70        80        90        100
ENERGY     KCAL   145.00    1.00    7     EEEEE                                                                                                *
VITAMIN A  IU       0.00    0.00    0     -                                                                                                   *
VITAMIN C  MG       0.00    0.00    0     -                                                                                                   *
THIAMIN    MG       0.00    0.00    0     -                                                                                                   *
RIBOFLAVN  MG       0.00    0.00    0     -                                                                                                   *
NIACIN     MG       0.00    0.00    0     -                                                                                                   *
IRON       MG       0.00    0.00    0     -                                                                                                   *
CALCIUM    MG       0.00    0.00    0     -                                                                                                   *
PHOSPHRUS  MG       0.00    0.00    0     -                                                                                                   *
POTASSIUM  MG       0.00    0.00    0     -                                                                                                   *
PROTEIN    G        0.00    0.00    0     -                                                                                                   *
CARBOHYDT  G       37.00    1.86   13     HHHHHH|HHHHH                                                                                         *
FAT        G        0.00    0.00    0     -                                                                                                   *
OLEIC A    G        0.00    0.00    0     -                                                                                                   *
LINOL A    G        0.00    0.00    0     -                                                                                                   *
SAT FAT A  G        0.00    0.00    0     -                                                                                                   *
*******************************************************************************
```

694 FRUIT-FLAVORED SODAS AND TOM COLLINS MIXER
ANALYSIS OF 372 GRAMS WHICH IS 12-FL OZ

```
NUTRIENT   UNIT   AMOUNT    INQ   % STD   0         10        20        30        40        50        60        70        80        90        100
ENERGY     KCAL   170.00    1.00    9     EEEEEE                                                                                              *
VITAMIN A  IU       0.00    0.00    0     -                                                                                                   *
VITAMIN C  MG       0.00    0.00    0     -                                                                                                   *
THIAMIN    MG       0.00    0.00    0     -                                                                                                   *
RIBOFLAVN  MG       0.00    0.00    0     -                                                                                                   *
NIACIN     MG       0.00    0.00    0     -                                                                                                   *
IRON       MG       0.00    0.00    0     -                                                                                                   *
CALCIUM    MG       0.00    0.00    0     -                                                                                                   *
PHOSPHRUS  MG       0.00    0.00    0     -                                                                                                   *
POTASSIUM  MG       0.00    0.00    0     -                                                                                                   *
PROTEIN    G        0.00    0.00    0     -                                                                                                   *
CARBOHYDT  G       45.00    1.93   16     HHHHHH|HHHHHH                                                                                        *
FAT        G        0.00    0.00    0     -                                                                                                   *
OLEIC A    G        0.00    0.00    0     -                                                                                                   *
LINOL A    G        0.00    0.00    0     -                                                                                                   *
SAT FAT A  G        0.00    0.00    0     -                                                                                                   *
*******************************************************************************
```

695 GINGER ALE
ANALYSIS OF 366 GRAMS WHICH IS 12-FL OZ

NUTRIENT	UNIT	AMOUNT	INQ	% STD	
ENERGY	KCAL	115.00	1.00	6	EEEEE
VITAMIN A	IU	0.00	0.00	0	
VITAMIN C	MG	0.00	0.00	0	
THIAMIN	MG	0.00	0.00	0	
RIBOFLAVN	MG	0.00	0.00	0	
NIACIN	MG	0.00	0.00	0	
IRON	MG	0.00	0.00	0	
CALCIUM	MG	0.00	0.00	0	
PHOSPHRUS	MG	0.00	0.00	0	
POTASSIUM	MG	0.00	0.00	0	
PROTEIN	G	0.00	0.00	0	
CARBOHYDT	G	29.00	1.83	11	HHHHIHHH
FAT	G	0.00	0.00	0	
OLEIC A	G	0.00	0.00	0	
LINOL A	G	0.00	0.00	0	
SAT FAT A	G	0.00	0.00	0	

696 ROOT BEER
ANALYSIS OF 370 GRAMS WHICH IS 12-FL OZ

NUTRIENT	UNIT	AMOUNT	INQ	% STD	
ENERGY	KCAL	150.00	1.00	8	EEEEE
VITAMIN A	IU	0.00	0.00	0	
VITAMIN C	MG	0.00	0.00	0	
THIAMIN	MG	0.00	0.00	0	
RIBOFLAVN	MG	0.00	0.00	0	
NIACIN	MG	0.00	0.00	0	
IRON	MG	0.00	0.00	0	
CALCIUM	MG	0.00	0.00	0	
PHOSPHRUS	MG	0.00	0.00	0	
POTASSIUM	MG	0.00	0.00	0	
PROTEIN	G	0.00	0.00	0	
CARBOHYDT	G	39.00	1.89	14	HHHHIHHHHH
FAT	G	0.00	0.00	0	
OLEIC A	G	0.00	0.00	0	
LINOL A	G	0.00	0.00	0	
SAT FAT A	G	0.00	0.00	0	

697 BITTER SWEET OR BAKING CHOCOLATE
ANALYSIS OF 28 GRAMS WHICH IS 1 OZ

NUTRIENT	UNIT	AMOUNT	INQ	% STD										
					0	10	20	30	40	50	60	70	80	90	100
ENERGY	KCAL	145.00	1.00	7	EEEEE									
VITAMIN A	IU	20.00	0.07	1	-									
VITAMIN C	MG	0.00	0.00	0	-									
THIAMIN	MG	0.01	0.14	1	T									
RIBOFLAVN	MG	0.07	0.80	6	RRRR									
NIACIN	MG	0.40	0.39	3	NN									
IRON	MG	1.90	1.64	12	IIIIIIIII									
CALCIUM	MG	22.00	0.34	2	KK									
PHOSPHRUS	MG	109.00	1.67	12	XXXXIXXXX									
POTASSIUM	MG	235.00	0.65	5	YYYY									
PROTEIN	G	3.00	0.83	6	PPPPP									
CARBOHYDT	G	8.00	0.40	3	HH									
FAT	G	15.00	2.65	19	FFFFFIFFFFFFFF									
OLEIC A	G	4.90	2.76	20	OOOOOIOOOOOOOOO									
LINOL A	G	0.40	0.28	2	LL									
SAT FAT A	G	8.90	4.31	31	SSSSSISSSSSSSSSSSSSSSSS									

****

698 GELATIN, DRY
ANALYSIS OF 7 GRAMS WHICH IS 1 ENVELOPE

NUTRIENT	UNIT	AMOUNT	INQ	% STD										
					0	10	20	30	40	50	60	70	80	90	100
ENERGY	KCAL	25.00	1.00	1	E									
VITAMIN A	IU	0.00	0.00	0	-									
VITAMIN C	MG	0.00	0.00	0	-									
THIAMIN	MG	0.00	0.00	0	-									
RIBOFLAVN	MG	0.00	0.00	0	-									
NIACIN	MG	0.00	0.00	0	-									
IRON	MG	0.00	0.00	0	-									
CALCIUM	MG	1.00	0.09	0	-									
PHOSPHRUS	MG	0.00	0.00	0	-									
POTASSIUM	MG	2.00	0.03	0	-									
PROTEIN	G	6.00	9.60	12	IPPPPPPPP									
CARBOHYDT	G	0.00	0.00	0	-									
FAT	G	0.00	0.00	0	-									
OLEIC A	G	0.00	0.00	0	-									
LINOL A	G	0.00	0.00	0	-									
SAT FAT A	G	0.00	0.00	0	-									

****

699 GELATIN DESSERT MADE WITH GELATIN POWDER AND WATER
ANALYSIS OF 240 GRAMS WHICH IS 1 CUP

NUTRIENT	UNIT	AMOUNT	INQ	% STD	0 ... 10 ... 20 ... 100
ENERGY	KCAL	140.00	1.00	7	EEEEE
VITAMIN A	IU	0.00	0.00	0	-
VITAMIN C	MG	0.00	0.00	0	-
THIAMIN	MG	0.00	0.00	0	-
RIBUFLAVN	MG	0.00	0.00	0	-
NIACIN	MG	0.00	0.00	0	-
IRON	MG	0.00	0.00	0	-
CALCIUM	MG	0.00	0.00	0	-
PHOSPHRUS	MG	0.00	0.00	0	-
POTASSIUM	MG	0.00	0.00	0	-
PROTEIN	G	4.00	1.14	8	PPPPP
CARBOHYDT	G	34.00	1.77	12	HHHHHIHHHH
FAT	G	0.00	0.00	0	-
OLEIC A	G	0.00	0.00	0	-
LINOL A	G	0.00	0.00	0	-
SAT FAT A	G	0.00	0.00	0	-

700 MUSTARD, YELLOW, PREPARED
ANALYSIS OF 5 GRAMS WHICH IS 1 TSP OR INDIVIDUAL SERVING POUCH

NUTRIENT	UNIT	AMOUNT	INQ	% STD	0 ... 10 ... 20 ... 100
ENERGY	KCAL	5.00	1.00	0	-
VITAMIN A	IU	0.00	0.00	0	-
VITAMIN C	MG	0.00	0.00	0	-
THIAMIN	MG	0.00	0.00	0	-
RIBUFLAVN	MG	0.00	0.00	0	-
NIACIN	MG	0.00	0.00	0	-
IRON	MG	0.10	2.50	1	I
CALCIUM	MG	4.00	1.78	0	-
PHOSPHRUS	MG	4.00	1.78	0	-
POTASSIUM	MG	7.00	0.56	0	-
PROTEIN	G	0.00	0.00	0	-
CARBOHYDT	G	0.00	0.00	0	-
FAT	G	0.00	0.00	0	-
OLEIC A	G	0.00	0.00	0	-
LINOL A	G	0.10	2.00	1	L
SAT FAT A	G	0.00	0.00	0	-

701 GREEN OLIVES, CANNED, PITTED
ANALYSIS OF 13 GRAMS WHICH IS 4 MEDIUM OR 3 EXTRA LARGE OR 2 GIANT

NUTRIENT	UNIT	AMOUNT	INQ	% STD		0	10	20	30	40	50	60	70	80	90	100
ENERGY	KCAL	15.00	1.00	1	E											
VITAMIN A	IU	40.00	1.33	1	A											
VITAMIN C	MG	0.00	0.00	0	-											
THIAMIN	MG	0.00	0.00	0	-											
RIBOFLAVN	MG	0.00	0.00	0	-											
NIACIN	MG	0.00	0.00	0	-											
IRON	MG	0.20	1.67	1	I											
CALCIUM	MG	8.00	1.19	1	K											
PHOSPHRUS	MG	2.00	0.30	0	-											
POTASSIUM	MG	7.00	0.19	0	-											
PROTEIN	G	0.00	0.00	0	-											
CARBOHYDT	G	0.00	0.00	0	IF											
FAT	G	2.00	3.42	3	1000											
OLEIC A	G	1.20	6.53	5	-											
LINOL A	G	0.10	0.67	1	S											
SAT FAT A	G	0.20	0.94	1												

702 RIPE OLIVES (MISSION), CANNED, PITTED
ANALYSIS OF 9 GRAMS WHICH IS 3 SMALL OR 2 LARGE

NUTRIENT	UNIT	AMOUNT	INQ	% STD		0	10	20	30	40	50	60	70	80	90	100
ENERGY	KCAL	15.00	1.00	1	E											
VITAMIN A	IU	10.00	0.33	0	-											
VITAMIN C	MG	0.00	0.00	0	-											
THIAMIN	MG	0.00	0.00	0	-											
RIBOFLAVN	MG	0.00	0.00	0	-											
NIACIN	MG	0.00	0.00	0	-											
IRON	MG	0.10	0.83	1	I											
CALCIUM	MG	9.00	1.33	1	K											
PHOSPHRUS	MG	1.00	0.15	0	-											
POTASSIUM	MG	2.00	0.05	0	-											
PROTEIN	G	0.00	0.00	0	-											
CARBOHYDT	G	0.00	0.00	0	IF											
FAT	G	2.00	3.42	3	1000											
OLEIC A	G	1.20	6.53	5	-											
LINOL A	G	0.10	0.67	1	S											
SAT FAT A	G	0.20	0.94	1												

703 DILL PICKLES
ANALYSIS OF 65 GRAMS WHICH IS 1 MEDIUM PICKEL 3 3/4-IN LONG, 1 1/4-IN DIAM

NUTRIENT	UNIT	AMOUNT	INQ	% STD		10	20	30	40	50	60	70	80	90	100
ENERGY	KCAL	5.00	1.00	0	-										
VITAMIN A	IU	70.00	7.00	2	A										
VITAMIN C	MG	4.00	26.67	7	CCCCC										
THIAMIN	MG	0.00	0.00	0											
RIBOFLAVN	MG	0.01	3.33	1	R										
NIACIN	MG	0.00	0.00	0											
IRON	MG	0.70	17.50	4	IIII										
CALCIUM	MG	17.00	7.56	2	KK										
PHOSPHRUS	MG	14.00	6.22	2	X										
POTASSIUM	MG	130.00	10.40	3	YY										
PROTEIN	G	1.00	1.45	0	-										
CARBOHYDT	G	0.00	0.00	0	-										
FAT	G	0.00	0.00	0	-										
OLEIC A	G	0.00	0.00	0	-										
LINOL A	G	0.00	0.00	0	-										
SAT FAT A	G	0.00	0.00	0	-										

704 PICKELS, FRESH-PACK SLICES
ANALYSIS OF 15 GRAMS WHICH IS 2 SLICES 1 1/2-IN DIAM, 1/4-IN THICK

NUTRIENT	UNIT	AMOUNT	INQ	% STD		10	20	30	40	50	60	70	80	90	100
ENERGY	KCAL	10.00	1.00	1	-										
VITAMIN A	IU	20.00	1.00	1	-										
VITAMIN C	MG	1.00	3.33	2	C										
THIAMIN	MG	0.00	0.00	0	-										
RIBOFLAVN	MG	0.00	0.00	0	-										
NIACIN	MG	0.00	0.00	0	-										
IRON	MG	0.30	3.75	2	II										
CALCIUM	MG	5.00	1.11	1	-										
PHOSPHRUS	MG	4.00	0.89	0	-										
POTASSIUM	MG	30.00	1.20	1	-										
PROTEIN	G	0.00	0.00	1	H										
CARBOHYDT	G	3.00	2.18	1	-										
FAT	G	0.00	0.00	0	-										
OLEIC A	G	0.00	0.00	0	-										
LINOL A	G	0.00	0.00	0	-										
SAT FAT A	G	0.00	0.00	0	-										

705 SWEET PICKLES, SMALL, WHOLE, GHERKINS
ANALYSIS OF 15 GRAMS WHICH IS 1 PICKEL, 2 1/2-IN LONG, 3/4-IN DIAM.

NUTRIENT	UNIT	AMOUNT	INQ	% STD	0	10	20	30	40	50	60	70	80	90	100
ENERGY	KCAL	20.00	1.00	1	E										*
VITAMIN A	IU	10.00	0.25	0											*
VITAMIN C	MG	1.00	1.67	2	C										*
THIAMIN	MG	0.00	0.00	0											*
RIBOFLAVN	MG	0.00	0.00	0											*
NIACIN	MG	0.00	0.00	0											*
IRON	MG	0.20	1.25	1	I										*
CALCIUM	MG	2.00	0.22	0											*
PHOSPHRUS	MG	2.00	0.22	0											*
POTASSIUM	MG	30.00	0.60	1											*
PROTEIN	G	0.00	0.00	0											*
CARBOHYDT	G	5.00	1.82	2	H										*
FAT	G	0.00	0.00	0											*
OLEIC A	G	0.00	0.00	0											*
LINOL A	G	0.00	0.00	0											*
SAT FAT A	G	0.00	0.00	0											*

706 SWEET PICKLE RELISH, FINELY CHOPPED
ANALYSIS OF 15 GRAMS WHICH IS 1 TBSP

NUTRIENT	UNIT	AMOUNT	INQ	% STD	0	10	20	30	40	50	60	70	80	90	100
ENERGY	KCAL	20.00	1.00	1	E										*
VITAMIN A	IU	20.00	0.50	1											*
VITAMIN C	MG	1.00	1.67	2	C										*
THIAMIN	MG	0.00	0.00	0											*
RIBOFLAVN	MG	0.00	0.00	0											*
NIACIN	MG	0.00	0.00	0											*
IRON	MG	0.10	0.63	1	I										*
CALCIUM	MG	3.00	0.33	0											*
PHOSPHRUS	MG	2.00	0.22	0											*
POTASSIUM	MG	30.00	0.60	1											*
PROTEIN	G	0.00	0.00	0											*
CARBOHYDT	G	5.00	1.82	2	H										*
FAT	G	0.00	0.00	0											*
OLEIC A	G	0.00	0.00	0											*
LINOL A	G	0.00	0.00	0											*
SAT FAT A	G	0.00	0.00	0											*

707 POPSICLE
ANALYSIS OF 95 GRAMS WHICH IS 3-FL OZ SIZE POPSICLE

NUTRIENT	UNIT	AMOUNT	INQ	% STD	0	10	20	30	40	50	60	70	80	90	100
ENERGY	KCAL	70.00	1.00	4	EEE										
VITAMIN A	IU	0.00	0.00	0											
VITAMIN C	MG	0.00	0.00	0											
THIAMIN	MG	0.00	0.00	0											
RIBOFLAVN	MG	0.00	0.00	0											
NIACIN	MG	0.00	0.00	0											
IRON	MG	0.00	0.00	0											
CALCIUM	MG	0.00	0.00	0											
PHOSPHRUS	MG	0.00	0.00	0											
POTASSIUM	MG	0.00	0.00	0											
PROTEIN	G	0.00	0.00	0											
CARBOHYDT	G	18.00	1.87	7	HH|HH										
FAT	G	0.00	0.00	0											
OLEIC A	G	0.00	0.00	0											
LINOL A	G	0.00	0.00	0											
SAT FAT A	G	0.00	0.00	0											

708 CREAM OF CHICKEN SOUP PREPARED WITH EQUAL VOLUME OF MILK, CANNED
ANALYSIS OF 245 GRAMS WHICH IS 1 CUP

NUTRIENT	UNIT	AMOUNT	INQ	% STD	0	10	20	30	40	50	60	70	80	90	100
ENERGY	KCAL	180.00	1.00	9	EEEEEE										
VITAMIN A	IU	610.00	1.69	15	AAAAAA|AAAAA										
VITAMIN C	MG	2.00	0.37	3	CCC										
THIAMIN	MG	0.05	0.56	5	TTT										
RIBOFLAVN	MG	0.27	2.50	23	RRRRR|RRRRRRRRRR										
NIACIN	MG	0.70	0.56	5	NNNN										
IRON	MG	0.50	0.35	3	III										
CALCIUM	MG	172.00	2.12	19	KKKKKK|KKKKKKK										
PHOSPHRUS	MG	152.00	1.88	17	XXXXXX|XXXXXXX										
POTASSIUM	MG	260.00	0.58	5	YYYY										
PROTEIN	G	7.00	1.56	14	PPPPP|PPPP										
CARBOHYDT	G	15.00	0.61	5	HHHH										
FAT	G	10.00	1.42	13	FFFFF|FFF										
OLEIC A	G	3.60	1.63	15	OOOOO|OOOOO										
LINOL A	G	1.30	0.72	7	LLLLL|L										
SAT FAT A	G	4.20	1.64	15	SSSSS|SSSSS										

709 CREAM OF MUSHROOM SOUP PREPARED WITH EQUAL VOLUME OF MILK, CANNED
ANALYSIS OF 245 GRAMS WHICH IS 1 CUP

```
NUTRIENT    UNIT  AMOUNT   INQ   % STD   0        10        20        30        40        50        60        70        80        90       100
ENERGY      KCAL  215.00   1.00   11     EEEEEEEE
VITAMIN A   IU    250.00   0.58    6     AAAAA |
VITAMIN C   MG      1.00   0.16    2     C     |
THIAMIN     MG      0.05   0.47    5     TTT   |
RIBOFLAVN   MG      0.34   2.64   28     RRRRRRRR|RRRRRRRRRRRR
NIACIN      MG      0.70   0.47    5     NNNN  |
IRON        MG      0.50   0.29    3     III   |
CALCIUM     MG    191.00   1.97   21     KKKKKKKK|KKKKKKKK
PHOSPHRUS   MG    169.00   1.75   19     XXXXXXXX|XXXXXX
POTASSIUM   MG    279.00   0.52    6     YYYY  |
PROTEIN     G       7.00   1.30   14     PPPPPPP|PP
CARBOHYDT   G      16.00   0.54    6     HHHH  |
FAT         G      14.00   1.67   18     FFFFFFFF|FFFFF
OLEIC A     G       2.90   1.10   12     OOOOOOOOO
LINOL A     G       4.60   2.14   23     LLLLLLLL|LLLLLLLLL
SAT FAT A   G       5.40   1.76   19     SSSSSSSS|SSSSSS
*****************************************************
```

710 TOMATO SOUP PREPARED WITH EQUAL VOLUME OF MILK, CANNED
ANALYSIS OF 250 GRAMS WHICH IS 1 CUP

```
NUTRIENT    UNIT  AMOUNT    INQ   % STD   0        10        20        30        40        50        60        70        80        90       100
ENERGY      KCAL  175.00    1.00    9     EEEEEEE
VITAMIN A   IU   1200.00    3.43   30     AAAAAAAA|AAAAAAAAAAAAAAAAAAAAAA
VITAMIN C   MG     15.00    2.86   25     CCCCCCC|CCCCCCCCCCCCCCCCC
THIAMIN     MG      0.10    1.14   10     TTTTTTTT
RIBOFLAVN   MG      0.25    2.38   21     RRRRRRRR|RRRRRRRRRRRR
NIACIN      MG      1.30    1.06    9     NNNNNNNN
IRON        MG      0.80    0.57    5     IIII  |
CALCIUM     MG    168.00    2.13   19     KKKKKKKK|KKKKKKKK
PHOSPHRUS   MG    155.00    1.97   17     XXXXXXXX|XXXXXXX
POTASSIUM   MG    418.00    0.96    8     YYYYYYY
PROTEIN     G       7.00    1.60   14     PPPPPPP|PPPP
CARBOHYDT   G      23.00    0.96    8     HHHHHHH
FAT         G       7.00    1.03    9     FFFFFFF
OLEIC A     G       1.70    0.79    7     OOOOOO
LINOL A     G       1.00    0.57    5     LLLL  |
SAT FAT A   G       3.40    1.36   12     SSSSSSS|SSS
*****************************************************
```

711 BEAN WITH PORK SOUP PREPARED WITH EQUAL VOLUME OF WATER, CANNED
ANALYSIS OF 250 GRAMS WHICH IS 1 CUP

NUTRIENT	UNIT	AMOUNT	INQ	% STD	0 10 20 30 40 50 60 70 80 90 100
ENERGY	KCAL	170.00	1.00	9	EEEEEEE
VITAMIN A	IU	650.00	1.91	16	AAAAAA|AAAAAA
VITAMIN C	MG	3.00	0.59	5	CCCC
THIAMIN	MG	0.13	1.53	13	TTTTT|TTT
RIBOFLAVN	MG	0.08	0.78	7	RRRR
NIACIN	MG	1.00	0.84	7	NNNNN
IRON	MG	2.30	1.69	14	IIIII|IIIII
CALCIUM	MG	63.00	0.82	7	KKKKK
PHOSPHRUS	MG	128.00	1.67	14	XXXXX|XXXX
POTASSIUM	MG	395.00	0.93	8	YYYYY|Y
PROTEIN	G	8.00	1.88	16	PPPPP|PPPPP
CARBOHYDT	G	22.00	0.94	8	HHHHHH
FAT	G	6.00	0.90	8	FFFFF
OLEIC A	G	1.80	0.86	7	OOOOOO
LINOL A	G	2.40	1.41	12	LLLLL|LLL
SAT FAT A	G	1.20	0.50	4	SSS

712 BEEF BROTH, BOUILLON, CONSOMME
ANALYSIS OF 240 GRAMS WHICH IS 1 CUP

NUTRIENT	UNIT	AMOUNT	INQ	% STD	0 10 20 30 40 50 60 70 80 90 100
ENERGY	KCAL	30.00	1.00	2	E
VITAMIN A	IU	0.00	0.00	0	-
VITAMIN C	MG	0.00	0.00	0	-
THIAMIN	MG	0.00	0.00	0	
RIBOFLAVN	MG	0.02	1.11	2	K
NIACIN	MG	1.20	5.71	9	NNNNNN
IRON	MG	0.50	2.08	3	II
CALCIUM	MG	0.00	0.00	0	
PHOSPHRUS	MG	31.00	2.30	3	XX
POTASSIUM	MG	130.00	1.73	3	Y
PROTEIN	G	5.00	6.67	10	PPPPPPP
CARBOHYDT	G	3.00	0.73	1	H
FAT	G	0.00	0.00	0	
OLEIC A	G	0.00	0.00	0	
LINOL A	G	0.00	0.00	0	
SAT FAT A	G	0.00	0.00	0	

713 BEEF NOODLE SOUP, PREPARED WITH EQUAL VOLUME OF WATER,CANNED
ANALYSIS OF 240 GRAMS WHICH IS 1 CUP

NUTRIENT	UNIT	AMOUNT	INQ	% STD	0 10 20 30 40 50 60 70 80 90 100
ENERGY	KCAL	65.00	1.00	3	EEE
VITAMIN A	IU	50.00	0.38	1	A	
VITAMIN C	MG	0.00	0.00	1	-	
THIAMIN	MG	0.05	1.54	5	TT|T
RIBOFLAVN	MG	0.07	1.79	6	RR|RR
NIACIN	MG	1.00	2.20	7	NN|NNN
IRON	MG	1.00	1.92	6	II|II
CALCIUM	MG	7.00	0.24	1	K	
PHOSPHRUS	MG	48.00	1.64	5	XX|X
POTASSIUM	MG	77.00	0.47	2	Y	
PROTEIN	G	4.00	2.46	8	PP|PPP
CARBOHYDT	G	7.00	0.78	3	HH|
FAT	G	3.00	1.18	4	FFF
OLEIC A	G	0.70	0.88	3	OOI
LINOL A	G	0.80	1.23	4	LLL
SAT FAT A	G	0.60	0.65	2	SSI

714 CLAM CHOWDER, MANHATTEN TYPE WITH TOMATOES AND WITH OUT MILK
ANALYSIS OF 245 GRAMS WHICH IS 1 CUP

NUTRIENT	UNIT	AMOUNT	INQ	% STD	0 10 20 30 40 50 60 70 80 90 100
ENERGY	KCAL	80.00	1.00	4	EEE
VITAMIN A	IU	880.00	5.50	22	AA|AAAAAAAAAAAAAAAA
VITAMIN C	MG	0.00	0.00	0	-	
THIAMIN	MG	0.02	0.50	2	IT|
RIBOFLAVN	MG	0.02	0.42	2	R	
NIACIN	MG	1.00	1.79	7	NN|NNN
IRON	MG	1.00	1.56	6	II|III
CALCIUM	MG	34.00	0.94	4	KKK
PHOSPHRUS	MG	47.00	1.31	5	XX|X
POTASSIUM	MG	184.00	0.92	4	YYY
PROTEIN	G	2.00	1.00	4	PPP
CARBOHYDT	G	12.00	1.09	4	HHH
FAT	G	3.00	0.96	4	FFF
OLEIC A	G	0.40	0.41	2	O	
LINOL A	G	1.30	1.63	7	LL|LLL
SAT FAT A	G	0.50	0.44	2	S	

715 CREAM OF CHICKEN SOUP PREPARED WITH EQUAL VOLUME OF WATER, CANNED
ANALYSIS OF 240 GRAMS WHICH IS 1 CUP

```
                                        0   10   20   30   40   50   60   70   80   90  100
                                                                                         ************************
NUTRIENT   UNIT   AMOUNT   INQ   % STD
ENERGY     KCAL    95.00   1.00    5   EEEE
VITAMIN A  IU     410.00   2.16   10   AAA|AAAA
VITAMIN C  MG       0.00   0.00    0   -|
THIAMIN    MG       0.02   0.42    2   TT|
RIBOFLAVN  MG       0.05   0.88    4   RRR|
NIACIN     MG       0.50   0.75    4   NNN|
IRON       MG       0.50   0.66    3   III|
CALCIUM    MG      24.00   0.56    3   KK|
PHOSPHRUS  MG      34.00   0.80    3   XXX|
POTASSIUM  MG      79.00   0.33    2   Y|
PROTEIN    G        3.00   1.26    6   PPP|P
CARBOHYDT  G        8.00   0.61    3   HH|
FAT        G        6.00   1.62    8   FFF|FF
OLEIC A    G        2.30   1.98    9   OOO1OOOO
LINOL A    G        1.10   1.16    6   LLLL
SAT FAT A  G        1.60   1.18    6   SSSS
*********************************************
```

716 CREAM OF MUSHROOM, PREPARED WITH EQUAL VOLUME OF WATER, CANNED
ANALYSIS OF 240 GRAMS WHICH IS 1 CUP

```
                                        0   10   20   30   40   50   60   70   80   90  100
                                                                                         ************************
NUTRIENT   UNIT   AMOUNT   INQ   % STD
ENERGY     KCAL   135.00   1.00    7   EEEEE
VITAMIN A  IU      70.00   0.26    2   A|
VITAMIN C  MG       0.00   0.00    0   -|
THIAMIN    MG       0.02   0.30    2   TT|
RIBOFLAVN  MG       0.12   1.48   10   RRRR|RRR
NIACIN     MG       0.70   0.74    5   NNNN|
IRON       MG       0.50   0.46    3   III|
CALCIUM    MG      41.00   0.67    5   KKKK|
PHOSPHRUS  MG      50.00   0.82    6   XXXX|
POTASSIUM  MG      98.00   0.29    2   YY|
PROTEIN    G        2.00   0.59    4   PPP|
CARBOHYDT  G       10.00   0.54    4   HHH|
FAT        G       10.00   1.90   13   FFF|FFFFF
OLEIC A    G        1.70   1.03    7   OOOOO|O
LINOL A    G        4.50   3.33   23   LLLLLLLLLLLLLLLLLL
SAT FAT A  G        2.60   1.35    9   SSSS|SS
*********************************************
```

717 MINESTRONE SOUP PREPARED WITH EQUAL VOLUME OF WATER, CANNED
ANALYSIS OF 245 GRAMS WHICH IS 1 CUP

NUTRIENT	UNIT	AMOUNT	INQ	% STD	0 10 20 30 40 50 60 70 80 90 100
ENERGY	KCAL	105.00	1.00	5	EEEE
VITAMIN A	IU	2350.00	11.19	59	AAA|AAAAAAAAAAAAAAAAAAAAAAAAAAAAAAAAAAAAAAAAAAAAAAAA
VITAMIN C	MG	0.00	0.00	0	-
THIAMIN	MG	0.07	1.33	7	TTT|TT
RIBOFLAVN	MG	0.05	0.79	4	RRR|
NIACIN	MG	1.00	1.36	7	NNN|NNN
IRON	MG	1.00	1.19	6	III|I
CALCIUM	MG	37.00	0.78	4	KKK|
PHOSPHRUS	MG	59.00	1.25	7	XXX|X
POTASSIUM	MG	314.00	1.20	6	YYY|Y
PROTEIN	G	5.00	1.90	10	PPP|PPPP
CARBOHYDT	G	14.00	0.97	5	HHH|
FAT	G	3.00	0.73	4	FFF|
OLEIC A	G	0.90	0.70	4	OOO|
LINOL A	G	1.30	1.24	7	LLL|L
SAT FAT A	G	0.70	0.47	2	SS |

718 SPLIT PEA SOUP PREPARED WITH EQUAL VOLUME OF WATER, CANNED
ANALYSIS OF 245 GRAMS WHICH IS 1 CUP

NUTRIENT	UNIT	AMOUNT	INQ	% STD	0 10 20 30 40 50 60 70 80 90 100
ENERGY	KCAL	145.00	1.00	7	EEEEEE
VITAMIN A	IU	440.00	1.52	11	AAAA|AAA
VITAMIN C	MG	1.00	0.23	2	C |
THIAMIN	MG	0.25	3.45	25	TTTTT|TTTTTTTTTTTTTTTT
RIBOFLAVN	MG	0.15	1.72	13	RRRR|RRRR
NIACIN	MG	1.50	1.48	11	NNNN|NNN
IRUN	MG	1.50	1.29	9	IIII|III
CALCIUM	MG	29.00	0.44	3	KKK|
PHOSPHRUS	MG	149.00	2.28	17	XXXXX|XXXXXXX
POTASSIUM	MG	270.00	0.74	5	YYYY|
PROTEIN	G	9.00	2.48	18	PPPPP|PPPPPPP
CARBOHYDT	G	21.00	1.05	8	HHHHH|
FAT	G	3.00	0.53	4	FFF|
OLEIC A	G	1.20	0.68	5	OOO|
LINOL A	G	0.40	0.28	2	LL |
SAT FAT A	G	1.10	0.53	4	SSS|

719 TOMATO SOUP PREPARED WITH EQUAL VOLUME OF WATER, CANNED
ANALYSIS OF 245 GRAMS WHICH IS 1 CUP

NUTRIENT	UNIT	AMOUNT	INQ	% STD	0 10 20 30 40 50 60 70 80 90 100
ENERGY	KCAL	90.00	1.00	5	EEEE
VITAMIN A	IU	1000.00	5.56	25	AAA|AAAAAAAAAAAAA
VITAMIN C	MG	12.00	4.44	20	CCC|CCCCCCCCCCC
THIAMIN	MG	0.05	1.11	5	T|T|T
RIBOFLAVN	MG	0.05	0.93	4	RRR|
NIACIN	MG	1.20	1.90	9	NNN|NNN
IRON	MG	0.70	0.97	4	III|
CALCIUM	MG	15.00	0.37	2	K|
PHOSPHRUS	MG	34.00	0.84	4	XXX|
POTASSIUM	MG	230.00	1.02	5	YYYY
PROTEIN	G	2.00	0.89	4	PPP|
CARBOHYDT	G	16.00	1.29	6	HHH|H
FAT	G	3.00	0.85	4	FFF|
OLEIC A	G	0.50	0.45	2	OO |
LINOL A	G	1.00	1.11	5	LLLL
SAT FAT A	G	0.50	0.39	2	S |

720 VEGETABLE BEEF SOUP PREPARED WITH EQUAL VOLUME OF WATER, CANNED
ANALYSIS OF 245 GRAMS WHICH IS 1 CUP

NUTRIENT	UNIT	AMOUNT	INQ	% STD	0 10 20 30 40 50 60 70 80 90 100
ENERGY	KCAL	80.00	1.00	4	EEE
VITAMIN A	IU	2700.00	16.88	68	AA|AAAAAAAAAAAAAAAAAAAAAAAAAAAAAAAAAAAAAAAAAAAAAAAAAAAAAAAAAAAAA
VITAMIN C	MG	0.00	0.00	0	- |
THIAMIN	MG	0.05	1.25	5	TT|T
RIBOFLAVN	MG	0.05	1.04	4	RRR|
NIACIN	MG	1.00	1.79	7	NNI|NNN
IRON	MG	0.70	1.09	4	III|
CALCIUM	MG	12.00	0.33	1	K |
PHOSPHRUS	MG	49.00	1.36	5	XX|X
POTASSIUM	MG	162.00	0.81	3	YYY|
PROTEIN	G	5.00	2.50	10	PP|PPPPP
CARBOHYDT	G	10.00	0.91	4	HHH|
FAT	G	2.00	0.64	3	FF|
OLEIC A	G	0.00	0.00	0	- |
LINOL A	G	0.00	0.00	0	- |
SAT FAT A	G	0.00	0.00	0	- |

721 VEGETARIAN SOUP PREPARED WITH EQUAL VOLUME OF WATER, CANNED
ANALYSIS OF 245 GRAMS WHICH IS 1 CUP

NUTRIENT	UNIT	AMOUNT	ING	% STD
ENERGY	KCAL	80.00	1.00	4
VITAMIN A	IU	2940.00	18.38	74
VITAMIN C	MG	0.00	0.00	0
THIAMIN	MG	0.05	1.25	5
RIBOFLAVN	MG	0.05	1.04	4
NIACIN	MG	1.00	1.79	7
IRON	MG	1.00	1.56	6
CALCIUM	MG	20.00	0.56	2
PHOSPHRUS	MG	39.00	1.08	3
POTASSIUM	MG	172.00	0.86	3
PROTEIN	G	2.00	1.00	4
CARBOHYDT	G	13.00	1.18	5
FAT	G	2.00	0.64	3
OLEIC A	G	0.00	0.00	0
LINOL A	G	0.00	0.00	0
SAT FAT A	G	0.00	0.00	0

722 BOUILLON CUBE
ANALYSIS OF 4 GRAMS WHICH IS 1/2-IN CUBE

NUTRIENT	UNIT	AMOUNT	ING	% STD
ENERGY	KCAL	5.00	1.00	0
VITAMIN A	IU	0.00	0.00	0
VITAMIN C	MG	0.00	0.00	0
THIAMIN	MG	0.00	0.00	0
RIBOFLAVN	MG	0.00	0.00	0
NIACIN	MG	0.00	0.00	0
IRON	MG	0.00	0.00	0
CALCIUM	MG	0.00	0.00	0
PHOSPHRUS	MG	0.00	0.00	0
POTASSIUM	MG	4.00	0.32	0
PROTEIN	G	1.00	8.00	2
CARBOHYDT	G	0.00	0.00	0
FAT	G	0.00	0.00	0
OLEIC A	G	0.10	1.63	0
LINOL A	G	0.00	0.00	0
SAT FAT A	G	0.00	0.00	0

723 ONION SOUP, UNPREPARED DRY MIX
ANALYSIS OF 43 GRAMS WHICH IS 1 1/2-OZ PKG

NUTRIENT	UNIT	AMOUNT	INQ	% STD
ENERGY	KCAL	150.00	1.00	8
VITAMIN A	IU	30.00	0.10	1
VITAMIN C	MG	6.00	1.33	10
THIAMIN	MG	0.05	0.67	5
RIBOFLAVN	MG	0.33	0.33	3
NIACIN	MG	0.29	0.50	2
IRON	MG	0.60	0.50	4
CALCIUM	MG	42.00	0.62	5
PHOSPHRUS	MG	49.00	0.73	5
POTASSIUM	MG	238.00	0.63	5
PROTEIN	G	6.00	1.60	12
CARBOHYDT	G	23.00	1.12	8
FAT	G	5.00	0.85	6
OLEIC A	G	2.30	1.25	9
LINOL A	G	1.00	0.67	5
SAT FAT A	G	1.10	0.51	4

724 CHICKEN NOODLE SOUP, PREPARED WITH WATER FROM DRY MIX
ANALYSIS OF 240 GRAMS WHICH IS 1 CUP

NUTRIENT	UNIT	AMOUNT	INQ	% STD
ENERGY	KCAL	55.00	1.00	3
VITAMIN A	IU	50.00	0.45	1
VITAMIN C	MG	0.00	0.00	0
THIAMIN	MG	0.07	2.55	7
RIBOFLAVN	MG	0.05	1.52	4
NIACIN	MG	0.50	1.30	4
IRON	MG	0.20	0.45	1
CALCIUM	MG	7.00	0.28	1
PHOSPHRUS	MG	19.00	0.77	2
POTASSIUM	MG	19.00	0.14	0
PROTEIN	G	2.00	1.45	4
CARBOHYDT	G	8.00	1.06	3
FAT	G	1.00	0.47	1
OLEIC A	G	0.00	0.00	0
LINOL A	G	0.00	0.00	0
SAT FAT A	G	0.00	0.00	0

725 ONION SOUP, PREPARED WITH WATER FROM DRY MIX
ANALYSIS OF 240 GRAMS WHICH IS 1 CUP

NUTRIENT	UNIT	AMOUNT	INQ	% STD	0
ENERGY	KCAL	35.00	1.00	2	E
VITAMIN A	IU	0.00	0.00	0	-
VITAMIN C	MG	2.00	1.90	3	ICC
THIAMIN	MG	0.00	0.00	0	-
RIBOFLAVN	MG	0.00	0.00	0	I
NIACIN	MG	0.00	0.00	1	I
IRON	MG	0.20	0.71	1	K
CALCIUM	MG	10.00	0.63	1	X
PHOSPHRUS	MG	12.00	0.76	1	Y
POTASSIUM	MG	58.00	0.66	1	IP
PROTEIN	G	1.00	1.14	2	IH
CARBOHYDT	G	6.00	1.25	2	IH
FAT	G	1.00	0.73	1	F
OLEIC A	G	0.00	0.00	0	I
LINOL A	G	0.00	0.00	0	I
SAT FAT A	G	0.00	0.00	0	I

726 TOMATO VEGETABLE WITH NOODLE SOUP PREPARED WITH WATER FROM DRY MIX
ANALYSIS OF 240 GRAMS WHICH IS 1 CUP

NUTRIENT	UNIT	AMOUNT	INQ	% STD	0
ENERGY	KCAL	65.00	1.00	3	EEE
VITAMIN A	IU	480.00	3.69	12	AAIAAAAAAA
VITAMIN C	MG	5.00	2.56	8	CCICCCC
THIAMIN	MG	0.05	1.54	5	TTIT
RIBOFLAVN	MG	0.02	0.51	2	R I
NIACIN	MG	0.50	1.10	4	NNN
IRON	MG	0.20	0.38	1	I
CALCIUM	MG	7.00	0.24	1	K I
PHOSPHRUS	MG	19.00	0.65	2	XX I
POTASSIUM	MG	29.00	0.18	1	I
PROTEIN	G	1.00	0.62	2	PPI
CARBOHYDT	G	12.00	1.34	4	HHH
FAT	G	1.00	0.39	1	F I
OLEIC A	G	0.00	0.00	0	I
LINOL A	G	0.00	0.00	0	I
SAT FAT A	G	0.00	0.00	0	I

727 VINEGAR, CIDER
ANALYSIS OF 15 GRAMS WHICH IS 1 TBSP

NUTRIENT	UNIT	AMOUNT	INQ	% STD
ENERGY	KCAL	0.00	0.00	0
VITAMIN A	IU	0.00	0.00	0
VITAMIN C	MG	0.00	0.00	0
THIAMIN	MG	0.00	0.00	0
RIBOFLAVN	MG	0.00	0.00	0
NIACIN	MG	0.00	0.00	0
IRON	MG	0.10	********	1
CALCIUM	MG	1.00	********	0
PHOSPHRUS	MG	1.00	********	0
POTASSIUM	MG	15.00	********	0
PROTEIN	G	1.00	********	0
CARBOHYDT	G	0.00	0.00	0
FAT	G	0.00	0.00	0
OLEIC A	G	0.00	0.00	0
LINOL A	G	0.00	0.00	0
SAT FAT A	G	0.00	0.00	0

728 WHITE SAUCE, MEDIUM WITH ENRICHED FLOUR
ANALYSIS OF 250 GRAMS WHICH IS 1 CUP

NUTRIENT	UNIT	AMOUNT	INQ	% STD
ENERGY	KCAL	405.00	1.00	20
VITAMIN A	IU	1150.00	1.42	29
VITAMIN C	MG	2.00	0.16	3
THIAMIN	MG	0.12	0.59	12
RIBOFLAVN	MG	0.43	1.77	36
NIACIN	MG	0.70	0.25	5
IRON	MG	0.50	0.15	3
CALCIUM	MG	288.00	1.58	32
PHOSPHRUS	MG	233.00	1.28	26
POTASSIUM	MG	348.00	0.34	7
PROTEIN	G	10.00	0.99	20
CARBOHYDT	G	22.00	0.40	8
FAT	G	31.00	1.96	40
OLEIC A	G	7.80	1.57	32
LINOL A	G	0.80	0.20	4
SAT FAT A	G	19.30	3.34	68

729 YEAST, BAKERS DRY ACTIVE
ANALYSIS OF 7 GRAMS WHICH IS 1 PACKAGE

NUTRIENT	UNIT	AMOUNT	INQ	% STD
ENERGY	KCAL	20.00	1.00	1
VITAMIN A	IU	0.00	0.00	0
VITAMIN C	MG	0.00	0.00	0
THIAMIN	MG	0.16	16.00	16
RIBOFLAVN	MG	0.38	31.67	32
NIACIN	MG	2.60	18.57	19
IRON	MG	1.10	6.88	7
CALCIUM	MG	3.00	0.33	0
PHOSPHRUS	MG	90.00	10.00	10
POTASSIUM	MG	140.00	2.80	3
PROTEIN	G	3.00	6.00	6
CARBOHYDT	G	3.00	1.09	1
FAT	G	0.00	0.00	0
OLEIC A	G	0.00	0.00	0
LINOL A	G	0.00	0.00	0
SAT FAT A	G	0.00	0.00	0

730 BREWER'S YEAST, DRY
ANALYSIS OF 8 GRAMS WHICH IS 1 TBSP

NUTRIENT	UNIT	AMOUNT	INQ	% STD
ENERGY	KCAL	25.00	1.00	1
VITAMIN A	IU	0.00	0.00	0
VITAMIN C	MG	0.00	0.00	0
THIAMIN	MG	1.25	100.00	125
RIBOFLAVN	MG	0.34	22.67	28
NIACIN	MG	3.00	17.14	21
IRON	MG	1.40	7.00	9
CALCIUM	MG	17.00	1.51	2
PHOSPHRUS	MG	140.00	12.44	16
POTASSIUM	MG	152.00	2.43	3
PROTEIN	G	3.00	4.80	6
CARBOHYDT	G	3.00	0.87	1
FAT	G	0.00	0.00	0
OLEIC A	G	0.00	0.00	0
LINOL A	G	0.00	0.00	0
SAT FAT A	G	0.00	0.00	0

PART III
Supplementary Foods Lists

13

Supplementary Foods Lists

As we have shown, the nutritional quality of any food or diet is a function of its nutrient components such as protein, vitamins and minerals as related to the specific nutrient needs of an individual. In the last section the concept called the Index of Nutritional Quality (INQ) was used to illustrate the nutritional content of foods. the INQ examines the nutritional quality of foods by relating the nutrients in foods to the kilocalories they contain. By using the INQ, an individual can simultaneously derive qualitative and quanitative evaluations of food and food combinations such as menus and diets.

An INQ of 1.0 or greater from any nutrients in a specified food indicates that the food supplies adequate amounts of that nutrient in comparison to the number of kilocalories it provides. If the food supplies a substantial number of nutrients with INQs for these nutrients of 1.0 or greater, it is of good nutritional quality. The nutrients that have INQs of less than 1.0, would have to be supplemented by other foods during the day. The Supplementary Foods Lists which follow identify foods relatively high in particular nutrients.

VITAMIN A VITAMIN A VITAMIN A VITAMIN A VITAMIN A VITAMIN A VITAMIN A VITAMIN A VITAMIN A VITAMIN A VITAMIN A VITAMIN A

FOODS WHICH PROVIDE A HIGH CONCENTRATION OF VITAMIN A RELATIVE TO CALORIES

(INQ AT LEAST 5.0)

AND AT LEAST 5 PERCENT OF THE RDA PER SERVING

(RDA FOR VITAMIN A = 4000.0 IU)

VITAMIN A VITAMIN A VITAMIN A VITAMIN A VITAMIN A VITAMIN A VITAMIN A VITAMIN A VITAMIN A VITAMIN A VITAMIN A VITAMIN A

*INDICATES FOODS WHICH PROVIDE AT LEAST 25 PERCENT OF THE RDA PER SERVING
**INDICATES FOODS WHICH PROVIDE AT LEAST 50 PERCENT OF THE RDA PER SERVING

HANDBOOK NUMBER	FOOD NAME / SERVING SIZE DESCRIPTION	GRAMS	KCAL	VITAMIN A IU	INQ	%RDA
177	*BEEF AND VEGETABLE STEW / 1 CUP	245	220	2400.00	5.45	60 **
188	**LIVER, BEEF, FRIED / 3 OZ	85	195	45390.00	116.38	1135 **
199	*BRAUNSCHWEIGER / 1 SLICE	28	90	1850.00	10.28	46 *
228	**APRICOTS, RAW, WITHOUT PITS / 3	107	55	2890.00	26.27	72 **
229	**APRICOTS CANNED IN HEAVY SIRUP / 1 CUP-HALVES AND SIRUP	258	220	4490.00	10.20	112 **
230	**APRICOTS,DRIED,UNCOOKED / 1 CUP-28 LARGE OR 37 MEDIUM HALVES	130	340	14170.00	20.84	354 **
231	**APRICOTS, DRIED, COOKED, UNSWEETENED / 1 CUP-FRUIT AND LIQUID	250	215	7500.00	17.44	188 **
232	**APRICOT NECTAR, CANNED / 1 CUP	251	145	2380.00	8.21	59 **
239	*CHERRIES, SOUR, RED, PITTED, CANNED, WATER PACK / 1 CUP	244	105	1660.00	7.90	42 *
246	GRAPEFRUIT, RAW, PINK OR RED, WT WITHOUT PEEL AND MEMBRANES / 1/2 MEDIUM (3 3/4-IN DIAM.) GRAPEFRUIT	123	50	540.00	5.40	14
271	**CANTALOUP, WT WITHOUT RIND AND SEEDS / 1/2 OF A 5-IN DIAM. MELON	272	80	9240.00	57.75	231 **
282	**PAPAYAS, RAW, 1/2 INCH CUBES / 1 CUP	140	55	2450.00	22.27	61 **
283	*PEACHES, RAW, WT FOR PEELED AND PITTED / 1--2 1/2-IN DIAM. PEACH	100	40	1330.00	16.63	33 *
284	**PEACHES, RAW, SLICED / 1 CUP	170	65	2260.00	17.38	57 **
286	*PEACHES, CANNED, WATER PACK / 1 CUP (SOLIDS AND LIQUID)	244	75	1100.00	7.33	28 *
287	**PEACHES, DRIED, UNCOOKED / 1 CUP	160	420	6240.00	7.43	156 **
288	**PEACHES, DRIED, COOKED, UNSWEETENED / 1 CUP (HALVES AND JUICE)	250	205	3050.00	7.44	76 **
302	**PLUMS, CANNED, HEAVY SYRUP PACK / 1 CUP (WITH PITS AND LIQUID)	272	215	3130.00	7.28	78 **
303	*PLUMS, CANNED, HEAVY SYRUP PACK / 3 PLUMS (WITH PITS) AND 2 3/4 TBSP LIQUID	140	110	1610.00	7.32	40 *
318	**WATERMELON, WT WITHOUT RIND AND SEEDS / 1/16 OF 33 LB MELON	426	110	2510.00	11.41	63 **
369	*BRAN FLAKES (40% BRAN), ADDED SUGAR, SALT, IRON AND VITAMINS / 1 CUP	35	105	1650.00	7.86	41 *
370	**BRAN FLAKES WITH RAISINS, ADDED SUGAR, SALT, IRON AND VITAMINS / 1 CUP	50	145	2350.00	8.10	59 **
371	*CORN FLAKES, PLAIN, ADDED SUGAR, SALT, IRON, VITAMINS / 1 CUP	25	95	1180.00	6.21	30 *

HANDBOOK NUMBER	FOOD NAME / SERVING SIZE DESCRIPTION	GRAMS	KCAL	VITAMIN A IU	INQ	%RDA
372	*CORN FLAKES, SUGAR-COATED, ADDED SALT, IRON, VITAMINS / 1 CUP	40	155	1880.00	6.06	47 *
373	PUFFED CORN, PLAIN, ADDED SUGAR, SALT, IRON, VITAMINS / 1 CUP	20	80	940.00	5.88	24
375	*PUFFED OATS, ADDED SUGAR, SALT, MINERALS, VITAMINS / 1 CUP	25	100	1180.00	5.90	30 *
377	*PUFFED RICE, PRESWEETENED, ADDED SALT, IRON, VITAMINS / 1 CUP	28	115	1250.00	5.43	31 *
378	*WHEAT FLAKES, ADDED SUGAR, SALT, IRON, VITAMINS / 1 CUP	30	105	1410.00	6.71	35 *
380	*PUFFED WHEAT, PRESWEETENED, ADDED SALT, IRON, VITAMINS / 1 CUP	38	140	1680.00	6.00	42 *
471	**PUMPKIN PIE / 1 PIE 9-IN DIAM	910	1920	22480.00	5.85	562 **
472	**PUMPKIN PIE / 1 SECTOR, 1/7 OF PIE	130	275	3210.00	5.84	80 **
564	*ASPARAGUS, COOKED,DRAINED,FROM RAW / 1 CUP (CUTS AND TIPS, 1 1/2 TO 2-IN LENGTHS)	145	30	1310.00	21.83	33 *
565	*ASPARAGUS, COOKED-DRAINED,FROM FROZEN / 1 CUP (CUTS AND TIPS, 1 1/2 TO 2-IN LENGTHS)	180	40	1530.00	19.13	38 *
566	ASPARAGUS, SPEARS 1/2-IN DIAM AT BASE FROM RAW / 4 SPEARS	60	10	540.00	27.00	14
567	ASPARAGUS, SPEARS 1/2-IN DIAM AT BASE FROM FROZEN / 4 SPEARS	60	15	470.00	15.67	12
568	ASPARAGUS, CANNED SPEARS / 4 SPEARS	80	15	640.00	21.33	16
571	GREEN SNAP BEANS, COOKED, DRAINED, FROM RAW / 1 CUP	125	30	680.00	11.33	17
572	GREEN SNAP BEANS, COOKED, DRAINED,CUTS FROM FROZEN / 1 CUP	135	35	780.00	11.14	20
573	GREEN SNAP BEANS, COOKED, DRAINED,FRENCH CUTS FROM FROZEN / 1 CUP	130	35	690.00	9.86	17
574	GREEN SNAP BEANS, CANNED, DRAINED SOLIDS (CUTS) / 1 CUP	135	30	630.00	10.50	16
584	**BEET GREENS, COOKED, DRAINED / 1 CUP	145	25	7400.00	148.00	185 **
587	**BROCCOLI, COOKED, DRAINED, FROM RAW / 1 WHOLE MEDIUM STALK	187	45	4500.00	50.00	113 **
588	**BROCCOLI, COOKED, DRAINED, FROM RAW / 1 CUP (STALKS CUT INTO 1/2-IN PIECES)	155	40	3880.00	48.50	97 **
589	BROCCOLI, FROM FROZEN, COOKED, DRAINED / 1 PIECE, 4 1/2 TO 5 IN LONG	30	10	570.00	28.50	14
590	**BROCCOLI, FROM FROZEN, CHOPPED, COOKED, DRAINED / 1 CUP	185	50	4810.00	48.10	120 **
591	BRUSSELS SPROUTS, COOKED, DRAINED, FROM RAW / 7-8 SPROUTS (1 1/4 TO 1 1/2-IN DIAM) 1 CUP	155	55	810.00	7.36	20

HANDBOOK NUMBER	FOOD NAME / SERVING SIZE DESCRIPTION	GRAMS	KCAL	VITAMIN A IU	INQ	%RDA
592	BRUSSELS SPROUTS, COOKED, DRAINED, FROM FROZEN 1 CUP	155	50	880.00	8.80	22
599	**WHITE MUSTARD CABBAGE, COOKED, DRAINED 1 CUP	170	25	5270.00	105.40	132 **
600	**CARROTS, RAW, PEELED 1 CARROT OR 18 STRIPS 2 1/2 TO 3-IN LONG	72	30	7930.00	132.17	198 **
601	**CARROTS, RAW, PEELED, GRATED 1 CUP	110	45	12100.00	134.44	302 **
602	**CARROTS (CROSSWISE CUTS) COOKED, DRAINED 1 CUP	155	50	16280.00	162.80	407 **
603	**CARROTS, CANNED, SLICED, DRAINED SOLIDS 1 CUP	155	45	23250.00	258.33	581 **
604	**CARROTS,STRAINED OR BABY FOOD 1 OZ (1 3/4 TO 2 TBSP)	28	10	3690.00	184.50	92 **
609	CELERY, RAW DICED 1 CUP	120	20	320.00	8.00	8
610	**COLLARDS, COOKED, DRAINED, FROM RAW 1 CUP	190	65	14820.00	114.00	371 **
611	**COLLARDS, COOKED DRAINED, FROM FROZEN 1 CUP	170	50	11560.00	115.60	289 **
620	**DANDELION GREENS, COOKED, DRAINED 1 CUP	105	35	12290.00	175.57	307 **
621	*ENDIVE,CURLY,RAW SMALL PIECES 1 CUP	50	10	1650.00	82.50	41 *
622	**KALE, COOKED, DRAINED, FROM RAW, LEAVES WITHOUT STEMS 1 CUP	110	45	9130.00	101.44	228 **
623	**KALE, COOKED, DRAINED, FROM FROZEN, LEAF STYLE 1 CUP	130	40	10660.00	133.25	266 **
624	*BUTTERHEAD LETTUCE, RAW 1 HEAD,5-IN DIAM.	220	25	1580.00	31.60	40 *
626	*ICEBERG LETTUCE (CRISPHEAD) 1 HEAD, 6-IN DIAM	567	70	1780.00	12.71	45 *
627	ICEBERG LETTUCE (CRISPHEAD) 1 WEDGE (1/4 HEAD)	135	20	450.00	11.25	11
629	*LOOSELEAF LETTUCE, CHOPPED OR SHREDDED 1 CUP	55	10	1050.00	52.50	26 *
631	**MUSTARD GREENS, COOKED, DRAINED, WITHOUT STEMS 1 CUP	140	30	8120.00	135.33	203 **
632	OKRA PODS, COOKED 10 PODS 3 BY 5/8 IN	106	30	520.00	8.67	13
637	PARSLEY, RAW, CHOPPED 1 TBSP	4	0	300.00	*********	8
642	*PEPPERS, HOT, RED, WITHOUT SEEDS, DRIED (GROUND CHILI PWDR ADDED SEASONING) 1 TSP	2	5	1300.00	130.00	33 *
643	SWEET PEPPERS, RAW 1 POD (5 PER LB)	74	15	310.00	10.33	8

HANDBOOK NUMBER	FOOD NAME SERVING SIZE DESCRIPTION	GRAMS	KCAL	VITAMIN A IU	INQ	%RDA
		73	15	310.00	10.33	8
644	SWEET PEPPERS, COOKED, DRAINED. 1 POD					
656	*PUMPKIN, CANNED 1 CUP	245	80	15680.00	98.00	392 **
659	**SPINACH, RAW, CHOPPED 1 CUP	55	15	4460.00	148.67	112 **
660	**SPINACH, COOKED, DRAINED FROM RAW 1 CUP	180	40	14580.00	182.25	365 **
661	**SPINACH, COOKED, DRAINED FROM FROZEN, CHOPPED 1 CUP	205	45	16200.00	180.00	405 **
662	*SPINACH, COOKED, DRAINED FROM FROZEN, LEAF. 1 CUP	190	45	15390.00	171.00	385 **
663	**SPINACH, CANNED, DRAINED SOLIDS 1 CUP	205	50	16400.00	164.00	410 **
664	SUMMER SQUASH, COOKED, DICED, DRAINED 1 CUP	210	30	820.00	13.67	21
665	**WINTER SQUASH, BAKED, MASHED 1 CUP	205	130	8610.00	33.12	215 **
666	**SWEETPOTATOES COOKED BAKED IN SKIN, PEELED. 1 POTATO (2 1/2 PER LB)	114	160	9230.00	28.84	231 **
667	**SWEETPOTATOES COOKED, BOILED IN SKIN, PEELED 1 POTATO (2 1/2 PER LB)	151	170	11940.00	35.12	299 **
668	**SWEETPOTATOES, CANDIED 1 PIECE (2 1/2 BY 2-IN)	105	175	6620.00	18.91	166 **
669	**SWEETPOTATOES, CANNED SOLID PACK, MASHED 1 CUP	255	275	19890.00	36.16	497 **
670	**SWEETPOTATOES, CANNED, VACUUM PACK 1 PIECE 2 3/4 BY 1-IN	40	45	3120.00	34.67	78 **
671	*TOMATOES, RAW 1 TOMATO 2 3/5-IN DIAM	135	25	1110.00	22.20	28 *
672	**TOMATOES, CANNED,SOLIDS AND LIQUIDS 1 CUP	241	50	2170.00	21.70	54 **
674	TOMATO CATSUP 1 TBSP	15	15	210.00	7.00	5
675	*TOMATO JUICE, CANNED 1 CUP	243	45	1940.00	21.56	49 *
676	*TOMATO JUICE, CANNED 1 GLASS 6 FL OZ	182	35	1460.00	20.86	37 *
678	**TURNIP GREENS, COOKED, DRAINED, FROM RAW (LEAVES AND STEMS) 1 CUP	145	30	8270.00	137.83	207 **
679	**TURNIP GREENS, COOKED, DRAINED, FROM FROZEN,CHOPPED 1 CUP	165	40	11390.00	142.38	285 **
680	**VEGETABLES, MIXED, FROZEN, COOKED, DRAINED. 1 CUP	182	115	9010.00	39.17	225 **
714	CLAM CHOWDER, MANHATTAN TYPE WITH TOMATOES AND WITHOUT MILK 1 CUP	245	80	880.00	5.50	22

VITAMIN C VITAMIN C VITAMIN C VITAMIN C VITAMIN C VITAMIN C VITAMIN C VITAMIN C VITAMIN C VITAMIN C

HANDBOOK				VITAMIN A		
NUMBER	FOOD NAME SERVING SIZE DESCRIPTION	GRAMS	KCAL	IU	INQ	%RDA
717	**MINESTRONE SOUP PREPARED WITH EQUAL VOLUME OF WATER, CANNED • • • • • 1 CUP	245	105	2350.00	11.19	59 **
719	*TOMATO SOUP PREPARED WITH EQUAL VOLUME OF WATER, CANNED • • • • • 1 CUP	245	90	1000.00	5.56	25 *
720	**VEGETABLE BEEF SOUP PREPARED WITH EQUAL VOLUME OF WATER, CANNED • • • 1 CUP	245	80	2700.00	16.88	68 **
721	**VEGETARIAN SOUP PREPARED WITH EQUAL VOLUME OF WATER, CANNED • • • • • 1 CUP	245	80	2940.00	18.38	74 **

FOODS WHICH PROVIDE A HIGH CONCENTRATION OF VITAMIN C RELATIVE TO CALORIES

(INQ AT LEAST 5.0)

AND AT LEAST 5 PERCENT OF THE RDA PER SERVING

(RDA FOR VITAMIN C = 60.0 MG)

VITAMIN C VITAMIN C VITAMIN C VITAMIN C VITAMIN C VITAMIN C VITAMIN C VITAMIN C VITAMIN C VITAMIN C

*INDICATES FOODS WHICH PROVIDE AT LEAST 25 PERCENT OF THE RDA PER SERVING

**INDICATES FOODS WHICH PROVIDE AT LEAST 50 PERCENT OF THE RDA PER SERVING

HANDBOOK NUMBER	FOOD NAME SERVING SIZE DESCRIPTION	GRAMS	KCAL	VITAMIN C MG	INQ	%RDA
152	**OYSTERS, RAW, MEAT ONLY / 1 CUP, 13-19 MEDIUM SELECTS	240	160	72.00	15.00	120 **
228	APRICOTS, RAW, WITHOUT PITS / 3	107	55	11.00	6.67	18
232	**APRICOT NECTAR, CANNED / 1 CUP	251	145	36.00	8.28	60 **
237	**BLACKBERRIES, RAW / 1 CUP	144	85	30.00	11.76	50 **
238	*BLUEBERRIES, RAW / 1 CUP	145	90	20.00	7.41	33 *
240	CHERRIES, SWEET, RAW, WITHOUT PITS AND STEMS / 10 CHERRIES	68	45	7.00	5.19	12
241	**CRANBERRY JUICE COCKTAIL, BOTTLED, SWEETENED / 1 CUP	253	165	81.00	16.36	135 **
246	**GRAPEFRUIT, RAW, PINK OR RED, WT WITHOUT PEEL AND MEMBRANES / 1/2 MEDIUM (3 3/4-IN DIAM.) GRAPEFRUIT	123	50	44.00	29.33	73 **
247	**GRAPEFRUIT, RAW, WHITE, WT WITHOUT PEEL AND MEMBRANES / 1/2 MEDIUM (3 3/4-IN DIAM.) GRAPEFRUIT	118	45	44.00	32.59	73 **
248	**GRAPEFRUIT, CANNED, SECTIONS WITH SIRUP / 1 CUP	254	180	76.00	14.07	127 **
249	**GRAPEFRUIT JUICE, RAW / 1 CUP	246	95	93.00	32.63	155 **
250	**GRAPEFRUIT JUICE, CANNED, UNSWEETENED / 1 CUP	247	100	84.00	28.00	140 **
251	**GRAPEFRUIT JUICE, CANNED, SWEETENED / 1 CUP	250	135	78.00	19.26	130 **
253	**GRAPEFRUIT JUICE, FROZEN, CONCENTRATE, UNSWEETENED, DILUTED / 1 CUP	247	100	96.00	32.00	160 **
254	**GRAPEFRUIT JUICE, DEHYDRATED CRYSTALS, PREPARED WITH WATER / 1 CUP	247	100	91.00	30.33	152 **
266	*LEMONADE CONCENTRATE, FROZEN, DILUTED / 1 CUP	248	105	17.00	5.40	28 *
271	**CANTALOUP, WT WITHOUT RIND AND SEEDS. / 1/2 OF A 5-IN DIAM. MELON	272	80	90.00	37.50	150 **
272	**HONEYDEW MELON, WT WITHOUT RIND AND SEEDS / 1/10 OF A 6 1/2-IN DIAM. MELON	149	50	34.00	22.67	57 **
273	**ORANGE, RAW, WT WITHOUT PEEL AND SEEDS / 1--2 5/8-IN DIAM.	131	65	66.00	33.85	110 **
274	**ORANGE SECTIONS WITHOUT MEMBRANES, RAW / 1 CUP	180	90	90.00	33.33	150 **
275	**ORANGE JUICE, FRESH / 1 CUP	248	110	124.00	37.58	207 **
276	**ORANGE JUICE, CANNED, UNSWEETENED / 1 CUP	249	120	100.00	27.78	167 **
278	**ORANGE JUICE, FROZEN CONCENTRATE, DILUTED / 1 CUP	249	120	120.00	33.33	200 **

HANDBOOK NUMBER	FOOD NAME / SERVING SIZE DESCRIPTION	GRAMS	KCAL	VITAMIN C MG	INQ	%RDA
279	**ORANGE JUICE, DEHYDRATED CRYSTALS, PREPARED WITH WATER. 1 CUP	248	115	109.00	31.59	182 **
281	**ORANGE AND GRAPEFRUIT JUICE, FROZEN CONCENTRATE, DILUTED 1 CUP	248	110	102.00	30.91	170 **
282	**PAPAYAS, RAW, 1/2 INCH CUBES 1 CUP	140	55	78.00	47.27	130 **
283	PEACHES, RAW, WT FOR PEELED AND PITTED 1--2 1/2-IN DIAM, PEACH	100	40	7.00	5.83	12
284	PEACHES, RAW, SLICED 1 CUP	170	65	12.00	6.15	20
290	**PEACHES, FROZEN, SLICED, SWEETENED 1 CUP	250	220	103.00	15.61	172 **
295	*PINEAPPLE, RAW, DICED 1 CUP	155	80	26.00	10.83	43 *
299	**PINEAPPLE JUICE, UNSWEETENED, CANNED. 1 CUP	250	140	80.00	19.05	133 **
309	**RASPBERRIES, RED, RAW, WHOLE 1 CUP	123	70	31.00	14.76	52 **
313	**STRAWBERRIES, RAW, WHOLE, CAPPED 1 CUP	149	55	88.00	53.33	147 **
316	*TANGERINE, RAW, WT WITHOUT PEEL 1 (2 3/8 IN DIAM.) TANGERINE	86	40	27.00	22.50	45 *
317	**TANGERINE JUICE, CANNED, SWEETENED 1 CUP	249	125	54.00	14.40	90 **
318	**WATERMELON, WT WITHOUT RIND AND SEEDS 1/16 OF 33 LB MELON	426	110	30.00	9.09	50 **
564	**ASPARAGUS, COOKED,DRAINED,FROM RAW 1 CUP (CUTS AND TIPS, 1 1/2 TO 2-IN LENGTHS)	145	30	38.00	42.22	63 **
565	**ASPARAGUS, COOKED,DRAINED,FROM FROZEN 1 CUP (CUTS AND TIPS, 1 1/2 TO 2-IN LENGTHS)	180	40	41.00	34.17	68 **
566	*ASPARAGUS, SPEARS 1/2-IN DIAM AT BASE FROM RAW 4 SPEARS	60	10	16.00	53.33	27 *
567	*ASPARAGUS, SPEARS 1/2-IN DIAM AT BASE FROM FROZEN 4 SPEARS	60	15	16.00	35.56	27 *
568	ASPARAGUS, CANNED SPEARS. 4 SPEARS	80	15	12.00	26.67	20
569	*LIMA BEANS,(FORDHOOKS),FROZEN,COOKED,DRAINED 1 CUP	170	170	29.00	5.69	48 *
571	*GREEN SNAP BEANS, COOKED, DRAINED, FROM RAW 1 CUP	125	30	15.00	16.67	25 *
572	GREEN SNAP BEANS, COOKED, DRAINED,CUTS FROM FROZEN 1 CUP	135	35	7.00	6.67	12
573	GREEN SNAP BEANS, COOKED, DRAINED,FRENCH CUTS FROM FROZEN 1 CUP	130	35	9.00	8.57	15
574	GREEN SNAP BEANS, CANNED, DRAINED SOLIDS (CUTS) 1 CUP	135	30	5.00	5.56	8

HANDBOOK NUMBER	FOOD NAME / SERVING SIZE DESCRIPTION	GRAMS	KCAL	VITAMIN C MG	INQ	%RDA
575	*YELLOW OR WAX BEANS, COOKED, DRAINED, FROM RAW / 1 CUP	125	30	16.00	17.78	27 *
576	YELLOW OR WAX BEANS, COOKED, DRAINED CUTS FROM FROZEN / 1 CUP	135	35	8.00	7.62	13
577	YELLOW OR WAX BEANS, CANNED, DRAINED SOLIDS (CUTS) / 1 CUP	135	30	7.00	7.78	12
578	*BEAN SPROUTS,(MUNG),RAW / 1 CUP	105	35	20.00	19.05	33 *
579	BEAN SPROUTS,(MUNG),COOKED, DRAINED / 1 CUP	125	35	8.00	7.62	13
580	BEETS, COOKED DRAINED, PEELED / 2 WHOLE BEETS, 2-IN DIAM.	100	30	6.00	6.67	10
581	BEETS, COOKED DRAINED,DICED OR SLICED / 1 CUP	170	55	10.00	6.06	17
584	*BEET GREENS, COOKED, DRAINED / 1 CUP	145	25	22.00	29.33	37 *
585	*BLACKEYE PEAS, COOKED, DRAINED, FROM RAW / 1 CUP	165	180	28.00	5.19	47 *
587	**BROCCOLI, COOKED, DRAINED, FROM RAW / 1 WHOLE MEDIUM STALK	187	45	162.00	120.00	270 **
588	**BROCCOLI, COOKED, DRAINED, FROM RAW. / 1 CUP (STALKS CUT INTO 1/2-IN PIECES)	155	40	140.00	116.67	233 **
589	*BROCCOLI, FROM FROZEN, COOKED, DRAINED / 1 PIECE, 4 1/2 TO 5 IN LONG	30	10	22.00	73.33	37 *
590	**BROCCOLI, FROM FROZEN, CHOPPED, COOKED, DRAINED / 1 CUP	185	50	105.00	70.00	175 **
591	**BRUSSELS SPROUTS, COOKED, DRAINED, FROM RAW / 7-8 SPROUTS (1 1/4 TO 1 1/2-IN DIAM) 1 CUP	155	55	135.00	81.82	225 **
592	**BRUSSELS SPROUTS, COOKED, DRAINED, FROM FROZEN / 1 CUP	155	50	126.00	84.00	210 **
593	**CABBAGE, RAW, COARSLY SHREDDED OR CHOPPED / 1 CUP	70	15	33.00	73.33	55 **
594	**CABBAGE,RAW, FINELY SHREDDED / 1 CUP	90	20	42.00	70.00	70 **
595	**CABBAGE, COOKED, DRAINED. / 1 CUP	145	30	48.00	53.33	80 **
596	**RED CABBAGE, RAW, COARSELY SHREDDED / 1 CUP	70	20	43.00	71.67	72 **
597	**SAVOY CABBAGE, RAW, COARSELY SHREDDED / 1 CUP	70	15	39.00	86.67	65 **
598	*CELERY CABBAGE (WONGBOK),RAW / 1 CUP (1-IN PIECES)	75	10	19.00	63.33	32 *
599	*WHITE MUSTARD CABBAGE, COOKED, DRAINED / 1 CUP	170	25	26.00	34.67	43 *
600	CARROTS, RAW, PEELED / 1 CARROT OR 18 STRIPS 2 1/2 TO 3-IN LONG	72	30	6.00	6.67	10

HANDBOOK NUMBER	FOOD NAME / SERVING SIZE DESCRIPTION	GRAMS	KCAL	VITAMIN C MG	INQ	%RDA
601	CARROTS, RAW, PEELED, GRATED / 1 CUP	110	45	9.00	6.67	15
602	CARROTS (CROSSWISE CUTS) COOKED, DRAINED / 1 CUP	155	50	9.00	6.00	15
605	**CAULIFLOWER, RAW, CHOPPED / 1 CUP	115	31	90.00	96.77	150 **
606	**CAULIFLOWER, COOKED, DRAINED FROM RAW / 1 CUP	125	30	69.00	76.67	115 **
607	**CAULIFLOWER, COOKED, DRAINED FROM FROZEN / 1 CUP	180	30	74.00	82.22	123 **
608	CELERY (PASCAL) RAW / 1 STALK, 8 BY 1 1/2 IN	40	5	4.00	26.67	7
609	CELERY, RAW DICED / 1 CUP	120	20	11.00	18.33	18
610	**COLLARDS, COOKED, DRAINED, FROM RAW / 1 CUP	190	65	144.00	73.85	240 **
611	**COLLARDS, COOKED DRAINED, FROM FROZEN / 1 CUP	170	50	56.00	37.33	93 **
618	CUCUMBER, WITH PEEL / 6 LARGE OR 8 SMALL SLICES	28	5	3.00	20.00	5
619	CUCUMBER, WITHOUT PEEL / 6 1/2 LARGE OR 9 SMALL SLICES	28	5	3.00	20.00	5
620	*DANDELION GREENS, COOKED, DRAINED / 1 CUP	105	35	19.00	18.10	32 *
621	ENDIVE,CURLY,RAW SMALL PIECES / 1 CUP	50	10	5.00	16.67	8
622	**KALE, COOKED, DRAINED, FROM RAW, LEAVES WITHOUT STEMS / 1 CUP	110	45	102.00	75.56	170 **
623	**KALE, COOKED, DRAINED, FROM FROZEN, LEAF STYLE / 1 CUP	130	40	49.00	40.83	82 **
624	BUTTERHEAD LETTUCE, RAW / 1 HEAD,5-IN DIAM,	220	25	13.00	17.33	22
626	**ICEBERG LETTUCE (CRISPHEAD) / 1 HEAD, 6-IN DIAM	567	70	32.00	15.24	53 **
627	ICEBERG LETTUCE (CRISPHEAD) / 1 WEDGE (1/4 HEAD)	135	20	8.00	13.33	13
628	ICEBERG LETTUCE, (CRISPHEAD), PIECES, CHOPPED OR SHREDDED / 1 CUP	55	5	3.00	20.00	5
629	LOOSELEAF LETTUCE, CHOPPED OR SHREDDED / 1 CUP	55	10	10.00	33.33	17
631	**MUSTARD GREENS, COOKED, DRAINED, WITHOUT STEMS / 1 CUP	140	30	67.00	74.44	112 **
632	*OKRA PODS, COOKED / 10 PODS 3 BY 5/8 IN	106	30	21.00	23.33	35 *
633	*ONIONS, MATURE, RAW, CHOPPED / 1 CUP	170	65	17.00	8.72	28 *

HANDBOOK NUMBER	FOOD NAME SERVING SIZE DESCRIPTION	GRAMS	KCAL	VITAMIN C MG	INQ	%RDA
634	ONIONS, MATURE,RAW SLICED 1 CUP	115	45	12.00	8.89	20
635	*ONIONS, MATURE, COOKED, DRAINED, WHOLE OR SLICED. 1 CUP	210	60	15.00	8.33	25 *
636	GREEN ONION 6 ONIONS (3/8-IN DIAM BULB)	30	15	8.00	17.78	13
637	PARSLEY, RAW, CHOPPED 1 TBSP	4	0	6.00********		*
638	*PARSNIPS, COOKED, DICED 1 CUP	155	100	16.00	5.33	27 *
640	GREEN PEAS, STRAINED (BABY FOOD) 1 OZ (1 3/4 TO 2 TBSP)	28	15	3.00	6.67	5
641	*GREEN PEAS, FROZEN, COOKED, DRAINED 1 CUP	160	110	21.00	6.36	35 *
643	**SWEET PEPPERS, RAW. 1 POD (5 PER LB)	74	15	94.00	208.89	157 **
644	**SWEET PEPPERS, COOKED, DRAINED. 1 POD	73	15	70.00	155.56	117 **
645	**BAKED POTATO, PEELED AFTER BAKING 1 POTATO (2 PER LB)	156	145	31.00	7.13	52 **
646	*BOILED POTATO, PEELED AFTER BOILING 1 POTATO (3 PER LB)	137	105	22.00	6.98	37 *
647	*BOILED POTATOES, PEELED BEFORE BOILING 1 POTATO (3 PER LB)	135	90	22.00	8.15	37 *
651	*MASHED POTATOES, PREPARED FROM RAW, MILK ADDED 1 CUP	210	135	21.00	5.19	35 *
656	PUMPKIN, CANNED 1 CUP	245	80	12.00	5.00	20
657	RADISHES,RAW. 4 RADISHES	18	5	5.00	33.33	8
658	**SAUERKRAUT, CANNED,SOLIDS AND LIQUIDS 1 CUP	235	40	33.00	27.50	55 **
659	*SPINACH, RAW, CHOPPED 1 CUP	55	15	28.00	62.22	47 *
660	**SPINACH, COOKED, DRAINED FROM RAW 1 CUP	180	40	50.00	41.67	83 **
661	**SPINACH, COOKED, DRAINED FROM FROZEN, CHOPPED 1 CUP	205	45	39.00	28.89	65 **
662	**SPINACH, COOKED, DRAINED FROM FROZEN, LEAF. 1 CUP	190	45	53.00	39.26	88 **
663	*SPINACH, CANNED, DRAINED SOLIDS 1 CUP	205	50	29.00	19.33	48 *
664	*SUMMER SQUASH, COOKED, DICED, DRAINED 1 CUP	210	30	21.00	23.33	35 *
665	*WINTER SQUASH, BAKED, MASHED 1 CUP	205	130	27.00	6.92	45 *

HANDBOOK NUMBER	FOOD NAME SERVING SIZE DESCRIPTION	GRAMS	KCAL	VITAMIN C MG	INQ	%RDA	
666	*SWEETPOTATOES COOKED BAKED IN SKIN, PEELED. 1 POTATO (2 1/2 PER LB)	114	160	25.00	5.21	42	*
667	*SWEETPOTATOES COOKED, BOILED IN SKIN, PEELED 1 POTATO (2 1/2 PER LB)	151	170	26.00	5.10	43	*
671	*TOMATOES, RAW 1 TOMATO 2 3/5-IN DIAM	135	25	28.00	37.33	47	*
672	**TOMATOES, CANNED,SOLIDS AND LIQUIDS 1 CUP	241	50	41.00	27.33	68	**
675	**TOMATO JUICE, CANNED 1 CUP	243	45	39.00	28.89	65	**
676	*TOMATO JUICE, CANNED 1 GLASS 6 FL OZ	182	35	29.00	27.62	48	*
677	**TURNIPS, COOKED, DICED 1 CUP	155	35	34.00	32.38	57	**
678	**TURNIP GREENS, COOKED, DRAINED, FROM RAW (LEAVES AND STEMS) 1 CUP	145	30	68.00	75.56	113	**
679	**TURNIP GREENS, COOKED, DRAINED, FROM FROZEN-CHOPPED 1 CUP	165	40	31.00	25.83	52	**
703	DILL PICKLES. 1 MEDIUM PICKLE 3 3/4-IN LONG, 1 1/4-IN DIAM	65	5	4.00	26.67	7	

THIAMIN THIAMIN THIAMIN THIAMIN THIAMIN THIAMIN THIAMIN THIAMIN THIAMIN

FOODS WHICH PROVIDE A HIGH CONCENTRATION OF THIAMIN RELATIVE TO CALORIES

(INQ AT LEAST 1.5)

AND AT LEAST 5 PERCENT OF THE RDA PER SERVING

(RDA FOR THIAMIN = 1.0 MG)

THIAMIN THIAMIN THIAMIN THIAMIN THIAMIN THIAMIN THIAMIN THIAMIN THIAMIN

*INDICATES FOODS WHICH PROVIDE AT LEAST 25 PERCENT OF THE RDA PER SERVING

**INDICATES FOODS WHICH PROVIDE AT LEAST 50 PERCENT OF THE RDA PER SERVING

HANDBOOK NUMBER	FOOD NAME / SERVING SIZE DESCRIPTION	GRAMS	KCAL	THIAMIN MG	INQ	%RDA
		3	10	0.30	60.00	30 *
35	*WHIPPED TOPPING, PRESSURIZED / 1 TBSP					
51	MILK, FLUID LOWFAT (2% FAT), NO MILK SOLIDS ADDED / 1 CUP	244	120	0.10	1.67	10
52	MILK, FLUID LOWFAT (2% FAT), LESS THAN 10 GRAMS OF PROTEIN PER CUP / 1 CUP	245	125	0.10	1.60	10
53	MILK, FLUID LOWFAT (2% FAT), MORE THAN 10 GRAMS OF PROTEIN PER CUP / 1 CUP	246	135	0.11	1.63	11
54	MILK, FLUID LOWFAT (1% FAT), NO MILK SOLIDS ADDED / 1 CUP	244	100	0.10	2.00	10
55	MILK, FLUID LOWFAT (1% FAT), LESS THAN 10 GRAMS OF PROTEIN PER CUP / 1 CUP	245	105	0.10	1.90	10
56	MILK, FLUID LOWFAT (1% FAT), MORE THAN 10 GRAMS OF PROTEIN PER CUP / 1 CUP	246	120	0.11	1.83	11
57	MILK, FLUID NONFAT (SKIM), NO MILK SOLIDS ADDED / 1 CUP	245	85	0.09	2.12	9
58	MILK, FLUID NONFAT (SKIM), LESS THAN 10 GRAMS OF PROTEIN PER CUP / 1 CUP	245	90	0.10	2.22	10
59	MILK, FLUID NONFAT (SKIM), MORE THAN 10 GRAMS OF PROTEIN PER CUP / 1 CUP	246	100	0.11	2.20	11
60	BUTTERMILK, FLUID / 1 CUP	245	100	0.08	1.60	8
72	NATURAL MALTED MILK (1CUP WHOLE MILK AND 3/4 OZ MALTED MILK POWDER) / 1 CUP PLUS POWDER	265	235	0.20	1.70	20
94	PLAIN YOGURT MADE WITH NONFAT MILK, WITH ADDED MILK SOLIDS / 8 OZ, NET WT.	227	125	0.11	1.76	11
146	CLAMS, RAW, MEAT ONLY / 3 OZ	85	65	0.08	2.46	8
148	CRABMEAT, CANNED / 1 CUP	135	135	0.11	1.63	11
152	*OYSTERS, RAW, MEAT ONLY / 1 CUP, 13-19 MEDIUM SELECTS	240	160	0.34	4.25	34 *
161	BACON, CRISP. / 2 SLICES	15	85	0.08	1.88	8
180	*CHOP SUEY WITH BEEF AND PORK(HOME RECIPE) / 1 CUP	250	300	0.28	1.87	28 *
181	HEART, BEEF, LEAN, BRAISED / 3 OZ	85	160	0.21	2.62	21
183	LAMB CHOP, BROILED, LEAN ONLY, BONE REMOVED / 2 OZ	57	120	0.09	1.50	9
185	LEG OF LAMB, ROASTED, LEAN ONLY / 2.5 OZ	71	130	0.12	1.85	12
187	LAMB SHOULDER, ROASTED, LEAN ONLY / 2.3 OZ	64	130	0.10	1.54	10
188	LIVER, BEEF, FRIED. / 3 OZ	85	195	0.22	2.26	22

HANDBOOK NUMBER	FOOD NAME / SERVING SIZE DESCRIPTION	GRAMS	KCAL	THIAMIN MG	INQ	%RDA
189	*HAM, LIGHT CURE, ROASTED, LEAN AND FAT / 3 OZ	85	245	0.40	3.27	40 *
190	LUNCHEON MEAT, BOILED HAM / 1 OZ	28	65	0.12	3.69	12
191	LUNCHEON MEAT, CANNED, SPICED OR UNSPICED / 1 OZ	60	175	0.19	2.17	19
192	**PORK CHOP, BROILED, LEAN AND FAT, BONE REMOVED / 1 SLICE (3 BY 2 BY 1/2 IN) 2.7 OZ	78	305	0.75	4.92	75 **
193	**PORK CHOP, BROILED, LEAN ONLY, BONE REMOVED / 2 OZ	56	150	0.63	8.40	63 **
194	**PORK ROAST, OVEN COOKED, LEAN AND FAT / 3 OZ	85	310	0.78	5.03	78 **
195	**PORK ROAST, OVEN COOKED, LEAN ONLY / 2.4 OZ	68	175	0.73	8.34	73 **
196	*PORK SHOULDER, SIMMERED, LEAN AND FAT / 3 OZ	85	320	0.46	2.88	46 *
197	*PORK SHOULDER, SIMMERED, LEAN ONLY / 2.2 OZ	63	135	0.42	6.22	42 *
200	BROWN AND SERVE SAUSAGES / 1 LINK (10-11 PER 8-OZ PKG.)	17	70	0.13	3.71	13
204	PORK LINK SAUSAGE / 1 LINK (16 PER 1-LB PKG.)	13	60	0.10	3.33	10
206	SALAMI, COOKED TYPE / 1 SLICE (8 PER 8-OZ PKG.)	28	90	0.07	1.56	7
234	*AVOCADOS, RAW, FLORIDA, WT. WITHOUT SKIN AND SEED / 1--3 5/8-IN DIAM.	304	390	0.33	1.69	33 *
246	GRAPEFRUIT, RAW, PINK OR RED, WT WITHOUT PEEL AND MEMBRANES / 1/2 MEDIUM (3 3/4-IN DIAM.) GRAPEFRUIT	123	50	0.05	2.00	5
247	GRAPEFRUIT, RAW, WHITE, WT WITHOUT PEEL AND MEMBRANES / 1/2 MEDIUM (3 3/4-IN DIAM.) GRAPEFRUIT	118	45	0.05	2.22	5
249	GRAPEFRUIT JUICE, RAW / 1 CUP	246	95	0.10	2.11	10
253	GRAPEFRUIT JUICE, FROZEN, CONCENTRATE, UNSWEETENED, DILUTED / 1 CUP	247	100	0.10	2.00	10
254	GRAPEFRUIT JUICE, DEHYDRATED CRYSTALS, PREPARED WITH WATER / 1 CUP	247	100	0.10	2.00	10
271	CANTALOUP, WT WITHOUT RIND AND SEEDS / 1/2 OF A 5-IN DIAM. MELON	272	80	0.11	2.75	11
272	HONEYDEW MELON, WT WITHOUT RIND AND SEEDS / 1/10 OF A 6 1/2-IN DIAM. MELON	149	50	0.06	2.40	6
273	ORANGE, RAW, WT WITHOUT PEEL AND SEEDS / 1--2 5/8-IN DIAM.	131	65	0.13	4.00	13
274	ORANGE SECTIONS WITHOUT MEMBRANES, RAW / 1 CUP	180	90	0.18	4.00	18
275	ORANGE JUICE, FRESH / 1 CUP	248	110	0.22	4.00	22

HANDBOOK NUMBER	FOOD NAME SERVING SIZE DESCRIPTION	GRAMS	KCAL	THIAMIN MG	INQ	%RDA
276	ORANGE JUICE, CANNED, UNSWEETENED 1 CUP	249	120	0.17	2.83	17
278	ORANGE JUICE, FROZEN CONCENTRATE, DILUTED 1 CUP	249	120	0.23	3.83	23
279	ORANGE JUICE, DEHYDRATED CRYSTALS, PREPARED WITH WATER 1 CUP	248	115	0.20	3.48	20
281	ORANGE AND GRAPEFRUIT JUICE, FROZEN CONCENTRATE, DILUTED 1 CUP	248	110	0.15	2.73	15
282	PAPAYAS, RAW, 1/2 INCH CUBES 1 CUP	140	55	0.06	2.18	6
295	PINEAPPLE, RAW, DICED 1 CUP	155	80	0.14	3.50	14
296	PINEAPPLE, CANNED, CRUSHED, CHUNKS, TIDBITS, HEAVY SYRUP PACK 1 CUP (SOLIDS AND LIQUID)	255	190	0.20	2.11	20
297	PINEAPPLE, CANNED, LARGE SLICE, HEAVY SYRUP PACK 1SLICE, 2 1/4 TBSP LIQUID	105	80	0.08	2.00	8
298	PINEAPPLE, CANNED, MEDIUM SLICE, HEAVY SYRUP PACK 1 SLICE, 1 1/4 TBSP LIQUID	58	45	0.05	2.22	5
299	PINEAPPLE JUICE, UNSWEETENED, CANNED 1 CUP	250	140	0.13	1.86	13
316	TANGERTNE, RAW, WT WITHOUT PEEL 1 (2 3/8 IN DIAM.) TANGERINE	86	40	0.05	2.50	5
317	TANGERINE JUICE, CANNED, SWEETENED 1 CUP	249	125	0.15	2.40	15
318	WATERMELON, WT WITHOUT RIND AND SEEDS 1/16 OF 33 LB MELON	426	110	0.13	2.36	13
319	BAGEL, MADE WITH EGG 1--3-IN DIAM.	55	165	0.14	1.70	14
320	BAGEL, MADE WITH WATER 1--3-IN DIAM.	55	165	0.15	1.82	15
322	BISCUITS, BAKING POWDER, HOME RECIPE. 2-IN DIAM. BISCUIT	28	105	0.08	1.52	8
323	BISCUITS, BAKING POWDER, MADE FROM MIX 2-IN DIAM. BISCUIT	28	90	0.09	2.00	9
327	CRACKED-WHEAT BREAD 1 SLICE (18 PER 1LB LOAF)	25	65	0.08	2.46	8
329	FRENCH BREAD 5 BY 2 1/2 BY 1 IN SLICE	35	100	0.14	2.80	14
330	VIENNA BREAD. 4 3/4 BY 4 BY 1/2 IN SLICE	25	75	0.10	2.67	10
332	ITALIAN BREAD 4 1/2 BY 3 1/4 BY 3/4 IN SLICE	30	85	0.12	2.82	12
334	RAISIN BREAD. 1 SLICE (18 PER 1LB LOAF)	25	65	0.09	2.77	9
336	RYE BREAD, AMERICAN, LIGHT 5 BY 4 BY 3/8 IN SLICE	25	60	0.07	2.33	7

HANDBOOK NUMBER	FOOD NAME SERVING SIZE DESCRIPTION	GRAMS	KCAL	THIAMIN MG	INQ	%RDA
338	RYE BREAD, PUMPERNICKEL. 5 BY 4 BY 3/8 IN SLICE	32	80	0.09	2.25	9
340	WHITE BREAD, SOFT-CRUMB TYPE 1 SLICE (18 PER 1LB LOAF)	25	70	0.10	2.86	10
352	WHITE BREAD, FIRM-CRUMB TYPE 1 SLICE (20 PER 1LB LOAF)	23	65	0.09	2.77	9
358	WHOLE-WHEAT BREAD, SOFT-CRUMB TYPE 1 SLICE (16 PER 1 LB LOAF)	28	65	0.09	2.77	9
363	CORN GRITS, COOKED, ENRICHED 1 CUP	245	125	0.10	1.60	10
365	FARINA, QUICK-COOKING, ENRICHED, COOKED 1 CUP	245	105	0.12	2.29	12
366	OATMEAL OR ROLLED OATS, COOKED. 1 CUP	240	130	0.19	2.92	19
367	WHEAT, ROLLED, COOKED 1 CUP	240	180	0.17	1.89	17
368	WHEAT, WHOLE-MEAL, COOKED 1 CUP	245	110	0.15	2.73	15
369	*BRAN FLAKES (40% BRAN), ADDED SUGAR, SALT, IRON AND VITAMINS. 1 CUP	35	105	0.41	7.81	41 *
370	**BRAN FLAKES WITH RAISINS, ADDED SUGAR, SALT, IRON AND VITAMINS 1 CUP	50	145	0.58	8.00	58 **
371	*CORN FLAKES, PLAIN, ADDED SUGAR, SALT, IRON, VITAMINS 1 CUP	25	95	0.29	6.11	29 *
372	*CORN FLAKES, SUGAR-COATED, ADDED SALT, IRON, VITAMINS 1 CUP	40	155	0.46	5.94	46 *
373	PUFFED CORN, PLAIN, ADDED SUGAR, SALT, IRON, VITAMINS. 1 CUP	20	80	0.23	5.75	23
374	SHREDDED CORN, ADDED SUGAR, SALT, IRON, THIAMIN, NIACIN 1 CUP	25	95	0.11	2.32	11
375	*PUFFED OATS, ADDED SUGAR, SALT, MINERALS, VITAMINS 1 CUP	25	100	0.29	5.80	29 *
376	PUFFED RICE, PLAIN, ADDED IRON, THIAMIN, NIACIN. 1 CUP	15	60	0.07	2.33	7
377	*PUFFED RICE, PRESWEETENED, ADDED SALT, IRON, VITAMINS 1 CUP	28	115	0.38	6.61	38 *
378	*WHEAT FLAKES, ADDED SUGAR, SALT, IRON, VITAMINS 1 CUP	30	105	0.35	6.67	35 *
379	PUFFED WHEAT, PLAIN, ADDED IRON, THIAMIN, NIACIN. 1 CUP	15	55	0.08	2.91	8
380	**PUFFED WHEAT, PRESWEETENED, ADDED SALT, IRON, VITAMINS 1 CUP	38	140	0.50	7.14	50 **
382	WHEAT GERM,WITHOUT SALT AND SUGAR,TOASTED 1 TBSP	6	25	0.11	8.80	11
418	GINGERSNAPS 4 COOKIES, 1/4-IN THICK	28	90	0.08	1.78	8

HANDBOOK NUMBER	FOOD NAME SERVING SIZE DESCRIPTION	GRAMS	KCAL	THIAMIN MG	INQ	%RDA
427	CORNMEAL,DEGERMED,ENRICHED,COOKED 1 CUP	240	120	0.14	2.33	14
432	SALTINES 4 CRACKERS OR 1 PACKET	11	50	0.05	2.00	5
438	MACARONI,ENRICHED, COOKED FIRM STAGE (HOT) 1 CUP	130	190	0.23	2.42	23
439	MACARONI,ENRICHED TENDER STAGE,COLD 1 CUP	105	115	0.15	2.61	15
440	MACARONI,ENRICHED,TENDER STAGE, HOT 1 CUP	140	155	0.20	2.58	20
443	BLUEBERRY MUFFINS, HOME RECIPE 1 MUFFIN, 2 3/8-IN DIAM, 1 1/2-IN HIGH	40	110	0.09	1.64	9
445	CORN MUFFINS, HOME RECIPE 1 MUFFIN 2 3/8IN DIAM, 1 1/2-IN HIGH	40	125	0.10	1.60	10
446	PLAIN MUFFIN, HOME RECIPE 1 MUFFIN, 3-IN DIAM, 1 1/2-IN HIGH	40	120	0.09	1.50	9
448	EGG NOODLES, ENRICHED, COOKED 1 CUP	160	200	0.22	2.20	22
451	PANCAKE MADE FROM HOME RECIPE 1 CAKE 4-IN DIAM	27	60	0.06	2.00	6
475	PIZZA(CHEESE), BAKED 1 SECTOR, 1/8 OF 12-IN DIAM PIE	60	145	0.16	2.21	16
478	POPCORN, SUGAR COATED 1 CUP	35	135	0.13	1.93	13
479	PRETZELS,DUTCH TWISTED 1 PRETZEL 2 3/4 BY 2 5/8-IN	16	60	0.05	1.67	5
480	PRETZELS,THIN TWISTED 10PRETZEL 3 1/4 BY 2 1/4 BY 1/4-IN	60	235	0.20	1.70	20
482	RICE,INSTANT, ENRICHED, COOKED 1 CUP	165	180	0.21	2.33	21
484	RICE,LONG GRAIN, ENRICHED, COOKED 1 CUP	205	225	0.23	2.04	23
486	RICE,PARBOILED, ENRICHED, COOKED 1 CUP	175	185	0.19	2.05	19
487	ROLLS,BROWN AND SERVE, BROWNED 1 ROLL	26	85	0.10	2.35	10
488	ROLLS,CLOVERLEAF OR PAN 1 ROLL 2 1/2-IN DIAM, 2-IN HIGH	28	85	0.11	2.59	11
489	HAMBURGER OR FRANKFURTER BUN 1 ROLL (8 PER 11 1/2-OZ PKG)	40	120	0.16	2.67	16
490	HARD ROLLS 1 ROLL 3 3/4-IN DIAM, 2-IN HIGH	50	155	0.20	2.58	20
491	**HOAGIE OR SUBMARINE BUNS 1 BUN (11 1/2 BY 3 BY 2 1/2 IN.)	135	390	0.54	2.77	54 **
492	CLOVERLEAF ROLLS FROM HOME RECIPE 1 ROLL (2 1/2-IN DIAM,,2-IN HIGH	35	120	0.12	2.00	12

HANDBOOK FOOD NAME NUMBER	SERVING SIZE DESCRIPTION	GRAMS	KCAL	THIAMIN MG	INQ	%RDA
495	*SPAGHETTI, ENRICHED, IN TOMATO SAUCE WITH CHEESE, HOME RECIPE, 1 CUP	250	260	0.25	1.92	25 *
496	*SPAGHETTI, ENRICHED, IN TOMATO SAUCE WITH CHEESE, CANNED, 1 CUP	250	190	0.35	3.68	35 *
497	*SPAGHETTI, ENRICHED, WITH MEAT BALLS IN TOMATO SAUCE, HOME RECIPE, 1 CUP	248	330	0.25	1.52	25 *
499	TOASTER PASTRIES, 1 PASTRY	50	200	0.16	1.60	16
500	WAFFLES FROM HOME RECIPE, 1 WAFFLE 7-IN DIAM	75	210	0.17	1.62	17
505	**SELF-RISING FLOUR,ENRICHED,UNSIFTED, SPOONED, 1 CUP	125	440	0.80	3.64	80 **
506	**WHOLE WHEAT FLOUR, 1 CUP	120	400	0.66	3.30	66 **
509	*DRY BEANS, GREAT NORTHERN COOKED, DRAINED, 1 CUP	180	210	0.25	2.38	25 *
510	*DRY BEANS, NAVY, COOKED, DRAINED, 1 CUP	190	225	0.27	2.40	27 *
515	*DRY LIMA BEANS, COOKED, DRAINED, 1 CUP	190	260	0.25	1.92	25 *
516	*BLACKEYE PEAS,DRY,COOKED, 1 CUP	250	190	0.40	4.21	40 *
517	*BRAZIL NUTS, 1 OZ. (6-8 LARGE KERNELS)	28	185	0.27	2.92	27 *
518	**CASHEW NUTS, ROASTED IN OIL, 1 CUP	140	785	0.60	1.53	60 **
525	*SPLIT PEAS, DRY,COOKED, 1 CUP	200	230	0.30	2.61	30 *
526	*PECANS, CHOPPED OR PIECES, 1 CUP (120 LARGE HALVES)	118	810	1.01	2.49	101 **
528	**SUNFLOWER SEEDS, DRY, HULLED, 1 CUP	145	810	2.84	7.01	284 **
564	ASPARAGUS, COOKED,DRAINED,FROM RAW, 1 CUP (CUTS AND TIPS, 1 1/2 TO 2-IN LENGTHS)	145	30	0.23	15.33	23
565	*ASPARAGUS, COOKED,DRAINED,FROM FROZEN, 1 CUP (CUTS AND TIPS, 1 1/2 TO 2-IN LENGTHS)	180	40	0.25	12.50	25 *
566	ASPARAGUS, SPEARS 1/2-IN DIAM AT BASE FROM RAW, 4 SPEARS	60	10	0.10	20.00	10
567	ASPARAGUS, SPEARS 1/2-IN DIAM AT BASE FROM FROZEN, 4 SPEARS	60	15	0.10	13.33	10
568	ASPARAGUS, CANNED SPEARS, 4 SPEARS	80	15	0.05	6.67	5
570	LIMA BEANS,(BABY LIMAS), FROZEN, COOKED, DRAINED, 1 CUP	180	210	0.16	1.52	16
571	GREEN SNAP BEANS, COOKED, DRAINED, FROM RAW, 1 CUP	125	30	0.09	6.00	9

HANDBOOK NUMBER	FOOD NAME SERVING SIZE DESCRIPTION	GRAMS	KCAL	THIAMIN MG	INQ	XRDA
572	GREEN SNAP BEANS, COOKED, DRAINED,CUTS FROM FROZEN • 1 CUP	135	35	0.09	5.14	9
573	GREEN SNAP BEANS, COOKED, DRAINED,FRENCH CUTS FROM FROZEN • 1 CUP	130	35	0.08	4.57	8
575	YELLOW OR WAX BEANS, COOKED, DRAINED, FROM RAW • 1 CUP	125	30	0.09	6.00	9
576	YELLOW OR WAX BEANS, COOKED, DRAINED CUTS FROM FROZEN • 1 CUP	135	35	0.09	5.14	9
578	BEAN SPROUTS,(MUNG),RAW • 1 CUP	105	35	0.14	8.00	14
579	BEAN SPROUTS,(MUNG),COOKED, DRAINED • 1 CUP	125	35	0.11	6.29	11
581	BEETS, COOKED DRAINED,DICED OR SLICED • 1 CUP	170	55	0.05	1.82	5
584	BEET GREENS, COOKED, DRAINED • 1 CUP	145	25	0.10	8.00	10
585	**BLACKEYE PEAS, COOKED, DRAINED, FROM RAW • 1 CUP	165	180	0.50	5.56	50 **
586	**BLACKEYE PEAS, COOKED, DRAINED, FROM FROZEN • 1 CUP	170	220	0.68	6.18	68 **
587	BROCCOLI, COOKED, DRAINED, FROM RAW • 1 WHOLE MEDIUM STALK	187	45	0.16	7.11	16
588	BROCCOLI, COOKED, DRAINED, FROM RAW • 1 CUP (STALKS CUT INTO 1/2-IN PIECES)	155	40	0.14	7.00	14
590	BROCCOLI, FROM FROZEN, CHOPPED, COOKED, DRAINED • 1 CUP	185	50	0.11	4.40	11
591	BRUSSELS SPROUTS, COOKED, DRAINED, FROM RAW • 7-8 SPROUTS (1 1/4 TO 1 1/2-IN DIAM) 1 CUP	155	55	0.12	4.36	12
592	BRUSSELS SPROUTS, COOKED, DRAINED, FROM FROZEN • 1 CUP	155	50	0.12	4.80	12
594	CABBAGE,RAW, FINELY SHREDDED • 1 CUP	90	20	0.05	5.00	5
595	CABBAGE, COOKED, DRAINED. • 1 CUP	145	30	0.06	4.00	6
596	RED CABBAGE, RAW, COARSELY SHREDDED • 1 CUP	70	20	0.06	6.00	6
599	WHITE MUSTARD CABBAGE, COOKED, DRAINED • 1 CUP	170	25	0.07	5.60	7
601	CARROTS, RAW, PEELED, GRATED • 1 CUP	110	45	0.07	3.11	7
602	CARROTS (CROSSWISE CUTS) COOKED, DRAINED • 1 CUP	155	50	0.08	3.20	8
605	CAULIFLOWER, RAW, CHOPPED • 1 CUP	115	31	0.13	8.39	13
606	CAULIFLOWER, COOKED, DRAINED FROM RAW • 1 CUP	125	30	0.11	7.33	11

HANDBOOK NUMBER	FOOD NAME / SERVING SIZE DESCRIPTION	GRAMS	KCAL	THIAMIN MG	INQ	%RDA
607	CAULIFLOWER, COOKED, DRAINED FROM FROZEN / 1 CUP	180	30	0.07	4.67	7
610	COLLARDS, COOKED, DRAINED, FROM RAW / 1 CUP	190	65	0.21	6.46	21
611	COLLARDS, COOKED DRAINED, FROM FROZEN / 1 CUP	170	50	0.10	4.00	10
612	CORN, COOKED, DRAINED FROM RAW, WT WITHOUT COB / 1 EAR (5 BY 1 3/4-IN)	77	70	0.09	2.57	9
613	CORN, COOKED, DRAINED FROM FROZEN, WT WITHOUT COB / 1 EAR (5-IN LONG)	126	120	0.18	3.00	18
614	CORN, COOKED, DRAINED FROM FROZEN / 1 CUP KERNELS	165	130	0.15	2.31	15
620	DANDELION GREENS, COOKED, DRAINED / 1 CUP	105	35	0.14	8.00	14
622	KALE, COOKED, DRAINED, FROM RAW, LEAVES WITHOUT STEMS / 1 CUP	110	45	0.11	4.89	11
623	KALE, COOKED, DRAINED, FROM FROZEN, LEAF STYLE / 1 CUP	130	40	0.08	4.00	8
624	BUTTERHEAD LETTUCE, RAW / 1 HEAD,5-IN DIAM.	220	25	0.10	8.00	10
626	*ICEBERG LETTUCE (CRISPHEAD) / 1 HEAD, 6-IN DIAM	567	70	0.32	9.14	32 *
627	ICEBERG LETTUCE (CRISPHEAD) / 1 WEDGE (1/4 HEAD)	135	20	0.08	8.00	8
630	MUSHROOMS, RAW, SLICED OR CHOPPED / 1 CUP	70	20	0.07	7.00	7
631	MUSTARD GREENS, COOKED, DRAINED, WITHOUT STEMS / 1 CUP	140	30	0.11	7.33	11
632	OKRA PODS, COOKED / 10 PODS 3 BY 5/8 IN	106	30	0.14	9.33	14
633	ONIONS, MATURE, RAW, CHOPPED / 1 CUP	170	65	0.05	1.54	5
635	ONIONS, MATURE, COOKED, DRAINED, WHOLE OR SLICED / 1 CUP	210	60	0.06	2.00	6
638	PARSNIPS, COOKED, DICED / 1 CUP	155	100	0.11	2.20	11
639	GREEN PEAS, CANNED, DRAINED SOLIDS / 1 CUP	170	150	0.15	2.00	15
641	*GREEN PEAS, FROZEN, COOKED, DRAINED / 1 CUP	160	110	0.43	7.82	43 *
643	SWEET PEPPERS, RAW / 1 POD (5 PER LB)	74	15	0.06	8.00	6
644	SWEET PEPPERS, COOKED, DRAINED / 1 POD	73	15	0.05	6.67	5
645	BAKED POTATO, PEELED AFTER BAKING / 1 POTATO (2 PER LB)	156	145	0.15	2.07	15

HANDBOOK NUMBER	FOOD NAME / SERVING SIZE DESCRIPTION	GRAMS	KCAL	THIAMIN MG	INQ	%RDA
646	BOILED POTATO, PEELED AFTER BOILING / 1 POTATO (3 PER LB)	137	105	0.12	2.29	12
647	BOILED POTATOES, PEELED BEFORE BOILING / 1 POTATO (3 PER LB)	135	90	0.12	2.67	12
651	MASHED POTATOES, PREPARED FROM RAW, MILK ADDED / 1 CUP	210	135	0.17	2.52	17
652	MASHED POTATOES, PREPARED FROM RAW, MILK AND BUTTER ADDED / 1 CUP	210	195	0.17	1.74	17
655	POTATO SALAD MADE WITH COOKED SALAD DRESSING / 1 CUP	250	250	0.20	1.60	20
656	PUMPKIN, CANNED / 1 CUP	245	80	0.07	1.75	7
658	SAUERKRAUT, CANNED, SOLIDS AND LIQUIDS / 1 CUP	235	40	0.07	3.50	7
659	SPINACH, RAW, CHOPPED / 1 CUP	55	15	0.06	8.00	6
660	SPINACH, COOKED, DRAINED FROM RAW / 1 CUP	180	40	0.13	6.50	13
661	SPINACH, COOKED, DRAINED FROM FROZEN, CHOPPED / 1 CUP	205	45	0.14	6.22	14
662	SPINACH, COOKED, DRAINED FROM FROZEN, LEAF / 1 CUP	190	45	0.15	6.67	15
664	SUMMER SQUASH, COOKED, DICED, DRAINED / 1 CUP	210	30	0.11	7.33	11
665	WINTER SQUASH, BAKED, MASHED / 1 CUP	205	130	0.10	1.54	10
667	SWEETPOTATOES COOKED, BOILED IN SKIN, PEELED / 1 POTATO (2 1/2 PER LB)	151	170	0.14	1.65	14
671	TOMATOES, RAW / 1 TOMATO 2 3/5-IN DIAM	135	25	0.07	5.60	7
672	TOMATOES, CANNED, SOLIDS AND LIQUIDS / 1 CUP	241	50	0.12	4.80	12
675	TOMATO JUICE, CANNED / 1 CUP	243	45	0.12	5.33	12
676	TOMATO JUICE, CANNED / 1 GLASS 6 FL OZ	182	35	0.09	5.14	9
677	TURNIPS, COOKED, DICED / 1 CUP	155	35	0.06	3.43	6
678	TURNIP GREENS, COOKED, DRAINED, FROM RAW (LEAVES AND STEMS) / 1 CUP	145	30	0.15	10.00	15
679	TURNIP GREENS, COOKED, DRAINED, FROM FROZEN, CHOPPED / 1 CUP	165	40	0.08	4.00	8
680	VEGETABLES, MIXED, FROZEN, COOKED, DRAINED / 1 CUP	182	115	0.22	3.83	22
711	BEAN WITH PORK SOUP PREPARED WITH EQUAL VOLUME OF WATER, CANNED / 1 CUP	250	170	0.13	1.53	13

HANDBOOK NUMBER	FOOD NAME SERVING SIZE DESCRIPTION	GRAMS	KCAL	THIAMIN MG	INQ	%RDA
713	BEEF NOODLE SOUP, PREPARED WITH EQUAL VOLUME OF WATER,CANNED. . . . . . 1 CUP	240	65	0.05	1.54	5
718	*SPLIT PEA SOUP PREPARED WITH EQUAL VOLUME OF WATER, CANNED . . . . . . 1 CUP	245	145	0.25	3.45	25 *
724	CHICKEN NOODLE SOUP, PREPARED WITH WATER FROM DRY MIX . . . . 1 CUP	240	55	0.07	2.55	7
726	TOMATO VEGETABLE WITH NOODLE SOUP PREPARED WITH WATER FROM DRY MIX. . . 1 CUP	240	65	0.05	1.54	5
730	**BREWER'S YEAST, DRY . . . . 1 TBSP	8	25	1.25	100.00	125 **

RIBOFLAVN RIBOFLAVN RIBOFLAVN RIBOFLAVN RIBOFLAVN RIBOFLAVN RIBOFLAVN RIBOFLAVN RIBOFLAVN

FOODS WHICH PROVIDE A HIGH CONCENTRATION OF RIBOFLAVN RELATIVE TO CALORIES

(INQ AT LEAST 1.5)

AND AT LEAST 5 PERCENT OF THE RDA PER SERVING

(RDA FOR RIBOFLAVN = 1.2 MG)

RIBOFLAVN RIBOFLAVN RIBOFLAVN RIBOFLAVN RIBOFLAVN RIBOFLAVN RIBOFLAVN RIBOFLAVN RIBOFLAVN

*INDICATES FOODS WHICH PROVIDE AT LEAST 25 PERCENT OF THE RDA PER SERVING

**INDICATES FOODS WHICH PROVIDE AT LEAST 50 PERCENT OF THE RDA PER SERVING

HANDBOOK NUMBER	FOOD NAME / SERVING SIZE DESCRIPTION	GRAMS	KCAL	RIBOFLAVN MG	INQ	%RDA
1	BLUE CHEESE / 1 OZ	28	100	0.11	1.83	9
2	CAMEMBERT CHEESE / 1 WEDGE	38	115	0.19	2.75	16 *
3	CHEDDAR CHEESE / 1 OZ	28	115	0.11	1.59	9
6	*COTTAGE CHEESE, CREAMED (4% FAT), LG CURD / 1 CUP	225	235	0.37	2.62	31 *
7	*COTTAGE CHEESE, CREAMED (4% FAT), SM CURD / 1 CUP	210	220	0.34	2.58	28 *
8	*COTTAGE CHEESE, 2% FAT / 1 CUP	226	205	0.42	3.41	35 *
9	*COTTAGE CHEESE, 1% FAT / 1 CUP	226	165	0.37	3.74	31 *
10	COTTAGE CHEESE, UNCREAMED (LESS THAN 0.5% FAT) / 1 CUP	145	125	0.21	2.80	17
13	MOZZARELLA CHEESE, MADE WITH SKIM MILK / 1 OZ	28	80	0.10	2.08	8
17	PROVOLONE CHEESE / 1 OZ	28	100	0.09	1.50	8
18	*RICOTTA CHEESE, MADE WITH WHOLE MILK / 1 CUP	246	428	0.48	1.87	40 *
19	*RICOTTA CHEESE, MADE WITH PART SKIM MILK / 1 CUP	246	340	0.46	2.25	38 *
20	ROMANO CHEESE / 1 OZ	28	110	0.11	1.67	9
21	SWISS CHEESE / 1 OZ	28	105	0.10	1.59	8
22	AMERICAN PASTEURIZED PROCESS CHEESE / 1 OZ	28	105	0.10	1.59	8
24	AMERICAN PASTEURIZED PROCESS CHEESE FOOD / 1 OZ	28	95	0.13	2.28	11
25	AMERICAN PASTEURIZED PROCESS CHEESE SPREAD / 1 OZ	28	82	0.12	2.44	10
50	*MILK, FLUID WHOLE (3.3% FAT) / 1 CUP	244	150	0.40	4.44	33 *
51	*MILK, FLUID LOWFAT (2% FAT), NO MILK SOLIDS ADDED / 1 CUP	244	120	0.40	5.56	33 *
52	*MILK, FLUID LOWFAT (2% FAT), LESS THAN 10 GRAMS OF PROTEIN PER CUP. / 1 CUP	245	125	0.42	5.60	35 *
53	*MILK, FLUID LOWFAT (2% FAT), MORE THAN 10 GRAMS OF PROTEIN PER CUP. / 1 CUP	246	135	0.48	5.93	40 *
54	*MILK, FLUID LOWFAT (1% FAT), NO MILK SOLIDS ADDED / 1 CUP	244	100	0.41	6.83	34 *
55	*MILK, FLUID LOWFAT (1% FAT), LESS THAN 10 GRAMS OF PROTEIN PER CUP. / 1 CUP	245	105	0.42	6.67	35 *

HANDBOOK NUMBER	FOOD NAME / SERVING SIZE DESCRIPTION	GRAMS	KCAL	RIBOFLAVN MG	INQ	%RDA
56	*MILK, FLUID LOWFAT (1% FAT), MORE THAN 10 GRAMS OF PROTEIN PER CUP. . . 1 CUP	246	120	0.47	6.53	39 *
57	*MILK, FLUID NONFAT (SKIM), NO MILK SOLIDS ADDED . . . 1 CUP	245	85	0.37	7.25	31 *
58	*MILK, FLUID NONFAT (SKIM), LESS THAN 10 GRAMS OF PROTEIN PER CUP . . . 1 CUP	245	90	0.43	7.96	36 *
59	*MILK, FLUID NONFAT (SKIM), MORE THAN 10 GRAMS OF PROTEIN PER CUP . . . 1 CUP	246	100	0.48	8.00	40 *
60	*BUTTERMILK, FLUID . . . 1 CUP	245	100	0.38	6.33	32 *
67	*CHOCOLATE MILK (COMMERCIAL) . . . 1 CUP	250	210	0.41	3.25	34 *
68	*CHOCOLATE MILK, LOWFAT (2%)(COMMERCIAL) . . . 1 CUP	250	180	0.42	3.89	35 *
69	*CHOCOLATE MILK, LOWFAT (1%)(COMMERCIAL) . . . 1 CUP	250	160	0.40	4.17	33 *
70	*EGGNOG (COMMERCIAL) . . . 1 CUP	254	340	0.48	2.35	40 *
71	*CHOCOLATE MALTED MILK (1 CUP WHOLE MILK AND 3/4 OZ MALTED MILK POWDER) 1 CUP PLUS POWDER	265	235	0.43	3.05	36 *
72	*NATURAL MALTED MILK (1CUP WHOLE MILK AND 3/4 OZ MALTED MILK POWDER) 1 CUP PLUS POWDER	265	235	0.54	3.83	45 *
73	**CHOCOLATE MILK SHAKE 10.6 OZ, NET WT.	300	355	0.67	3.15	56 **
74	**VANILLA MILK SHAKE, 11 OZ, NET WT.	313	350	0.61	2.90	51 **
76	*ICE CREAM, REGULAR (11% FAT), HARDENED 1 CUP	133	270	0.33	2.04	28 *
77	ICE CREAM, REGULAR (11% FAT), HARDENED 3-FL OZ	50	100	0.12	2.00	10
78	*ICE CREAM, REGULAR (11% FAT), SOFT SERVE 1 CUP	173	375	0.45	2.00	38 *
82	*ICE MILK, HARDENED (4.3% FAT) 1 CUP	131	185	0.35	3.15	29 *
83	*ICE MILK, SOFT SERVE (2.6% FAT) 1 CUP	175	225	0.54	4.00	45 *
86	*CUSTARD, BAKED . . . 1 CUP	265	305	0.50	2.73	42 *
87	*CHOCOLATE PUDDING, HOME RECIPE, STARCH BASE 1 CUP	260	385	0.36	1.56	30 *
88	*VANILLA PUDDING (BLANCMANGE), HOME RECIPE, STARCH BASE. 1 CUP	255	285	0.41	2.40	34 *
89	*TAPIOCA CREAM PUDDING, HOME RECIPE . . . 1 CUP	165	220	0.30	2.27	25 *
90	*CHOCOLATE PUDDING, COOKED FROM A MIX. 1 CUP	260	320	0.39	2.03	33 *

HANDBOOK FOOD NUMBER	FOOD NAME SERVING SIZE DESCRIPTION	GRAMS	KCAL	RIBOFLAVN MG	INQ	%RDA
91	*CHOCOLATE PUDDING, INSTANT 1 CUP	260	325	0.39	2.00	33 *
92	*FRUIT-FLAVORED YOGURT MADE WITH LOWFAT MILK, WITH ADDED MILK SOLIDS 8 OZ, NET WT.	227	230	0.40	2.90	33 *
93	*PLAIN YOGURT MADE WITH LOWFAT MILK, WITH ADDED MILK SOLIDS 8 OZ, NET WT.	227	145	0.49	5.63	41 *
94	*PLAIN YOGURT MADE WITH NONFAT MILK, WITH ADDED MILK SOLIDS 8 OZ, NET WT.	227	125	0.53	7.07	44 *
95	*PLAIN YOGURT MADE WITH WHOLE MILK, WITHOUT ADDED MILK SOLIDS 8 OZ, NET WT.	227	140	0.32	3.81	27 *
99	EGG, FRIED IN BUTTER (LARGE) 1 EGG	46	85	0.13	2.55	11
100	EGG, HARD-COOKED (LARGE), WITHOUT SHELL 1 EGG	50	80	0.14	2.92	12
101	EGG, POACHED (LARGE) 1 EGG	50	80	0.13	2.71	11
102	EGG, SCRAMBLED (MILK ADDED) IN BUTTER (LARGE) 1 EGG	64	95	0.16	2.81	13
146	CLAMS, RAW, MEAT ONLY 3 OZ	85	65	0.15	3.85	13
147	CLAMS, CANNED, SOLIDS AND LIQUIDS 3 OZ	85	45	0.09	3.33	8
152	*OYSTERS, RAW, MEAT ONLY 1 CUP, 13-19 MEDIUM SELECTS	240	160	0.43	4.48	36 *
153	SALMON, PINK, CANNED, SOLIDS AND LIQUIDS 3 OZ	85	120	0.16	2.22	13
154	SARDINES, ATLANTIC, CANNED IN OIL, DRAINED SOLIDS 3 OZ	85	175	0.17	1.62	14
156	SHAD, BAKED WITH FAT 3 OZ	85	170	0.22	2.16	18
163	BEEF CUTS COOKED, LEAN ONLY 2.5 OZ	72	140	0.17	2.02	14
164	GROUND BEEF, BROILED, LEAN WITH 10% FAT 3 OZ OR 3 BY 5/8 IN PATTY	85	185	0.20	1.80	17
168	ROAST BEEF, OVEN COOKED, RELATIVELY LEAN, LEAN AND FAT 3 OZ	85	165	0.19	1.92	16
169	ROAST BEEF, OVEN COOKED, RELATIVELY LEAN, LEAN ONLY 2.8 OZ	78	125	0.18	2.40	15
171	STEAK, SIRLOIN, BROILED, LEAN ONLY, BONE REMOVED 2 OZ	56	115	0.14	2.03	12
173	STEAK, ROUND, BRAISED, LEAN ONLY, BONE REMOVED 2.4 OZ	68	130	0.16	2.05	13
174	CORNED BEEF CANNED 3 OZ	85	185	0.20	1.80	17
176	CHIPPED BEEF, DRIED 2 1/2 OZ JAR	71	145	0.23	2.64	19

HANDBOOK FOOD NAME NUMBER — SERVING SIZE DESCRIPTION	GRAMS	KCAL	RIBOFLAVN MG	INQ	%RDA
180 *CHOP SUEY WITH BEEF AND PORK(HOME RECIPE) — 1 CUP	250	300	0.38	2.11	32 *
181 **HEART, BEEF, LEAN, BRAISED — 3 OZ	85	160	1.04	10.83	87 **
183 LAMB CHOP, BROILED, LEAN ONLY, BONE REMOVED — 2 OZ	57	120	0.15	2.08	13
184 LEG OF LAMB, ROASTED, LEAN AND FAT — 3 OZ	85	235	0.23	1.63	19
185 LEG OF LAMB, ROASTED, LEAN ONLY — 2.5 OZ	71	130	0.21	2.69	17
187 LAMB SHOULDER, ROASTED, LEAN ONLY — 2.3 OZ	64	130	0.18	2.31	15
188 **LIVER, BEEF, FRIED — 3 OZ	85	195	3.56	30.43	297 **
193 PORK CHOP, BROILED, LEAN ONLY, BONE REMOVED — 2 OZ	56	150	0.18	2.00	15
195 PORK ROAST, OVEN COOKED, LEAN ONLY — 2.4 OZ	68	175	0.21	2.00	17
197 PORK SHOULDER, SIMMERED, LEAN ONLY — 2.2 OZ	63	135	0.19	2.35	16
199 *BRAUNSCHWEIGER — 1 SLICE	28	90	0.41	7.59	34 *
208 VEAL CUTLET, BRAISED OR BROILED, BONE REMOVED — 3 OZ	85	185	0.21	1.89	17
209 VEAL RIB, ROASTED, BONE REMOVED — 3 OZ	85	230	0.26	1.88	22
210 CHICKEN BREAST, FRIED, BONES REMOVED — 2.8 OZ	79	160	0.17	1.77	14
211 CHICKEN DRUMSTICK, FRIED, BONES REMOVED — 1.3 OZ	38	90	0.15	2.78	13
212 *CHICKEN, HALF BROILER, BONES REMOVED — 6.2 OZ	176	240	0.34	2.36	28 *
216 CHICKEN CHOW MEIN, CANNED — 1 CUP	250	95	0.10	1.75	8
217 CHICKEN CHOW MEIN (HOME RECIPE) — 1 CUP	250	255	0.23	1.50	19
219 TURKEY, DARK MEAT, FLESH ONLY, ROASTED — 4 PIECES (2 1/2 BY 1 5/8 BY 1/4 IN.)	85	175	0.20	1.90	17
221 TURKEY, LIGHT AND DARK MEAT CHOPPED — 1 CUP	140	265	0.25	1.57	21
222 TURKEY, LIGHT AND DARK — 1.5 OZ EACH	85	160	0.15	1.56	13
233 *AVOCADOS, RAW, CALIFORNIA, WT. WITHOUT SKIN AND SEED — 1--3 1/8-IN DIAM.	216	370	0.43	1.94	36 *
234 **AVOCADOS, RAW, FLORIDA, WT. WITHOUT SKIN AND SEED — 1--3 5/8-IN DIAM.	304	390	0.61	2.61	51 **

HANDBOOK NUMBER	FOOD NAME / SERVING SIZE DESCRIPTION	GRAMS	KCAL	RIBOFLAVN MG	INQ	%RDA
238	BLUEBERRIES, RAW / 1 CUP	145	90	0.09	1.67	6
271	CANTALOUP, WT WITHOUT RIND AND SEEDS / 1/2 OF A 5-IN DIAM. MELON	272	80	0.08	1.67	7
282	PAPAYAS, RAW, 1/2 INCH CUBES / 1 CUP	140	55	0.06	1.82	5
284	PEACHES, RAW, SLICED / 1 CUP	170	65	0.09	2.31	8
286	PEACHES, CANNED, WATER PACK / 1 CUP (SOLIDS AND LIQUID)	244	75	0.07	1.56	6
309	RASPBERRIES, RED, RAW, WHOLE / 1 CUP	123	70	0.11	2.62	9
313	STRAWBERRIES, RAW, WHOLE, CAPPED / 1 CUP	149	55	0.10	3.03	8
318	WATERMELON, WT WITHOUT RIND AND SEEDS / 1/16 OF 33 LB MELON	426	110	0.13	1.97	11
327	CRACKED-WHEAT BREAD / 1 SLICE (18 PER 1LB LOAF)	25	65	0.06	1.54	5
334	RAISIN BREAD / 1 SLICE (18 PER 1LB LOAF)	25	65	0.06	1.54	5
352	WHITE BREAD, FIRM-CRUMB TYPE / 1 SLICE (20 PER 1LB LOAF)	23	65	0.06	1.54	5
369	*BRAN FLAKES (40% BRAN), ADDED SUGAR, SALT, IRON AND VITAMINS. / 1 CUP	35	105	0.49	7.78	41 *
370	**BRAN FLAKES WITH RAISINS, ADDED SUGAR, SALT, IRON AND VITAMINS / 1 CUP	50	145	0.71	8.16	59 **
371	*CORN FLAKES, PLAIN, ADDED SUGAR, SALT, IRON, VITAMINS / 1 CUP	25	95	0.35	6.14	29 *
372	*CORN FLAKES, SUGAR-COATED, ADDED SALT, IRON, VITAMINS / 1 CUP	40	155	0.56	6.02	47 *
373	PUFFED CORN, PLAIN, ADDED SUGAR, SALT, IRON, VITAMINS. / 1 CUP	20	80	0.28	5.83	23
375	*PUFFED OATS, ADDED SUGAR, SALT, MINERALS, VITAMINS / 1 CUP	25	100	0.35	5.83	29 *
377	*PUFFED RICE, PRESWEETENED, ADDED SALT, IRON, VITAMINS / 1 CUP	28	115	0.43	6.23	36 *
378	*WHEAT FLAKES, ADDED SUGAR, SALT, IRON, VITAMINS / 1 CUP	30	105	0.42	6.67	35 *
380	*PUFFED WHEAT, PRESWEETENED, ADDED SALT, IRON, VITAMINS. / 1 CUP	38	140	0.57	6.79	48 *
430	GRAHAM CRACKERS PLAIN / 2 CRACKERS	14	55	0.08	2.42	7
441	MACARONI (ENRICHED) AND CHEESE, CANNED / 1 CUP	240	230	0.24	1.74	20
442	*MACARONI (ENRICHED) AND CHEESE, HOME RECIPE / 1 CUP	200	430	0.40	1.55	33 *

HANDBOOK NUMBER	FOOD NAME SERVING SIZE DESCRIPTION	GRAMS	KCAL	RIBOFLAVN MG	INQ	%RDA
443	BLUEBERRY MUFFINS, HOME RECIPE / 1 MUFFIN, 2 3/8-IN DIAM., 1 1/2-IN HIGH	40	110	0.10	1.52	8
444	BRAN MUFFINS, HOME RECIPE / 1 MUFFIN 2 3/8-IN DIAM., 1 1/2-IN HIGH	40	105	0.10	1.59	8
446	PLAIN MUFFIN, HOME RECIPE / 1 MUFFIN, 3-IN DIAM, 1 1/2-IN HIGH	40	120	0.12	1.67	10
451	PANCAKE MADE FROM HOME RECIPE / 1 CAKE 4-IN DIAM	27	60	0.07	1.94	6
452	PANCAKE MADE FROM MIX / 1 CAKE 4-IN DIAM	27	60	0.06	1.67	5
462	CUSTARD PIE / 1 SECTOR, 1/7 OF PIE	130	285	0.27	1.58	23
475	PIZZA(CHEESE), BAKED / 1 SECTOR, 1/8 OF 12-IN DIAM PIE	60	145	0.18	2.07	15
492	CLOVERLEAF ROLLS FROM HOME RECIPE / 1 ROLL (2 1/2-IN DIAM.,2-IN HIGH	35	120	0.12	1.67	10
496	SPAGHETTI, ENRICHED, IN TOMATO SAUCE WITH CHEESE, CANNED / 1 CUP	250	190	0.28	2.46	23
497	*SPAGHETTI, ENRICHED, WITH MEAT BALLS IN TOMATO SAUCE, HOME RECIPE / 1 CUP	248	330	0.30	1.52	25 *
500	WAFFLES FROM HOME RECIPE / 1 WAFFLE 7-IN DIAM	75	210	0.23	1.83	19
501	WAFFLES FROM MIX,EGG AND MILK ADDED / 1 WAFFLE 7-IN. DIAM	75	205	0.22	1.79	18
505	*SELF-RISING FLOUR,ENRICHED,UNSIFTED, SPOONED / 1 CUP	125	440	0.50	1.89	42 *
507	**ALMONDS, CHOPPED / 1 CUP (130 ALMONDS)	130	775	1.20	2.58	100 **
508	**ALMONDS, SLIVERED / 1 CUP (115 NUTS)	115	690	1.06	2.56	88 **
546	CHOCOLATE FLAVORED BEVERAGE POWDER WITH NONFAT DRY MILK / 1 OZ (4 HEAPING TSP)	28	100	0.21	3.50	17
564	ASPARAGUS, COOKED,DRAINED,FROM RAW / 1 CUP (CUTS AND TIPS, 1 1/2 TO 2-IN LENGTHS)	145	30	0.26	14.44	22
565	ASPARAGUS, COOKED,DRAINED,FROM FROZEN / 1 CUP (CUTS AND TIPS, 1 1/2 TO 2-IN LENGTHS)	180	40	0.23	9.58	19
566	ASPARAGUS, SPEARS 1/2-IN DIAM AT BASE FROM RAW / 4 SPEARS	60	10	0.11	18.33	9
567	ASPARAGUS, SPEARS 1/2-IN DIAM AT BASE FROM FROZEN / 4 SPEARS	60	15	0.08	8.89	7
568	ASPARAGUS, CANNED SPEARS / 4 SPEARS	80	15	0.08	8.89	7
571	GREEN SNAP BEANS, COOKED, DRAINED, FROM RAW / 1 CUP	125	30	0.11	6.11	9
572	GREEN SNAP BEANS, COOKED, DRAINED,CUTS FROM FROZEN / 1 CUP	135	35	0.12	5.71	10

HANDBOOK FOOD NUMBER	FOOD NAME SERVING SIZE DESCRIPTION	GRAMS	KCAL	RIBOFLAVN MG	INQ	%RDA
573	GREEN SNAP BEANS, COOKED, DRAINED,FRENCH CUTS FROM FROZEN 1 CUP	130	35	0.10	4.76	8
574	GREEN SNAP BEANS, CANNED, DRAINED SOLIDS (CUTS) 1 CUP	135	30	0.07	3.89	6
575	YELLOW OR WAX BEANS, COOKED, DRAINED, FROM RAW 1 CUP	125	30	0.11	6.11	9
576	YELLOW OR WAX BEANS, COOKED, DRAINED CUTS FROM FROZEN 1 CUP	135	35	0.11	5.24	9
577	YELLOW OR WAX BEANS, CANNED, DRAINED SOLIDS (CUTS) 1 CUP	135	30	0.07	3.89	6
578	BEAN SPROUTS,(MUNG),RAW 1 CUP	105	35	0.14	6.67	12
579	BEAN SPROUTS,(MUNG),COOKED, DRAINED 1 CUP	125	35	0.13	6.19	11
581	BEETS, COOKED DRAINED,DICED OR SLICED 1 CUP	170	55	0.07	2.12	6
584	BEET GREENS, COOKED, DRAINED 1 CUP	145	25	0.22	14.67	18
585	BLACKEYE PEAS, COOKED, DRAINED, FROM RAW 1 CUP	165	180	0.18	1.67	15
587	*BROCCOLI, COOKED, DRAINED, FROM RAW 1 WHOLE MEDIUM STALK	187	45	0.36	13.33	30 *
588	*BROCCOLI, COOKED, DRAINED, FROM RAW 1 CUP (STALKS CUT INTO 1/2-IN PIECES)	155	40	0.31	12.92	26 *
590	BROCCOLI, FROM FROZEN, CHOPPED, COOKED, DRAINED 1 CUP	185	50	0.22	7.33	18
591	BRUSSELS SPROUTS, COOKED, DRAINED, FROM RAW 7-8 SPROUTS (1 1/4 TO 1 1/2-IN DIAM) 1 CUP	155	55	0.22	6.67	18
592	BRUSSELS SPROUTS, COOKED, DRAINED, FROM FROZEN 1 CUP	155	50	0.16	5.33	13
595	CABBAGE, COOKED, DRAINED 1 CUP	145	30	0.06	3.33	5
597	SAVOY CABBAGE, RAW, COARSELY SHREDDED 1 CUP	70	15	0.06	6.67	5
599	WHITE MUSTARD CABBAGE, COOKED, DRAINED 1 CUP	170	25	0.14	9.33	12
601	CARROTS, RAW, PEELED, GRATED 1 CUP	110	45	0.06	2.22	5
602	CARROTS (CROSSWISE CUTS) COOKED, DRAINED 1 CUP	155	50	0.08	2.67	7
605	CAULIFLOWER, RAW, CHOPPED 1 CUP	115	31	0.12	6.45	10
606	CAULIFLOWER, COOKED, DRAINED FROM RAW 1 CUP	125	30	0.10	5.56	8
607	CAULIFLOWER, COOKED, DRAINED FROM FROZEN 1 CUP	180	30	0.09	5.00	8

HANDBOOK NUMBER	FOOD NAME SERVING SIZE DESCRIPTION	GRAMS	KCAL	RIBOFLAVN MG	INQ	%RDA
610	*COLLARDS, COOKED, DRAINED, FROM RAW. 1 CUP	190	65	0.38	9.74	32 *
611	COLLARDS, COOKED DRAINED, FROM FROZEN 1 CUP	170	50	0.24	8.00	20
612	CORN, COOKED, DRAINED FROM RAW, WT WITHOUT COB 1 EAR (5 BY 1 3/4-IN)	77	70	0.08	1.90	7
620	DANDELION GREENS, COOKED, DRAINED 1 CUP	105	35	0.17	8.10	14
621	ENDIVE,CURLY,RAW SMALL PIECES 1 CUP	50	10	0.07	11.67	6
622	KALE, COOKED, DRAINED, FROM RAW, LEAVES WITHOUT STEMS 1 CUP	110	45	0.20	7.41	17
623	KALE, COOKED, DRAINED, FROM FROZEN, LEAF STYLE 1 CUP	130	40	0.20	8.33	17
624	BUTTERHEAD LETTUCE, RAW 1 HEAD,5-IN DIAM.	220	25	0.10	6.67	8
626	*ICEBERG LETTUCE (CRISPHEAD) 1 HEAD,6-IN DIAM	567	70	0.32	7.62	27 *
627	ICEBERG LETTUCE (CRISPHEAD) 1 WEDGE (1/4 HEAD)	135	20	0.08	6.67	7
630	*MUSHROOMS, RAW, SLICED OR CHOPPED 1 CUP	70	20	0.32	26.67	27 *
631	MUSTARD GREENS, COOKED, DRAINED, WITHOUT STEMS 1 CUP	140	30	0.20	11.11	17
632	OKRA PODS, COOKED 10 PODS 3 BY 5/8 IN	106	30	0.19	10.56	16
633	ONIONS, MATURE, RAW, CHOPPED 1 CUP	170	65	0.07	1.79	6
635	ONIONS, MATURE, COOKED, DRAINED, WHOLE OR SLICED. 1 CUP	210	60	0.06	1.67	5
638	PARSNIPS, COOKED, DICED 1 CUP	155	100	0.12	2.00	10
641	GREEN PEAS, FROZEN, COOKED, DRAINED 1 CUP	160	110	0.14	2.12	12
643	SWEET PEPPERS, RAW. 1 POD (5 PER LB)	74	15	0.06	6.67	5
656	PUMPKIN, CANNED 1 CUP	245	80	0.12	2.50	10
658	SAUERKRAUT, CANNED,SOLIDS AND LIQUIDS 1 CUP	235	40	0.09	3.75	8
659	SPINACH, RAW, CHOPPED 1 CUP	55	15	0.11	12.22	9
660	SPINACH, COOKED, DRAINED FROM RAW 1 CUP	180	40	0.25	10.42	21
661	*SPINACH, COOKED, DRAINED FROM FROZEN, CHOPPED 1 CUP	205	45	0.31	11.48	26 *

HANDBOOK NUMBER	FOOD NAME SERVING SIZE DESCRIPTION	GRAMS	KCAL	RIBOFLAVN MG	INQ	%RDA
662	SPINACH, COOKED, DRAINED FROM FROZEN, LEAF. 1 CUP	190	45	0.27	10.00	23
663	SPINACH, CANNED, DRAINED SOLIDS 1 CUP	205	50	0.25	8.33	21
664	SUMMER SQUASH, COOKED, DICED, DRAINED 1 CUP	210	30	0.17	9.44	14
665	WINTER SQUASH, BAKED, MASHED 1 CUP	205	130	0.27	3.46	23
672	TOMATOES, CANNED, SOLIDS AND LIQUIDS 1 CUP	241	50	0.07	2.33	6
675	TOMATO JUICE, CANNED 1 CUP	243	45	0.07	2.59	6
677	TURNIPS, COOKED, DICED 1 CUP	155	35	0.08	3.81	7
678	*TURNIP GREENS, COOKED, DRAINED, FROM RAW (LEAVES AND STEMS) 1 CUP	145	30	0.33	18.33	28 *
679	TURNIP GREENS, COOKED, DRAINED, FROM FROZEN, CHOPPED 1 CUP	165	40	0.15	6.25	13
680	VEGETABLES, MIXED, FROZEN, COOKED, DRAINED 1 CUP	182	115	0.13	1.88	11
708	CREAM OF CHICKEN SOUP PREPARED WITH EQUAL VOLUME OF MILK, CANNED 1 CUP	245	180	0.27	2.50	23
709	*CREAM OF MUSHROOM SOUP PREPARED WITH EQUAL VOLUME OF MILK, CANNED 1 CUP	245	215	0.34	2.64	28 *
710	TOMATO SOUP PREPARED WITH EQUAL VOLUME OF MILK, CANNED 1 CUP	250	175	0.25	2.38	21
713	BEEF NOODLE SOUP, PREPARED WITH EQUAL VOLUME OF WATER, CANNED 1 CUP	240	65	0.07	1.79	6
718	SPLIT PEA SOUP PREPARED WITH EQUAL VOLUME OF WATER, CANNED 1 CUP	245	145	0.15	1.72	13
730	*BREWER'S YEAST, DRY 1 TBSP	8	25	0.34	22.67	28 *

FOODS WHICH PROVIDE A HIGH CONCENTRATION OF NIACIN RELATIVE TO CALORIES
(INQ AT LEAST 1.5) AND AT LEAST 5 PERCENT OF THE RDA PER SERVING
(RDA FOR NIACIN = 14.0 MG)

*INDICATES FOODS WHICH PROVIDE AT LEAST 25 PERCENT OF THE RDA PER SERVING
**INDICATES FOODS WHICH PROVIDE AT LEAST 50 PERCENT OF THE RDA PER SERVING

HANDBOOK FOOD NUMBER	FOOD NAME / SERVING SIZE DESCRIPTION	GRAMS	KCAL	NIACIN MG	INQ	%RDA
145	BLUEFISH, BAKED WITH BUTTER OR MARGARINE 3 OZ	85	135	1.60	1.69	11
146	CLAMS, RAW, MEAT ONLY 3 OZ	85	65	1.10	2.42	8
147	CLAMS, CANNED, SOLIDS AND LIQUIDS 3 OZ	85	45	0.90	2.86	6
148	CRABMEAT, CANNED 1 CUP	135	135	2.60	2.75	19
150	HADDOCK, BREADED, FRIED 3 OZ	85	140	2.70	2.76	19
152	*OYSTERS, RAW, MEAT ONLY 1 CUP, 13-19 MEDIUM SELECTS	240	160	6.00	5.36	43 *
153	*SALMON, PINK, CANNED, SOLIDS AND LIQUIDS 3 OZ	85	120	6.80	8.10	49 *
154	*SARDINES, ATLANTIC, CANNED IN OIL, DRAINED SOLIDS 3 OZ	85	175	4.60	3.76	33 *
156	**SHAD, BAKED WITH FAT 3 OZ	85	170	7.30	6.13	52 **
157	SHRIMP, CANNED 3 OZ	85	100	1.50	2.14	11
158	SHRIMP, FRENCH FRIED 3 OZ	85	190	2.30	1.73	16
159	**TUNA, CANNED IN OIL, DRAINED SOLIDS 3 OZ	85	170	10.10	8.49	72 **
160	**TUNA SALAD(WITH CELERY, MAYONNAISE TYPE DRESSING, PICKLE, ONION, EGG) 1 CUP	205	350	10.30	4.20	74 **
162	*BEEF CUTS COOKED, LEAN AND FAT. 3 OZ - 2 1/2 BY 2 1/2 BY 3/4 IN	85	245	3.60	2.10	26 *
163	BEEF CUTS COOKED, LEAN ONLY 2.5 OZ	72	140	3.30	3.37	24
164	*GROUND BEEF, BROILED, LEAN WITH 10% FAT 3 OZ OR 3 BY 5/8 IN PATTY	85	185	5.10	3.94	36 *
165	*GROUND BEEF, BROILED, LEAN WITH 21% FAT 2.9 OZ OR 3 BY 5/8 IN PATTY	82	235	4.40	2.67	31 *
167	ROAST BEEF, OVEN COOKED, LEAN ONLY 1.8 OZ	51	125	2.60	2.97	19
168	*ROAST BEEF, OVEN COOKED, RELATIVELY LEAN, LEAN AND FAT. 3 OZ	85	165	4.50	3.90	32 *
169	*ROAST BEEF, OVEN COOKED, RELATIVELY LEAN, LEAN ONLY 2.8 OZ	78	125	4.30	4.91	31 *
170	*STEAK, SIRLOIN, BROILED, LEAN AND FAT, BONE REMOVED 3 OZ	85	330	4.00	1.73	29 *
171	*STEAK, SIRLOIN, BROILED, LEAN ONLY, BONE REMOVED 2 OZ	56	115	3.60	4.47	26 *
172	*STEAK, ROUND, BRAISED, LEAN AND FAT, BONE REMOVED 3 OZ	85	220	4.80	3.12	34 *

HANDBOOK NUMBER	FOOD NAME / SERVING SIZE DESCRIPTION	GRAMS	KCAL	NIACIN MG	INQ	%RDA	
173	*STEAK, ROUND, BRAISED, LEAN ONLY, BONE REMOVED • 2.4 OZ	68	130	4.10	4.51	29	*
174	CORNED BEEF CANNED. • 3 OZ	85	185	2.90	2.24	21	
175	*CORNED BEEF HASH • 1 CUP	220	400	4.60	1.64	33	*
176	CHIPPED BEEF, DRIED • 2 1/2 OZ JAR	71	145	2.70	2.66	19	
177	*BEEF AND VEGETABLE STEW • 1 CUP	245	220	4.70	3.05	34	*
178	*BEEF POTPIE (HOME RECIPE) 1/3 OF 9-IN DIAM. PIE	210	515	5.50	1.53	39	*
180	*CHOP SUEY WITH BEEF AND PORK(HOME RECIPE) • 1 CUP	250	300	5.00	2.38	36	*
181	*HEART, BEEF, LEAN, BRAISED • 3 OZ	85	160	6.50	5.80	46	*
182	*LAMB CHOP, BROILED, LEAN AND FAT, BONE REMOVED 3.1 OZ	89	360	4.10	1.63	29	*
183	LAMB CHOP, BROILED, LEAN ONLY, BONE REMOVED 2 OZ	57	120	3.40	4.05	24	
184	*LEG OF LAMB, ROASTED, LEAN AND FAT • 3 OZ	85	235	4.70	2.86	34	*
185	*LEG OF LAMB, ROASTED, LEAN ONLY • 2.5 OZ	71	130	4.40	4.84	31	*
186	*LAMB SHOULDER, ROASTED, LEAN AND FAT. • 3 OZ	85	285	4.00	2.01	29	*
187	*LAMB SHOULDER, ROASTED, LEAN ONLY • 2.3 OZ	64	130	3.70	4.07	26	*
188	**LIVER, BEEF, FRIED. • 3 OZ	85	195	14.00	10.26	100	**
189	HAM, LIGHT CURE, ROASTED, LEAN AND FAT • 3 OZ	85	245	3.10	1.81	22	
190	LUNCHEON MEAT, BOILED HAM • 1 OZ	28	65	0.70	1.54	5	
192	*PORK CHOP, BROILED, LEAN AND FAT, BONE REMOVED 2.7 OZ	78	305	4.50	2.11	32	*
193	*PORK CHOP, BROILED, LEAN ONLY, BONE REMOVED 2 OZ	56	150	3.80	3.62	27	*
194	*PORK ROAST, OVEN COOKED, LEAN AND FAT • 3 OZ	85	310	4.80	2.21	34	*
195	*PORK ROAST, OVEN COOKED, LEAN ONLY • 2.4 OZ	68	175	4.40	3.59	31	*
196	*PORK SHOULDER, SIMMERED, LEAN AND FAT • 3 OZ	85	320	4.10	1.83	29	*
197	*PORK SHOULDER, SIMMERED, LEAN ONLY • 2.2 OZ	63	135	3.70	3.92	26	*

HANDBOOK FOOD NAME NUMBER SERVING SIZE DESCRIPTION	GRAMS	KCAL	NIACIN MG	INQ	XRDA
199 BRAUNSCHWEIGER, 1 SLICE	28	90	2.30	3.65	16
206 SALAMI, COOKED TYPE, 1 SLICE (8 PER 8-OZ PKG.)	28	90	1.20	1.90	9
208 *VEAL CUTLET, BRAISED OR BROILED, BONE REMOVED, 3 OZ	85	185	4.60	3.55	33 *
209 *VEAL RIB, ROASTED, BONE REMOVED, 3 OZ	85	230	6.60	4.10	47 *
210 **CHICKEN BREAST, FRIED, BONES REMOVED, 2.8 OZ	79	160	11.60	10.36	83 **
211 CHICKEN DRUMSTICK, FRIED, BONES REMOVED, 1.3 OZ	38	90	2.70	4.29	19
212 **CHICKEN, HALF BROILER, BONES REMOVED, 6.2 OZ	176	240	15.50	9.23	111 **
213 *CHICKEN, CANNED, BONELESS, 3 OZ	85	170	3.70	3.11	26 *
214 *CHICKEN A LA KING (HOME RECIPE), 1 CUP	245	470	5.40	1.64	39 *
215 *CHICKEN AND NOODLES (HOME RECIPE), 1 CUP	240	365	4.30	1.68	31 *
216 CHICKEN CHOW MEIN, CANNED, 1 CUP	250	95	1.00	1.50	7
217 *CHICKEN CHOW MEIN (HOME RECIPE), 1 CUP	250	255	4.30	2.41	31 *
219 *TURKEY, DARK MEAT, FLESH ONLY, ROASTED, 4 PIECES (2 1/2 BY 1 5/8 BY 1/4 IN.)	85	175	3.60	2.94	26 *
220 **TURKEY, LIGHT MEAT, FLESH ONLY, ROASTED, 2 PIECES (4 BY 2 BY 1/4 IN.)	85	150	9.40	8.95	67 **
221 **TURKEY, LIGHT AND DARK MEAT CHOPPED, 1 CUP	140	265	10.80	5.82	77 **
222 *TURKEY, LIGHT AND DARK, 1.5 OZ EACH	85	160	6.50	5.80	46 *
230 *APRICOTS, DRIED, UNCOOKED, 1 CUP-28 LARGE OR 37 MEDIUM HALVES	130	340	4.30	1.81	31 *
231 APRICOTS, DRIED, COOKED, UNSWEETENED, 1 CUP-FRUIT AND LIQUID	250	215	2.50	1.66	18
234 *AVOCADOS, RAW, FLORIDA, WT. WITHOUT SKIN AND SEED, 1--3 5/8-IN DIAM.	304	390	4.90	1.79	35 *
271 CANTALOUP, WT WITHOUT RIND AND SEEDS, 1/2 OF A 5-IN DIAM. MELON	272	80	1.60	2.86	11
272 HONEYDEW MELON, WT WITHOUT RIND AND SEEDS, 1/10 OF A 6 1/2-IN DIAM. MELON	149	50	0.90	2.57	6
283 PEACHES, RAW, WT FOR PEELED AND PITTED, 1--2 1/2-IN DIAM. PEACH	100	40	1.00	3.57	7
284 PEACHES, RAW, SLICED, 1 CUP	170	65	1.70	3.74	12

HANDBOOK NUMBER	FOOD NAME / SERVING SIZE DESCRIPTION	GRAMS	KCAL	NIACIN MG	INQ	%RDA
			75	1.50	2.86	11
286	PEACHES, CANNED, WATER PACK / 1 CUP (SOLIDS AND LIQUID)	244				
287	**PEACHES, DRIED, UNCOOKED. / 1 CUP	160	420	8.50	2.89	61 **
288	*PEACHES, DRIED, COOKED, UNSWEETENED / 1 CUP (HALVES AND JUICE)	250	205	3.80	2.65	27 *
309	RASPBERRIES, RED, RAW, WHOLE / 1 CUP	123	70	1.10	2.24	8
313	STRAWBERRIES, RAW, WHOLE, CAPPED / 1 CUP	149	55	0.90	2.34	6
327	CRACKED-WHEAT BREAD / 1 SLICE (18 PER 1LB LOAF)	25	65	0.80	1.76	6
329	FRENCH BREAD. / 5 BY 2 1/2 BY 1 IN SLICE	35	100	1.20	1.71	9
330	VIENNA BREAD. / 4 3/4 BY 4 BY 1/2 IN SLICE	25	75	0.80	1.52	6
332	ITALIAN BREAD / 4 1/2 BY 3 1/4 BY 3/4 IN SLICE	30	85	1.00	1.68	7
336	RYE BREAD, AMERICAN, LIGHT / 5 BY 4 BY 3/8 IN SLICE	25	60	0.70	1.67	5
340	WHITE BREAD, SOFT-CRUMB TYPE / 1 SLICE (18 PER 1LB LOAF)	25	70	0.80	1.63	6
352	WHITE BREAD, FIRM-CRUMB TYPE / 1 SLICE (20 PER 1LB LOAF)	23	65	0.80	1.76	6
358	WHOLE-WHEAT BREAD, SOFT-CRUMB TYPE / 1 SLICE (16 PER 1 LB LOAF)	28	65	0.80	1.76	6
367	WHEAT, ROLLED, COOKED / 1 CUP	240	180	2.20	1.75	16
368	WHEAT, WHOLE-MEAL, COOKED / 1 CUP	245	110	1.50	1.95	11
369	*BRAN FLAKES (40% BRAN), ADDED SUGAR, SALT, IRON AND VITAMINS. / 1 CUP	35	105	4.10	5.58	29 *
370	*BRAN FLAKES WITH RAISINS, ADDED SUGAR, SALT, IRON AND VITAMINS / 1 CUP	50	145	5.80	5.71	41 *
371	CORN FLAKES, PLAIN, ADDED SUGAR, SALT, IRON, VITAMINS / 1 CUP	25	95	2.90	4.36	21
372	*CORN FLAKES, SUGAR-COATED, ADDED SALT, IRON, VITAMINS / 1 CUP	40	155	4.60	4.24	33 *
373	PUFFED CORN, PLAIN, ADDED SUGAR, SALT, IRON, VITAMINS. / 1 CUP	20	80	2.30	4.11	16
375	PUFFED OATS, ADDED SUGAR, SALT, MINERALS, VITAMINS / 1 CUP	25	100	2.90	4.14	21
376	PUFFED RICE, PLAIN, ADDED IRON, THIAMIN, NIACIN. / 1 CUP	15	60	0.70	1.67	5
377	*PUFFED RICE, PRESWEETENED, ADDED SALT, IRON, VITAMINS / 1 CUP	28	115	5.00	6.21	36 *

HANDBOOK NUMBER	FOOD NAME / SERVING SIZE DESCRIPTION	GRAMS	KCAL	NIACIN MG	INQ	%RDA
378	*WHEAT FLAKES, ADDED SUGAR, SALT, IRON, VITAMINS / 1 CUP	30	105	3.50	4.76	25 *
379	PUFFED WHEAT, PLAIN, ADDED IRON, THIAMIN, NIACIN / 1 CUP	15	55	1.20	3.12	9
380	*PUFFED WHEAT, PRESWEETENED, ADDED SALT, IRON, VITAMINS / 1 CUP	38	140	6.70	6.84	46 *
381	SHREDDED WHEAT, PLAIN / 1 LARGE BISCUIT OR 1/2 CUP SMALL BISCUITS	25	90	1.10	1.75	8
444	BRAN MUFFINS, HOME RECIPE / 1 MUFFIN 2 3/8-IN DIAM., 1 1/2-IN HIGH	40	105	1.70	2.31	12
475	PIZZA(CHEESE), BAKED / 1 SECTOR, 1/8 OF 12-IN DIAM PIE	60	145	1.60	1.58	11
479	PRETZELS, DUTCH TWISTED / 1 PRETZEL 2 3/4 BY 2 5/8-IN	16	60	0.70	1.67	5
480	PRETZELS, THIN TWISTED / 10 PRETZEL 3 1/4 BY 2 1/4 BY 1/4-IN.	60	235	2.50	1.52	18
486	RICE, PARBOILED, ENRICHED, COOKED / 1 CUP	175	185	2.10	1.62	15
487	ROLLS, BROWN AND SERVE, BROWNED / 1 ROLL	26	85	0.90	1.51	6
488	ROLLS, CLOVERLEAF OR PAN / 1 ROLL 2 1/2-IN DIAM, 2-IN HIGH	28	85	0.90	1.51	6
489	HAMBURGER OR FRANKFURTER BUN / 1 ROLL (8 PER 11 1/2-OZ PKG)	40	120	1.30	1.55	9
490	HARD ROLLS / 1 ROLL 3 3/4-IN DIAM, 2-IN HIGH	50	155	1.70	1.57	12
491	*HOAGIE OR SUBMARINE BUNS / 1 BUN (11 1/2 BY 3 BY 2 1/2 IN.)	135	390	4.50	1.65	32 *
496	*SPAGHETTI, ENRICHED, IN TOMATO SAUCE WITH CHEESE, CANNED / 1 CUP	250	190	4.50	3.38	32 *
497	*SPAGHETTI, ENRICHED, WITH MEAT BALLS IN TOMATO SAUCE, HOME RECIPE / 1 CUP	248	330	4.00	1.73	29 *
499	TOASTER PASTRIES / 1 PASTRY	50	200	2.10	1.50	15
505	*SELF-RISING FLOUR, ENRICHED, UNSIFTED, SPOONED / 1 CUP	125	440	6.60	2.14	47 *
506	*WHOLE WHEAT FLOUR / 1 CUP	120	400	5.20	1.86	37 *
523	**PEANUTS, ROASTED IN OIL, SALTED / 1 CUP (WHOLE, HALVES, CHOPPED)	144	840	24.80	4.22	177 **
524	PEANUT BUTTER / 1 TBSP	16	95	2.40	3.61	17
540	CHOCOLATE COATED PEANUTS / 1 OZ	28	160	2.10	1.88	15
564	ASPARAGUS, COOKED, DRAINED, FROM RAW / 1 CUP (CUTS AND TIPS, 1 1/2 TO 2-IN LENGTHS)	145	30	2.00	9.52	14

HANDBOOK NUMBER	FOOD NAME SERVING SIZE DESCRIPTION	GRAMS	KCAL	NIACIN MG	INQ	%RDA
565	ASPARAGUS, COOKED,DRAINED,FROM FROZEN 1 CUP (CUTS AND TIPS, 1 1/2 TO 2-IN LENGTHS)	180	40	1.80	6.43	13
566	ASPARAGUS, SPEARS 1/2-IN DIAM AT BASE FROM RAW 4 SPEARS	60	10	0.80	11.43	6
567	ASPARAGUS, SPEARS 1/2-IN DIAM AT BASE FROM FROZEN 4 SPEARS	60	15	0.70	6.67	5
578	BEAN SPROUTS,(MUNG),RAW 1 CUP	105	35	0.80	3.27	6
579	BEAN SPROUTS,(MUNG),COOKED, DRAINED 1 CUP	125	35	0.90	3.67	6
585	BLACKEYE PEAS, COOKED, DRAINED, FROM RAW 1 CUP	165	180	2.30	1.83	16
586	BLACKEYE PEAS, COOKED, DRAINED, FROM FROZEN 1 CUP	170	220	2.40	1.56	17
587	BROCCOLI, COOKED, DRAINED, FROM RAW 1 WHOLE MEDIUM STALK	187	45	1.40	4.44	10
588	BROCCOLI, COOKED, DRAINED, FROM RAW 1 CUP (STALKS CUT INTO 1/2-IN PIECES)	155	40	1.20	4.29	9
590	BROCCOLI, FROM FROZEN, CHOPPED, COOKED, DRAINED 1 CUP	185	50	0.90	2.57	6
591	BRUSSELS SPROUTS, COOKED, DRAINED, FROM RAW 7-8 SPROUTS (1 1/4 TO 1 1/2-IN DIAM) 1 CUP	155	55	1.20	3.12	9
592	BRUSSELS SPROUTS, COOKED, DRAINED, FROM FROZEN 1 CUP	155	50	0.90	2.57	6
599	WHITE MUSTARD CABBAGE, COOKED, DRAINED 1 CUP	170	25	1.20	6.86	9
601	CARROTS, RAW, PEELED, GRATED 1 CUP	110	45	0.70	2.22	5
602	CARROTS (CROSSWISE CUTS) COOKED, DRAINED 1 CUP	155	50	0.80	2.29	6
605	CAULIFLOWER, RAW, CHOPPED 1 CUP	115	31	0.80	3.69	6
606	CAULIFLOWER, COOKED, DRAINED FROM RAW 1 CUP	125	30	0.80	3.81	6
607	CAULIFLOWER, COOKED, DRAINED FROM FROZEN 1 CUP	180	30	0.70	3.33	5
610	COLLARDS, COOKED, DRAINED, FROM RAW 1 CUP	190	65	2.30	5.05	16
611	COLLARDS, COOKED DRAINED, FROM FROZEN 1 CUP	170	50	1.00	2.86	7
612	CORN, COOKED, DRAINED FROM RAW, WT WITHOUT COB 1 EAR (5 BY 1 3/4-IN)	77	70	1.10	2.24	8
613	CORN, COOKED, DRAINED FROM FROZEN, WT WITHOUT COB 1 EAR (5-IN LONG)	126	120	2.10	2.50	15
614	CORN, COOKED, DRAINED FROM FROZEN 1 CUP KERNELS	165	130	2.50	2.75	18

HANDBOOK NUMBER	FOOD NAME SERVING SIZE DESCRIPTION	GRAMS	KCAL	NIACIN MG	INQ	%RDA
		256	210	2.60	1.77	19
615	CORN, CANNED CREAM STYLE. 1 CUP	256	210	2.60	1.77	19
616	CORN, CANNED, WHOLE KERNAL, VACUUM PACK 1 CUP	210	175	2.30	1.88	16
617	CORN, CANNED, WET PACK, DRAINED SOLIDS 1 CUP	165	140	1.50	1.53	11
622	KALE, COOKED, DRAINED, FROM RAW, LEAVES WITHOUT STEMS 1 CUP	110	45	1.80	5.71	13
623	KALE, COOKED, DRAINED, FROM FROZEN, LEAF STYLE 1 CUP	130	40	0.90	3.21	6
626	ICEBERG LETTUCE (CRISPHEAD) 1 HEAD, 6-IN DIAM	567	70	1.60	3.27	11
630	MUSHROOMS, RAW, SLICED OR CHOPPED 1 CUP	70	20	2.90	20.71	21
631	MUSTARD GREENS, COOKED, DRAINED, WITHOUT STEMS 1 CUP	140	30	0.80	3.81	6
632	OKRA PODS, COOKED. 10 PODS 3 BY 5/8 IN	106	30	1.00	4.76	7
641	GREEN PEAS, FROZEN, COOKED, DRAINED 1 CUP	160	110	2.70	3.51	19
645	BAKED POTATO, PEELED AFTER BAKING 1 POTATO (2 PER LB)	156	145	2.70	2.66	19
646	BOILED POTATO, PEELED AFTER BOILING 1 POTATO (3 PER LB)	137	105	2.00	2.72	14
647	BOILED POTATOES, PEELED BEFORE BOILING 1 POTATO (3 PER LB)	135	90	1.60	2.54	11
648	FRENCH FRIED POTATOES, PREPARED FROM RAW 10 STRIPS 2 TO 3 1/2 IN LONG	50	135	1.60	1.69	11
649	FRENCH FRIED POTATOES, FROZEN, OVEN HEATED. 10 STRIPS	50	110	1.30	1.69	9
651	MASHED POTATOES, PREPARED FROM RAW, MILK ADDED 1 CUP	210	135	2.10	2.22	15
652	MASHED POTATOES, PREPARED FROM RAW, MILK AND BUTTER ADDED 1 CUP	210	195	2.10	1.54	15
655	POTATO SALAD MADE WITH COOKED SALAD DRESSING 1 CUP	250	250	2.80	1.60	20
656	PUMPKIN, CANNED 1 CUP	245	80	1.50	2.68	11
660	SPINACH, COOKED, DRAINED FROM RAW 1 CUP	180	40	0.90	3.21	6
661	SPINACH, COOKED, DRAINED FROM FROZEN, CHOPPED 1 CUP	205	45	0.80	2.54	6
662	SPINACH, COOKED, DRAINED FROM FROZEN, LEAF. 1 CUP	190	45	1.00	3.17	7
664	SUMMER SQUASH, COOKED, DICED, DRAINED 1 CUP	210	30	1.70	8.10	12

HANDBOOK NUMBER	FOOD NAME SERVING SIZE DESCRIPTION	GRAMS	KCAL	NIACIN MG	INQ	%RDA
721	VEGETARIAN SOUP PREPARED WITH EQUAL VOLUME OF WATER, CANNED . . . . 1 CUP	245	80	1.00	1.79	7
730	BREWER'S YEAST, DRY . . . . . 1 TBSP	8	25	3.00	17.14	21
665	WINTER SQUASH, BAKED, MASHED . . . . 1 CUP	205	130	1.40	1.54	10
671	TOMATOES, RAW . . . . . 1 TOMATO 2 3/5-IN DIAM	135	25	0.90	5.14	6
672	TOMATOES, CANNED,SOLIDS AND LIQUIDS . . . . 1 CUP	241	50	1.70	4.86	12
675	TOMATO JUICE, CANNED . . . . . 1 CUP	243	45	1.90	6.03	14
676	TOMATO JUICE, CANNED . . . . . 1 GLASS 6 FL OZ	182	35	1.50	6.12	11
678	TURNIP GREENS, COOKED, DRAINED, FROM RAW (LEAVES AND STEMS) . . 1 CUP	145	30	0.70	3.33	5
679	TURNIP GREENS, COOKED, DRAINED, FROM FROZEN,CHOPPED . . . . 1 CUP	165	40	0.70	2.50	5
680	VEGETABLES, MIXED, FROZEN, COOKED, DRAINED. . . . . 1 CUP	182	115	2.00	2.48	14
686	BEER . . . . . 12 FL OZ	360	150	2.20	2.10	16
712	BEEF BROTH, BOUILLON, CONSOMME. . . . . 1 CUP	240	30	1.20	5.71	9
713	BEEF NOODLE SOUP, PREPARED WITH EQUAL VOLUME OF WATER,CANNED. . . 1 CUP	240	65	1.00	2.20	7
714	CLAM CHOWDER, MANHATTEN TYPE WITH TOMATOES AND WITH OUT MILK. . . 1 CUP	245	80	1.00	1.79	7
719	TOMATO SOUP PREPARED WITH EQUAL VOLUME OF WATER, CANNED . . . . 1 CUP	245	90	1.20	1.90	9
720	VEGETABLE BEEF SOUP PREPARED WITH EQUAL VOLUME OF WATER, CANNED . . 1 CUP	245	80	1.00	1.79	7

IRON   IRON   IRON   IRON   IRON   IRON   IRON   IRON

IRON   IRON   IRON   IRON   IRON   IRON   IRON   IRON

FOODS WHICH PROVIDE A HIGH CONCENTRATION OF IRON RELATIVE TO CALORIES

(INQ AT LEAST 1.5)

AND AT LEAST 5 PERCENT OF THE RDA PER SERVING

(RDA FOR IRON = 18.0 MG)

*INDICATES FOODS WHICH PROVIDE AT LEAST 25 PERCENT OF THE RDA PER SERVING

**INDICATES FOODS WHICH PROVIDE AT LEAST 50 PERCENT OF THE RDA PER SERVING

HANDBOOK NUMBER	FOOD NAME / SERVING SIZE DESCRIPTION	GRAMS	KCAL	IRON MG	INQ	%RDA
100	EGG, HARD-COOKED (LARGE), WITHOUT SHELL / 1 EGG	50	80	1.00	1.56	6
101	EGG, POACHED (LARGE) / 1 EGG	50	80	1.00	1.56	6
146	*CLAMS, RAW, MEAT ONLY / 3 OZ	85	65	5.20	10.00	33 *
147	CLAMS, CANNED, SOLIDS AND LIQUIDS / 3 OZ	85	45	3.50	9.72	22
152	**OYSTERS, RAW, MEAT ONLY / 1 CUP, 13-19 MEDIUM SELECTS	240	160	13.20	10.31	83 **
154	SARDINES, ATLANTIC, CANNED IN OIL, DRAINED SOLIDS / 3 OZ	85	175	2.50	1.79	16
155	SCALLOPS, FROZEN, BREADED, FRIED, REHEATED / 6 SCALLOPS	90	175	3.20	2.29	20
157	SHRIMP, CANNED / 3 OZ	85	100	2.60	3.25	16
163	BEEF CUTS COOKED, LEAN ONLY / 2.5 OZ	72	140	2.70	2.41	17
164	GROUND BEEF, BROILED, LEAN WITH 10% FAT / 3 OZ OR 3 BY 5/8 IN PATTY	85	185	3.00	2.03	19
167	ROAST BEEF, OVEN COOKED, LEAN ONLY / 1.8 OZ	51	125	1.80	1.80	11
168	ROAST BEEF, OVEN COOKED, RELATIVELY LEAN, LEAN AND FAT / 3 OZ	85	165	3.20	2.42	20
169	ROAST BEEF, OVEN COOKED, RELATIVELY LEAN, LEAN ONLY / 2.8 OZ	78	125	3.00	3.00	19
171	STEAK, SIRLOIN, BROILED, LEAN ONLY, BONE REMOVED / 2 OZ	56	115	2.20	2.39	14
172	STEAK, ROUND, BRAISED, LEAN AND FAT, BONE REMOVED / 3 OZ	85	220	3.00	1.70	19
173	STEAK, ROUND, BRAISED, LEAN ONLY, BONE REMOVED / 2.4 OZ	68	130	2.50	2.40	16
174	CORNED BEEF CANNED / 3 OZ	85	185	3.70	2.50	23
176	CHIPPED BEEF, DRIED / 2 1/2 OZ JAR	71	145	3.60	3.10	23
177	BEEF AND VEGETABLE STEW / 1 CUP	245	220	2.90	1.65	18
179	*CHILI CON CARNE WITH BEANS, CANNED / 1 CUP	255	340	4.30	1.58	27 *
180	*CHOP SUEY WITH BEEF AND PORK(HOME RECIPE) / 1 CUP	250	300	4.80	2.00	30 *
181	*HEART, BEEF, LEAN, BRAISED / 3 OZ	85	160	5.00	3.91	31 *
188	*LIVER, BEEF, FRIED / 3 OZ	85	195	7.50	4.61	47 *

HANDBOOK NUMBER	FOOD NAME SERVING SIZE DESCRIPTION	GRAMS	KCAL	IRON MG	INQ	%RDA
190	LUNCHEON MEAT, BOILED HAM, 1 OZ	28	65	0.80	1.54	5
193	PORK CHOP, BROILED, LEAN ONLY, BONE REMOVED, 2 OZ	56	150	2.20	1.83	14
195	PORK ROAST, OVEN COOKED, LEAN ONLY, 2.4 OZ	68	175	2.60	1.86	16
197	PORK SHOULDER, SIMMERED, LEAN ONLY, 2.2 OZ	63	135	2.30	2.13	14
199	BRAUNSCHWEIGER, 1 SLICE, 2.2 OZ	28	90	1.70	2.36	11
208	VEAL CUTLET, BRAISED OR BROILED, BONE REMOVED, 3 OZ	85	185	2.70	1.82	17
209	VEAL RIB, ROASTED, BONE REMOVED, 3 OZ	85	230	2.90	1.58	18
212	CHICKEN, HALF BROILER, BONES REMOVED, 6.2 OZ	176	240	3.00	1.56	19
216	CHICKEN CHOW MEIN, CANNED, 1 CUP	250	95	1.30	1.71	8
225	APPLEJUICE, BOTTLED OR CANNED, 1 CUP	248	120	1.50	1.56	9
227	APPLESAUCE, UNSWEETENED, 1 CUP	244	100	1.20	1.50	7
230	*APRICOTS,DRIED, UNCOOKED, 1 CUP=28 LARGE OR 37 MEDIUM HALVES	130	340	7.20	2.65	45 *
231	*APRICOTS, DRIED, COOKED, UNSWEETENED, 1 CUP—FRUIT AND LIQUID	250	215	4.50	2.62	28 *
237	BLACKBERRIES, RAW, 1 CUP	144	85	1.30	1.91	8
238	BLUEBERRIES, RAW, 1 CUP	145	90	1.50	2.08	9
271	CANTALOUP, WT WITHOUT RIND AND SEEDS, 1/2 OF A 5-IN DIAM. MELON	272	80	1.10	1.72	7
284	PEACHES, RAW, SLICED, 1 CUP	170	65	0.90	1.73	6
287	**PEACHES, DRIED, UNCOOKED, 1 CUP	160	420	9.60	2.86	60 **
288	*PEACHES, DRIED, COOKED, UNSWEETENED, 1 CUP (HALVES AND JUICE)	250	205	4.80	2.93	30 *
304	PRUNES, DRIED, "SOFTENIZED," WITH PITS, UNCOOKED, 4 EXTRA LARGE OR 5 LARGE PRUNES	49	110	1.70	1.93	11
305	PRUNES, DRIED, "SOFTENIZED," WITH PITS, COOKED, UNSWEETENED, 1 CUP (FRUIT AND LIQUID)	250	255	3.80	1.86	24
309	RASPBERRIES, RED, RAW, WHOLE, 1 CUP	123	70	1.10	1.96	7
313	STRAWBERRIES, RAW, WHOLE, CAPPED, 1 CUP	149	55	1.50	3.41	9

HANDBOOK NUMBER	FOOD NAME / SERVING SIZE DESCRIPTION	GRAMS	KCAL	IRON MG	INQ	%RDA
318	WATERMELON, WT WITHOUT RIND AND SEEDS / 1/16 OF 33 LB MELON	426	110	2.10	2.59	13
358	WHOLE-WHEAT BREAD, SOFT-CRUMB TYPE / 1 SLICE (16 PER 1 LB LOAF)	28	65	0.80	1.54	5
369	*BRAN FLAKES (40% BRAN), ADDED SUGAR, SALT, IRON AND VITAMINS. / 1 CUP	35	105	5.60	6.67	35 *
370	*BRAN FLAKES WITH RAISINS, ADDED SUGAR, SALT, IRON AND VITAMINS / 1 CUP	50	145	6.90	5.95	43 *
373	PUFFED CORN, PLAIN, ADDED SUGAR, SALT, IRON, VITAMINS. / 1 CUP	20	80	2.30	3.59	14
375	PUFFED OATS, ADDED SUGAR, SALT, MINERALS, VITAMINS / 1 CUP	25	100	2.90	3.63	18
444	BRAN MUFFINS, HOME RECIPE. / 1 MUFFIN 2 3/8-IN DIAM.,, 1 1/2-IN HIGH	40	105	1.50	1.79	9
496	SPAGHETTI, ENRICHED, IN TOMATO SAUCE WITH CHEESE, CANNED / 1 CUP	250	190	2.80	1.84	18
498	SPAGHETTI, ENRICHED, WITH MEAT BALLS IN TOMATO SAUCE, CANNED. / 1 CUP	250	260	3.30	1.59	21
509	*DRY BEANS, GREAT NORTHERN COOKED, DRAINED / 1 CUP	180	210	4.90	2.92	31 *
510	*DRY BEANS, NAVY, COOKED, DRAINED / 1 CUP	190	225	5.10	2.83	32 *
511	*BEANS WITH FRANKFURTERS,CANNED. / 1 CUP	255	365	4.80	1.64	30 *
512	*PORK AND BEANS IN TOMATO SAUCE. / 1 CUP	255	310	4.60	1.85	29 *
513	*PORK AND BEANS IN SWEET SAUCE / 1 CUP	255	385	5.90	1.92	37 *
514	*RED KIDNEY BEANS, CANNED. / 1 CUP	255	230	4.60	2.50	29 *
515	*DRY LIMA BEANS, COOKED, DRAINED / 1 CUP	190	260	5.90	2.84	37 *
516	BLACKEYE PEAS,DRY,COOKED. / 1 CUP	250	190	3.30	2.17	21
522	*LENTILS, WHOLE, COOKED / 1 CUP	200	210	4.20	2.50	26 *
525	SPLIT PEAS, DRY,COOKED / 1 CUP	200	230	3.40	1.85	21
527	**PUMPKIN AND SQUASH SEEDS, DRY, HULLED / 1 CUP	140	775	15.70	2.53	98 **
528	**SUNFLOWER SEEDS, DRY, HULLED / 1 CUP	145	810	10.30	1.59	64 **
555	MOLASSES, LIGHT CANE / 1 TBSP.	20	50	0.90	2.25	6
556	BLACKSTRAP MOLASSES / 1 TBSP.	20	45	3.20	8.89	20

HANDBOOK NUMBER	FOOD NAME SERVING SIZE DESCRIPTION	GRAMS	KCAL	IRON MG	INQ	%RDA	
557	SORGHUM 1 TBSP	21	55	2.60	5.91	16	
558	TABLE BLEND SYRUPS (CHIEFLY CORN) LIGHT AND DARK. 1 TBSP	21	60	0.80	1.67	5	
564	ASPARAGUS, COOKED, DRAINED, FROM RAW 1 CUP (CUTS AND TIPS, 1 1/2 TO 2-IN LENGTHS)	145	30	0.90	3.75	6	
565	ASPARAGUS, COOKED, DRAINED, FROM FROZEN 1 CUP (CUTS AND TIPS, 1 1/2 TO 2-IN LENGTHS)	180	40	2.20	6.88	14	
568	ASPARAGUS, CANNED SPEARS. 4 SPEARS	80	15	1.50	12.50	9	
569	LIMA BEANS, (FORDHOOKS), FROZEN, COOKED, DRAINED 1 CUP	170	170	2.90	2.13	18	
570	*LIMA BEANS, (BABY LIMAS), FROZEN, COOKED, DRAINED. 1 CUP	180	210	4.70	2.80	29	*
571	GREEN SNAP BEANS, COOKED, DRAINED, FROM RAW 1 CUP	125	30	0.80	3.33	5	
572	GREEN SNAP BEANS, COOKED, DRAINED, CUTS FROM FROZEN 1 CUP	135	35	0.90	3.21	6	
573	GREEN SNAP BEANS, COOKED, DRAINED, FRENCH CUTS FROM FROZEN 1 CUP	130	35	1.20	4.29	7	
574	GREEN SNAP BEANS, CANNED, DRAINED SOLIDS (CUTS) 1 CUP	135	30	2.00	8.33	13	
575	YELLOW OR WAX BEANS, COOKED, DRAINED, FROM RAW 1 CUP	125	30	0.80	3.33	5	
576	YELLOW OR WAX BEANS, COOKED, DRAINED CUTS FROM FROZEN 1 CUP	135	35	0.90	3.21	6	
577	YELLOW OR WAX BEANS, CANNED, DRAINED SOLIDS (CUTS) 1 CUP	135	30	2.00	8.33	13	
578	BEAN SPROUTS, (MUNG), RAW 1 CUP	105	35	1.40	5.00	9	
579	BEAN SPROUTS, (MUNG), COOKED, DRAINED 1 CUP	125	35	1.10	3.93	7	
581	BEETS, COOKED DRAINED, DICED OR SLICED 1 CUP	170	55	0.90	2.05	6	
582	BEETS, CANNED, DRAINED SOLIDS, WHOLE SMALL BEETS. 1 CUP	160	60	1.10	2.29	7	
583	BEETS, CANNED, DRAINED SOLIDS, DICED OR SLICED 1 CUP	170	65	1.20	2.31	7	
584	BEET GREENS, COOKED, DRAINED CUP	145	25	2.80	14.00	18	
585	BLACKEYE PEAS, COOKED, DRAINED, FROM RAW 1 CUP	165	180	3.50	2.43	22	
586	*BLACKEYE PEAS, COOKED, DRAINED, FROM FROZEN 1 CUP	170	220	4.80	2.73	30	*
587	BROCCOLI, COOKED, DRAINED, FROM RAW 1 WHOLE MEDIUM STALK	187	45	1.40	3.89	9	

HANDBOOK NUMBER	FOOD NAME / SERVING SIZE DESCRIPTION	GRAMS	KCAL	IRON MG	INQ	%RDA
588	BROCCOLI, COOKED, DRAINED, FROM RAW. 1 CUP (STALKS CUT INTO 1/2-IN PIECES)	155	40	1.20	3.75	7
590	BROCCOLI, FROM FROZEN, CHOPPED, COOKED, DRAINED. 1 CUP	185	50	1.30	3.25	8
591	BRUSSELS SPROUTS, COOKED, DRAINED, FROM RAW. 7-8 SPROUTS (1 1/4 TO 1 1/2-IN DIAM) 1 CUP	155	55	1.70	3.86	11
592	BRUSSELS SPROUTS, COOKED, DRAINED, FROM FROZEN. 1 CUP	155	50	1.20	3.00	7
599	WHITE MUSTARD CABBAGE, COOKED, DRAINED	170	25	1.00	5.00	6
601	CARROTS, RAW, PEELED, GRATED. 1 CUP	110	45	0.80	2.22	5
602	CARROTS (CROSSWISE CUTS) COOKED, DRAINED. 1 CUP	155	50	0.90	2.25	6
603	CARROTS, CANNED, SLICED, DRAINED SOLIDS. 1 CUP	155	45	1.10	3.06	7
605	CAULIFLOWER, RAW, CHOPPED. 1 CUP	115	31	1.30	5.24	8
606	CAULIFLOWER, COOKED, DRAINED FROM RAW. 1 CUP	125	30	0.90	3.75	6
607	CAULIFLOWER, COOKED, DRAINED FROM FROZEN. 1 CUP	180	30	0.90	3.75	6
610	COLLARDS, COOKED, DRAINED, FROM RAW. 1 CUP	190	65	1.50	2.88	9
611	COLLARDS, COOKED DRAINED, FROM FROZEN. 1 CUP	170	50	1.70	4.25	11
620	DANDELION GREENS, COOKED, DRAINED. 1 CUP	105	35	1.90	6.79	12
621	ENDIVE, CURLY, RAW SMALL PIECES. 1 CUP	50	10	0.90	11.25	6
622	KALE, COOKED, DRAINED, FROM RAW, LEAVES WITHOUT STEMS. 1 CUP	110	45	1.80	5.00	11
623	KALE, COOKED, DRAINED, FROM FROZEN, LEAF STYLE. 1 CUP	130	40	1.30	4.06	8
624	BUTTERHEAD LETTUCE, RAW. 1 HEAD, 5-IN DIAM.	220	25	3.30	16.50	21
626	ICEBERG LETTUCE (CRISPHEAD). 1 HEAD, 6-IN DIAM	567	70	2.70	4.82	17
629	LOOSELEAF LETTUCE, CHOPPED OR SHREDDED. 1 CUP	55	10	0.80	10.00	5
631	MUSTARD GREENS, COOKED, DRAINED, WITHOUT STEMS. 1 CUP	140	30	2.50	10.42	16
633	ONIONS, MATURE, RAW, CHOPPED. 1 CUP	170	65	0.90	1.73	6
635	ONIONS, MATURE, COOKED, DRAINED, WHOLE OR SLICED. 1 CUP	210	60	0.80	1.67	5

HANDBOOK NUMBER	FOOD NAME / SERVING SIZE DESCRIPTION	GRAMS	KCAL	IRON MG	INQ	%RDA
639	GREEN PEAS, CANNED, DRAINED SOLIDS / 1 CUP	170	150	3.20	2.67	20
641	GREEN PEAS, FROZEN, COOKED, DRAINED / 1 CUP	160	110	3.00	3.41	19
656	PUMPKIN, CANNED / 1 CUP	245	80	1.00	1.56	6
658	SAUERKRAUT, CANNED, SOLIDS AND LIQUIDS / 1 CUP	235	40	1.20	3.75	7
659	SPINACH, RAW, CHOPPED / 1 CUP	55	15	1.70	14.17	11
660	*SPINACH, COOKED, DRAINED FROM RAW / 1 CUP	180	40	4.00	12.50	25 *
661	*SPINACH, COOKED, DRAINED FROM FROZEN, CHOPPED / 1 CUP	205	45	4.30	11.94	27 *
662	*SPINACH, COOKED, DRAINED FROM FROZEN, LEAF / 1 CUP	190	45	4.80	13.33	30 *
663	*SPINACH, CANNED, DRAINED SOLIDS / 1 CUP	205	50	5.30	13.25	33 *
664	SUMMER SQUASH, COOKED, DICED, DRAINED / 1 CUP	210	30	0.80	3.33	5
665	WINTER SQUASH, BAKED, MASHED / 1 CUP	205	130	1.60	1.54	10
672	TOMATOES, CANNED, SOLIDS AND LIQUIDS / 1 CUP	241	50	1.20	3.00	7
675	TOMATO JUICE, CANNED / 1 CUP	243	45	2.20	6.11	14
676	TOMATO JUICE, CANNED / 1 GLASS 6 FL OZ	182	35	1.60	5.71	10
678	TURNIP GREENS, COOKED, DRAINED, FROM RAW (LEAVES AND STEMS) / 1 CUP	145	30	1.50	6.25	9
679	TURNIP GREENS, COOKED, DRAINED, FROM FROZEN, CHOPPED / 1 CUP	165	40	2.60	8.13	16
680	VEGETABLES, MIXED, FROZEN, COOKED, DRAINED / 1 CUP	182	115	2.40	2.61	15
697	BITTER SWEET OR BAKING CHOCOLATE / 1 OZ	28	145	1.90	1.64	12
711	BEAN WITH PORK SOUP PREPARED WITH EQUAL VOLUME OF WATER, CANNED / 1 CUP	250	170	2.30	1.69	14
713	BEEF NOODLE SOUP, PREPARED WITH EQUAL VOLUME OF WATER, CANNED / 1 CUP	240	65	1.00	1.92	6
714	CLAM CHOWDER, MANHATTEN TYPE WITH TOMATOES AND WITH OUT MILK / 1 CUP	245	80	1.00	1.56	6
721	VEGETARIAN SOUP PREPARED WITH EQUAL VOLUME OF WATER, CANNED / 1 CUP	245	80	1.00	1.56	6
730	BREWER'S YEAST, DRY / 1 TBSP	8	25	1.40	7.00	9

CALCIUM CALCIUM CALCIUM CALCIUM CALCIUM CALCIUM CALCIUM CALCIUM CALCIUM CALCIUM

FOODS WHICH PROVIDE A HIGH CONCENTRATION OF CALCIUM RELATIVE TO CALORIES

(INQ AT LEAST 1.5)

AND AT LEAST 5 PERCENT OF THE RDA PER SERVING

(RDA FOR CALCIUM = 900.0 MG)

CALCIUM CALCIUM CALCIUM CALCIUM CALCIUM CALCIUM CALCIUM CALCIUM

*INDICATES FOODS WHICH PROVIDE AT LEAST 25 PERCENT OF THE RDA PER SERVING

**INDICATES FOODS WHICH PROVIDE AT LEAST 50 PERCENT OF THE RDA PER SERVING

HANDBOOK FOOD NAME NUMBER	SERVING SIZE DESCRIPTION	GRAMS	KCAL	CALCIUM MG	INQ	XRDA
1	BLUE CHEESE, 1 OZ	28	100	150.00	3.33	17
2	CAMEMBERT CHEESE, 1 WEDGE	38	115	147.00	2.84	16
3	CHEDDAR CHEESE, 1 OZ	28	115	204.00	3.94	23
4	CHEDDAR CHEESE, 1 CUBIC INCH	17	70	124.00	3.94	14
8	COTTAGE CHEESE, 2X FAT, 1 CUP	226	205	155.00	1.68	17
9	COTTAGE CHEESE, 1X FAT, 1 CUP	226	165	138.00	1.86	15
12	MOZZARELLA CHEESE, MADE WITH WHOLE MILK, 1 OZ	28	90	163.00	4.02	18
13	MOZZARELLA CHEESE, MADE WITH SKIM MILK, 1 OZ	28	80	207.00	5.75	23
15	PARMESAN CHEESE, GRATED, 1 TBSP	5	25	69.00	6.13	8
16	*PARMESAN CHEESE, GRATED, 1 OZ	28	130	390.00	6.67	43 *
17	PROVOLONE CHEESE, 1 OZ	28	100	214.00	4.76	24
18	**RICOTTA CHEESE, MADE WITH WHOLE MILK, 1 CUP	246	428	509.00	2.64	57 **
19	**RICOTTA CHEESE, MADE WITH PART SKIM MILK, 1 CUP	246	340	669.00	4.37	74 **
20	*ROMANO CHEESE, 1 OZ	28	110	302.00	6.10	34 *
21	*SWISS CHEESE, 1 OZ	28	105	272.00	5.76	30 *
22	AMERICAN PASTEURIZED PROCESS CHEESE, 1 OZ	28	105	174.00	3.68	19
23	SWISS PASTEURIZED PROCESS CHEESE, 1 OZ	28	95	219.00	5.12	24
24	AMERICAN PASTEURIZED PROCESS CHEESE FOOD, 1 OZ	28	95	163.00	3.81	18
25	AMERICAN PASTEURIZED PROCESS CHEESE SPREAD, 1 OZ	28	82	159.00	4.31	18
50	*MILK, FLUID WHOLE (3.3% FAT), 1 CUP	244	150	291.00	4.31	32 *
51	*MILK, FLUID LOWFAT (2% FAT), NO MILK SOLIDS ADDED, 1 CUP	244	120	297.00	5.50	33 *
52	*MILK, FLUID LOWFAT (2% FAT), LESS THAN 10 GRAMS OF PROTEIN PER CUP, 1 CUP	245	125	313.00	5.56	35 *
53	*MILK, FLUID LOWFAT (2% FAT), MORE THAN 10 GRAMS OF PROTEIN PER CUP, 1 CUP	246	135	352.00	5.79	39 *

HANDBOOK NUMBER	FOOD NAME SERVING SIZE DESCRIPTION	GRAMS	KCAL	CALCIUM MG	INQ	%RDA
54	*MILK, FLUID LOWFAT (1% FAT), NO MILK SOLIDS ADDED • • • 1 CUP	244	100	300.00	6.67	33 *
55	*MILK, FLUID LOWFAT (1% FAT), LESS THAN 10 GRAMS OF PROTEIN PER CUP. • • 1 CUP	245	105	313.00	6.62	35 *
56	*MILK, FLUID LOWFAT (1% FAT), MORE THAN 10 GRAMS OF PROTEIN PER CUP. • • 1 CUP	246	120	349.00	6.46	39 *
57	*MILK, FLUID NONFAT (SKIM), NO MILK SOLIDS ADDED • • • 1 CUP	245	85	302.00	7.90	34 *
58	*MILK, FLUID NONFAT (SKIM), LESS THAN 10 GRAMS OF PROTEIN PER CUP • • • 1 CUP	245	90	316.00	7.80	35 *
59	*MILK, FLUID NONFAT (SKIM), MORE THAN 10 GRAMS OF PROTEIN PER CUP • • • 1 CUP	246	100	352.00	7.82	39 *
60	*BUTTERMILK, FLUID • • • • 1 CUP	245	100	285.00	6.33	32 *
67	*CHOCOLATE MILK (COMMERCIAL) • • • • 1 CUP	250	210	280.00	2.96	31 *
68	*CHOCOLATE MILK, LOWFAT (2%)(COMMERICIAL) • • • • 1 CUP	250	180	284.00	3.51	32 *
69	*CHOCOLATE MILK, LOWFAT (1%)(COMMERCIAL) • • • • 1 CUP	250	160	287.00	3.99	32 *
70	*EGGNOG (COMMERCIAL) • • • • 1 CUP	254	340	330.00	2.16	37 *
71	*CHOCOLATE MALTED MILK (1 CUP WHOLE MILK AND 3/4 OZ MALTED MILK POWDER) 1 CUP PLUS POWDER	265	235	304.00	2.87	34 *
72	*NATURAL MALTED MILK (1CUP WHOLE MILK AND 3/4 OZ MALTED MILK POWDER) 1 CUP PLUS POWDER	265	235	347.00	3.28	39 *
73	*CHOCOLATE MILK SHAKE • • • • 10.6 OZ, NET WT.	300	355	396.00	2.48	44 *
74	**VANILLA MILK SHAKE. • • • • 11 OZ, NET WT.	313	350	457.00	2.90	51 **
82	ICE MILK, HARDENED (4.3% FAT) • • • • 1 CUP	131	185	176.00	2.11	20
83	*ICE MILK, SOFT SERVE (2.6% FAT) • • • • 1 CUP	175	225	274.00	2.71	30 *
86	*CUSTARD, BAKED • • • • 1 CUP	265	305	297.00	2.16	33 *
88	*VANILLA PUDDING (BLANCMANGE), HOME RECIPE, STARCH BASE. • • • 1 CUP	255	285	298.00	2.32	33 *
89	TAPIOCA CREAM PUDDING, HOME RECIPE • • • • 1 CUP	165	220	173.00	1.75	19
90	*CHOCOLATE PUDDING, COOKED FROM A MIX. • • • • 1 CUP	260	320	265.00	1.84	29 *
91	*CHOCOLATE PUDDING, INSTANT • • • • 1 CUP	260	325	374.00	2.56	42 *
92	*FRUIT-FLAVORED YOGURT MADE WITH LOWFAT MILK, WITH ADDED MILK SOLIDS 8 OZ, NET WT.	227	230	343.00	3.31	38 *

HANDBOOK NUMBER	FOOD NAME / SERVING SIZE DESCRIPTION	GRAMS	KCAL	CALCIUM MG	INQ	%RDA
93	*PLAIN YOGURT MADE WITH LOWFAT MILK, WITH ADDED MILK SOLIDS, 8 OZ, NET WT.	227	145	415.00	6.36	46 *
94	**PLAIN YOGURT MADE WITH NONFAT MILK, WITH ADDED MILK SOLIDS, 8 OZ, NET WT.	227	125	452.00	8.04	50 **
95	*PLAIN YOGURT MADE WITH WHOLE MILK, WITHOUT ADDED MILK SOLIDS, 8 OZ, NET WT.	227	140	274.00	4.35	30 *
146	CLAMS, RAW, MEAT ONLY, 3 OZ	85	65	59.00	2.02	7
147	CLAMS, CANNED, SOLIDS AND LIQUIDS, 3 OZ	85	45	47.00	2.32	5
152	*OYSTERS, RAW, MEAT ONLY, 1 CUP, 13-19 MEDIUM SELECTS	240	160	226.00	3.14	25 *
153	SALMON, PINK, CANNED, SOLIDS AND LIQUIDS, 3 OZ	85	120	167.00	3.09	19
154	*SARDINES, ATLANTIC, CANNED IN OIL, DRAINED SOLIDS, 3 OZ	85	175	372.00	4.72	41 *
157	SHRIMP, CANNED, 3 OZ	85	100	98.00	2.18	11
273	ORANGE, RAW, WT WITHOUT PEEL AND SEEDS, 1--2 5/8-IN DIAM.	131	65	54.00	1.85	6
274	ORANGE SECTIONS WITHOUT MEMBRANES, RAW, 1 CUP	180	90	74.00	1.83	8
365	FARINA, QUICK-COOKING, ENRICHED, COOKED, 1 CUP	245	105	147.00	3.11	16
441	MACARONI (ENRICHED) AND CHEESE, CANNED, 1 CUP	240	230	199.00	1.92	22
442	*MACARONI (ENRICHED) AND CHEESE, HOME RECIPE, 1 CUP	200	430	362.00	1.87	40 *
447	CORN MUFFIN MIX, EGG, MILK, 1 MUFFIN, 2 3/8-IN DIAM., 1 1/2 IN HIGH	40	130	96.00	1.64	11
450	BUCKWHEAT PANCAKES MADE FROM MIX, 1 CAKE 4-IN DIAM	27	55	59.00	2.38	7
452	PANCAKE MADE FROM MIX, 1 CAKE 4-IN DIAM	27	60	58.00	2.15	6
501	WAFFLES FROM MIX, EGG AND MILK ADDED, 1 WAFFLE 7-IN. DIAM	75	205	179.00	1.94	20
505	*SELF-RISING FLOUR, ENRICHED, UNSIFTED, SPOONED, 1 CUP	125	440	331.00	1.67	37 *
546	CHOCOLATE FLAVORED BEVERAGE POWDER WITH NONFAT DRY MILK, 1 OZ (4 HEAPING TSP)	28	100	167.00	3.71	19
556	BLACKSTRAP MOLASSES, 1 TBSP.	20	45	137.00	6.77	15
571	GREEN SNAP BEANS, COOKED, DRAINED, FROM RAW, 1 CUP	125	30	63.00	4.67	7
572	GREEN SNAP BEANS, COOKED, DRAINED, CUTS FROM FROZEN, 1 CUP	135	35	54.00	3.43	6

HANDBOOK NUMBER	FOOD NAME SERVING SIZE DESCRIPTION	GRAMS	KCAL	CALCIUM MG	INQ	XRDA
573	GREEN SNAP BEANS, COOKED, DRAINED,FRENCH CUTS FROM FROZEN 1 CUP	130	35	49.00	3.11	5
574	GREEN SNAP BEANS, CANNED, DRAINED SOLIDS (CUTS) 1 CUP	135	30	61.00	4.52	7
575	YELLOW OR WAX BEANS, COOKED, DRAINED, FROM RAW 1 CUP	125	30	63.00	4.67	7
576	YELLOW OR WAX BEANS, COOKED, DRAINED CUTS FROM FROZEN 1 CUP	135	35	47.00	2.98	5
577	YELLOW OR WAX BEANS, CANNED, DRAINED SOLIDS (CUTS) 1 CUP	135	30	61.00	4.52	7
584	BEET GREENS, COOKED, DRAINED 1 CUP	145	25	144.00	12.80	16
587	BROCCOLI, COOKED, DRAINED, FROM RAW 1 WHOLE MEDIUM STALK	187	45	158.00	7.80	18
588	BROCCOLI, COOKED, DRAINED, FROM RAW 1 CUP (STALKS CUT INTO 1/2-IN PIECES)	155	40	136.00	7.56	15
590	BROCCOLI, FROM FROZEN, CHOPPED, COOKED, DRAINED 1 CUP	185	50	100.00	4.44	11
591	BRUSSELS SPROUTS, COOKED, DRAINED, FROM RAW 7-8 SPROUTS (1 1/4 TO 1 1/2-IN DIAM) 1 CUP	155	55	50.00	2.02	6
595	CABBAGE, COOKED, DRAINED 1 CUP	145	30	64.00	4.74	7
597	SAVOY CABBAGE, RAW, COARSELY SHREDDED 1 CUP	70	15	47.00	6.96	5
599	*WHITE MUSTARD CABBAGE, COOKED, DRAINED 1 CUP	170	25	252.00	22.40	28 *
602	CARROTS (CROSSWISE CUTS) COOKED, DRAINED 1 CUP	155	50	51.00	2.27	6
603	CARROTS, CANNED, SLICED, DRAINED SOLIDS 1 CUP	155	45	47.00	2.32	5
609	CELERY, RAW DICED 1 CUP	120	20	47.00	5.22	5
610	*COLLARDS, COOKED, DRAINED, FROM RAW 1 CUP	190	65	357.00	12.21	40 *
611	*COLLARDS, COOKED DRAINED, FROM FROZEN 1 CUP	170	50	299.00	13.29	33 *
620	DANDELION GREENS, COOKED, DRAINED 1 CUP	105	35	147.00	9.33	16
622	KALE, COOKED, DRAINED, FROM RAW, LEAVES WITHOUT STEMS 1 CUP	110	45	206.00	10.17	23
623	KALE, COOKED, DRAINED, FROM FROZEN, LEAF STYLE 1 CUP	130	40	157.00	8.72	17
624	BUTTERHEAD LETTUCE, RAW 1 HEAD,5-IN DIAM.	220	25	57.00	5.07	6
626	ICEBERG LETTUCE (CRISPHEAD) 1 HEAD, 6-IN DIAM	567	70	108.00	3.43	12

HANDBOOK NUMBER	FOOD NAME SERVING SIZE DESCRIPTION	GRAMS	KCAL	CALCIUM MG	INQ	%RDA
631	MUSTARD GREENS, COOKED, DRAINED, WITHOUT STEMS 1 CUP	140	30	193.00	14.30	21
632	OKRA PODS, COOKED 10 PODS 3 BY 5/8 IN	106	30	98.00	7.26	11
633	ONIONS, MATURE, RAW, CHOPPED 1 CUP	170	65	46.00	1.57	5
635	ONIONS, MATURE, COOKED, DRAINED, WHOLE OR SLICED 1 CUP	210	60	50.00	1.85	6
638	PARSNIPS, COOKED, DICED 1 CUP	155	100	70.00	1.56	8
656	PUMPKIN, CANNED 1 CUP	245	80	61.00	1.69	7
658	SAUERKRAUT, CANNED, SOLIDS AND LIQUIDS 1 CUP	235	40	85.00	4.72	9
659	SPINACH, RAW, CHOPPED 1 CUP	55	15	51.00	7.56	6
660	SPINACH, COOKED, DRAINED FROM RAW 1 CUP	180	40	167.00	9.28	19
661	*SPINACH, COOKED, DRAINED FROM FROZEN, CHOPPED 1 CUP	205	45	232.00	11.46	26 *
662	SPINACH, COOKED, DRAINED FROM FROZEN, LEAF 1 CUP	190	45	200.00	9.88	22
663	*SPINACH, CANNED, DRAINED SOLIDS 1 CUP	205	50	242.00	10.76	27 *
664	SUMMER SQUASH, COOKED, DICED, DRAINED 1 CUP	210	30	53.00	3.93	6
677	TURNIPS, COOKED, DICED 1 CUP	155	35	54.00	3.43	6
678	*TURNIP GREENS, COOKED, DRAINED, FROM RAW (LEAVES AND STEMS) 1 CUP	145	30	252.00	18.67	28 *
679	TURNIP GREENS, COOKED, DRAINED, FROM FROZEN, CHOPPED 1 CUP	165	40	195.00	10.83	22
708	CREAM OF CHICKEN SOUP PREPARED WITH EQUAL VOLUME OF MILK, CANNED 1 CUP	245	180	172.00	2.12	19
709	CREAM OF MUSHROOM SOUP PREPARED WITH EQUAL VOLUME OF MILK, CANNED 1 CUP	245	215	191.00	1.97	21
710	TOMATO SOUP PREPARED WITH EQUAL VOLUME OF MILK, CANNED 1 CUP	250	175	168.00	2.13	19

PHOSPHRUS PHOSPHRUS PHOSPHRUS PHOSPHRUS PHOSPHRUS PHOSPHRUS PHOSPHRUS PHOSPHRUS PHOSPHRUS PHOSPHRUS PHOSPHRUS

FOODS WHICH PROVIDE A HIGH CONCENTRATION OF PHOSPHRUS RELATIVE TO CALORIES

(INQ AT LEAST 1.5)

AND AT LEAST 5 PERCENT OF THE RDA PER SERVING

(RDA FOR PHOSPHRUS = 900.0 MG)

PHOSPHRUS PHOSPHRUS PHOSPHRUS PHOSPHRUS PHOSPHRUS PHOSPHRUS PHOSPHRUS PHOSPHRUS PHOSPHRUS PHOSPHRUS PHOSPHRUS

*INDICATES FOODS WHICH PROVIDE AT LEAST 25 PERCENT OF THE RDA PER SERVING

**INDICATES FOODS WHICH PROVIDE AT LEAST 50 PERCENT OF THE RDA PER SERVING

HANDBOOK NUMBER	FOOD NAME SERVING SIZE DESCRIPTION	GRAMS	KCAL	PHOSPHRUS MG	INQ	SRDA
1	BLUE CHEESE . . . . . 1 OZ	28	100	110.00	2.44	12
2	CAMEMBERT CHEESE . . . . 1 WEDGE	38	115	132.00	2.55	15
3	CHEDDAR CHEESE . . . . 1 OZ	28	115	145.00	2.80	16
4	CHEDDAR CHEESE . . . . 1 CUBIC INCH	17	70	86.00	2.79	10
6	*COTTAGE CHEESE, CREAMED (4% FAT), LG CURD . . . 1 CUP	225	235	297.00	2.81	33 *
7	*COTTAGE CHEESE, CREAMED (4% FAT), SM CURD . . . 1 CUP	210	220	277.00	2.80	31 *
8	*COTTAGE CHEESE, 2% FAT . . . . 1 CUP	226	205	340.00	3.69	38 *
9	*COTTAGE CHEESE, 1% FAT . . . . 1 CUP	226	165	302.00	4.07	34 *
10	COTTAGE CHEESE, UNCREAMED (LESS THAN 0.5% FAT) . . 1 CUP	145	125	151.00	2.68	17
12	MOZZARELLA CHEESE, MADE WITH WHOLE MILK . . 1 OZ	28	90	117.00	2.89	13
13	MOZZARELLA CHEESE, MADE WITH SKIM MILK . . 1 OZ	28	80	149.00	4.14	17
16	*PARMESAN CHEESE, GRATED . . . . 1 OZ	28	130	229.00	3.91	25 *
17	PROVOLONE CHEESE . . . . . 1 OZ	28	100	141.00	3.13	16
18	*RICOTTA CHEESE, MADE WITH WHOLE MILK. . . . 1 CUP	246	428	389.00	2.02	43 *
19	*RICOTTA CHEESE, MADE WITH PART SKIM MILK . . 1 CUP	246	340	449.00	2.93	50 *
20	ROMANO CHEESE . . . . . 1 OZ	28	110	215.00	4.34	24
21	SWISS CHEESE. . . . . . 1 OZ	28	105	171.00	3.62	19
22	AMERICAN PASTEURIZED PROCESS CHEESE . . . 1 OZ	28	105	211.00	4.47	23
23	SWISS PASTEURIZED PROCESS CHEESE . . . 1 OZ	28	95	216.00	5.05	24
24	AMERICAN PASTEURIZED PROCESS CHEESE FOOD . . 1 OZ	28	95	130.00	3.04	14
25	AMERICAN PASTEURIZED PROCESS CHEESE SPREAD. . . 1 OZ	28	82	202.00	5.47	22
50	*MILK, FLUID WHOLE (3.3% FAT) . . . 1 CUP	244	150	228.00	3.38	25 *
51	*MILK, FLUID LOWFAT (2% FAT), NO MILK SOLIDS ADDED . 1 CUP	244	120	232.00	4.30	26 *

HANDBOOK NUMBER	FOOD NAME / SERVING SIZE DESCRIPTION	GRAMS	KCAL	PHOSPHRUS MG	INQ	%RDA	*
52	*MILK, FLUID LOWFAT (2% FAT), LESS THAN 10 GRAMS OF PROTEIN PER CUP. 1 CUP	245	125	245.00	4.36	27	*
53	*MILK, FLUID LOWFAT (2% FAT), MORE THAN 10 GRAMS OF PROTEIN PER CUP. 1 CUP	246	135	276.00	4.54	31	*
54	*MILK, FLUID LOWFAT (1% FAT), NO MILK SOLIDS ADDED. 1 CUP	244	100	235.00	5.22	26	*
55	*MILK, FLUID LOWFAT (1% FAT), LESS THAN 10 GRAMS OF PROTEIN PER CUP. 1 CUP	245	105	245.00	5.19	27	*
56	*MILK, FLUID LOWFAT (1% FAT), MORE THAN 10 GRAMS OF PROTEIN PER CUP. 1 CUP	246	120	273.00	5.06	30	*
57	*MILK, FLUID NONFAT (SKIM), NO MILK SOLIDS ADDED. 1 CUP	245	85	247.00	6.46	27	*
58	*MILK, FLUID NONFAT (SKIM), LESS THAN 10 GRAMS OF PROTEIN PER CUP. 1 CUP	245	90	255.00	6.30	28	*
59	*MILK, FLUID NONFAT (SKIM), MORE THAN 10 GRAMS OF PROTEIN PER CUP. 1 CUP	246	100	275.00	6.11	31	*
60	BUTTERMILK, FLUID. 1 CUP	245	100	219.00	4.87	24	*
67	*CHOCOLATE MILK (COMMERCIAL). 1 CUP	250	210	251.00	2.66	28	*
68	*CHOCOLATE MILK, LOWFAT (2%)(COMMERCIAL). 1 CUP	250	180	254.00	3.14	28	*
69	*CHOCOLATE MILK, LOWFAT (1%)(COMMERCIAL). 1 CUP	250	160	257.00	3.57	29	*
70	*EGGNOG (COMMERCIAL). 1 CUP	254	340	278.00	1.82	31	*
71	*CHOCOLATE MALTED MILK (1 CUP WHOLE MILK AND 3/4 OZ MALTED MILK POWDER). 1 CUP PLUS POWDER	265	235	265.00	2.51	29	*
72	*NATURAL MALTED MILK (1CUP WHOLE MILK AND 3/4 OZ MALTED MILK POWDER). 1 CUP PLUS POWDER	265	235	307.00	2.90	34	*
73	*CHOCOLATE MILK SHAKE. 10.6 OZ, NET WT.	300	355	378.00	2.37	42	*
74	*VANILLA MILK SHAKE. 11 OZ, NET WT.	313	350	361.00	2.29	40	*
82	ICE MILK, HARDENED (4.3% FAT). 1 CUP	131	185	129.00	1.55	14	*
83	ICE MILK, SOFT SERVE (2.6% FAT). 1 CUP	175	225	202.00	2.00	22	*
86	*CUSTARD, BAKED. 1 CUP	265	305	310.00	2.26	34	*
88	*VANILLA PUDDING (BLANCMANGE), HOME RECIPE, STARCH BASE. 1 CUP	255	285	232.00	1.81	26	*
89	TAPIOCA CREAM PUDDING, HOME RECIPE. 1 CUP	165	220	180.00	1.82	20	*
90	*CHOCOLATE PUDDING, COOKED FROM A MIX. 1 CUP	260	320	247.00	1.72	27	*

HANDBOOK NUMBER	FOOD NAME SERVING SIZE DESCRIPTION	GRAMS	KCAL	PHOSPHRUS MG	INQ	%RDA
91	*CHOCOLATE PUDDING, INSTANT 1 CUP	260	325	237.00	1.62	26 *
92	*FRUIT-FLAVORED YOGURT MADE WITH LOWFAT MILK, WITH ADDED MILK SOLIDS 8 OZ, NET WT.	227	230	269.00	2.60	30 *
93	*PLAIN YOGURT MADE WITH LOWFAT MILK, WITH ADDED MILK SOLIDS 8 OZ, NET WT.	227	145	326.00	5.00	36 *
94	*PLAIN YOGURT MADE WITH NONFAT MILK, WITH ADDED MILK SOLIDS 8 OZ, NET WT.	227	125	355.00	6.31	39 *
95	PLAIN YOGURT MADE WITH WHOLE MILK, WITHOUT ADDED MILK SOLIDS 8 OZ, NET WT.	227	140	215.00	3.41	24
99	EGG, FRIED IN BUTTER (LARGE) 1 EGG	46	85	80.00	2.09	9
100	EGG, HARD-COOKED (LARGE), WITHOUT SHELL 1 EGG	50	80	90.00	2.50	10
101	EGG, POACHED (LARGE) 1 EGG	50	80	90.00	2.50	10
102	EGG, SCRAMBLED (MILK ADDED) IN BUTTER (LARGE) 1 EGG	64	95	97.00	2.27	11
145	*BLUEFISH, BAKED WITH BUTTER OR MARGARINE 3 OZ	85	135	244.00	4.02	27 *
146	CLAMS, RAW, MEAT ONLY 3 OZ	85	65	138.00	4.72	15
147	CLAMS, CANNED, SOLIDS AND LIQUIDS 3 OZ	85	45	116.00	5.73	13
148	*CRABMEAT, CANNED 1 CUP	135	135	246.00	4.05	27 *
149	FISH STICKS, BREADED, COOKED 14 BY 1 BY 1/2 IN) STICK OR 1 OZ	28	50	47.00	2.09	5
150	HADDOCK, BREADED, FRIED 3 OZ	85	140	210.00	3.33	23
151	OCEAN PERCH, BREADED, FRIED 1 FILLET	85	195	192.00	2.19	21
152	*OYSTERS, RAW, MEAT ONLY 1 CUP, 13-19 MEDIUM SELECTS	240	160	343.00	4.76	38 *
153	*SALMON, PINK, CANNED, SOLIDS AND LIQUIDS 3 OZ	85	120	243.00	4.50	27 *
154	*SARDINES, ATLANTIC, CANNED IN OIL, DRAINED SOLIDS 3 OZ	85	175	424.00	5.38	47 *
155	SCALLOPS, FROZEN, BREADED, FRIED, REHEATED. 6 SCALLOPS	90	175	176.00	2.23	20
156	*SHAD, BAKED WITH FAT 3 OZ	85	170	266.00	3.48	30 *
157	SHRIMP, CANNED 3 OZ	85	100	224.00	4.98	25
158	SHRIMP, FRENCH FRIED 3 OZ	85	190	162.00	1.89	18

HANDBOOK NUMBER	FOOD NAME / SERVING SIZE DESCRIPTION	GRAMS	KCAL	PHOSPHRUS MG	ING	%RDA
159	TUNA, CANNED IN OIL, DRAINED SOLIDS / 3 OZ	85	170	199.00	2.60	22
160	*TUNA SALAD(WITH CELERY, MAYONNAISE TYPE DRESSING, PICKLE, ONION, EGG) / 1 CUP	205	350	291.00	1.85	32 *
163	BEEF CUTS COOKED, LEAN ONLY / 2.5 OZ	72	140	108.00	1.71	12
164	GROUND BEEF, BROILED, LEAN WITH 10% FAT / 3 OZ OR 3 BY 5/8 IN PATTY	85	185	196.00	2.35	22
165	GROUND BEEF, BROILED, LEAN WITH 21% FAT / 2.9 OZ OR 3 BY 5/8 IN PATTY	82	235	159.00	1.50	18
167	ROAST BEEF, OVEN COOKED, LEAN ONLY / 1.8 OZ	51	125	131.00	2.33	15
168	ROAST BEEF, OVEN COOKED, RELATIVELY LEAN, LEAN AND FAT. / 3 OZ	85	165	208.00	2.80	23
169	ROAST BEEF, OVEN COOKED, RELATIVELY LEAN, LEAN ONLY / 2.8 OZ	78	125	199.00	3.54	22
171	STEAK, SIRLOIN, BROILED, LEAN ONLY, BONE REMOVED. / 2 OZ	56	115	146.00	2.82	16
172	STEAK, ROUND, BRAISED, LEAN AND FAT, BONE REMOVED / 3 OZ	85	220	213.00	2.15	24
173	STEAK, ROUND, BRAISED, LEAN ONLY, BONE REMOVED / 2.4 OZ	68	130	182.00	3.11	20
176	*CHIPPED BEEF, DRIED / 2 1/2 OZ JAR	71	145	287.00	4.40	32 *
177	BEEF AND VEGETABLE STEW / 1 CUP	245	220	184.00	1.86	20
179	*CHILI CON CARNE WITH BEANS, CANNED / 1 CUP	255	340	321.00	2.10	36 *
180	*CHOP SUEY WITH BEEF AND PORK(HOME RECIPE) / 1 CUP	250	300	248.00	1.84	28 *
181	HEART, BEEF, LEAN, BRAISED / 3 OZ	85	160	154.00	2.14	17
183	LAMB CHOP, BROILED, LEAN ONLY, BONE REMOVED / 2 OZ	57	120	121.00	2.24	13
184	LEG OF LAMB, ROASTED, LEAN AND FAT / 3 OZ	85	235	177.00	1.67	20
185	LEG OF LAMB, ROASTED, LEAN ONLY / 2.5 OZ	71	130	169.00	2.89	19
187	LAMB SHOULDER, ROASTED, LEAN ONLY / 2.3 OZ	64	130	140.00	2.39	16
188	*LIVER, BEEF, FRIED. / 3 OZ	85	195	405.00	4.62	45 *
190	LUNCHEON MEAT, BOILED HAM / 1 OZ	28	65	47.00	1.61	5
192	PORK CHOP, BROILED, LEAN AND FAT, BONE REMOVED / 2.7 OZ	78	305	209.00	1.52	23

HANDBOOK NUMBER	FOOD NAME SERVING SIZE DESCRIPTION	GRAMS	KCAL	PHOSPHRUS MG	INQ	%RDA
193	PORK CHOP, BROILED, LEAN ONLY, BONE REMOVED 2 OZ	56	150	181.00	2.68	20
194	PORK ROAST, OVEN COOKED, LEAN AND FAT 3 OZ	85	310	218.00	1.56	24
195	PORK ROAST, OVEN COOKED, LEAN ONLY 2.4 OZ	68	175	211.00	2.68	23
197	PORK SHOULDER, SIMMERED, LEAN ONLY 2.2 OZ	63	135	111.00	1.83	12
199	BRAUNSCHWEIGER 1 SLICE	28	90	69.00	1.70	8
208	VEAL CUTLET, BRAISED OR BROILED, BONE REMOVED 3 OZ	85	185	196.00	2.35	22
209	VEAL RIB, ROASTED, BONE REMOVED 3 OZ	85	230	211.00	2.04	23
210	CHICKEN BREAST, FRIED, BONES REMOVED 2.8 OZ	79	160	218.00	3.03	24
211	CHICKEN DRUMSTICK, FRIED, BONES REMOVED 1.3 OZ	38	90	89.00	2.20	10
212	*CHICKEN, HALF BROILER, BONES REMOVED 6.2 OZ	176	240	355.00	3.29	39 *
213	CHICKEN, CANNED, BONELESS 3 OZ	85	170	210.00	2.75	23
214	*CHICKEN A LA KING (HOME RECIPE) 1 CUP	245	470	358.00	1.69	40 *
215	*CHICKEN AND NOODLES (HOME RECIPE) 1 CUP	240	365	247.00	1.50	27 *
216	CHICKEN CHOW MEIN, CANNED 1 CUP	250	95	85.00	1.99	9
217	*CHICKEN CHOW MEIN (HOME RECIPE) 1 CUP	250	255	293.00	2.55	33 *
220	*TURKEY, LIGHT MEAT, FLESH ONLY, ROASTED 2 PIECES (4 BY 2 BY 1/4 IN.)	85	150	225.00	3.33	25 *
221	*TURKEY, LIGHT AND DARK MEAT CHOPPED 1 CUP	140	265	351.00	2.94	39 *
222	TURKEY, LIGHT AND DARK 1.5 OZ EACH	85	160	213.00	2.96	24
323	BISCUITS, BAKING POWDER, MADE FROM MIX 2-IN DIAM. BISCUIT	28	90	65.00	1.60	7
325	BOSTON BROWN BREAD, CANNED 1-3 1/4 BY 1/2 IN. SLICE	45	95	72.00	1.68	8
338	RYE BREAD, PUMPERNICKEL 5 BY 4 BY 3/8 IN SLICE	32	80	73.00	2.03	8
358	WHOLE-WHEAT BREAD, SOFT-CRUMB TYPE 1 SLICE (16 PER 1 LB LOAF)	28	65	71.00	2.43	8
365	FARINA, QUICK-COOKING, ENRICHED, COOKED 1 CUP	245	105	113.00	2.39	13

HANDBOOK NUMBER	FOOD NAME / SERVING SIZE DESCRIPTION	GRAMS	KCAL	PHOSPHORUS MG	INQ	%RDA
366	OATMEAL OR ROLLED OATS, COOKED. 1 CUP	240	130	137.00	2.34	15
367	WHEAT, ROLLED, COOKED 1 CUP	240	180	182.00	2.25	20
368	WHEAT, WHOLE-MEAL, COOKED 1 CUP	245	110	127.00	2.57	14
369	BRAN FLAKES (40% BRAN), ADDED SUGAR, SALT, IRON AND VITAMINS. 1 CUP	35	105	125.00	2.65	14
370	BRAN FLAKES WITH RAISINS, ADDED SUGAR, SALT, IRON AND VITAMINS 1 CUP	50	145	146.00	2.24	16
375	PUFFED OATS, ADDED SUGAR, SALT, MINERALS, VITAMINS 1 CUP	25	100	102.00	2.27	11
378	WHEAT FLAKES, ADDED SUGAR, SALT, IRON, VITAMINS 1 CUP	30	105	83.00	1.76	9
379	PUFFED WHEAT, PLAIN, ADDED IRON, THIAMIN, NIACIN. 1 CUP	15	55	48.00	1.94	5
381	SHREDDED WHEAT, PLAIN 1 LARGE BISCUIT OR 1/2 CUP SMALL BISCUITS	25	90	97.00	2.40	11
382	WHEAT GERM, WITHOUT SALT AND SUGAR, TOASTED 1 TBSP	6	25	70.00	6.22	8
431	RYE WAFERS, WHOLE GRAIN, 1 7/8 BY 3 1/2-IN. 2 WAFERS	13	45	50.00	2.47	6
441	MACARONI (ENRICHED) AND CHEESE, CANNED 1 CUP	240	230	182.00	1.76	20
442	*MACARONI (ENRICHED) AND CHEESE, HOME RECIPE 1 CUP	200	430	322.00	1.66	36 *
444	BRAN MUFFINS, HOME RECIPE 1 MUFFIN 2 3/8-IN DIAM., 1 1/2-IN HIGH	40	105	162.00	3.43	18
447	CORN MUFFIN MIX, EGG, MILK 1 MUFFIN, 2 3/8-IN DIAM., 11/2 IN HIGH	40	130	152.00	2.60	17
450	BUCKWHEAT PANCAKES MADE FROM MIX 1 CAKE 4-IN DIAM	27	55	91.00	3.68	10
452	PANCAKE MADE FROM MIX 1 CAKE 4-IN DIAM	27	60	70.00	2.59	8
497	*SPAGHETTI, ENRICHED, WITH MEAT BALLS IN TOMATO SAUCE, HOME RECIPE 1 CUP	248	330	236.00	1.59	26 *
501	*WAFFLES FROM MIX, EGG AND MILK ADDED 1 WAFFLE 7-IN, DIAM	75	205	257.00	2.79	29 *
505	**SELF-RISING FLOUR, ENRICHED, UNSIFTED, SPOONED 1 CUP	125	440	583.00	2.94	65 **
506	**WHOLE WHEAT FLOUR 1 CUP	120	400	446.00	2.48	50 *
507	**ALMONDS, CHOPPED 1 CUP (130 ALMONDS)	130	775	655.00	1.88	73 **
508	**ALMONDS, SLIVERED 1 CUP (115 NUTS)	115	690	580.00	1.67	64 **

HANDBOOK NUMBER	FOOD NAME SERVING SIZE DESCRIPTION	GRAMS	KCAL	PHOSPHRUS MG	INQ	%RDA	
509	*DRY BEANS, GREAT NORTHERN COOKED, DRAINED 1 CUP	180	210	266.00	2.81	30	*
510	*DRY BEANS, NAVY, COOKED, DRAINED 1 CUP	190	225	281.00	2.78	31	*
511	**BEANS WITH FRANKFURTERS,CANNED. 1 CUP	255	365	303.00	1.84	34	*
512	*PORK AND BEANS IN TOMATO SAUCE. 1 CUP	255	310	235.00	1.68	26	*
513	*PORK AND BEANS IN SWEET SAUCE 1 CUP	255	385	291.00	1.68	32	*
514	*RED KIDNEY BEANS, CANNED. 1 CUP	255	230	278.00	2.69	31	*
515	*DRY LIMA BEANS, COOKED, DRAINED 1 CUP	190	260	293.00	2.50	33	*
516	**BLACKEYE PEAS,DRY,COOKED. 1 CUP	250	190	238.00	2.78	26	*
517	BRAZIL NUTS 1 OZ. (6-8 LARGE KERNALS)	28	185	196.00	2.35	22	
522	*LENTILS, WHOLE, COOKED 1 CUP	200	210	238.00	2.52	26	*
523	**PEANUTS, ROASTED IN OIL, SALTED 1 CUP (WHOLE, HALVES, CHOPPED)	144	840	577.00	1.53	64	**
525	SPLIT PEAS, DRY,COOKED 1 CUP	200	230	178.00	1.72	20	
527	**PUMPKIN AND SQUASH SEEDS, DRY, HULLED 1 CUP	140	775	1602.00	4.59	178	**
528	**SUNFLOWER SEEDS, DRY, HULLED 1 CUP	145	810	1214.00	3.33	135	**
529	**BLACK WALNUTS, CHOPPED 1 CUP	125	785	713.00	2.02	79	**
530	**BLACK WALNUTS, GROUND 1 CUP	80	500	456.00	2.03	51	**
546	CHOCOLATE FLAVORED BEVERAGE POWDER WITH NONFAT DRY MILK 1 OZ (4 HEAPING TSP)	28	100	155.00	3.44	17	
564	ASPARAGUS, COOKED,DRAINED,FROM RAW 1 CUP(CUTS AND TIPS, 1 1/2 TO 2-IN LENGTHS)	145	30	73.00	5.41	8	
565	ASPARAGUS, COOKED,DRAINED,FROM FROZEN 1 CUP (CUTS AND TIPS, 1 1/2 TO 2-IN LENGTHS)	180	40	115.00	6.39	13	
569	LIMA BEANS,(FORDHOOKS),FROZEN,COOKED,DRAINED 1 CUP	170	170	153.00	2.00	17	
570	*LIMA BEANS,(BABY LIMAS), FROZEN, COOKED, DRAINED. 1 CUP	180	210	227.00	2.40	25	*
571	GREEN SNAP BEANS, COOKED, DRAINED, FROM RAW 1 CUP	125	30	46.00	3.41	5	
575	YELLOW OR WAX BEANS, COOKED, DRAINED, FROM RAW 1 CUP	125	30	46.00	3.41	5	

HANDBOOK NUMBER	FOOD NAME / SERVING SIZE DESCRIPTION	GRAMS	KCAL	PHOSPHRUS MG	INQ	%RDA
		105	35	67.00	4.25	7
578	BEAN SPROUTS,(MUNG),RAW / 1 CUP	105	35	67.00	4.25	7
579	BEAN SPROUTS,(MUNG),COOKED, DRAINED / 1 CUP	125	35	60.00	3.81	7
585	*BLACKEYE PEAS, COOKED, DRAINED, FROM RAW / 1 CUP	165	180	241.00	2.98	27 *
586	*BLACKEYE PEAS, COOKED, DRAINED, FROM FROZEN / 1 CUP	170	220	286.00	2.89	32 *
587	BROCCOLI, COOKED, DRAINED, FROM RAW / 1 WHOLE MEDIUM STALK	187	45	112.00	5.53	12
588	BROCCOLI, COOKED, DRAINED, FROM RAW / 1 CUP (STALKS CUT INTO 1/2-IN PIECES)	155	40	96.00	5.33	11
590	BROCCOLI, FROM FROZEN, CHOPPED, COOKED, DRAINED / 1 CUP	185	50	104.00	4.62	12
591	BRUSSELS SPROUTS, COOKED, DRAINED, FROM RAW / 7-8 SPROUTS (1 1/4 TO 1 1/2-IN DIAM) 1 CUP	155	55	112.00	4.53	12
592	BRUSSELS SPROUTS, COOKED, DRAINED, FROM FROZEN / 1 CUP	155	50	95.00	4.22	11
599	WHITE MUSTARD CABBAGE, COOKED, DRAINED / 1 CUP	170	25	56.00	4.98	6
602	CARROTS (CROSSWISE CUTS) COOKED, DRAINED / 1 CUP	155	50	48.00	2.13	5
605	CAULIFLOWER, RAW, CHOPPED / 1 CUP	115	31	64.00	4.59	7
606	CAULIFLOWER, COOKED, DRAINED FROM RAW / 1 CUP	125	30	53.00	3.93	6
607	CAULIFLOWER, COOKED, DRAINED FROM FROZEN / 1 CUP	180	30	68.00	5.04	8
610	COLLARDS, COOKED, DRAINED, FROM RAW / 1 CUP	190	65	99.00	3.38	11
611	COLLARDS, COOKED DRAINED, FROM FROZEN / 1 CUP	170	50	87.00	3.87	10
612	CORN, COOKED, DRAINED FROM RAW, WT WITHOUT COB / 1 EAR (5 BY 1 3/4=IN)	77	70	69.00	2.19	8
613	CORN, COOKED, DRAINED FROM FROZEN, WT WITHOUT COB / 1 EAR (5-IN LONG)	126	120	121.00	2.24	13
614	CORN, COOKED, DRAINED FROM FROZEN / 1 CUP KERNELS	165	130	120.00	2.05	13
615	CORN, CANNED CREAM STYLE / 1 CUP	256	210	143.00	1.51	16
616	CORN, CANNED, WHOLE KERNEL, VACUUM PACK / 1 CUP	210	175	153.00	1.94	17
622	KALE, COOKED, DRAINED, FROM RAW, LEAVES WITHOUT STEMS / 1 CUP	110	45	64.00	3.16	7
623	KALE, COOKED, DRAINED, FROM FROZEN, LEAF STYLE / 1 CUP	130	40	62.00	3.44	7

HANDBOOK NUMBER	FOOD NAME SERVING SIZE DESCRIPTION	GRAMS	KCAL	PHOSPHRUS MG	INQ	%RDA
626	ICEBERG LETTUCE (CRISPHEAD) 1 HEAD, 6-IN DIAM	567	70	118.00	3.75	13
630	MUSHROOMS, RAW, SLICED OR CHOPPED 1 CUP	70	20	81.00	9.00	9
631	MUSTARD GREENS, COOKED, DRAINED, WITHOUT STEMS 1 CUP	140	30	45.00	3.33	5
633	ONIONS, MATURE, RAW, CHOPPED 1 CUP	170	65	61.00	2.09	7
635	ONIONS, MATURE, COOKED, DRAINED, WHOLE OR SLICED 1 CUP	210	60	61.00	2.26	7
638	PARSNIPS, COOKED, DICED 1 CUP	155	100	96.00	2.13	11
639	GREEN PEAS, CANNED, DRAINED SOLIDS 1 CUP	170	150	129.00	1.91	14
641	GREEN PEAS, FROZEN, COOKED, DRAINED 1 CUP	160	110	138.00	2.79	15
645	BAKED POTATO, PEELED AFTER BAKING 1 POTATO (2 PER LB)	156	145	101.00	1.55	11
646	BOILED POTATO, PEELED AFTER BOILING 1 POTATO (3 PER LB)	137	105	72.00	1.52	8
651	MASHED POTATOES, PREPARED FROM RAW, MILK ADDED 1 CUP	210	135	103.00	1.70	11
656	PUMPKIN, CANNED 1 CUP	245	80	64.00	1.78	7
660	SPINACH, COOKED, DRAINED FROM RAW 1 CUP	180	40	68.00	3.78	8
661	SPINACH, COOKED, DRAINED FROM FROZEN, CHOPPED 1 CUP	205	45	90.00	4.44	10
662	SPINACH, COOKED, DRAINED FROM FROZEN, LEAF 1 CUP	190	45	84.00	4.15	9
663	SPINACH, CANNED, DRAINED SOLIDS 1 CUP	205	50	53.00	2.36	6
664	SUMMER SQUASH, COOKED, DICED, DRAINED 1 CUP	210	30	53.00	3.93	6
665	WINTER SQUASH, BAKED, MASHED 1 CUP	205	130	98.00	1.68	11
672	TOMATOES, CANNED, SOLIDS AND LIQUIDS 1 CUP	241	50	46.00	2.04	5
678	TURNIP GREENS, COOKED, DRAINED, FROM RAW (LEAVES AND STEMS) 1 CUP	145	30	49.00	3.63	5
679	TURNIP GREENS, COOKED, DRAINED, FROM FROZEN, CHOPPED 1 CUP	165	40	64.00	3.56	7
680	VEGETABLES, MIXED, FROZEN, COOKED, DRAINED 1 CUP	182	115	115.00	2.22	13
686	BEER 12 FL OZ	360	150	108.00	1.60	12

HANDBOOK NUMBER	FOOD NAME SERVING SIZE DESCRIPTION	GRAMS	KCAL	PHOSPHRUS MG	INQ	%RDA
697	BITTER SWEET OR BAKING CHOCOLATE . . . . 1 OZ	28	145	109.00	1.67	12
708	CREAM OF CHICKEN SOUP PREPARED WITH EQUAL VOLUME OF MILK, CANNED . . . 1 CUP	245	180	152.00	1.88	17
709	CREAM OF MUSHROOM SOUP PREPARED WITH EQUAL VOLUME OF MILK, CANNED . . . 1 CUP	245	215	169.00	1.75	19
710	TOMATO SOUP PREPARED WITH EQUAL VOLUME OF MILK, CANNED. . . . . . . 1 CUP	250	175	155.00	1.97	17
711	BEAN WITH PORK SOUP PREPARED WITH EQUAL VOLUME OF WATER, CANNED . . . 1 CUP	250	170	128.00	1.67	14
713	BEEF NOODLE SOUP, PREPARED WITH EQUAL VOLUME OF WATER,CANNED. . . . . 1 CUP	240	65	48.00	1.64	5
718	SPLIT PEA SOUP PREPARED WITH EQUAL VOLUME OF WATER, CANNED . . . . . 1 CUP	245	145	149.00	2.28	17
730	BREWER'S YEAST, DRY . . . . 1 TBSP	8	25	140.00	12.44	16

POTASSIUM POTASSIUM POTASSIUM POTASSIUM POTASSIUM POTASSIUM POTASSIUM POTASSIUM POTASSIUM POTASSIUM POTASSIUM

FOODS WHICH PROVIDE A HIGH CONCENTRATION OF POTASSIUM RELATIVE TO CALORIES

(INQ AT LEAST 1.5)

AND AT LEAST 5 PERCENT OF THE RDA PER SERVING

(RDA FOR POTASSIUM = 5000.0 MG)

POTASSIUM POTASSIUM POTASSIUM POTASSIUM POTASSIUM POTASSIUM POTASSIUM POTASSIUM POTASSIUM POTASSIUM POTASSIUM

*INDICATES FOODS WHICH PROVIDE AT LEAST 25 PERCENT OF THE RDA PER SERVING

**INDICATES FOODS WHICH PROVIDE AT LEAST 50 PERCENT OF THE RDA PER SERVING

HANDBOOK NUMBER	FOOD NAME SERVING SIZE DESCRIPTION	GRAMS	KCAL	POTASSIUM MG	ING	%RDA
54	MILK, FLUID LOWFAT (1% FAT), NO MILK SOLIDS ADDED / 1 CUP	244	100	361.00	1.52	8
55	MILK, FLUID LOWFAT (1% FAT), LESS THAN 10 GRAMS OF PROTEIN PER CUP / 1 CUP	245	105	397.00	1.51	8
57	MILK, FLUID NONFAT (SKIM), NO MILK SOLIDS ADDED / 1 CUP	245	85	406.00	1.91	8
58	MILK, FLUID NONFAT (SKIM), LESS THAN 10 GRAMS OF PROTEIN PER CUP / 1 CUP	245	90	418.00	1.86	8
59	MILK, FLUID NONFAT (SKIM), MORE THAN 10 GRAMS OF PROTEIN PER CUP / 1 CUP	246	100	446.00	1.78	9
94	PLAIN YOGURT MADE WITH NONFAT MILK, WITH ADDED MILK SOLIDS / 8 OZ, NET WT.	227	125	579.00	1.85	12
216	CHICKEN CHOW MEIN, CANNED / 1 CUP	250	95	418.00	1.76	8
228	APRICOTS, RAW, WITHOUT PITS / 3	107	55	301.00	2.19	6
234	*AVOCADOS, RAW, FLORIDA, WT. WITHOUT SKIN AND SEED / 1--3 5/8-IN DIAM.	304	390	1836.00	1.88	37 *
235	BANANA, RAW, WITHOUT PEEL / 1--2.6 PER LB WITH PEEL	119	100	440.00	1.76	9
249	GRAPEFRUIT JUICE, RAW / 1 CUP	246	95	399.00	1.68	8
250	GRAPEFRUIT JUICE, CANNED, UNSWEETENED / 1 CUP	247	100	400.00	1.60	8
253	GRAPEFRUIT JUICE, FROZEN, CONCENTRATE, UNSWEETENED, DILUTED / 1 CUP	247	100	420.00	1.68	8
254	GRAPEFRUIT JUICE, DEHYDRATED CRYSTALS, PREPARED WITH WATER / 1 CUP	247	100	412.00	1.65	8
271	CANTALOUP, WT WITHOUT RIND AND SEEDS / 1/2 OF A 5-IN DIAM. MELON	272	80	682.00	3.41	14
272	HONEYDEW MELON, WT WITHOUT RIND AND SEEDS / 1/10 OF A 6 1/2-IN DIAM. MELON	149	50	374.00	2.99	7
273	ORANGE, RAW, WT WITHOUT PEEL AND SEEDS / 1--2 5/8-IN DIAM.	131	65	263.00	1.62	5
274	ORANGE SECTIONS WITHOUT MEMBRANES, RAW / 1 CUP	180	90	360.00	1.60	7
275	ORANGE JUICE, FRESH / 1 CUP	248	110	496.00	1.80	10
276	ORANGE JUICE, CANNED, UNSWEETENED / 1 CUP	249	120	496.00	1.65	10
278	ORANGE JUICE, FROZEN CONCENTRATE, DILUTED / 1 CUP	249	120	503.00	1.68	10
279	ORANGE JUICE, DEHYDRATED CRYSTALS, PREPARED WITH WATER / 1 CUP	248	115	518.00	1.80	10
281	ORANGE AND GRAPEFRUIT JUICE, FROZEN CONCENTRATE, DILUTED / 1 CUP	248	110	459.00	1.60	9

HANDBOOK NUMBER	FOOD NAME / SERVING SIZE DESCRIPTION	GRAMS	KCAL	POTASSIUM MG	INQ	%RDA
282	PAPAYAS, RAW, 1/2 INCH CUBES, 1 CUP	140	55	326.00	2.39	7
284	PEACHES, RAW, SLICED, 1 CUP	170	65	343.00	2.11	7
286	PEACHES, CANNED, WATER PACK, 1 CUP (SOLIDS AND LIQUID)	244	75	334.00	1.78	7
318	WATERMELON, WT WITHOUT RIND AND SEEDS, 1/16 OF 33 LB MELON	426	110	426.00	1.55	9
515	DRY LIMA BEANS, COOKED, DRAINED, 1 CUP	190	260	1163.00	1.79	23
556	BLACKSTRAP MOLASSES, 1 TBSP	20	45	585.00	5.20	12
564	ASPARAGUS, COOKED,DRAINED,FROM RAW, 1 CUP (CUTS AND TIPS, 1 1/2 TO 2-IN LENGTHS)	145	30	265.00	3.53	5
565	ASPARAGUS, COOKED,DRAINED,FROM FROZEN, 1 CUP (CUTS AND TIPS, 1 1/2 TO 2-IN LENGTHS)	180	40	396.00	3.96	8
569	LIMA BEANS,(FORDHOOKS),FROZEN,COOKED,DRAINED, 1 CUP	170	170	724.00	1.70	14
581	BEETS, COOKED DRAINED,DICED OR SLICED, 1 CUP	170	55	354.00	2.57	7
582	BEETS, CANNED, DRAINED SOLIDS, WHOLE SMALL BEETS, 1 CUP	160	60	267.00	1.78	5
583	BEETS, CANNED, DRAINED SOLIDS, DICED OR SLICED, 1 CUP	170	65	284.00	1.75	6
584	BEET GREENS, COOKED, DRAINED, 1 CUP	145	25	481.00	7.70	10
587	BROCCOLI, COOKED, DRAINED, FROM RAW, 1 WHOLE MEDIUM STALK	187	45	481.00	4.28	10
588	BROCCOLI, COOKED, DRAINED, FROM RAW, 1 CUP (STALKS CUT INTO 1/2-IN PIECES)	155	40	414.00	4.14	8
590	BROCCOLI, FROM FROZEN, CHOPPED, COOKED, DRAINED, 1 CUP	185	50	392.00	3.14	8
591	BRUSSELS SPROUTS, COOKED, DRAINED, FROM RAW, 7-8 SPROUTS (1 1/4 TO 1 1/2-IN DIAM) 1 CUP	155	55	423.00	3.08	8
592	BRUSSELS SPROUTS, COOKED, DRAINED, FROM FROZEN, 1 CUP	155	50	457.00	3.66	9
599	WHITE MUSTARD CABBAGE, COOKED, DRAINED, 1 CUP	170	25	364.00	5.82	7
601	CARROTS, RAW, PEELED, GRATED, 1 CUP	110	45	375.00	3.33	8
602	CARROTS (CROSSWISE CUTS) COOKED, DRAINED, 1 CUP	155	50	344.00	2.75	7
605	CAULIFLOWER, RAW, CHOPPED, 1 CUP	115	31	339.00	4.37	7
606	CAULIFLOWER, COOKED, DRAINED FROM RAW, 1 CUP	125	30	258.00	3.44	5

HANDBOOK NUMBER	FOOD NAME / SERVING SIZE DESCRIPTION	GRAMS	KCAL	POTASSIUM MG	INQ	%RDA
607	CAULIFLOWER, COOKED, DRAINED FROM FROZEN · 1 CUP	180	30	375.00	4.97	7
609	CELERY, RAW DICED · 1 CUP	120	20	409.00	8.18	8
610	COLLARDS, COOKED, DRAINED, FROM RAW · 1 CUP	190	65	498.00	3.06	10
611	COLLARDS, COOKED DRAINED, FROM FROZEN · 1 CUP	170	50	401.00	3.21	8
623	KALE, COOKED, DRAINED, FROM FROZEN, LEAF STYLE · 1 CUP	130	40	251.00	2.51	5
624	BUTTERHEAD LETTUCE, RAW · 1 HEAD, 5-IN DIAM.	220	25	430.00	6.88	9
626	ICEBERG LETTUCE (CRISPHEAD) · 1 HEAD, 6-IN DIAM	567	70	943.00	5.39	19
630	MUSHROOMS, RAW, SLICED OR CHOPPED · 1 CUP	70	20	290.00	5.80	6
631	MUSTARD GREENS, COOKED, DRAINED, WITHOUT STEMS · 1 CUP	140	30	308.00	4.11	6
633	ONIONS, MATURE, RAW, CHOPPED · 1 CUP	170	65	267.00	1.64	5
638	PARSNIPS, COOKED, DICED · 1 CUP	155	100	587.00	2.35	12
645	BAKED POTATO, PEELED AFTER BAKING · 1 POTATO (2 PER LB)	156	145	782.00	2.16	16
646	BOILED POTATO, PEELED AFTER BOILING · 1 POTATO (3 PER LB)	137	105	556.00	2.12	11
647	BOILED POTATOES, PEELED BEFORE BOILING · 1 POTATO (3 PER LB)	135	90	385.00	1.71	8
651	MASHED POTATOES, PREPARED FROM RAW, MILK ADDED · 1 CUP	210	135	548.00	1.62	11
656	PUMPKIN, CANNED · 1 CUP	245	80	588.00	2.94	12
658	SAUERKRAUT, CANNED, SOLIDS AND LIQUIDS · 1 CUP	235	40	329.00	3.29	7
659	SPINACH, RAW, CHOPPED · 1 CUP	55	15	259.00	6.91	5
660	SPINACH, COOKED, DRAINED FROM RAW · 1 CUP	180	40	583.00	5.83	12
661	SPINACH, COOKED, DRAINED FROM FROZEN, CHOPPED · 1 CUP	205	45	683.00	6.07	14
662	SPINACH, COOKED, DRAINED FROM FROZEN, LEAF · 1 CUP	190	45	688.00	6.12	14
663	SPINACH, CANNED, DRAINED SOLIDS · 1 CUP	205	50	513.00	4.10	10
664	SUMMER SQUASH, COOKED, DICED, DRAINED · 1 CUP	210	30	296.00	3.95	6

HANDBOOK NUMBER	FOOD NAME SERVING SIZE DESCRIPTION	GRAMS	KCAL	POTASSIUM MG	ING	%RDA
665	WINTER SQUASH, BAKED, MASHED . . . . 1 CUP	205	130	945.00	2.91	19
671	TOMATOES, RAW . . . . 1 TOMATO 2 3/5-IN DIAM	135	25	300.00	4.80	6
672	TOMATOES, CANNED, SOLIDS AND LIQUIDS . . . . . . 1 CUP	241	50	523.00	4.18	10
675	TOMATO JUICE, CANNED . . . . 1 CUP	243	45	552.00	4.91	11
676	TOMATO JUICE, CANNED . . . . 1 GLASS 6 FL OZ	182	35	413.00	4.72	8
677	TURNIPS, COOKED, DICED . . . . 1 CUP	155	35	291.00	3.33	6
678	TURNIP GREENS, COOKED, DRAINED, FROM RAW (LEAVES AND STEMS) . . . . . 1 CUP	145	30	470.00	6.27	9

PROTEIN PROTEIN PROTEIN PROTEIN PROTEIN PROTEIN PROTEIN PROTEIN PROTEIN PROTEIN

FOODS WHICH PROVIDE A HIGH CONCENTRATION OF PROTEIN RELATIVE TO CALORIES

(INQ AT LEAST 1.5)

AND AT LEAST 5 PERCENT OF THE RDA PER SERVING

(RDA FOR PROTEIN = 50.0 G)

PROTEIN PROTEIN PROTEIN PROTEIN PROTEIN PROTEIN PROTEIN PROTEIN PROTEIN PROTEIN

*INDICATES FOODS WHICH PROVIDE AT LEAST 25 PERCENT OF THE RDA PER SERVING

**INDICATES FOODS WHICH PROVIDE AT LEAST 50 PERCENT OF THE RDA PER SERVING

HANDBOOK NUMBER	FOOD NAME / SERVING SIZE DESCRIPTION	GRAMS	KCAL	PROTEIN G	INU	%RDA
1	BLUE CHEESE / 1 OZ	28	100	6.00	2.40	12
2	CAMEMBERT CHEESE / 1 WEDGE	38	115	8.00	2.78	16
3	CHEDDAR CHEESE / 1 OZ	28	115	7.00	2.43	14
4	CHEDDAR CHEESE / 1 CUBIC INCH	17	70	4.00	2.29	8
6	**COTTAGE CHEESE, CREAMED (4% FAT), LG CURD / 1 CUP	225	235	28.00	4.77	56 **
7	**COTTAGE CHEESE, CREAMED (4% FAT), SM CURD / 1 CUP	210	220	26.00	4.73	52 **
8	**COTTAGE CHEESE, 2% FAT / 1 CUP	226	205	31.00	6.05	62 **
9	**COTTAGE CHEESE, 1% FAT / 1 CUP	226	165	28.00	6.79	56 **
10	**COTTAGE CHEESE, UNCREAMED (LESS THAN 0.5% FAT) / 1 CUP	145	125	25.00	8.00	50 **
12	MOZZARELLA CHEESE, MADE WITH WHOLE MILK / 1 OZ	28	90	6.00	2.67	12
13	MOZZARELLA CHEESE, MADE WITH SKIM MILK / 1 OZ	28	80	8.00	4.00	16
16	PARMESAN CHEESE, GRATED / 1 OZ	28	130	12.00	3.69	24
17	PROVOLONE CHEESE / 1 OZ	28	100	7.00	2.80	14
18	**RICOTTA CHEESE, MADE WITH WHOLE MILK / 1 CUP	246	428	28.00	2.62	56 **
19	**RICOTTA CHEESE, MADE WITH PART SKIM MILK / 1 CUP	246	340	28.00	3.29	56 **
20	ROMANO CHEESE / 1 OZ	28	110	9.00	3.27	18
21	SWISS CHEESE / 1 OZ	28	105	8.00	3.05	16
22	AMERICAN PASTEURIZED PROCESS CHEESE / 1 OZ	28	105	6.00	2.29	12
23	SWISS PASTEURIZED PROCESS CHEESE / 1 OZ	28	95	7.00	2.95	14
24	AMERICAN PASTEURIZED PROCESS CHEESE FOOD / 1 OZ	28	95	6.00	2.53	12
25	AMERICAN PASTEURIZED PROCESS CHEESE SPREAD / 1 OZ	28	82	5.00	2.44	10
50	MILK, FLUID WHOLE (3.3% FAT) / 1 CUP	244	150	8.00	2.13	16
51	MILK, FLUID LOWFAT (2% FAT), NO MILK SOLIDS ADDED / 1 CUP	244	120	8.00	2.67	16

HANDBOOK NUMBER	FOOD NAME SERVING SIZE DESCRIPTION	GRAMS	KCAL	PROTEIN G	INQ	%RDA
52	MILK, FLUID LOWFAT (2% FAT), LESS THAN 10 GRAMS OF PROTEIN PER CUP 1 CUP	245	125	9.00	2.88	18
53	MILK, FLUID LOWFAT (2% FAT), MORE THAN 10 GRAMS OF PROTEIN PER CUP 1 CUP	246	135	10.00	2.96	20
54	MILK, FLUID LOWFAT (1% FAT), NO MILK SOLIDS ADDED 1 CUP	244	100	8.00	3.20	16
55	MILK, FLUID LOWFAT (1% FAT), LESS THAN 10 GRAMS OF PROTEIN PER CUP 1 CUP	245	105	9.00	3.43	18
56	MILK, FLUID LOWFAT (1% FAT), MORE THAN 10 GRAMS OF PROTEIN PER CUP 1 CUP	246	120	10.00	3.33	20
57	MILK, FLUID NONFAT (SKIM), NO MILK SOLIDS ADDED 1 CUP	245	85	8.00	3.76	16
58	MILK, FLUID NONFAT (SKIM), LESS THAN 10 GRAMS OF PROTEIN PER CUP 1 CUP	245	90	9.00	4.00	18
59	MILK, FLUID NONFAT (SKIM), MORE THAN 10 GRAMS OF PROTEIN PER CUP 1 CUP	246	100	10.00	4.00	20
60	BUTTERMILK, FLUID 1 CUP	245	100	8.00	3.20	16
67	CHOCOLATE MILK (COMMERCIAL) 1 CUP	250	210	8.00	1.52	16
68	CHOCOLATE MILK, LOWFAT (2%)(COMMERICIAL) 1 CUP	250	180	8.00	1.78	16
69	CHOCOLATE MILK, LOWFAT (1%)(COMMERCIAL) 1 CUP	250	160	8.00	2.00	16
71	CHOCOLATE MALTED MILK (1 CUP WHOLE MILK AND 3/4 OZ MALTED MILK POWDER) 1 CUP PLUS POWDER	265	235	9.00	1.53	18
72	NATURAL MALTED MILK (1CUP WHOLE MILK AND 3/4 OZ MALTED MILK POWDER) 1 CUP PLUS POWDER	265	235	11.00	1.87	22
86	*CUSTARD, BAKED 1 CUP	265	305	14.00	1.84	28 *
92	FRUIT-FLAVORED YOGURT MADE WITH LOWFAT MILK, WITH ADDED MILK SOLIDS 8 OZ, NET WT.	227	230	10.00	1.74	20
93	PLAIN YOGURT MADE WITH LOWFAT MILK, WITH ADDED MILK SOLIDS 8 OZ, NET WT.	227	145	12.00	3.31	24
94	*PLAIN YOGURT MADE WITH NONFAT MILK, WITH ADDED MILK SOLIDS 8 OZ, NET WT.	227	125	13.00	4.16	26 *
95	PLAIN YOGURT MADE WITH WHOLE MILK, WITHOUT ADDED MILK SOLIDS. 8 OZ, NET WT.	227	140	8.00	2.29	16
99	EGG, FRIED IN BUTTER (LARGE) 1 EGG	46	85	5.00	2.35	10
100	EGG, HARD-COOKED (LARGE), WITHOUT SHELL 1 EGG	50	80	6.00	3.00	12
101	EGG, POACHED (LARGE) 1 EGG	50	80	6.00	3.00	12
102	EGG, SCRAMBLED (MILK ADDED) IN BUTTER (LARGE) 1 EGG	64	95	6.00	2.53	12

HANDBOOK NUMBER	FOOD NAME / SERVING SIZE DESCRIPTION	GRAMS	KCAL	PROTEIN G	IND	IHDA
145	*BLUEFISH, BAKED WITH BUTTER OR MARGARINE / 3 OZ	85	135	22.00	6.52	44 *
146	CLAMS, RAW, MEAT ONLY / 3 OZ	85	65	11.00	6.77	22 *
147	CLAMS, CANNED, SOLIDS AND LIQUIDS / 3 OZ	85	45	7.00	6.22	14 *
148	*CRABMEAT, CANNED / 1 CUP	135	135	24.00	7.11	48 *
149	FISH STICKS, BREADED, COOKED / 1(4 BY 1 BY 1/2 IN) STICK OR 1 OZ	28	50	5.00	4.00	10 *
150	*HADDOCK, BREADED, FRIED / 3 OZ	85	140	17.00	4.86	34 *
151	*OCEAN PERCH, BREADED, FRIED / 1 FILLET	85	195	16.00	3.28	32 *
152	*OYSTERS, RAW, MEAT ONLY / 1 CUP, 13-19 MEDIUM SELECTS	240	160	20.00	5.00	40 *
153	*SALMON, PINK, CANNED, SOLIDS AND LIQUIDS / 3 OZ	85	120	17.00	5.67	34 *
154	*SARDINES, ATLANTIC, CANNED IN OIL, DRAINED SOLIDS / 3 OZ	85	175	20.00	4.57	40 *
155	*SCALLOPS, FROZEN, BREADED, FRIED, REHEATED / 6 SCALLOPS	90	175	16.00	3.66	32 *
156	*SHAD, BAKED WITH FAT / 3 OZ	85	170	20.00	4.71	40 *
157	*SHRIMP, CANNED / 3 OZ	85	100	21.00	8.40	42 *
158	*SHRIMP, FRENCH FRIED / 3 OZ	85	190	17.00	3.58	34 *
159	*TUNA, CANNED IN OIL, DRAINED SOLIDS / 3 OZ	85	170	24.00	5.65	48 *
160	**TUNA SALAD(WITH CELERY, MAYONNAISE TYPE DRESSING, PICKLE, ONION, EGG) / 1 CUP	205	350	30.00	3.43	60 **
161	BACON, CRISP / 2 SLICES	15	85	4.00	1.88	8
162	*BEEF CUTS COOKED, LEAN AND FAT / 3 OZ - 2 1/2 BY 2 1/2 BY 3/4 IN	85	245	23.00	3.76	46 *
163	*BEEF CUTS COOKED, LEAN ONLY / 2.5 OZ	72	140	22.00	6.29	44 *
164	*GROUND BEEF, BROILED, LEAN WITH 10% FAT / 3 OZ OR 3 BY 5/8 IN PATTY	85	185	23.00	4.97	46 *
165	*GROUND BEEF, BROILED, LEAN WITH 21% FAT / 2.9 OZ OR 3 BY 5/8 IN PATTY	82	235	20.00	3.40	40 *
166	*ROAST BEEF, OVEN COOKED, MODERATELY FAT, LEAN AND FAT / 3 OZ	85	375	17.00	1.81	34 *
167	*ROAST BEEF, OVEN COOKED, LEAN ONLY / 1.8 OZ	51	125	14.00	4.48	28 *

HANDBOOK FOOD NAME NUMBER / SERVING SIZE DESCRIPTION	GRAMS	KCAL	PROTEIN G	INQ	%RDA
168 **ROAST BEEF, OVEN COOKED, RELATIVELY LEAN, LEAN AND FAT. 3 OZ	85	165	25.00	6.06	50 **
169 *ROAST BEEF, OVEN COOKED, RELATIVELY LEAN, LEAN ONLY 2.8 OZ	78	125	24.00	7.68	48 *
170 *STEAK, SIRLOIN, BROILED, LEAN AND FAT, BONE REMOVED 3 OZ	85	330	20.00	2.42	40 *
171 *STEAK, SIRLOIN, BROILED, LEAN ONLY, BONE REMOVED. 2 OZ	56	115	18.00	6.26	36 *
172 *STEAK, ROUND, BRAISED, LEAN AND FAT, BONE REMOVED 3 OZ	85	220	24.00	4.36	48 *
173 *STEAK, ROUND, BRAISED, LEAN ONLY, BONE REMOVED 2.4 OZ	68	130	21.00	6.46	42 *
174 *CORNED BEEF CANNED. 3 OZ	85	185	22.00	4.76	44 *
175 *CORNED BEEF HASH 1 CUP	220	400	19.00	1.90	38 *
176 *CHIPPED BEEF, DRIED 2 1/2 OZ JAR	71	145	24.00	6.62	48 *
177 *BEEF AND VEGETABLE STEW 1 CUP	245	220	16.00	2.91	32 *
178 *BEEF POTPIE (HOME RECIPE) 1/3 OF 9-IN DIAM. PIE	210	515	21.00	1.63	42 *
179 *CHILI CON CARNE WITH BEANS, CANNED 1 CUP	255	340	19.00	2.24	38 *
180 **CHOP SUEY WITH BEEF AND PORK(HOME RECIPE) 1 CUP	250	300	26.00	3.47	52 **
181 **HEART, BEEF, LEAN, BRAISED 3 OZ	85	160	27.00	6.75	54 **
182 *LAMB CHOP, BROILED, LEAN AND FAT, BONE REMOVED 3.1 OZ	89	360	18.00	2.00	36 *
183 *LAMB CHOP, BROILED, LEAN ONLY, BONE REMOVED 2 OZ	57	120	16.00	5.33	32 *
184 *LEG OF LAMB, ROASTED, LEAN AND FAT 3 OZ	85	235	22.00	3.74	44 *
185 *LEG OF LAMB, ROASTED, LEAN ONLY 2.5 OZ	71	130	20.00	6.15	40 *
186 *LAMB SHOULDER, ROASTED, LEAN AND FAT. 3 OZ	85	285	18.00	2.53	36 *
187 *LAMB SHOULDER, ROASTED, LEAN ONLY 2.3 OZ	64	130	17.00	5.23	34 *
188 *LIVER, BEEF, FRIED. 3 OZ	85	195	22.00	4.51	44 *
189 *HAM, LIGHT CURE, ROASTED, LEAN AND FAT 3 OZ	85	245	18.00	2.94	36 *
190 LUNCHEON MEAT, BOILED HAM 1 OZ	28	65	5.00	3.08	10

HANDBOOK NUMBER	FOOD NAME / SERVING SIZE DESCRIPTION	GRAMS	KCAL	PROTEIN G	INQ	%XMDA	
191	LUNCHEON MEAT, CANNED, SPICED OR UNSPICED 1 SLICE (3 BY 2 BY 1/2 IN)	60	175	9.00	2.06	18	
192	*PORK CHOP, BROILED, LEAN AND FAT, BONE REMOVED 2.7 OZ	78	305	19.00	2.49	38	*
193	*PORK CHOP, BROILED, LEAN ONLY, BONE REMOVED 2 OZ	56	150	17.00	4.53	34	*
194	*PORK ROAST, OVEN COOKED, LEAN AND FAT 3 OZ	85	310	21.00	2.71	42	*
195	*PORK ROAST, OVEN COOKED, LEAN ONLY 2.4 OZ	68	175	20.00	4.57	40	*
196	*PORK SHOULDER, SIMMERED, LEAN AND FAT 3 OZ	85	320	20.00	2.50	40	*
197	*PORK SHOULDER, SIMMERED, LEAN ONLY 2.2 OZ	63	135	18.00	5.33	36	*
199	BRAUNSCHWEIGER 1 SLICE	28	90	4.00	1.78	8	
200	BROWN AND SERVE SAUSAGES 1 LINK (10-11 PER 8-OZ PKG.)	17	70	3.00	1.71	6	
202	FRANKFURTER 1 FRANKFURTER (8 PER 1-LB PKG.)	56	170	7.00	1.65	14	
206	SALAMI, COOKED TYPE 1 SLICE (8 PER 8-OZ PKG.)	28	90	5.00	2.22	10	
208	*VEAL CUTLET, BRAISED OR BROILED, BONE REMOVED 3 OZ	85	185	23.00	4.97	46	*
209	*VEAL RIB, ROASTED, BONE REMOVED 3 OZ	85	230	23.00	4.00	46	*
210	**CHICKEN BREAST, FRIED, BONES REMOVED. 2.8 OZ	79	160	26.00	6.50	52	**
211	CHICKEN DRUMSTICK, FRIED, BONES REMOVED 1.3 OZ	38	90	12.00	5.33	24	
212	**CHICKEN, HALF BROILER, BONES REMOVED. 6.2 OZ	176	240	42.00	7.00	84	**
213	*CHICKEN, CANNED, BONELESS 3 OZ	85	170	18.00	4.24	36	*
214	**CHICKEN A LA KING (HOME RECIPE) 1 CUP	245	470	27.00	2.30	54	**
215	*CHICKEN AND NOODLES (HOME RECIPE) 1 CUP	240	365	22.00	2.41	44	*
216	CHICKEN CHOW MEIN, CANNED 1 CUP	250	95	7.00	2.95	14	
217	**CHICKEN CHOW MEIN (HOME RECIPE) 1 CUP	250	255	31.00	4.86	62	**
218	*CHICKEN POTPIE (HOME RECIPE) 1 PIECE OR 1/3 OF 9-IN DIAM. PIE	232	545	23.00	1.69	46	*
219	**TURKEY, DARK MEAT, FLESH ONLY, ROASTED 4 PIECES (2 1/2 BY 1 5/8 BY 1/4 IN.)	85	175	26.00	5.94	52	**

HANDBOOK NUMBER	FOOD NAME SERVING SIZE DESCRIPTION	GRAMS	KCAL	PROTEIN G	INQ	%RDA
220	**TURKEY, LIGHT MEAT, FLESH ONLY, ROASTED 2 PIECES (4 BY 2 BY 1/4 IN.)	85	150	28.00	7.47	56 **
221	**TURKEY, LIGHT AND DARK MEAT CHOPPED 1 CUP	140	265	44.00	6.64	88 **
222	**TURKEY, LIGHT AND DARK 1.5 OZ EACH	85	160	27.00	6.75	54 **
338	RYE BREAD, PUMPERNICKEL 5 BY 4 BY 3/8 IN SLICE	32	80	3.00	1.50	6
358	WHOLE-WHEAT BREAD, SOFT-CRUMB TYPE 1 SLICE (16 PER 1 LB LOAF)	28	65	3.00	1.85	6
366	OATMEAL OR ROLLED OATS, COOKED 1 CUP	240	130	5.00	1.54	10
369	BRAN FLAKES (40% BRAN), ADDED SUGAR, SALT, IRON AND VITAMINS 1 CUP	35	105	4.00	1.52	8
441	MACARONI (ENRICHED) AND CHEESE, CANNED 1 CUP	240	230	9.00	1.57	18
442	*MACARONI (ENRICHED) AND CHEESE, HOME RECIPE 1 CUP	200	430	17.00	1.58	34 *
475	PIZZA(CHEESE), BAKED 1 SECTOR, 1/8 OF 12-IN DIAM PIE	60	145	6.00	1.66	12
497	*SPAGHETTI, ENRICHED, WITH MEAT BALLS IN TOMATO SAUCE, HOME RECIPE 1 CUP	248	330	19.00	2.30	38 *
498	SPAGHETTI, ENRICHED, WITH MEAT BALLS IN TOMATO SAUCE, CANNED 1 CUP	250	260	12.00	1.85	24
506	*WHOLE WHEAT FLOUR 1 CUP	120	400	16.00	1.60	32 *
509	*DRY BEANS, GREAT NORTHERN COOKED, DRAINED 1 CUP	180	210	14.00	2.67	28 *
510	*DRY BEANS, NAVY, COOKED, DRAINED 1 CUP	190	225	15.00	2.67	30 *
511	*BEANS WITH FRANKFURTERS,CANNED 1 CUP	255	365	19.00	2.08	38 *
512	*PORK AND BEANS IN TOMATO SAUCE 1 CUP	255	310	16.00	2.06	32 *
513	*PORK AND BEANS IN SWEET SAUCE 1 CUP	255	385	16.00	1.66	32 *
514	*RED KIDNEY BEANS, CANNED 1 CUP	255	230	15.00	2.61	30 *
515	*DRY LIMA BEANS, COOKED, DRAINED 1 CUP	190	260	16.00	2.46	32 *
516	*BLACKEYE PEAS,DRY,COOKED 1 CUP	250	190	13.00	2.74	26 *
522	*LENTILS, WHOLE, COOKED 1 CUP	200	210	16.00	3.05	32 *
523	**PEANUTS, ROASTED IN OIL, SALTED 1 CUP (WHOLE, HALVES, CHOPPED)	144	840	37.00	1.76	74 **

HANDBOOK NUMBER	FOOD NAME SERVING SIZE DESCRIPTION	GRAMS	KCAL	PROTEIN G	INQ	%RDA
524	PEANUT BUTTER, 1 TBSP	16	95	4.00	1.68	8
525	*SPLIT PEAS, DRY,COOKED, 1 CUP	200	230	16.00	2.78	32 *
527	**PUMPKIN AND SQUASH SEEDS, DRY, HULLED, 1 CUP	140	775	41.00	2.12	82 **
528	**SUNFLOWER SEEDS, DRY, HULLED, 1 CUP	145	810	35.00	1.73	70 **
546	CHOCOLATE FLAVORED BEVERAGE POWDER WITH NONFAT DRY MILK, 1 OZ (4 HEAPING TSP)	28	100	5.00	2.00	10
564	ASPARAGUS, COOKED,DRAINED,FROM RAW, 1 CUP (CUTS AND TIPS, 1 1/2 TO 2-IN LENGTHS)	145	30	3.00	4.00	6
565	ASPARAGUS, COOKED,DRAINED,FROM FROZEN, 1 CUP (CUTS AND TIPS, 1 1/2 TO 2-IN LENGTHS)	180	40	6.00	6.00	12
569	LIMA BEANS,(FORDHOOKS),FROZEN,COOKED,DRAINED, 1 CUP	170	170	10.00	2.35	20
570	*LIMA BEANS,(BABY LIMAS), FROZEN, COOKED, DRAINED, 1 CUP	180	210	13.00	2.48	26 *
578	BEAN SPROUTS,(MUNG),RAW, 1 CUP	105	35	4.00	4.57	8
579	BEAN SPROUTS,(MUNG),COOKED, DRAINED, 1 CUP	125	35	4.00	4.57	8
585	*BLACKEYE PEAS, COOKED, DRAINED, FROM RAW, 1 CUP	165	180	13.00	2.89	26 *
586	*BLACKEYE PEAS, COOKED, DRAINED, FROM FROZEN, 1 CUP	170	220	15.00	2.73	30 *
587	BROCCOLI, COOKED, DRAINED, FROM RAW, 1 WHOLE MEDIUM STALK	187	45	6.00	5.33	12
588	BROCCOLI, COOKED, DRAINED, FROM RAW, 1 CUP (STALKS CUT INTO 1/2-IN PIECES)	155	40	5.00	5.00	10
590	BROCCOLI, FROM FROZEN, CHOPPED, COOKED, DRAINED, 1 CUP	185	50	5.00	4.00	10
591	BRUSSELS SPROUTS, COOKED, DRAINED, FROM RAW, 7-8 SPROUTS (1 1/4 TO 1 1/2-IN DIAM) 1 CUP	155	55	7.00	5.09	14
592	BRUSSELS SPROUTS, COOKED, DRAINED, FROM FROZEN, 1 CUP	155	50	5.00	4.00	10
605	CAULIFLOWER, RAW, CHOPPED, 1 CUP	115	31	3.00	3.87	6
606	CAULIFLOWER, COOKED, DRAINED FROM RAW, 1 CUP	125	30	3.00	4.00	6
607	CAULIFLOWER, COOKED, DRAINED FROM FROZEN, 1 CUP	180	30	3.00	4.00	6
610	COLLARDS, COOKED, DRAINED, FROM RAW, 1 CUP	190	65	7.00	4.31	14
611	COLLARDS, COOKED DRAINED, FROM FROZEN, 1 CUP	170	50	5.00	4.00	10

HANDBOOK NUMBER	FOOD NAME SERVING SIZE DESCRIPTION	GRAMS	KCAL	PROTEIN G	INQ	%RDA
614	CORN, COOKED, DRAINED FROM FROZEN, 1 CUP KERNELS	165	130	5.00	1.54	10
622	KALE, COOKED, DRAINED, FROM RAW, LEAVES WITHOUT STEMS, 1 CUP	110	45	5.00	4.44	10
623	KALE, COOKED, DRAINED, FROM FROZEN, LEAF STYLE, 1 CUP	130	40	4.00	4.00	8
626	ICEBERG LETTUCE (CRISPHEAD), 1 HEAD, 6-IN DIAM	567	70	5.00	2.86	10
631	MUSTARD GREENS, COOKED, DRAINED, WITHOUT STEMS, 1 CUP	140	30	3.00	4.00	6
633	ONIONS, MATURE, RAW, CHOPPED, 1 CUP	170	65	3.00	1.85	6
635	ONIONS, MATURE, COOKED, DRAINED, WHOLE OR SLICED, 1 CUP	210	60	3.00	2.00	6
639	GREEN PEAS, CANNED, DRAINED SOLIDS, 1 CUP	170	150	8.00	2.13	16
641	GREEN PEAS, FROZEN, COOKED, DRAINED, 1 CUP	160	110	8.00	2.91	16
660	SPINACH, COOKED, DRAINED FROM RAW, 1 CUP	180	40	5.00	5.00	10
661	SPINACH, COOKED, DRAINED FROM FROZEN, CHOPPED, 1 CUP	205	45	6.00	5.33	12
662	SPINACH, COOKED, DRAINED FROM FROZEN, LEAF, 1 CUP	190	45	6.00	5.33	12
663	SPINACH, CANNED, DRAINED SOLIDS, 1 CUP	205	50	6.00	4.80	12
678	TURNIP GREENS, COOKED, DRAINED, FROM RAW (LEAVES AND STEMS), 1 CUP	145	30	3.00	4.00	6
679	TURNIP GREENS, COOKED, DRAINED, FROM FROZEN,CHOPPED, 1 CUP	165	40	4.00	4.00	8
680	VEGETABLES, MIXED, FROZEN, COOKED, DRAINED, 1 CUP	182	115	6.00	2.09	12
698	GELATIN, DRY, 1 ENVELOPE	7	25	6.00	9.60	12
708	CREAM OF CHICKEN SOUP PREPARED WITH EQUAL VOLUME OF MILK, CANNED, 1 CUP	245	180	7.00	1.56	14
710	TOMATO SOUP PREPARED WITH EQUAL VOLUME OF MILK, CANNED, 1 CUP	250	175	7.00	1.60	14
711	BEAN WITH PORK SOUP PREPARED WITH EQUAL VOLUME OF WATER, CANNED, 1 CUP	250	170	8.00	1.88	16
712	BEEF BROTH, BOUILLON, CONSOMME, 1 CUP	240	30	5.00	6.67	10
713	BEEF NOODLE SOUP, PREPARED WITH EQUAL VOLUME OF WATER,CANNED, 1 CUP	240	65	4.00	2.46	8
717	MINESTRONE SOUP PREPARED WITH EQUAL VOLUME OF WATER, CANNED, 1 CUP	245	105	5.00	1.90	10

| HANDBOOK | FOOD NAME | | | | |
NUMBER	SERVING SIZE DESCRIPTION	GRAMS	KCAL	PROTEIN G	INQ	%RDA
718	SPLIT PEA SOUP PREPARED WITH EQUAL VOLUME OF WATER, CANNED	245	145	9.00	2.48	18
	1 CUP					
720	VEGETABLE BEEF SOUP PREPARED WITH EQUAL VOLUME OF WATER, CANNED	245	80	5.00	2.50	10
	1 CUP					
730	BREWER'S YEAST, DRY	8	25	3.00	4.80	6
	1 TBSP					

LINOL A   LINOL A   LINOL A   LINOL A   LINOL A   LINOL A   LINOL A   LINOL A

FOODS WHICH PROVIDE A HIGH CONCENTRATION OF LINOL A   RELATIVE TO CALORIES

(INQ AT LEAST 1.5)

AND AT LEAST 5 PERCENT OF THE RDA PER SERVING

(RDA FOR LINOL A = 20.0 G)

LINOL A   LINOL A   LINOL A   LINOL A   LINOL A   LINOL A   LINOL A   LINOL A

*INDICATES FOODS WHICH PROVIDE AT LEAST 25 PERCENT OF THE RDA PER SERVING

**INDICATES FOODS WHICH PROVIDE AT LEAST 50 PERCENT OF THE RDA PER SERVING

HANDBOOK NUMBER	FOOD NAME SERVING SIZE DESCRIPTION	GRAMS	KCAL	LINOL A G	INQ	%RDA
		13	110	3.10	2.82	16
110	VEGETABLE SHORTENINGS					
	1 TBSP					
114	MARGARINE, REGULAR.	14	100	3.10	3.10	16
	1 TBSP					
115	MARGARINE, REGULAR.	5	35	1.10	3.14	6
	1 PAT (90 PER LB)					
117	MARGARINE, SOFT.	14	100	4.10	4.10	21
	1 TBSP					
119	MARGARINE, WHIPPED.	9	70	2.10	3.00	11
	1 TBSP					
121	*CORN OIL	14	120	7.80	6.50	39 *
	1 TBSP					
125	PEANUT OIL	14	120	4.20	3.50	21
	1 TBSP					
127	**SAFFLOWER OIL	14	120	10.00	8.33	50 **
	1 TBSP					
129	SOYBEAN OIL, HYDROGENATED	14	120	4.70	3.92	24
	1 TBSP					
131	*SOYBEAN-COTTONSEED OIL BLEND, HYDROGENATED.	14	120	6.20	5.17	31 *
	1 TBSP					
132	BLUE CHEESE REGULAR SALAD DRESSING	15	75	3.80	5.07	19
	1 TBSP					
134	FRENCH REGULAR SALAD DRESSING	16	65	3.20	4.92	16
	1 TBSP					
136	ITALIAN REGULAR SALAD DRESSING.	15	85	4.70	5.53	24
	1 TBSP					
138	*MAYONNAISE	14	100	5.60	5.60	28 *
	1 TBSP					
139	MAYONNAISE TYPE SALAD DRESSING.	15	65	3.20	4.92	16
	1 TBSP					
140	MAYONNAISE TYPE LOW CALORIE SALAD DRESSING.	16	20	1.00	5.00	5
	1 TBSP					
141	TARTAR SAUCE.	14	75	4.10	5.47	21
	1 TBSP					
142	THOUSAND ISLAND REGULAR SALAD DRESSING	16	80	4.00	5.00	20
	1 TBSP					
143	THOUSAND ISLAND LOW CALORIE SALAD DRESSING.	15	25	1.00	4.00	5
	1 TBSP					
160	*TUNA SALAD(WITH CELERY, MAYONNAISE TYPE DRESSING, PICKLE, ONION, EGG)	205	350	6.70	1.91	33 *
	1 CUP					
216	CHICKEN CHOW MEIN, CANNED	250	95	3.40	3.58	17
	1 CUP					
413	BROWNIES WITH NUTS, COMMERCIAL RECIPE.	20	85	1.30	1.53	7
	1 BROWNIE, 1 3/4 BY 1 3/4 BY 7/8 IN					
437	DOUGHNUTS, YEAST-LEAVENED, GLAZED,	50	205	3.30	1.61	17
	1 DOUGHNUT, 3 3/4-IN DIAM., 1 1/4-IN HIGH					

HANDBOOK NUMBER	FOOD NAME / SERVING SIZE DESCRIPTION	GRAMS	KCAL	LINOL A G	IN3	XHDA
498	SPAGHETTI, ENRICHED, WITH MEAT BALLS IN TOMATO SAUCE, CANNED. 1 CUP	250	260	3.90	1.50	20
507	**ALMONDS, CHOPPED. 1 CUP (130 ALMONDS)	130	775	12.80	1.65	64 **
508	**ALMONDS, SLIVERED. 1 CUP (115 NUTS)	115	690	11.30	1.64	57 **
517	*BRAZIL NUTS. 1 OZ. (6-8 LARGE KERNALS)	28	185	7.10	3.84	36 *
523	**PEANUTS, ROASTED IN OIL, SALTED. 1 CUP (WHOLE, HALVES, CHOPPED)	144	840	20.70	2.46	104 **
524	PEANUT BUTTER. 1 TBSP	16	95	2.30	2.42	12
526	**PECANS, CHOPPED OR PIECES. 1 CUP (120 LARGE HALVES)	118	810	20.00	2.47	100 **
527	**PUMPKIN AND SQUASH SEEDS, DRY, HULLED. 1 CUP	140	775	27.50	3.55	138 **
528	*SUNFLOWER SEEDS, DRY, HULLED. 1 CUP	145	810	43.20	5.33	216 **
529	**BLACK WALNUTS, CHOPPED. 1 CUP	125	765	45.70	5.82	229 **
530	**BLACK WALNUTS, GROUND. 1 CUP	80	500	29.20	5.84	146 **
531	**PERSIAN OR ENGLISH WALNUTS, CHOPPED. 1 CUP (60 HALVES)	120	780	42.20	5.41	211 **
648	FRENCH FRIED POTATOES, PREPARED FROM RAW. 10 STRIPS 2 TO 3 1/2 IN LONG	50	135	3.30	2.44	17
649	FRENCH FRIED POTATOES, FROZEN, OVEN HEATED. 10 STRIPS	50	110	2.10	1.91	11
650	*HASHBROWN POTATOES, PREPARED FROM FROZEN. 1 CUP	155	345	9.00	2.61	45 *
654	POTATO CHIPS. 10 CHIPS 1 3/4 BY 2 1/2-IN	20	115	4.00	3.48	20
709	CREAM OF MUSHROOM SOUP PREPARED WITH EQUAL VOLUME OF MILK, CANNED. 1 CUP	245	215	4.60	2.14	23
714	CLAM CHOWDER, MANHATTEN TYPE WITH TOMATOES AND WITH OUT MILK. 1 CUP	245	80	1.30	1.63	7
716	CREAM OF MUSHROOM, PREPARED WITH EQUAL VOLUME OF WATER, CANNED. 1 CUP	240	135	4.50	3.33	23

Food Item Index

625

Index

Other AVI Books

DIETARY NUTRIENT GUIDE
Pennington

ECONOMICS OF FOOD PROCESSING
Greig

ECONOMICS OF NEW FOOD PRODUCT DEVELOPMENT
Desrosier and Desrosier

FOOD AND ECONOMICS
Hungate and Sherman

FOOD AND THE CONSUMER
Kramer

FOOD FOR THOUGHT
2nd Edition   *Labuza and Sloan*

FOOD SERVICE FACILITIES PLANNING
Kazarian

FOOD SERVICE SCIENCE
Smith and Minor

MENU PLANNING
2nd Edition   *Eckstein*

PACKAGING REGULATIONS
Sacharow

QUALITY CONTROL IN FOOD SERVICE
Thorner and Manning

SCHOOL FOODSERVICE
Van Egmond

WORK ANALYSIS AND DESIGN FOR HOTELS, RESTAURANTS
& INSTITUTIONS, 2nd Edition   *Kazarian*